Clinical Neuroimmunology

CURRENT CLINICAL NEUROLOGY

Daniel Tarsy, MD, SERIES EDITOR

For further volumes:
http://www.springer.com/series/7630

Clinical Neuroimmunology

Multiple Sclerosis and Related Disorders

Edited by

Syed A. Rizvi, MD
Associate Professor of Neurology (Clinical)
Department of Clinical Neuroscience
Brown University
Providence, RI, USA

Patricia K. Coyle, MD
Professor and Acting Chair
Department of Neurology
Stony Brook Medical Center
East Setauket, NY, USA

✵ Humana Press

Editors
Syed A. Rizvi, MD
Associate Professor
of Neurology (Clinical)
Department of Clinical Neuroscience
Brown University
2 Dudley Street
Suite 555
Providence, RI 02905
USA
SRizvi@Lifespan.org

Patricia K. Coyle, MD
Professor and Acting Chair
Department of Neurology
Stony Brook Medical Center
179 Belle Meade Rd.
East Setauket, NY 11733
USA
pcoyle@notes.cc.sunysb.edu

ISBN 978-1-60327-859-1   e-ISBN 978-1-60327-860-7
DOI 10.1007/978-1-60327-860-7
Springer New York Dordrecht Heidelberg London

Library of Congress Control Number: 2011934049

© Springer Science+Business Media, LLC 2011
All rights reserved. This work may not be translated or copied in whole or in part without
the written permission of the publisher (Humana Press, c/o Springer Science+Business Media,
LLC, 233 Spring Street, New York, NY 10013, USA), except for brief excerpts in connection
with reviews or scholarly analysis. Use in connection with any form of information storage and
retrieval, electronic adaptation, computer software, or by similar or dissimilar methodology now
known or hereafter developed is forbidden.
The use in this publication of trade names, trademarks, service marks, and similar terms, even if
they are not identified as such, is not to be taken as an expression of opinion as to whether or not
they are subject to proprietary rights.
While the advice and information in this book are believed to be true and accurate at the date
of going to press, neither the authors nor the editors nor the publisher can accept any legal
responsibility for any errors or omissions that may be made. The publisher makes no warranty,
express or implied, with respect to the material contained herein.

Printed on acid-free paper

Humana Press is a part of Springer Science+Business Media (www.springer.com)

Series Editor's Introduction

The role of the immune system in the pathophysiology of neurological disorders is a topic of longstanding interest among clinicians and investigators in the field. As stated by Drs Rizvi and Coyle, editors of *Clinical Neuroimmunology: Multiple Sclerosis and Related Disorders*, much new information has accumulated in recent years which is beginning to influence the diagnosis and treatment of many of these disorders. This book serves the very useful purpose of making recent important developments in the field accessible, as well as understandable, to the general neurologist dealing with these disorders in the clinic.

The volume begins with a thorough overview of neuroimmunology and targeted immunotherapies followed by several chapters on the genetics, immunology, epidemiology, clinical and laboratory features, and treatment of multiple sclerosis. Subsequent sections deal with inflammatory disorders of the central nervous system, immune-mediated disorders of the peripheral nervous system, and systemic disorders with presumed autoimmune manifestations which affect the central and peripheral nervous system. Particular topics which are often not emphasized elsewhere are pediatric multiple sclerosis, the immunology of cortical diseases, and immunological aspects of movement disorders. Other chapters deal with the topical issues of neuromyelitis optica and the question of whether there is evidence for a vascular basis of multiple sclerosis. Of particular interest is the chapter by Dr. Howard Weiner predicting that the next 20 years in multiple sclerosis research will provide new and more effective treatments of progressive forms of multiple sclerosis, better biomarkers and an improved understanding of nervous system repair. The reader of this volume will discover that the quantity of knowledge gained in recent years is worthy of this new and comprehensive summary of the field.

Daniel Tarsy, MD
Beth Israel Deaconess Medical Center
Harvard Medical School
Boston, MA

Preface

Immune activation of the central or peripheral nervous system (CNS or PNS) has been shown to play a key role in the pathogenesis of many neurological disorders. Basic concepts in Clinical Neuroimmunology have changed significantly during the last 10 years, and are constantly evolving. New data has driven treatment concepts for a large number of autoimmune diseases, none more so than multiple sclerosis. As this area of research has become increasingly active and productive, the need for a comprehensive up-to-date handbook has become apparent.

Clinical Neuroimmunology: Multiple Sclerosis and Related Disorders has been written with the clinician in mind and targets residents, fellows, internists, nurse practitioners, as well as general neurologists. The aim of this book is to make recent developments in neuroimmunology accessible to the clinician who feels daunted by such advances, and requires a clear explanation of the scientific and clinical issues. The chapters have been written by experts in their fields. The introduction, *Part I* is written by Patricia K. Coyle and Lloyd Kasper and provides a logical and straightforward overview of neuroimmunology. *Part II* consists of eight chapters focused on multiple sclerosis. It includes a chapter on Chronic Cerebrospinal Venous Insufficiency (CCSVI), a topic currently getting a great deal of attention in the media. CCSVI is under investigation for its possible association with MS. Another chapter written by Howard Weiner envisions MS 20 years in the future. *Part III* has seven chapters and focuses on other CNS inflammatory disorders including neuromyelitis optica, ADEM, CNS infections, and immunological aspects of cancer. *Part IV* includes two chapters that describe autoimmune disorders of the PNS. The final *(V) part* includes a single chapter that focuses on various systemic diseases with prominent autoimmune CNS and PNS manifestations such as Behcet's disease, Sarcoidosis, and Systemic Lupus Erythematosis. We hope health professionals who are interested in neuroimmunological disorders will find this book useful.

Finally, we would like to thank our contributing authors, for their hard work and guidance.

Providence, RI   Syed A. Rizvi
Stony Brook, NY   Patricia K. Coyle

Contents

1. Introduction to Neuroimmunology 1
   Patricia K. Coyle

2. Principles of Immunotherapy.. 15
   Jennifer L. Joscelyn and Lloyd Kasper

Part I   Multiple Sclerosis

3. MS: Pathology and Immunology 43
   Patricia K. Coyle

4. MS: Epidemiology and Genetics 71
   Robert H. Gross and Philip L. De Jager

5. MS: Clinical Features, Symptom Management, and Diagnosis 89
   James M. Stankiewicz and Guy J. Buckle

6. Advances in Magnetic Resonance
   Imaging of Multiple Sclerosis... 111
   Robert Zivadinov

7. Disease Modifying Agents in the
   Treatment of Multiple Sclerosis... 131
   Syed A. Rizvi

8. Pediatric Multiple Sclerosis 157
   Lauren Krupp, Yashma Patel, and Vikram Bhise

9. Is Multiple Sclerosis a Vascular Disease?...................................... 179
   Mahesh V. Jayaraman and Syed A. Rizvi

10. Multiple Sclerosis: The Next 20 Years 191
    Howard L. Weiner

Part II   Other CNS Inflammatory Disorders

11.   Acute Disseminated Encephalomyelitis 203
      Patricia K. Coyle

12.   Neuromyelitis Optica Spectrum Disorders 219
      Dean M. Wingerchuk

13.   The Neuroimmunology of Cancer 233
      Enrico C. Lallana, William F. Hickey, and Camilo E. Fadul

14.   Infections of the Central Nervous System 255
      Najam Zaidi, Melissa Gaitanis, John N. Gaitanis,
      Karl Meisel, and Syed A. Rizvi

15.   The Neuroimmunology of Cortical Disease
      (Dementia, Epilepsy, and Autoimmune Encephalopathies) 275
      Julie L. Roth, Brian R. Ott, John N. Gaitanis,
      and Andrew S. Blum

16.   Autoimmune Movement Disorders... 291
      Victoria C. Chang

17.   CNS Vasculitis 307
      David S. Younger and Adam P.J. Younger

Part III   Peripheral Nervous System Disorders

18.   Immunologic Disorders of Neuromuscular
      Junction and Muscle 333
      Kara A. Chisholm, James M. Gilchrist, and John E. Donahue

19.   Autoimmune Neuropathies 349
      George Sachs

Part IV   Systemic Disorders

20.   Systemic Autoimmune Diseases with
      Neurological Manifestations.. 375
      Richard Choi, Valarie Gendron, Mac McLaughlin,
      Jonathan Cahill, Fathima Qadeer, and Syed A. Rizvi

Index 391

Contributors

Vikram Bhise
Department of Neurology, Stony Brook University Medical Center,
Stony Brook, NY, USA

Andrew S. Blum, MD, PhD
Comprehensive Epilepsy Program, Department of Neurology,
Rhode Island Hospital, The Warren Alpert Medical School at Brown
University, Providence, RI, USA

Guy J. Buckle, MD
Partners MS Center, Brigham & Women's Hospital,
Harvard Medical School, Brookline, MA, USA

Jonathan Cahill, MD
UMASS Medical School, Worcester, MA, USA

Victoria C. Chang, MD
Department of Medicine, Division of Neurology, Providence VA Medical
Center, Providence, RI, USA; The Movement Disorders Program,
Butler Hospital, Providence, RI; USA; Department of Clinical Neurosciences,
The Warren Alpert School of Medicine at Brown University,
Providence, RI, USA

Kara A. Chisholm, MD
Department of Neurology, Rhode Island Hospital, Warren Alpert Medical
School at Brown University, Providence, RI, USA

Richard Choi
Department of Neurology, Rhode Island Hospital, Providence, RI, USA

Patricia K. Coyle, MD
Professor and Acting Chair, Department of Neurology,
Stony Brook Medical Center, East Setauket, NY, USA

John E. Donahue, MD
Department of Pathology, Division of Neuropathology, Rhode Island
Hospital, Department of Pathology and Laboratory Medicine,
Warren Alpert Medical School at Brown University, Providence, RI, USA

Camilo E. Fadul, MD
Neuro-Oncology Program, Norris Cotton Cancer Center,
Departments of Medicine and Neurology, Dartmouth Medical School,
Dartmouth-Hitchcock Medical Center, Lebanon, NH, USA

Melissa Gaitanis
Infectious Disease-Department of Medicine, Warren Alpert Medical School
at Brown University, Providence, RI, USA

John N. Gaitanis
Department of Clinical Neurosciences, Warren Alpert Medical School
at Brown University, Providence, RI, USA

Valarie Gendron
Department of Neurology, Rhode Island Hospital,
Providence, RI, USA

James M. Gilchrist, MD
Department of Neurology, Rhode Island Hospital, Warren Alpert Medical
School at Brown University, Providence, RI, USA

Robert H. Gross, MD
Department of Neurology, Center for Neurologic Diseases, Brigham &
Women's Hospital, Boston, MA, USA; Harvard Medical School, Boston,
MA, USA; Partners Center for Personalized Genetic Medicine, Boston, MA,
USA; Program in Medical & Population Genetics, Broad Institute of Harvard
University and Massachusetts Institute of Technology, Cambridge, MA, USA

William F. Hickey, MD
Department of Pathology, Dartmouth Medical School, Dartmouth-Hitchcock
Medical Center, Lebanon, NH, USA

Philip L. De Jager, MD, PhD
Department of Neurology, Center for Neurologic Diseases,
Brigham & Women's Hospital, Boston, MA, USA; Harvard Medical School,
Boston, MA, USA; Partners Center for Personalized Genetic Medicine,
Boston, MA, USA; Program in Medical & Population Genetics,
Broad Institute of Harvard University and Massachusetts Institute
of Technology, Cambridge, MA, USA

Mahesh V. Jayaraman, MD
Warren Alpert Medical School at Brown University,
Interventional Neuroradiology, Rhode Island Hospital, Providence, RI, USA

Jennifer L. Joscelyn, MS
100 Merrimack Street, Hooksett, NH, USA

Lloyd Kasper
Dartmouth Medical School, Lebanon, NH, USA

Lauren Krupp
Department of Neurology, Stony Brook University Medical Center,
Stony Brook, NY, USA

Enrico C. Lallana, MD
Neuro-Oncology Program, Norris Cotton Cancer Center,
Departments of Medicine and Neurology, Dartmouth Medical School,
Dartmouth-Hitchcock Medical Center, Lebanon, NH, USA

Mac McLaughlin, MD
UMASS Medical School, Worcester, MA, USA

Karl Meisel
Department of Neurology, Rhode Island Hospital,
Providence, RI, USA

Brian R. Ott
Alzheimer's Disease & Memory Disorders Center, Department of Neurology,
Rhode Island Hospital, The Warren Alpert Medical School
at Brown University, Providence, RI, USA

Yashma Patel
Department of Neurology, Stony Brook University Medical Center,
Stony Brook, NY, USA

Fathima Qadeer, MD
Rhode Island Hospital, Providence, RI, USA

Syed A. Rizvi, MD
Associate Professor of Neurology (Clinical), Department of Clinical
Neuroscience, Brown University, Providence, RI, USA

Julie L. Roth
Comprehensive Epilepsy Program, Department of Neurology,
Rhode Island Hospital, The Warren Alpert Medical School
at Brown University, Providence, RI, USA

George Sachs, MD, PhD
Alpert Medical School of Brown University, EMG Laboratory,
Rhode Island Hospital, Providence, RI, USA

James M. Stankiewicz, MD
Partners MS Center, Brigham & Women's Hospital,
Harvard Medical School, Brookline, MA, USA

Howard L. Weiner, MD
Partners Multiple Sclerosis Center, Center for Neurologic Diseases,
Brigham and Women's Hospital, Harvard Medical School, Boston, MA, USA

Dean M. Wingerchuk, MD, MSc, FRCP(C)
Division of Multiple Sclerosis and Autoimmune Neurology,
Mayo Clinic College of Medicine, Scottsdale, AZ, USA

David S. Younger, MD
Department of Neurology, New York University School of Medicine,
New York, NY, USA

Adam P.J. Younger, MD
College of Arts and Sciences, Case Western Reserve University,
Cleveland, OH, USA

Najam Zaidi, MD
Warren Alpert Medical School at Brown University, Providence, RI,
USA and Department of Medicine, Kent Hospital, Warwick, RI, USA

Robert Zivadinov, MD
Department of Neurology, Buffalo Neuroimaging Analysis Center,
The Jacobs Neurological Institute, State University of New York, Buffalo,
NY, USA

Introduction to Neuroimmunology

Patricia K. Coyle

Keywords: Neuroimmunology, Inflammation, Immunity, Astrocytes, Microglia, Cytokine

Introduction

Neuroimmunology is the neuroscience specialty that focuses on interactions between the nervous system and immune system. It encompasses both basic science fields, as well as clinical disciplines which deal with a special set of central (CNS) and peripheral nervous system (PNS) disorders (Table 1.1) [1–3]. These disorders result from immune-mediated damage, and require diagnostic and therapeutic approaches that recognize and address this fact.

The nervous system involves both the CNS (brain and spinal cord) and the PNS (peripheral nerves, neuromuscular junction, skeletal muscle). The autonomic nervous system can be considered a functional subdivision, with both CNS and PNS components.

Historically, the CNS has been described as a sequestered compartment protected from the systemic immune system, and without its own immune components or response system. This image is based on a variety of factors (Table 1.2). When examined more closely, however, the CNS is better characterized as an immunologically privileged site [4].

Unique Anatomy

CNS anatomy is unique. Because the CNS is encased by bone, with a relatively inelastic dura lining, small volume changes can result in injury. The brain and spinal cord are encased in the bony protective skull and vertebral column, as well as a three-part membranous covering (pia, arachnoid, dura). The pia and arachnoid membranes form the subarachnoid space, which is filled with cerebrospinal fluid (CSF). In essence, the brain and spinal cord float in a water bath, since CSF is 99% water [5, 6]. It acts as a buoyancy

From: *Clinical Neuroimmunology: Multiple Sclerosis and Related Disorders*, Current Clinical Neurology,
Edited by: S.A. Rizvi and P.K. Coyle, DOI 10.1007/978-1-60327-860-7_1,
© Springer Science+Business Media, LLC 2011

Table 1.1 Neuroimmune disorders.

CNS

- Acute disseminated encephalomyelitis/postinfectious encephalomyelitis
- Multiple sclerosis
- Neuromyelitis optica-Devic's disease
- Acute transverse myelitis
- Optic neuritis
- Tropical spastic paraparesis – HTLV1-associated myelopathy
- Rasmussen encephalitis
- Stiff Person syndrome
- Poststreptococcal movement disorders
- Pediatric Autoimmune Neuropsychiatric Disorders (PANDAS)
- Hashimoto's and other misc. autoimmune encephalopathy/encephalitis
- Paraneoplastic syndromes (can involve PNS)
- CNS vasculitis

PNS

- Guillain–Barre syndrome
- Chronic relapsing/inflammatory demyelinating polyneuropathy
- Multifocal motor neuropathy
- Other immune polyneuropathies (anti-MAG, anti-sulfatide, GALOP, POEMS, etc.)

Neuromuscular junction

- Myasthenia gravis
- Lambert–Easton myasthenic syndrome
- Arthrogryposis multiplex congenital

Muscle

- Polymyositis
- Dermatomyositis
- Inclusion body myositis (degenerative plus inflammation components)

Table 1.2 Basis for CNS consideration as an immune privileged site.

- Unique anatomic isolation
- Blood–brain and blood–CSF barriers
- Lack of a typical lymphatic drainage system
- Lack of fully operational antigen-presenting cells
- Lack of rejection of foreign graft tissue
- Little constitutive expression of major histocompatibility complex molecules

fluid. CSF is an active product of the secretory epithelium of the choroid plexus, but up to 40% also represents extracellular fluid from the CNS parenchyma. This extracellular fluid is added to CSF at virtually all points along the neuraxis. CSF circulates from within the ventricles (where the choroid plexi are situated) into the subarachnoid space, flowing down the spinal axis and back up, to be resorbed into the venous blood system via the arachnoid villi.

These arachnoid villi are outpouchings of the arachnoid membrane that extend into the venous sinuses of the cerebral hemispheres. CSF is made continually, at approximately 20 cc per hour. The total volume (125–150 cc in a typical adult), is completely turned over 4½ times every 24 h.

Since the ependymal cells which line the ventricles lack tight junctions, there is essentially free communication between CNS white matter extracellular fluid and ventricular CSF. CNS gray matter fluid at the brain surface also communicates with CSF via the Virchow Robin spaces, specialized perivascular spaces associated with penetrating arteries that are continuous with the subarachnoid space.

CSF leukocyte count in normal controls ranges up to 5 WBCs per mm³. WBCs are largely (80%) CD4+ memory T cells [7]. About 5% are monocytes, while <1% are B cells. CSF T cells express CD27 and CD45 RO, markers of central memory T cells. Very late antigen-4 (VLA-4) expression is also increased compared to peripheral T cells. CSF T cells show higher expression of CXC chemokine receptor 3, compared to other chemokines. CSF memory T cells can encounter potential antigen-presenting cells (APCs) cells at several sites, including the ependyma, Virchow Robin spaces, and choroid plexus.

Blood–Brain and Blood–CSF Barriers

The blood–brain barrier can be demonstrated by inhibition of entry of intravenous dyes into the CNS [8, 9]. It is formed by specialized features unique to CNS blood vessels. CNS capillaries not only lack fenestrae, but they have interendothelial cell tight junctions which prevent cell migration. They also do not pinocytose effectively. The blood–brain barrier is not absolute. It is actually relative or even selective, limiting entry of large hydrophilic proteins, but allowing smaller lipophilic compounds and small gaseous molecules [10]. The endothelial basement membrane and perivascular glia limitans do not seem to play a role in the blood–brain barrier.

Although the choroid plexus capillaries are fenestrated, with 80 nm openings [4], the choroid plexus epithelium has tight junctions. This is the anatomic basis for the blood–CSF barrier. There are specific CNS regions which do not have a barrier. The circumventricular organs (area postrema, organum vasculosum of the lamina terminalis, median eminence, subfornical organ) lack tight junctions between capillary endothelial cells. At these sites molecules can diffuse very easily into the CNS. The nasal barrier is another leaky site, where there is continuing turnover of olfactory receptor neurons allowing access to CSF and olfactory bulbs [11].

The blood–brain and blood–CSF barriers, along with the CSF circulation, provide bidirectional control of flow. Damaging CNS factors can be removed via efflux transporters into the blood, while influx transporters can promote nutrients into the CNS. The PNS has a similar blood–nerve barrier in peripheral nerve, but this is absent in spinal roots and at the dorsal root ganglia.

CNS Lymphatics

The CNS has no conventional lymphatic system (H). However, cervical lymph nodes may be involved in B- and T-cell-mediated CNS immune responses [12, 13]. In animals such as rodents and ruminants, CSF drains into cervical lymph nodes [14–17], and CSF has several drainage pathways. The subarachnoid space surrounding the olfactory bulb does cross the cribriform plate at the base of the ethmoid bone, into nasal submucosal lymphatics [13]. In animals, CSF drains from the subarachnoid space along cranial and spinal nerve roots, and to a lesser extent the dura mater, to cervical and lumbar lymph nodes [13]. This route is present in humans [12]. CSF also moves directly into venous circulation through the arachnoid villi granulations in the walls of the venous sinuses. CNS soluble antigens within the CSF can access lymphoid tissue via both cervical lymphatics and venous drainage [4].

It is likely that not only CSF, but also interstitial fluid drains into cervical lymph nodes. CNS interstitial fluid, which is estimated at 280 cc, drains along capillary and artery walls, along the tunica media and adventitia of leptomeningeal and major cerebral arteries, and out the base of the skull to deep cervical nodes. This is demonstrable in animal models using tracer studies, and indirect evidence supports a similar pathway in humans [13].

CNS Immunity

The CNS is composed of neurons, glia, blood vessels, and meninges. Neurons contain dendritic, somatic, axonal, and synaptic regions. Glia consists of neuroectodermal cells (astrocytes, oligodendrocytes, ependymal cells) as well as bone marrow-derived cells (microglia).

The CNS does have a resident immune system. Both microglia and astrocytes play key roles in CNS innate immune responses. They are complemented by infiltrating monocytes and dendritic cells from the blood, that accumulate at nonparenchymal CNS sites [16]. Innate immune responses can be neuroprotective or neurotoxic.

In contrast, acquired immune responses are more difficult to initiate within the CNS. Activated T cells (regardless of antigen specificity) are believed to penetrate into the CNS as a normal phenomenon, but then rapidly exit. CD4+ and CD8+ T cells penetrate by different mechanisms [17]. Usually T cells accumulate in the perivascular Virchow Robin spaces and subarachnoid spaces. These T cells cause problems only if they recognize specific antigens in the context of MHC. CD4+ T cells recognize antigen in the context of MHC Class II, while CD8+ T cells recognize antigen in the context of MHC Class I. Normally, the CNS has low level of MHC expression. Since microglia and astrocytes are nonprofessional APCs, they express low levels of MHC and costimulatory molecules. They are more likely to induce T-cell anergy, rather than activate naïve T cells [16].

Dendritic cells are recognized as the most potent professional APCs. There are no resident dendritic cells within the CNS, although recent reports describe a resident population in mouse brain [18, 19]. Dendritic cells can infiltrate into CSF, choroid plexus, meninges, perivascular spaces, and CNS parenchyma as part of a neuroinflammatory response [20]. Along with macrophages, they probably reactivate T cells which enter the CNS [17]. Diverse chronic inflammatory processes can result in peripheral dendritic cells entering the brain [21]. Dendritic cells can be derived from monocytes or lymphoid precursors. Both myeloid and lymphoid dendritic cells are capable of entering the CNS under inflammatory conditions.

The CNS immune/inflammatory response differs from that in other organ systems. CNS neurons are largely postmitotic and nonregenerating. Neuronal necrosis induced by neurotoxin injection does not elicit a typical inflammatory response. Virus inoculated into the parenchyma is cleared slowly and inefficiently [22].

There are three distinct routes of entry for WBCs into the CNS [4, 23]. The first pathway involves cells moving from blood vessels into the stroma of the choroid plexus, and then crossing the blood–CSF barrier into CSF. This appears to be the most likely site for physiologic entry of leukocytes into CSF. A second route of cell entry is also across the blood–CSF barrier, into the subarachnoid space, involving postcapillary venules at the pia into the subarachnoid space and the Virchow–Robin perivascular spaces. The endothelial cells express adhesion molecules, which promote T-cell adherence, allowing direct exchange between circulating leukocytes and perivascular cells [24, 25]. The third route involves activated T cells moving from blood to the parenchymal perivascular space, across the blood–brain barrier [17].

Leukocyte transmigration into tissue, including the CNS, involves a coordinated stepwise process [26]. There is initial contact, then tethering/rolling (involving selectins and glycoprotein ligands), activation (involving chemokines and G protein-coupled receptors), adhesion (involving integrins and adhesion molecules) and diapedesis with migration to vascular junctions, penetration into the subendothelial compartment, and breach of the vascular basement membrane into tissue [26]. T-cell migration into the CNS under inflammatory conditions involves $\alpha4\beta1$ integrin expressed on T cells, interacting with vascular cell adhesion molecule1 on activated endothelial cells. Expression of chemokines and chemokine receptors also plays a role in T-cell trafficking. The rate-limiting step in transmigration is crossing the basement membrane laminins. T cells migrate across laminin 411 but not laminin 511. Laminen $\alpha4$ (a component of laminin 411) preferentially involves CD4+ T-cell migration, but not CD8+ T cells, macrophages, or dendritic cells.

It has been suggested that WBC extravasation into the spinal cord may differ somewhat from that into the brain, but very little work has been done in this area [27].

CNS immune surveillance may occur primarily within the subarachnoid space [17]. This is thought to be the initial site of T-cell infiltration, where cells can be reactivated by MHC Class II APCs, with T-cell proliferation and formation of large cellular aggregates. There can be a rapid T-cell response within the subarachnoid space to antigen challenge. This reactivation of T cells promotes further inflammation, and cell entry into the perivascular space and then the brain parenchyma.

Major Histocompatibility Molecule Expression

In the CNS resting state, there is absent or minimal expression of MHC Class I and II molecules [28, 29]. MHC expression is generally limited to low level expression on microglia, but can be induced in a variety of CNS components. Interferon gamma (IFNγ) induces MHC expression on neurons [16].

CNS Cell Components

Microglia

Microglia are the resident immune cells of the CNS, with myelomonocytic lineage [30]. They are the tissue macrophages of the CNS, responsible for innate immune responses and immune surveillance within the brain [31, 32]. Microglia make up 10% of the total glial population, and are as numerous as neurons [33]. They are usually in a resting state. They are present throughout the CNS but enriched in certain areas, with more cells in gray matter than white matter [34]. Circulating precursor mesodermal hematopoietic cells enter the CNS during perinatal development, to transform into microglia [35]. Mature cells express macrophage-specific markers including toll-like receptors (TLR), CD11b integrin, and the F4/80 glycoprotein, but show lower expression of CD45. Based on morphology, microglia are classified as resting ramified, activated, or ameboid phagocytic cells [30]. Ameboid phagocytic microglia predominate in the perinatal brain, but become ramified resting microglia during postnatal development. They can be activated by injury, infection, or neurodegenerative processes [32].

Microglia monitor their microenvironment and conduct routine surveillance of the CNS via pinocytosis and neuronal interaction [33, 36]. They respond to a complex mix of excitatory and inhibitory input, including cell–cell contact and soluble factor exposures. Activation by inflammatory or injury factors provokes a pre-programmed response designed to both kill, as well as promote recovery and repair. Classical activation, alternative activation, and acquired deactivation are all going on, but may differ within regional areas. As examples, substance P neurotransmitter causes activation, while neuronal activity inhibits MHC class II expression to IFNγ. A neuronal surface molecule (CD200) appears to be an important regulator of microglial function. Soluble factors such as granulocyte-macrophage colony-stimulating factor (GM-CSF) and macrophage-CSF (MO-CSF) affect microglia function and development.

Resting ramified microglia are activated by detecting lipopolysaccharides, amyloid beta, thrombin, IFNγ, and other proinflammatory cytokines [37]. Microglia express TLR. They can initiate innate immune responses by producing cytokines such as interleukin-1 (IL-1), IL-6, and tumor necrosis factor α (TNFα); chemokines such as monocyte chemoattractant protein-1 (MCP-1), macrophage inflammatory protein-1, and RANTES; and nitric oxide (NO). The net result is local cell production of more proinflammatory cytokines and chemokines, and upregulation of immunomodulatory surface markers, with injury to the blood–brain barrier and subsequent entry of soluble factors and systemic immune cells. Microglial activation precedes this systemic cell entry. CNS injury results in phagocytic and cytotoxic activities of microglia. Complement and Fc gamma receptors are upregulated, leading to enhanced phagocytic ability. Cytotoxic superoxide radicals and NO are released into the microenvironment.

Resting microglia are very poor APCs. However, activation causes marked expression of MHC and costimulatory molecules [38, 39]. The activation state involves morphological changes as well as gene expression changes, migratory and proliferative responses, and phagocytic behavior. Activated microglia will express CD40, CD80, CD86, and MHC class II molecules. Subsequent interaction with T cells leads to microglial release of nitric synthase. IFNγ promotes MHC class II as well as adhesion and costimulatory molecule expression.

Table 1.3 Activated microglia products.

- Chemokines
- Complement proteins
- Cytokines
- Neurotrophic factors
- Prostaglandins
- Proteinases
- Reactive oxygen species/reactive nitrogen species (nitric oxide, peroxynitrite, superoxide)

Microglia also play an important role in regulation. Microglia express Fas ligand, which can bind to Fas receptor on T cells, leading to activation-induced T-cell apoptosis. Cytotoxic microglial products, such as NO, can lead to death of immune cells (Table 1.3). Thus, activation of microglia can be self limited, as it leads ultimately to removal of effector immune cells.

Microglia dynamically modulate neurons and astrocytes, share receptors, and produce factors that activate these surrounding cells. Microglia modulate glutamate levels and can protect or injure neurons [40]. They are a central immune system player in the CNS.

Astrocytes

Astrocytes are the most abundant cells in the CNS, making up 90% of the brain [41]. Protoplasmic astrocytes are found in gray matter, and have numerous ramified branches contacting neurons and blood vessels [10]. Fibrous astrocytes within white matter have longer, thinner processes. All astrocytes express intermediate filament glial fibrillary acidic protein (GFAP). Activation results in upregulation of GFAP as part of gliosis. Astrocytes have multiple functions (Table 1.4).

Astrocytes play an important role in regulating CNS inflammation and cell trafficking. In vitro, they can produce proinflammatory cytokines and chemokines, and reactive oxygen species (ROS) to enhance inflammation, as well as regulatory cytokines and ROS scavengers to limit inflammation [42]. Astrocytes have important interactions with blood vessels. Reactive astrocytes can act as perivascular barriers to restrict leukocyte entry during pathologic states.

With regard to the role of the astrocyte as an immune cell, they appear to function in both innate and acquired immunity, both in the normal and inflamed CNS. Astrocytes have dual actions, both beneficial and injurious. Astrocytes can express a variety of pattern recognition receptors, including TLRs, dsRNA-dependent protein kinase, complement receptors, mannose receptors, and scavenger receptors. Astrocytes also show APC-like function in vitro. They can be induced to express MHC class I and II molecules, to upregulate costimulatory molecules CD80 and CD86, to activate CD4+ and CD8+ T cells, and to present antigen to CD4+ T cells [1, 10]. During inflammation astrocytes release a variety of cytokines (IL-1, IL-6, and IL-10; TNFα; TGFβ) that influence T-cell responses. Astrocytes can contribute to lymphocyte penetration into the CNS in three ways: by a blood–brain barrier effect, by expression of adhesion molecules such as ICAM-1 and VCAM-1,

Table 1.4 Role of astrocytes.

- Neuronal support
  - Microenvironmental ion, pH homeostasis
  - Glycogen storage
  - Clearance of toxic waste products
- Synaptic transmission modulation
  - Glutamate uptake
  - Release of neuromodulatory factors
  - Astrocyte neuron gap junction
- Neuron and glial survival
  - Production of neurotrophins: brain-derived neurotrophic factor (BDNF), neurotrophin-3 (NT-3), at baseline; BDNF, nerve growth factor (NGF) on injury
  - Astrocyte-mediated growth factor production
- Maintenance of blood–brain barrier
  - Astrocyte endfeet surround CNS capillaries and perivascular macrophages
  - Astrocyte products can increase or tighten permeability
- Immune function
  - Contribute to both innate and acquired immunity

and by release of chemokines such as CCL5, CCL2, CXCL8, and CXCL10. Therefore, astrocytes can participate in amplifying CNS inflammatory responses, but also appear to suppress T-cell activation by upregulating cytotoxic T lymphocyte antigen (CTLA)-4 on activated T cells [10]. Astrocytes can also induce regulatory T cells exhibiting suppressor activity. Activated astrocytes release IL-17 to suppress Th17 cells.

Astrocytes both impede and promote CNS repair mechanisms. By forming a glial scar there is an additional physical barrier producing multiple biochemical changes, including expression of molecules on the astrocyte surface, that can block axon regeneration as well as oligodendrocyte precursor cells. By production of certain chemokines, cytokines, and matrix metalloproteinases (MMPs), as well as their tissue inhibitors, repair is promoted

Oligodendrocytes

Oligodendrocytes are the glial cells responsible for CNS myelination. Oligodendrocytes form a myelin sheath around multiple axons to electrically insulate them. This results in sodium channel clustering at the nodes of Ranvier, to allow saltatory conduction. Normal axonal transport and neuronal viability seems to require proper myelination, which also boosts axon diameter. Oligodendrocytes provide trophic support to neurons via neurotrophic factors such as glial-derived (GDNF), brain-derived (BDNF), and insulin-like 1 (IGF-1) growth factors [43].

Oligodendrocytes show extremely high metabolic rates and consume large quantities of oxygen and ATP, leading to high levels of intracellular hydrogen peroxide and ROS [44, 45]. The numerous myelin synthesis enzymes, which require iron as a cofactor, results in oligodendrocytes and oligodendrocyte precursor cells (OPCs) containing the highest intracellular iron stores in the brain [43]. This can result in free radical formation and lipid peroxidation. Oligodendrocytes also have only low concentrations of the anti-oxidative enzyme glutathione.

The capacity of the oligodendrocyte's endoplasmic reticulum to produce and fold proteins is also quite susceptible to minimum changes causing marked disturbances. All of this makes oligodendrocytes particularly vulnerable to oxidative damage and mitochondrial injury, and more vulnerable to bystander damage than neurons or astrocytes.

Oligodendrocyts are vulnerable to excitotoxic cell damage; they express glutamate AMPA, kainate, and NMDA receptors, and the ATP receptor P2x7. Proinflammatory cytokines such as TNFα induce oligodendrocyte apoptosis by binding to the p55 TNF receptor [45]. Although IFNγ has no negative effect on mature oligodendrocytes, it is highly toxic for proliferating OPCs and mildly toxic for immature oligodendrocytes. A variety of proinflammatory cytokines can induce mitochondrial injury, indirectly damaging the more vulnerable oligodendrocyte population. Autoantibodies which bind to surface myelin or oligodendrocyte epitopes can lead to damage via complement activation, or Fc receptor recognition on activated neurophages.

Oligodendrocytes do not express MHC antigens, but in vitro exposure to IFNγ results in MHC class I induction.

Neurons

Although neurons have been said not to express MHC, recent work indicates they most likely do express MHC class I that can be up or downregulated by various factors [46]. This would make them vulnerable to attack by CD8+ T cells. Natural killer (NK) cells can also lead to neuronal destruction.

Neurons can regulate T-cell activities either directly or indirectly, using a variety of contact-dependent and independent mechanisms. They release soluble factors (neurotransmitters, neuropeptide, neurotrophins, cytokines, soluble Fas ligand, soluble ICAM-5) that can reduce microglial and T-cell activation. This downregulation occurs predominantly within the perivascular and subarachnoid spaces [16]. Neurons can also interact directly with microglia and T cells via contact-dependent mechanisms involving neuronal glycoproteins such as CD22, CD47, CD200, neural cell adhesion molecule, and semaphorins [16].

Endothelial Cells

CNS endothelial cells express MHC class I but not class II antigen. Brain capillary endothelium contain enzymes not otherwise found in the CNS (alkaline phosphatase and γ-glutamyl transpeptidase). They have much fewer cytoplasmic vesicles than non-CNS endothelium, which will contribute to lower penetration into the CNS. Pericytes are found along the length of the cerebral capillaries and partially surround the endothelium, and contribute to the basal lamina [8, 47]. (C,E). Astrocytes have integrins on their end feet, that bind to laminin in the basal membrane to provide an additional seal to the blood–brain barrier. There is actually a dual basement membrane surrounding the endothelium, a three-dimensional mesh as thick as 200 nm, consisting of proteins including integrins, dystroglycans, collagens, and laminins. Disruption of extracellular matrix increases blood–brain barrier permeability [48].

Other Immunologic Factors

Cytokines

Immune system cells produce cytokines that can have important effects on the nervous system. Cytokines such as IL-1, IL-6, and tumor necrosis factor (TNF) cross the blood–brain barrier around the hypothalamus, due to fenestration as well as active transport mechanisms. They have direct impact on the hypothalamic neurons which regulate temperature, appetite, and sleep [2].

Matrix Metalloproteinases

MMPs are a family of zinc-dependent endopeptidases that degrade extracellular matrix to increase capillary permeability and permit cell penetration. They are divided into four groups of enzymes: collagenases, stromelysins, gelatinases, and membrane-type metalloproteinases [40]. They are activated by cleavage, plasmin, or reactive oxygen radicals. MMP-2 (Gelatinase A) is normally present in brain tissue and CSF. MMP-9 (Gelatinase B), MMP-3, and MMP-12 are induced during an inflammatory response involving immediate early genes (c-FOS; c-JUNE) and cytokines such as TNFα and IL-1B. Astrocytes stain for MMP-2. MMP-9 appears in endothelial cells and neutrophils during CNS injury. MMP-3 has been detected in microglia and neurons during ischemia, while MMP-12 is expressed by activated microglia and macrophages.

Toll-Like Receptors

TLR are part of the innate immune system. They are pathogen recognition receptors, type I transmembrane glycoprotein receptors with a highly variable extracellular region, and a highly conserved intracellular tail, localized to the cell surface or within endosomes [49]. They protect the host against pathogens. Many different TLRs are expressed by microglia [50]. They trigger a standardized cytokine and chemokines response, regardless of the inciting antigen, that can be beneficial or harmful. Activation of astrocytes, oligodendrocytes, and neurons can also result in TLR expression. These TLRs play various roles which are cell specific, and include cell migration and differentiation, limiting inflammation, and mounting repair processes.

Nervous, Immune, and Endocrine System Network

There is a strong reciprocal relationship between the nervous, immune, and endocrine systems. These three systems participate in an extensive tridirectional network that involves both cell to cell contact, as well as soluble factors (cytokines/chemokines, growth factors, hormones, neurotransmitters/neuropeptides). Sharing regulatory molecules allows coordinated responses to homeostatis disturbance produced by inflammation, infection, or stress [51]. These three body organ systems are anatomically and functionally connected. Neuroimmune activation and neuroinflammation play an important role even in diseases not considered to be classically neuroimmune, such as stroke, Alzheimer disease, and Parkinson disease.

Neurotransmitters help regulate the host response to injury and infection. Immune cells express neurotransmitter receptors. Catecholamine can affect antigen presentation by dendritic cells, enhance antibody responses, suppress cellular immune responses, clonal lymphocyte expansion, and cell migration and trafficking [52]. Net effects reflect whether α or β adrenergic receptors are activated.

The brain helps control immune activation. The cholinergic vagus nerve excites sympathetic neurons that innervate the spleen and synapse directly on immune cells [53]. Immune cells express receptors for pituitary hormones (prolactin, human growth hormone, thyroid stimulating hormone, insulin-like growth factor 1) as well as neurotransmitters (acetylcholine, glutamate, norepinephrine, endorphins). In turn, MHC Class I molecules modulate neural synapse formation during brain development, and can regulate these synapses as well in the mature brain [54]. Cytokines such as TNF regulate the AMPA class of glutamatergic receptors.

The brain and immune system communicate via the hypothalamic–pituitary–adrenal gland (HPA) axis, and the sympathetic nervous system. The HPA axis maintains homeostasis by regulating the neuroendocrine, sympathetic nervous system, and immune system. Abnormalities in HPA axis have been implicated in autoimmune/immune-mediated disorders [55]. It is an important feedback loop, and a major component of how the nervous and endocrine systems communicate. The paraventricular nucleus of the hypothalamus secretes two peptides, vasopressin and corticotrophin-releasing hormone (CRH). They in turn act on the anterior lobe of the pituitary gland to secrete adrenocorticotropic hormone (ACTH). In turn, ACTH acts on the adrenal gland cortex to produce glucocorticoid hormones (chiefly cortisol), which in a negative feedback loop suppress CRH and ACTH release. CRH synthesis is influenced by stress cortisol blood levels, and the diurnal sleep–wake cycle. Cortisol normally rises 30–45 min after awakening in the morning, and in the late afternoon, and is lowest in the middle of the night.

Psychoneuroimmunology is a reflection of the organ system links outlined above. It studies the interactions between psychological processes, such as stress and anxiety, and the nervous and immune systems. Traumatic life events, personality traits, coping mechanisms, and strong emotions can impact on nervous and immune function. For example, cell-mediated immunity can be impaired in individuals who lose a loved one. Stress can make individuals more vulnerable to infections. Psychoneuroimmunology evaluates models such as sickness behavior, neuropsychiatric disorders, and the effects of stress on the nervous system.

Conclusion

The immune system plays a pivotal role in neuroimmune disorders. In addition, it is increasingly recognized to be a factor in most major neurologic diseases. It also determines how the body responds behaviorally to external factors. Practicing Neurologists who are familiar with basic neuroimmunology concepts will have a better understanding of current and future advances in understanding and treating nervous system disorders.

References

1. Pender MP. An introduction to neuroimmunology. In: Pender MP, McCombe PA, editors. Autoimmune neurological disease. Cambridge: Cambridge University Press; 1995. p. 14–25.
2. Bhat R, Steinman L. Innate and adaptive autoimmunity directed to the central nervous system. Neuron. 2009;64:123–32.

 3. Diamond B, Huerta PT, Mina-Osorio P, et al. Losing your nerves? Maybe it's the antibodies. Nat Rev Immunol. 2009;9:449–56.
 4. Ransohoff RM, Kivisakk P, Kidd G. Three or more routes for leukocyte migration into the central nervous system. Nat Rev Immunol. 2003;3:569–81.
 5. Regeniter A, Kuhle J, Mehling M, et al. A modern approach to CSF analysis: pathophysiology, clinical application, proof of concept and laboratory reporting. Clin Neurol Neurosurg. 2009;111:313–8.
 6. Maurer MH. Proteomics of brain extracellular fluid (ECF) and cerebrospinal fluid (CSF). Mass Spectrom Rev. 2010;29:17–28.
 7. Svenningsson A et al. Adhesion molecule expression on cerebrospinal fluid T lymphocytes: evidence for common recruitment mechanisms in multiple sclerosis, aseptic meningitis, and normal controls. Ann Neurol. 1993;34:155–61.
 8. Engehardt B, Sorokin L. The blood-brain and the blood-cerebrospinal fluid barriers: function and dysfunction. Semin Immunopathol. 2009;31:497–511.
 9. Palmer AM. The role of the blood-CNS barrier in CNS disorders and their treatment. Neurobiol Dis. 2010;37:3–12.
10. Nair A, Frederick TJ, Miller SD. Astrocytes in multiple sclerosis: a product of their environment. Cell Mol Life Sci. 2008;65:2702–20.
11. Dhuria SV, Hanson LR, Frey II WH. Intranasal delivery to the central nervous system: mechanisms and experimental considerations. J Pharm Sci. 2010;99(4): 1654–73.
12. Johnston M, Zakharov A, Papaiconomou G, et al. Evidence of connections between cerebrospinal fluid and nasal lymphatic vessels in humans, non-human primates and other mammalian species. Cerebrospinal Fluid Res. 2004;1:2–15.
13. Weller RO, Kida S, Zhang ET. Pathways of fluid drainage from the brain: morphological aspects and immunological significance in rat and man. Brain Pathol. 1992;2:277–84.
14. Cserr HF, Knopf PM. Cervical lymphatics, the blood-brain barrier and the immunoreactivity of the brain: a new view. Immunol Today. 1992;13:507–12.
15. Widner H, Moller G, Johansson BB. Immune response in deep cervical lymph nodes and spleen in the mouse after antigen deposition in different intracerebral sites. Scand J Immunol. 1988;28:563–71.
16. Tian L, Rauvala H, Gahmberg CG. Neuronal regulation of immune responses in the central nervous system. Trends Immunol. 2009;30:91–9.
17. Goverman J, Autoimmune T. cell responses in the central nervous system. Nat Rev Immunol. 2009;9:393–407.
18. Bulloch K, Miller MM, Gal-Toth J, et al. CD11c/EYFP transgene illuminated a discrete network of dendritic cells within the embryonic, neonatal, adult, and injured mouse brain. J Comp Neurol. 2008;508:687–710.
19. Felger JC, Abe T, Kaunzner UW, et al. Brain dendritic cells in ischemic stroke: time course, activation state, and origin. Brain Behav Immun. 2010;24(5):724–37.
20. Hatterer E, Touret M, Belin MF, et al. Cerebrospinal fluid dendritic cells infiltrate the brain parenchyma and target the cervical lymph nodes under neuroinflammatory conditions. PLoS One. 2008;3:1–15.
21. Gottfried-Blackmore A, Kaunzner UW, Idoyaga J, et al. Acute in vivo exposure to interferon-γ enables resident brain dendritic cells to become effective antigen presenting cells. Proc Natl Acad Sci USA. 2009;106(49):20918–23.
22. Stevenson PG, Austyn JM, Hawke S. Uncoupling of virus-induced inflammation and anti-viral immunity in the brain parenchyma. J Gen Virol. 2002;83:1735–43.
23. Kivisakk P, Mahad DJ, Callahan MK, et al. Human cerebrospinal fluid central memory CD4+ T cells: evidence by trafficking through choroid plexus and meninges via P-selectin. Proc Natl Acad Sci USA. 2003;100:8389–94.
24. Lassman H, Schmied M, Vass K, et al. Bone marrow derived elements and resident microglia in brain inflammation. Glia. 1993;7:19–24.

25. Hickey WF. Leukocyte traffic in the central nervous system: the participants and their roles. Semin Immunol. 1999;11:125–37.
26. Lee BPL, Imhof BA. Lymphocyte transmigration in the brain: a new way of thinking. Nat Immunol. 2008;9:117–8.
27. Vajkoczy P, Laschinger M, Engelhardt B. α4-integrin-VCAM-1 binding mediates G protein-independent capture of encephalitogenic T cell blasts to CNS white matter microvessels. J Clin Invest. 2001;108:557–65.
28. Yang I, Kremen TJ, Giovannone AJ, et al. Modulation of major histocompatibility complex Class I molecules and major histocompatibility complex-bound immunogenic peptides induced by interferon-alpha and interferon-gamma treatment of human glioblastoma multiforme. J Neurosurg. 2004;100:310–9.
29. Stoll M, Capper D, Dietz K, et al. Differential microglial regulation in the human spinal cord under normal and pathological conditions. Neuropathol Appl Neurobiol. 2006;32:650–61.
30. Ling EA, Wong WC. The origin and nature of ramified and amoeboid microglia: a historical review and current concepts. Glia. 1993;7:9–18.
31. van Rossum D, Hanisch UK. Microglia. Metab Brain Dis. 2004;19:393–411.
32. Block ML, Hong JS. Microglia and inflammation-mediated neurodegeneration: multiple triggers with a common mechanism. Prog Neurobiol. 2005;76:77–98.
33. Barres BA. The mystery and magic of glia: a perspective on their roles in health and disease. Neuron. 2008;60:430–40.
34. Rivest S. Regulation of innate immune responses in the brain. Nat Rev Immunol. 2009;9:429–39.
35. Yang I, Han SJ, Kaur G, et al. The role of microglia in central nervous system immunity and glioma immunology. J Clin Neurosci. 2010;17:6–10.
36. Nimmerjahn A, Kirchhoff F, Helmchen F. Resting microglial cells are highly dynamic surveillants of brain parenchyma in vivo. Science. 2005;308:1314–8.
37. Bsibsi M, Ravid R, Gveric D, et al. Broad expression of Toll-like receptors in the human central nervous system. J Neuropathol Exp Neurol. 2002;61:1013–21.
38. De Simone R, Giampaolo A, Giometto B, et al. The costimulatory molecule B7 is expressed on human microglia in culture and in multiple sclerosis acute lesions. J Neuropathol Exp Neurol. 1995;54:175–87.
39. Kreutzberg GW. Microglia: a sensor for pathological events in the CNS. Trends Neurosci. 1996;19:312–8.
40. Wang J, Tsirka SE. Contribution of extracellular proteolysis and microglia to intracerebral hemorrhage. Neurocrit Care. 2005;3:77–85.
41. He F, Sun YE. Glial cells more than support cells? Int J Biochem Cell Biol. 2007; 39:661–5.
42. Voskuhl RR, Peterson RS, Song B, et al. Reactive astrocytes form scar-like perivascular barriers to leukocytes during adaptive immune inflammation of the CNS. J Neurosci. 2009;37:11511–22.
43. Bradl M, Lassmann H. Oligodendrocytes: biology and pathology. Acta Neuropathol. 2010;119:37–53.
44. McTigue DM, Tripathi RB. The life, death, and replacement of oligodendrocytes in the adult CNS. J Neurochem. 2008;107:1–19.
45. Jurewicz A, Matysiak M, Tybor K, et al. Tumour necrosis factor-induced death of adult human oligodendrocytes is mediated by apoptosis inducing factor. Brain. 2005;128:2675–88.
46. Shatz CJ. MHC Class I: an unexpected role in neuronal plasticity. Neuron. 2009; 64:40–5.
47. Krueger M, Bechmann I. CNS pericytes: concepts, misconceptions, and a way out. Glia. 2010;58:1–10.
48. Abbott NJ, Patagbendige AAK, Dolman DEM, et al. Structure and function of the blood-brain-barrier. Neurobiol Dis. 2010;37:13–25.

49. Fukata M, Vamadevan AS, Abreu MT. Toll-like receptors (TLRs) and Nod-like receptors (NLRs) in inflammatory disorders. Semin Immunol. 2009;21:242–53.
50. Van Noort JM, Bsibsi M. Toll-like receptors in the CNS: implications for neurodegeneration and repair. Prog Brain Res. 2009;175:139–48.
51. Chesnokova V, Melmed S. Minireview: neuro-immuno-endocrine modulation of the hypothalamic-pituitary-adrenal (HPA) axis by gp130 signaling molecules. Endocrinology. 2002;14:1571–4.
52. Tracey KJ. Reflex control of immunity. Nat Rev Immunol. 2009;9:418–28.
53. Pavlov VA et al. Brain acetylcholinesterase activity controls systemic cytokine levels through the cholinergic anti-inflammatory pathway. Brain Behav Immun. 2009;23:41–5.
54. Goddard CA, Butts DA, Shatz CJ. Regulation of CNS synapses by neuronal MHC class I. Proc Natl Acad Sci USA. 2007;104:6828–33.
55. Morale C, Brouwer J, Testa N, et al. Stress, glucocorticoids and the susceptibility to develop autoimmune disorders of the central nervous system. Neurol Sci. 2001; 2:159–62.

2

Principles of Immunotherapy

Jennifer L. Joscelyn and Lloyd Kasper

Keywords: Autoimmunity, Lymphocytes, NK cells, Chemokines, Receptors, Blood–brain barrier

Introduction

Immunotherapeutic intervention varies from immunomodulation, which adjusts the immune system back toward a state of homeostasis, to immunosuppression, which ablates specific compartments or pathways involved in the pathologic process. These approaches carry both benefit and risk. This chapter will discuss current and future principles of immunotherapeutic approaches.

Autoimmunity

Autoimmune disease results from failure of tolerance, the ability to discriminate between self and non-self. The immune system may then attack the individual's own cells and tissues. An inflammatory state may arise due to, excessive activation of effector cells (resulting in a proinflammatory state), or insufficient regulatory cells leading to a loss of immune tolerance [1]. Several mechanisms work together to prevent autoimmunity. These mechanisms include central and peripheral tolerance, including T-cell depletion, clonal anergy, and immune suppression provided by an important subpopulation of T regulatory (Treg) cells. These cells may carry either a CD4+ or CD8+ phenotype, and include CD25+FoxP3+Tregs. Immunologic tolerance is controlled by this population of T cells [2]. Restoration of tolerance may be critical to the effective resolution of autoimmune disease processes.

In addition to the loss of immune homeostatic balance in those with autoimmune conditions, genetic predisposition provides a further complex association. Multiple gene loci, most importantly the MHC/HLA haplotypes, are fundamental for the presentation of peptide antigens to T cells. Environmental variables such as geography, exposure, commensal microbiota, and infection also play a key role. Infections may activate self-reactive

From: *Clinical Neuroimmunology: Multiple Sclerosis and Related Disorders*, Current Clinical Neurology,
Edited by: S.A. Rizvi and P.K. Coyle, DOI 10.1007/978-1-60327-860-7_2,
© Springer Science+Business Media, LLC 2011

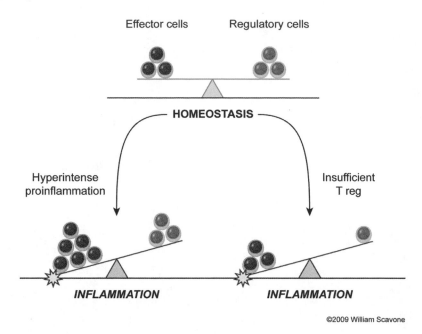

Figure 2.1 Homeostatic balance of immune system

lymphocytes, and lead to the development of autoimmune diseases in predisposed individuals (Figure 2.1).

Many autoimmune diseases follow a relapsing–remitting course, with periods of exacerbation followed by stability. This may relate to infection-triggered immune changes. The initiating response amplifies rapidly via activation of the innate immune system, but is soon followed by a more target-specific response via the adaptive immune system. This includes antigen-specific T cells and antibody-producing B cells. Cytotoxic T cells and antibodies lead to efficient destruction of the invading microbe by eliciting specific inflammatory molecules, such as the interleukins that further activate the immune system and destroy the target in a variety of ways (including direct cell to target contact and oxidative molecules such as nitric oxide). Once the invading organism is eliminated reduction in the immune response is rapid, limiting the damage to host tissue. Memory cells persist and provide the basis for secondary antigen-specific response. In autoimmune disorders the tissue damage and immunological response does not completely subside, although clinical remissions are commonplace [3].

Clinical autoimmunity arises as a result of an altered balance between autoreactive effector cells and regulatory [1, 4]. The goal in treating autoimmune disease is to re-establish immune homeostasis and restore balance between effector and regulatory T lymphocytes. Current immunotherapies are primarily used to intervene early and reduce epitope spread, induce and support the "quiescent" stage, and prevent future exacerbations.

The immune system may often seem overwhelming and too complex for the non-immunologist to fully understand, but there are recognized patterns to make organizing the information and concepts easier. The immune system is always trying to maintain balance, so for each action there is an equal and opposite reaction. Cell lineage and generative lymphoid organs form a second pattern (Figure 2.2).

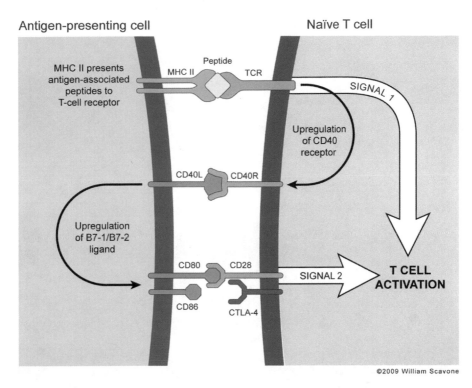

Figure 2.2 Adaptive immune activation. Co-stimulation and T-cell activation: full activation of T cells in the periphery is dependent on the recognition of co-stimulation factors on antigen-presenting cells (APCs), and completion of the two-signal activation. The first signal is comprised of antigen recognition: the APC presents MHC-associated antigenic peptides to the T-cell receptor (TCR) on the naive T cell. Chemokines are released from the APC that react with the G-protein-coupled receptor (GPCR) on the T cell, increasing the affinity and avidity of the T-cell/APC adhesion. Once the first signal is complete another set of molecules participate in increasing co-stimulatory signaling and secreting polarizing cytokines, for example, CD40 receptor is upregulated on the APC and engages with the constitutively expressed CD40 ligand on the T cell. The second signal is comprised of an upregulation of B7-1/B7-2 (CD80/CD86) ligand on the APC, following antigen recognition, that bind to the CD28 receptor on the T cell. Once the second signal is complete, the T cell is activated leading to clonal expansion and differentiation into effector functions. It is important to note that without the completion of second signal the T cells become functionally inactive, anergic

T Cells

In T-cell-mediated autoimmunity one of the most important players is the CD4+ T cell. Emerging from the thymus, naïve CD4+ cells differentiate into subtypes based on the cytokines they encounter in the periphery and/or within the CNS. Each CD4+ T-cell subtype exhibits unique functions largely based on the cytokines they produce [5]. CD4+ T cells are both effector and regulatory. Effector CD4+ T cells can be categorized as either Th1 or Th2 T cells by their cytokine production. The signature cytokine for Th1 cells is interferon (IFN)-γ, and for Th2 cells is IL-4 (Figure 2.3). Upon encounter with antigen/ MHC complexes, naive T cells become activated and can polarize into either a Th1 or Th2 cell. The process is influenced by a variety of factors, the most important of which is the cytokine milieu. The principal cytokines produced by antigen-presenting cells (APCs) for influencing Th1 cell polarization is IL-12, and for the TH2 it is IL-4 (Figure 2.3). Once polarized, on the single

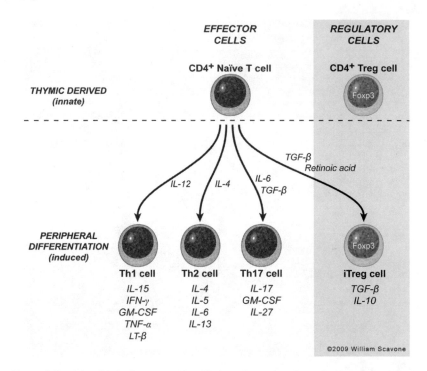

Figure 2.3 Naive CD4+ lineage. Naive CD4+ cells emerge from the thymus and further differentiate into subtypes based on the cytokine microenvironment. Each subtype of CD4 T cells exhibit unique functions largely based on the cytokines that they produce. Treg cells are both thymic derived and induced in the periphery (iTreg)

cell level the CD4+ Th1 and Th2 cells are committed and cannot revert back to a naive phenotype or convert to the other lineage. Using the early definition of T-cell functions, IFN-γ facilitates macrophage activation and IL-4 facilitates the production of certain immunoglobulin subtypes. However, the lines between Th1 and Th2 functions have become blurred. IFN-γ is also required for the production of certain immunoglobulin (Ig) subtypes, and IL-4 can also be involved in macrophage activation [5]. The Igs induced by IL-4 serve specific functions, separating the activity of the two T cells. IL-4 is required for production of IgG1 and IgE. IgE sensitizes mast cells, a consequence of which can be allergic reactions; IgG1 is involved in opsonization of pathogens. The IFN-γ-induced or classically activated macrophages produce nitric oxide (NO), which is proinflammatory and drives chronic inflammation and tissue injury. Other cytokines produced by Th2 cells that influence the immune response include IL-5, IL-6, and IL-13 (Figure 2.3). Th1 T cells also produce IL-2, IL-15, granulocyte macrophage colony-stimulating factor (GM-CSF), tumor necrosis factor (TNF)-α and other cytokines (Figure 2.3). Like CD8+ T cells, Th1 cells also have the capacity to induce cytotoxicity of target cells by several different mechanisms. The immune response can be shaped by controlling the phenotype of the responding CD4 T cell [5].

Recently, an important subpopulation of immune lymphocytes has been recognized. Treg cells are essential in the everyday control of immune responses and maintaining peripheral tolerance [6, 7]. Two populations of T$_{regs}$ control inflammation: natural (constitutive) Treg cells and induced Treg cells (iT$_{reg}$) (Figure 2.3). Natural T$_{reg}$ cells are a population of CD4+ lymphocytes residing in the thymus that express the interleukin (IL)-2 receptor CD25 and the transcription repression factor FoxP3. These cells constitute 5–12% of the entire CD4+ cell population, and represent a very small proportion of the circulating WBC population. Specific populations of natural T$_{reg}$ cells are generated principally by interaction with immature APCs in the periphery. They recognize major histocompatibility complex (MHC) molecules in association with autoantigens with high specificity. These natural T$_{reg}$ cells are normally anergic, but can be activated by exposure to antigens or to high concentrations of IL-2 released from activated TH1 cells. Induced T$_{reg}$ cells are derived from either naïve CD8+ or CD4+ precursor cells in the thymus in response to the local antigen or cytokine environment. Three subpopulations of iT$_{reg}$ cells can be distinguished on the basis of surface markers: CD8+ T$_{reg}$ cells, TH3 cells and TR1 cells. The latter two are derived from CD4+ precursors. In autoimmune disease autoantigens can stimulate the differentiation of these iT$_{reg}$ cells. iT$_{reg}$ cells release cytokines such as IL-10 and TGF-β (Figure 2.3) that suppress the activity of effector T cells as well as of APCs. Effector cells and APCs may be inhibited by direct contact with natural and induced T$_{reg}$ cells and involve interactions of cell surface proteins. This helps prevent the development of hypersensitivity reactions of allergies, autoimmune disease, and promotes long-term graft tolerance. On the other hand, there may also be detrimental effects of inhibition of immune function by T$_{reg}$ cells, it attenuates immunity to pathogens and reduces both immunological surveillance and prevention of tumorogenesis.

The best-studied T$_{reg}$ cell to date is the Foxp3+ CD4+ T cell, a key regulatory molecule in the development and function of T$_{reg}$ cells. FoxP3, is a transcriptional repression factor of the Forkhead/winged box family. It is expressed by all functional T$_{reg}$ cells except the TR1 class. Mutations in FoxP3 impair development of T$_{reg}$ cells in the thymus and are associated with inherited autoimmune diseases, such as Scurfy in the mouse and IPEX (an X-linked fatal autoimmune disorder) in humans [8, 9]. Seminal experiments have demonstrated that depletion of CD4+CD25+ suppressor cells results in the onset of systemic autoimmune disease in mice [10]. The defining influence of these cells in the control of autoimmunity was recently demonstrated in an experimental murine model. Foxp3 expressing cells were specifically depleted in adult mice, resulting in the development of rapidly fatal autoimmunity that involved a variety of host tissue beyond the lymphatic system [2]. Although the exact mechanisms by which T$_{reg}$ cells regulate and suppress immune responses are not always clear, one method is through the production of the anti-inflammatory cytokine IL-10 [11]. IL-10 controls inflammation by regulating expression of cytokines and molecules involved in antigen presentation. T$_{reg}$ cells mediate peripheral tolerance by suppressing proliferation and cytokine production of autoreactive effector T cells that cause tissue damage and inflammation [12]. CD4 T cell population heterogeneity is essential for a properly functioning inflammatory response, and their differential production of cytokines is one method by which they exert their unique functions. As noted above, iT$_{reg}$ can be derived from naïve CD8+ cells as well as CD4+ cells. The possibility that CD8+ T cells may also possess regulatory functions has received less attention, despite earlier studies [13]. CD8+ T cells can suppress the response of activated CD4+ cells. FoxP3 Treg cells inhibit the proliferation and cytokine production by both Th1 and Th2 cells and may suppressing B cells [14].

NK Cells

Natural killer (NK) cells are a subset of bone marrow-derived lymphocytes, distinct from B and T cells, that function in innate response to kill microbe-infected cells and to activate phagocytes by secreting IFN-γ, they enhance the adaptive response against infectious agents [15]. NK cells do not express clonally distributed antigen receptors such as Ig or TCRs. Their activation is regulated by a combination of stimulatory and inhibitory cell surface receptors. The inhibitory cell surface receptors are responsible for recognizing self MHC molecules [15]. The ability of NK cells to protect against infections is enhanced by IL-12 produced by macrophages, as well as antibody-mediated targeting. NK cells and other leukocytes may bind to antibody-coated cells and destroy them by opsonization. NK cells express an Fc receptor, FcγRIII (CD16), that binds to IgG antibody arrays attached to a cell [15]. As a result, NK cells are activated and kill the opsonized target, via antibody-dependent cellular cytotoxicity (ADCC). Although NK cell-mediated ADCC is not as important as phagocytosis of microbes in defense against most bacterial and viral infections [15], in autoimmunity the connection between infections and initiation/amplification of the aberrant immune response is key. NK cells play opposing roles in autoimmunity, as they function as both regulators and inducers of autoimmune diseases, dependent on the cytokine milieu and cell–cell interactions. NK cells comprise about 10% of the lymphocytes in the blood and peripheral organs.

IL-15 appears to play pivotal roles in the differentiation of NK cells from their progenitors, and their survival and activation. CD56bright NK cells are an important NK cell subset that exert immunoregulatory effects [16]. In vivo, blockade of the human IL-2R by monoclonal antibody (Daclizumab) has been used for immunosuppression in transplantation, to treat leukemia and autoimmune diseases. In one study, in uveitis patients, administration of a humanized IL-2R blocking mAb induced a 4- to 20-fold expansion of CD56bright regulatory NK cells. The induced CD56bright regulatory NK cells from patients exhibited similar phenotype to naturally occurring CD56bright cells. Patients with active uveitis had a significantly lower level of CD56bright NK cells compared with normal donors. In addition, the induced CD56bright cells, but not CD56dim cells, could secrete large amounts of immunosuppressive cytokine IL-10. This suggests that the induction of the CD56bright cells might lead to the remission of active uveitis [17]. This observation may have implications for IL-2R blockade therapy, and for the potential role of CD56bright regulatory NK cells in autoimmune diseases. By blocking the IL-2Rα chain the mAb can limit T-cell expansion and direct the co-stimulated cell toward NK production (CD56bright) through the heterodimer IL2Rβ, inducing IL-15. Antibodies to IL-2Rα do not inhibit the action of IL-15 [18]. The IL-15 receptor includes IL-2/15R and γc subunits, which are shared with IL-2, and an IL-15-specific receptor subunit, IL-15R [18]. The induced expansion of NK cells produced similar phenotype and function as naturally occurring NK cells, and correlated highly to the reduction of inflammatory activity in human and animal studies. These beneficial outcomes still need to be completely understood.

NKT Cells

Natural Killer T (NKT) cells share characteristics of both T and NK cells and play a regulatory role in autoimmunity. NKT cells are thymically derived innate lymphocytes that express the TCR and receptors of the NK lineage, NK1.1. The TCR on the majority of the NKT cells expresses an invariant Va-Ja combination that translates into Va14 Ja281 (also called Ja18) in the mouse, and Va24 JaQ in humans [19]. NKT cells recognize glycolipids, such as α-galactosylceramide (α-GalCer), presented by the CD1d molecule on APCs [20, 21]. Unlike the classical MHC molecule that presents protein to lymphocytes, the CD1d molecule presents glycolipids to the TCR on the NKT cell [22]. Because of TCR chain characteristics on classical NKT cells, they are also called invariant (i)NKT cells [19]. Invariant NKT cells (iNKT) are regulatory T lymphocytes that are CD1d reactive with an invariant TCRα chain, Vα24-JαQVβ11 [21]. The regulatory function of iNKT cells is related to their rapid and diverse secretion of cytokines like IFNγ, IL-4, IL-5, and IL-10 upon TCR stimulation. iNKTs play a dual role in the modulation of T-cell-mediated immunity. They provide frontline defense against parasites, bacteria, and viruses, and induce tolerance for the prevention of autoimmune diseases (similar to that of classical T_{regs}). Balancing the two functions of adjuvant and regulation is related to the microenvironment, either to build an effective inflammatory immune response (upregulation of IL-12/IL-23 by APC or effector cells), or prevent autoimmunity with regulation/counter-regulation (upregulation of CD1d or IL-10 by APCs or effector cells). In EAE, it was noted that the lipid structure of the CD1 ligands influence the duration of interaction between APCs and iNKT cells and thus the cytokine secretion by the activated iNKT cell. A shortened glycolipid and TCR contact time produced TH2 cytokine profile, while a longer glycolipid and TCR contact time resulted in a pronounced TH1 cytokine profile of iNKT cells [19]. Concerted interactions between iNKT cells and CD1d+ cells, DCs, macrophages, and B cells, are involved in rendering autoreactive T cells unresponsive [19]. A primary goal in treatment of autoimmune disorders is to find a therapeutic regime that inhibits reactive T cells while improving regulatory cell function. iNKT cells represent an important cellular bridge between the innate and adaptive arms of the immune system.

B Cells

The role of B cells in normal immunity is well understood. The role of B cells is less clear in autoimmune diseases and historically associated with antibody production, the antibody-dependent role. Lymphocytes are the main immune cells. As discussed earlier, T lymphocytes dictate cell-mediated immunity. B lymphocytes are responsible for humoral immunity, the host defense mediated by secreted antibodies that protect against extracellular microbes and their toxins [15]. Humoral immunity is important to prevent infection. Generation of the mature B cell pool involves stepwise development of hematopoietic

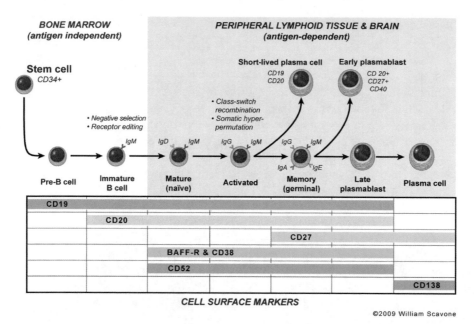

BONE MARROW
(antigen independent)

PERIPHERAL LYMPHOID TISSUE & BRAIN
(antigen-dependent)

©2009 William Scavone

Figure 2.4 B-Cell maturation and humoral immune response. The maturation of B lymphocytes proceeds through sequential steps. Many of which occur within the bone marrow. There is receptor editing and negative selection prior to maturation. Once mature, the naïve IgM+IgD+ B cell is able to recognize antigen, undergo activation upon engagement with T lymphocytes and stimuli within the microenvironment. The activated, antigen-specific, effector cells can undergo class switching and affinity maturation, improving the capacity to identify and bind to identified antigen. The expression of cell surface receptors are important to the understanding of B-cell therapeutic targets for autoimmunity

stem cells into pro-B cells, which mature into pre-B cells and then immature B cells [15, 23] (Figure 2.4). Immature B cells are then exported to the periphery as transitional B cells, which undergo further selection and development. When mature IgM+IgD+ B cells encounter T-cell-dependent antigen (Ag), they differentiate into high-affinity effector cells, namely memory B cells and immunoglobulin (Ig)-secreting cells (plasma cells) within the secondary lymphoid tissue of germinal centers [15, 23] (Figure 2.4). Mature B cells are responsible for the generation of humoral immunity and long-lived serological memory. The coordinated differentiation of B cells at these different stages of development and maturation is influenced by multiple factors, such as stromal cells and cytokines provided within the bone marrow environment, Ag exposure, and interactions between B cells, Ig-specific T cells, and dendritic cells (DC) in the periphery [15, 24, 25]. Accumulating evidence strongly supports an increased involvement of B cells in autoimmune neurological diseases, with noted antibody-dependent and antibody-independent roles.

B-cell development is complex and a multiple-step process. Differentiation of mature B cells into effector cells must be strictly regulated to ensure sufficient specific humoral immunity, while simultaneously avoiding production of autoantibodies. Receptor–ligand pairs of the tumor necrosis factor receptor (TNF-R/TNF) superfamily play critical roles in humoral immunity by regulating activated B-cell responses [26]. Two members of the TNF family; B-cell-activating factor (BAFF) and a proliferation-inducing ligand (APRIL) have been identified in recent years as crucial factors for B-cell survival, differentiation, germinal center formation, and antibody production [27]. BAFF binds three receptors, which all belong to the TNF-R superfamily – BAFF receptor (BAFF-R) [28], transmembrane activator of and calcium modulator and cyclophilin ligand interactor (TACI), and B cell maturation antigen (BCMA) [29, 30]; the latter two receptors also bind APRIL [27]. BAFF is predominately produced by myeloid cells such as macrophages, monocytes, dendritic cells, and astrocytes [31, 32] and neutrophils [33]. However, production can be further induced by cytokines (INF-γ and IL-10) [32, 34]. Pathogen-associated molecular patterns (PAMPs) molecules and toll-like receptors (TLR) can also induce production of BAFF in B cells, in response to microbial components such as peptidoglycan, CpG dsDNA, and lipopolysaccharide (LPS) when they are within contact [35, 36]. BAFF is required for late B-cell development and maintenance of B-cell homeostasis. Normal human B cells first express BAFF receptors at the transitional stage of development, and remain capable of receiving BAFF-dependent signals at least until they terminally differentiate into plasma cells (PC) (Figure 2.4). Dysregulation of BAFF has been observed in patients with many systemic autoimmune diseases. The serum levels of BAFF are notably increased in these patients, and correlated with severity of their symptoms [37–41]. It is speculated that BAFF protects self-reactive B cells from deletion by modifying expression of pro-and anti-apoptotic molecules; it reduces the pro-apoptotic molecules while increasing the anti-apoptotic molecules [24, 26]; and impairs B-cell self-tolerance. Normally, BAFF provides survival signals for B cells involved in immune defenses against infection. Elevated BAFF levels are involved in the survival of self-reactive B cells and autoimmune diseases. BAFF does not affect the central self-tolerance of B cells during their early development in bone marrow, but influences the peripheral self-tolerance of B cells, especially in later transitional stages of B-cell development (Figure 2.4) [26, 42]. The relationship between BAFF and toll-like receptor (TLR) signaling is strong in mouse models of autoimmunity [36] and therefore another potential area of therapeutic opportunity, as TLR signaling is also implicated in the pathogenesis of human autoimmune diseases [26]. Antagonists of BAFF are promising therapeutic agents to treat autoimmune diseases [26, 27].

Many organ-specific autoimmune diseases in humans are believed to be caused by T cells. Antibodies that cause disease are most often autoantibodies against self-antigens, and less commonly are specific for foreign antigens. Autoantibodies may bind to self-antigens in tissues or they may form immune complexes with circulating self-antigens [15], such as in Myasthenia Gravis (MG). The contribution of activated B cells has traditionally been viewed as a secondary consequence of breakdown of T-cell tolerance. In certain neurological diseases, including Myasthenia Gravis and specific neuropathies, autoantibodies are pathogenic and exert a direct effect on self-antigens either by functioning as neutralizing antibodies, or by activating and fixing complement on the targeted tissues (Figure 2.5a) [27]. Normally the complement system helps eliminate microbes during innate and adaptive immune responses. Opsonization is probably the most important function of complement activation. However, during the membrane attack small peptide fragments are produced by proteolysis. These fragments are chemotactic for neutrophils, and stimulate release of inflammatory mediators from various leukocytes. Neutrophils also act on endothelium to enhance movement of leukocytes and plasma proteins

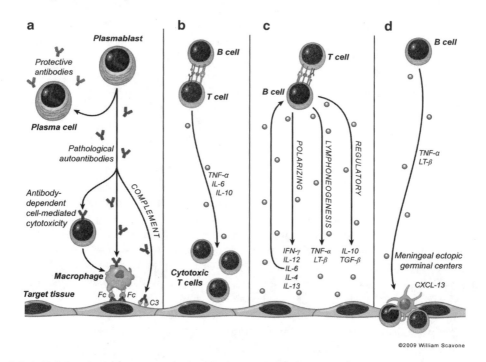

©2009 William Scavone

Figure 2.5 B-Cell functions in autoimmunity: (**a**) Antibody-producing cells–plasma cells. (**b**) Antigen-presenting cells (autoreactive T cells with a specific antigen; regulatory with low levels of nonspecific antigen). (**c**) Cytokine-producing cells; regulatory (B-cell activation with isolated CD40 stimulation), polarizing (B-cell activation with dual stimulation of BCR and CD40), lymphoneogenesis (memory B cells, primarily produce proinflammatory cytokines, TNFα/LT following dual stimulation of BCR and CD40). (**d**) Development of tertiary/ectopic germinal centers

into affected tissues to eliminate microbes. In normal individuals B cells are tightly controlled and prevented from making autoantibodies, perhaps via their interaction with T_{regs}. In autoimmune disorders this process of activating and fixing complement by autoantibodies leads to activation of ADCC (Figure 2.5a) [27]. In ADCC, NK cells and other leukocytes may bind to antibody-coated cells and destroy them.

Another mechanism of B-cell involvement in autoimmune disorders involves presentation of antigenic peptides, with clonal expansion of either autoreactive or regulatory T cells (Figure 2.5b) [27, 43–45]. Divergence of T-cell phenotypes and functions relates once again to the environment and specificity of antigens. B cells present specific antigens to cognate CD4+ T cells with extremely high efficiency to drive autoreactivity, so that they obtain help from CD4+ T cells for the production of high-affinity antibodies. Nonspecific antigens derived from low levels of endogenous proteins are also presented by B cells, but the outcome of presentation of nonspecific antigens is T-cell tolerance [43]. B cells are 100–1,000 times more potent in antigen presentation than other postulated APCs, including dendritic cells [27, 46, 47]. B lymphocytes that bind protein antigens by their specific antigen receptors endocytose these antigens, process them in endosomal vesicles, and display MHC II-associated peptides for recognition. They are also effective at presenting low concentrations of antigen. The membrane Ig of the B cell is a high-affinity receptor that specifically binds a particular antigen, even when the extracellular concentration of the antigen is very low [15]. Affinity maturation is in response to an antigen, and increases with prolonged or repeated exposure. In addition to presenting antigen via MHCII, B cells also express co-stimulatory factors (such as B7) that activate, via two-signal co-stimulation, the autoreactive T lymphocyte. This in turn activates T cells by expressing CD40 ligand and secreting cytokines. This promotes clonal expansion, proliferation, and differentiation. As this co-activation between B cell (APC) and T cell occurs, heavy chain class switching and affinity maturation are also stimulated, demonstrating further that B cells play an important role in magnifying and sustaining the T-cell response. Although the antigens are unknown, modulating/suppressing B cells and the ensuing co-stimulation of T cells may contribute to the treatment effects noted with early treatment of many neurological autoimmune disorders.

Cytokine-producing B cells influence the initiation of immune responses and regulate T-cell responses. As noted in Figure 2.5c, another antibody-independent function of B cells is to production of a diverse array of cytokines, including regulatory (IL-10, TGFβ), polarizing (IL-4, IL-13, IFNγ, IL-12), and lymphoid tissue-organizing cytokines (TNFα, LTβ) [47, 48]. B-cell-derived cytokines are produced and dictated by the balance of stimulatory signals via the B-cell receptor (BCR) and CD40 [49]. CD40 is constitutively expressed on all B cells [50] and therefore B cells are capable of activation via BCR/CD40 ligation or singularly with CD40L via local immune responsive T cells [49]. Cytokines produced by B cells, including IL-6, play important roles in regulating autoimmune responses. IL-6 produced by activated (BCR/CD40 stimulated) B cells functions in an autocrine fashion. It induces differentiation of IL-6 receptor (IL-6R) expressing B cells into antibody-secreting plasma cells, and by enhances the long-term survival of the IL6-R+ plasma cells [47]. In normal B cells the IL-6/IL-6R autocrine loop is tightly regulated. Dysregulation of B-cell-derived IL-6 has been suggested to contribute to formation of autoantibodies, and development and magnification of autoimmune disorders [47, 49]. IL-10 is a suppressive cytokine produced by normal B cells and B cells associated with autoimmune disorders. IL-10 producing B cells, in EAE, have the ability to downregulate the ongoing type 1 autoimmune response [51, 52], and suppress the expansion of autoimmune type 1 cells [53]. Duddy and colleagues demonstrated that naïve (CD19+CD27−) and memory (CD19+CD27+) human B cells express distinct profiles of effector cytokines, and reconfirmed earlier findings of context-dependent cytokine production of IL-10 and TNFα/LT [2]. Regulatory B cells control active CNS demyelination in a murine EAE model [54]. Naïve B cells (CD19+CD27−) almost exclusively produce IL-10, specifically after B-cell activation with isolated CD40 stimulation ex vivo [2, 49]. As a well-established regulatory cytokine that suppresses APC and T-cell activation, B cell IL-10 likely decreases inappropriate immune responses by limiting undesirable polyclonal expansion and inducing apoptosis [49]. Memory B cells (CD19+Cd27+) primarily produce proinflammatory cytokines, TNFα/LT following dual stimulation of BCR and CD40 [2, 49]. It is important to remember the homeostatic function of the immune system; IL-10 producing B cells may ameliorate T-cell-mediated autoimmune disease, while activated B cells are proficient producers of inflammatory cytokines, such as lymphotoxin (LT) and TNFα (Figure 2.5d). Current and future therapeutics are focused on selective B-cell depletion (anti-CD20 mAb) and chemoablative techniques (anti-CD52 mAb, autologous stem cell therapy [2].

Lymphotoxins and TNFα produced by B cells are responsible for organizing secondary and tertiary/ectopic lymphoid structures (Figure 2.5d) [27] in autoimmune disorders. Ectopic lymphoid structures could represent a critical step in sustaining humoral autoimmunity and disease exacerbation in neurological autoimmune disorders [55]. In a healthy immune response, peripheral lymphoid organs are organized to concentrate antigen, APCs, and lymphocytes in a way that optimizes interactions among the cells and produces appropriate adaptive response. An example of this organization would be in lymph nodes (LNs), specialized organs for trapping antigen from local tissue supplied by lymphatic vessels. LNs can be divided into three regions: cortex, paracortex, and medulla [15]. Naïve mature B cells are drawn into developing LNs by expression of the chemokine CXCL13. These B cells are then organized into follicles containing follicular dendritic cells (FDCs), located in the cortex of LNs, surrounded by T lymphocytes within the paracortex-containing dendritic cells (DCs). The organization of the T and B cells adjacent to one another enables the two cells to migrate toward each other, and interact to help B cells differentiate into antibody-producing cells. Normally affinity maturation occurs in the germinal centers of lymphoid follicles, as a result of somatic hypermutation of the Ig genes [15]. In autoimmune disorders, LT produced by B cells facilitates the development of tertiary structures, referred to as lymphoid neogenesis, occurring in the intermeningeal spaces of patients with MS, the thymus of Myasthenia Gravis patients, and in the target organs associated with RA, Sjogren's and Thyroditis [15, 47]. Ectopic germinal centers of the thymus have also been found to develop preferentially in patients with early onset Myasthenia Gravis (EOMG) [56, 57]. In other autoimmune diseases it has been demonstrated that ectopic follicles are found in tissues with the highest degree of inflammation, indicating that formation of ectopic lymphoid tissue requires a strong immune activation via autoimmune dysregulation and/ or infectious stimulus (viral/bacterial) that results in a persistent inflammatory microenvironment [58, 59]. Formation of ectopic lymphoid tissue is viewed as part of an adaptive response against infection. It may also have the potential to support autoimmunity through expansion and activation of autoreactive B and T lymphocytes, and further destruction of tissue [68]. Therapeutic targets (possibly B-cell depletion, chemokine antagonists, or LTβR-Ig) should be focused on prevention or eradication of such tertiary lymphoid structures nested within the CNS and other target organs of autoimmunity.

Trafficking Molecules

The central nervous system (CNS) is characterized by an immune-specialized environment as a result of limited lymphatic drainage, resident DC's, and MHC expression [15, 60]. Under normal conditions the CNS strictly controls immunosurveillance, localized to the perivascular and subarachnoid spaces, as it is crucial for host defense [60]. Often the blood–brain barrier (BBB) is the only site of leukocyte transmigration. There are three potential sites for leukocytes to enter into the CNS: the BBB, the blood–CSF barrier (BCSFB), and the blood–spinal cord barrier (BSpCB) [60, 61]. The remaining discussion will focus on the BBB, which should be thought to include both capillary and post-capillary venules (they show equal restriction of molecules, with no differential characteristics) [60]. Slight differences between BBB meningeal and parenchymal microvessels have been identified. The meningeal microvessels lack astrocytic ensheathment, [62] while the parenchymal microvessels lack P-selectin [63]. The choroid plexus epithelium establishes the Brain–CSF Barrier (BCSFB). Data suggests that lymphocytes enter the CSF across the BCSFB during normal immunosurveillance to monitor the subarachnoid space. They retain the capacity to initiate a local immune reaction if needed, or return to secondary lymphoid organs, via CCR7 and L-selectin [63]. Ventricular and lumbar CSF from healthy patients is uniformly composed of CD4+ central-memory T cells [64]. What guides autoreactive leukocytes (lymphocytes, macrophages, monocytes, eosinophils, neutrophils) into the CNS in neuroimmune inflammation disorders is still unclear. Whether antigen presentation takes place in the cervical or lumbar lymph nodes, as both are specific lymphatic drainage sites for CNS solutes (molecular mimicry) and antigens (neuro-specific antigens) [65] is not yet clarified. There are chemokine gradients between brain parenchyma and circulation that could be initiated by a viral or bacterial infection, that would then trigger TLRs in innate immune cells of the brain (microglia and astrocytes) [66]. Could prolonged inflammation and/or specific BBB transmigration thru post-capillary venules give way to ectopic germinal center formation and amplification of the disease process? Understanding the mechanisms of leukocyte trafficking into the brain might provide insight into how to modulate pathologic immune responses with specific therapeutic targets.

Leukocyte transmigration is governed by chemoattractant cytokines, chemokines, and adhesion molecules, and is a multistep well-orchestrated response to injury and inflammation (Figure 2.6). It requires specific adhesion molecules (AMs), selectins, to make transient contact with the endothelium cells. Autoreactive leukocytes loosely tether and roll along the endothelial cells due to the low-affinity binding of selectins and associated ligands (Figure 2.6A) [60, 61]. There are three types of selectins: L-selectin is expressed on most circulating leukocytes, while P- and E-selectin expressions are inducible on endothelial cells involved in acute and chronic inflammatory processes. The shear forces of the blood flow continue the autoreactive leukocyte in a rolling motion, while it senses activating factors on the endothelial surface [60, 61]. Luminal chemokines are immobilized on endothelial surfaces to trigger activation of integrins from circulating leukocytes (Figure 2.6A) [61].

Once the rolling leukocyte slows in velocity it reacts to chemokines on the endothelial surface via G-protein-coupled receptor, resulting in activation and conformational changes of integrins on the leukocyte surface (Figure 2.6B). Integrins are a large family of $\alpha\beta$ heterodimeric transmembrane proteins that provide a physical linkage, mediating cell–cell and cell–extracellular matrix interactions, and help to regulate cell behavior through discrete regulatory cues [15]. Upregulated integrins on the autoagressive leukocytes include P-selectin glycoproteinligand-1 (PSGP-1), and very late antigen-4 (VLA-4)/α-4 integrin ($\alpha4\beta7$). G-protein-dependent activation leads to secure lymphocyte fixation, due to increased affinity and avidity of integrins for endothelial ligands vascular cell adhesion molecule-1 (VCAM-1) and intracellular adhesion molecule-1 (ICAM-1) (Figure 2.6C). Newly identified adhesion molecules, junctional adhesion molecule-A (JAM-A) and platelet-endothelial cell adhesion molecule-1 (PECAM-1), are involved in the permeability and transmigration of the BBB [60]. They may be future therapeutic targets.

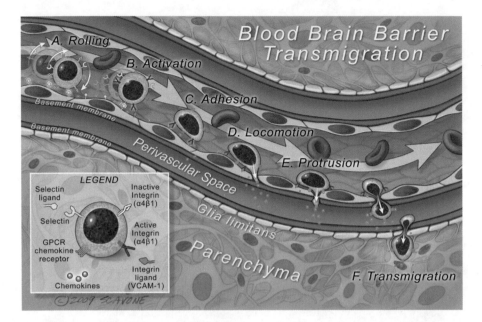

Figure 2.6 Blood–brain barrier transmigration: Multistep recruitment of leukocytes across the blood and CSF barriers in the inflamed brain. (**A**) Rolling: autoreactive leukocytes loosely tether and roll along the endothelial cells due to the binding of selectins and associated ligands. The shear forces of the blood flow continue the autoreactive leukocyte in a rolling motion while sensing activating factors. (**B**) Activation: once the rolling leukocyte slows in velocity it reacts to chemokines on the endothelial surface via G-protein-coupled receptor, resulting in activation and conformational changes of integrins on the leukocyte surface. (**C**) Adhesion: activation leads to an increased affinity and avidity for endothelial ligands and arrest of the leukocytes rolling motion. Only activated leukocytes are able to mediate firm adhesion. (**D**) Locomotion: arrested leukocytes move across the endothelial surface until the tight junctions of the endothelium, interendothelial junctions, are identified. (**E**) Protrusion: activated leukocytes extend protrusions through the tight junctions sensing chemokines that serve as guides. (**F**) Transmigration: diapedesis of leukocytes through the endothelial barrier between the endothelial basement membrane and the basement membrane of the glia limitans within the perivascular space. Matrix Metalloproteinases (MMPs) facilitate the leukocytes migrating both basement membranes and the glia limitans, providing entry into the parenchyma

Only activated leukocytes mediate firm adhesion and arrest of rolling. They then travel across endothelial surfaces until they identify interendothelial tight junctions (Figure 2.6D) [67]. Activated leukocytes extend protrusions through the tight junctions in response to chemokines (Figure 2.6E) [61]. Chemokines are a large family of low-molecular weight chemotactic cytokines that direct cells to specific sites of inflammation or injury and play an important role in leukocyte homing [68]. Chemokines secreted by lymph node cells attract B cells to germinal centers, DCs and T cells to T-cell areas. The chemokine family is comprised of approximately 50 molecules and 20 receptors [68, 69]. The chemokine ligand superfamily is divided into subgroups, the largest being CC chemokines (28 members), CXC chemokines (16 members), and CX3C chemokines (1 member) [68, 70]. Subgroup members are functionally related, and signal to corresponding families of chemokine G-protein-coupled receptors (GPCRs). Most of the receptors bind several different chemokines, and many chemokines bind different receptors. Chemokine receptors are localized to various cell types, direct adaptive immune responses, and contribute to the pathogenesis of many diseases. In the CNS, specific chemokine receptors have been detected on microglia, astrocytes, oligodendrocytes, neurons, and brain microvasulature [68]. Chemokines are implicated in many autoimmune disorders as they regulate a multitude of effector cells by governing their departure from the bloodstream into tissues, their migration through lesions, and their effector functions. Assigning roles to individual receptors is critical to the identification of relevant therapeutic targets.

Transmigration (diapedesis) occurs as leukocytes extravagate thru the endothelial barrier, between the endothelial basement membrane and the basement membrane of the glia limitans within the perivascular space (Figure 2.6F). Activated cells (including monocytes, macrophages, T lymphocytes, neutrophils, endothelial cells, microglia, astrocytes, oligodendrocytes) secrete matrix metalloproteinases (MMPs). MMPs are enzymes that digest various collagen components of the extracellular matrix and basement membrane [71]. Tissue inhibitor of metalloproteinases (TIMP) controls the activity of MMPs. MMPs in coordination with TIMP facilitate the final step of leukocytes migrating the basement membrane and glia limitans, providing entry into the parenchyma [61]. There are many immunological targets to halt leukocyte trafficking into the parenchyma including, but not limited to, G-coupled protein receptor, adhesion molecules, chemokines, and MMP/TIMP.

S1P1

A newer therapeutic paradigm to affect leukocyte transmigration in involves blocking leukocyte lymphoid and thymic egress, thru sphingosine 1-phosphate (S1P). S1P is an important signaling molecule produced inside cells by sphingosine kinase driven phosphorylation [72]. Once the S1P cells are transported and externalized into blood and interstitial fluids, they actively engage with associated GPCRs, regulated by cellular activation, on a multitude of cells. Both sphingolipid metabolites, S1P, and ceramide, have been identified as critical regulators of cell survival and death [73]. S1P is associated with decreased apoptosis, while ceramide conversely is associated with pro-apoptosis. Not only do these two sphingolipid metabolites exert opposing roles, they are also interconvertible. This suggests the dynamic ratio between S1P and ceramide is responsible for cell fate [74], and ultimately health or disease, in a wide distribution of systems. S1P receptors 1–5 are ubiquitously expressed, but show differential cell association and physiological action [72]. In the context of neurological autoimmunity, S1P1 normally transduces S1P effects on lymph node (LN) egress and tissue migration of naive lymphocytes, S1P4 has been detected primarily in the immune compartments and leukocytes [75] and it has been postulated that S1P4 may participate in cytokine production by T lymphocytes [76]; S1P5 is expressed primarily in the CNS white matter tracts, specifically in the oligodendrocytes [77]. S1P1 receptor regulates the mobilization of NKT cells to inflammation within the periphery [78]. S1P1 agonist prevents lymphocyte egress from secondary lymphoid tissues, resulting in a reduction of peripheral lymphocytes and therefore limiting potential recirculation into the CNS. Recently, a small molecule pro-ligand (agonist) for sphingosine 1-phosphate type 1 receptor (S1P1) (FTY720) was approved for relapsing forms of MS. The T1IFNb protein, CD69, also impairs the function of S1P1 in a similar function [79]. S1P is a clear therapeutic target for many serious medical conditions such as cancer, inflammation, and immune-mediated disorders such as MS.

Dendritic Cells

DCs are bone marrow-derived cells (HPCs) (Figure 2.7), found in epithelia and most organs, morphologically characterized by thin membranous projections, dendrites. DCs are specialized to capture and process antigens, to present their peptides to lymphocyte. They are found in all peripheral tissues, blood/circulatory system, and lymphoid organs [4, 80]. DCs play a pivotal role in orchestrating the immune response. The activation status and cytokine secretion profile of DCs control both activation and tolerization of immune responses against self and non-self-antigens. They function as "professional" APCs for naïve T lymphocytes, and are important for the initiation of adaptive immune response

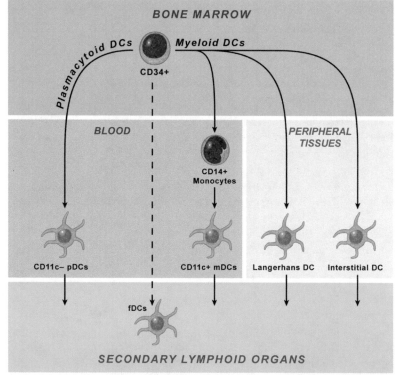

©2009 William Scavone

Figure 2.7 Dendritic cell lineage and subtypes: two main pathways of dendritic cells (DCs) originate from bone marrow hematopoietic progenitor cells (HPCs), into myeloid DC (mDCs) and plasmacytoid DC (pDCs). Resident DCs are mature and found in the secondary lymphoid tissues. Follicular DCs (fDCs) are unique and found within the germinal centers of lymph nodes with the primary role of presenting antigen to B cells, not T cells. pDC exist in the blood/circulatory compartment. mDCs exist in the peripheral tissues, blood, and secondary lymphoid compartments. Within the peripheral tissues there are two additional subtypes; interstitial DCs (intDCs), located within the dermis and responsible for humoral immunity; and Langerhans DCs (LCs), located within the epidermis and responsible for cell-mediated immunity to protein antigens [15]. Integral to specific autoimmune diseases is an imbalance in the production of a particular cytokine (i.e., Rheumatoid Arthritis, TNF-α; Systemic Lupus Erythematosus (SLE), T1IFN; MS, IL-12/23, IL-17) that are dependent upon DC interactions. In MS, it is well known that the cytokine profiles of CD4+ T lymphocytes are dictated by the ability of APCs (such as DCs) to secrete either IL-12/IL-23, for a Th1 response, or the combination of TGFβ and IL-6, for a Th17 response. In addition, DCs secreting IL-10 have been shown to induce IL-10-producing Tregs [81, 82]. The immune system is a dynamic system of cytokine vectors. Equilibrium maintains health and protective immunity, while a predominant skewing leads to autoimmunity and immunopathology. DC maturation and subsets play a critical role in stimulating immune responses as well as maintaining tolerance. This understanding has led to the potential of DCs as a distinct therapeutic target for various inflammatory and autoimmune diseases [4].

Dendritic Cells Subtype and Maturation

The maturation and subtypes of DCs are presumably a response to the encountered pathogen and the cytokine milieu, either in the peripheral lymph nodes via the lymph, or in the spleen via the circulatory system. Non-activated immature DCs are thought to continuously present self-antigen to autoreactive T cells in the absence of co-stimulation. This induces anergy or deletion of potentially harmful T cells (Figure 2.8) [83]. If a microbe breaches the epithelium to enter connective tissue and parenchymal organs, it can be captured by an immature DC that reside in these tissues, and be transported to the peripheral lymph nodes for antigen presentation to T lymphocytes. Recent studies indicate that soluble antigens directly diffuse into draining LNs via lymphatics and conduits, thereby reaching the resident DCs [84]. Despite their proficiency as APCs, during this process of migration into the lymph nodes the activated DCs can undergo semi-maturation into tolerogenic DCs. Semi-mature DCs, in a steady state, have demonstrated tolerogenic functions by skewing TH1/TH2 balance as well generating and interacting with regulatory T lymphocytes (CD4+CD25+FOXP3), to suppress autoimmunity (Figure 2.8) [85]. DCs become activated following the capture of antigens, triggering of toll-like receptors (TLRs) and the innate proinflammatory cytokine production. Activated DCs lose adhesiveness for epithelial tissue, but express surface receptors for homing chemokines that direct the DCs into the lymph and peripheral lymph nodes. Antigen presentation of both MHC I and II, as well as expression of co-stimulatory molecules (CD80/CD86), and proinflammatory cytokines efficiently activate T-lymphocyte effector functions and cytokine production of TNFα and IL-2 (Figure 2.8) [86]. Traditionally, DCs have been referred to as mobile sentinels due to their capacity to capture antigen, migrate to LNs, and present to and activate lymphocytes. However, recent research has uncovered that DCs have the ability to minimize autoimmunity. Once these processes are better understood, they may be used to induce tolerance in autoimmune diseases.

Cytokines

Cytokines represent critical mediators of the autoimmune process. They are generally small molecular weight soluble proteins that are secreted and responsible for communication between leukocytes and between leukocytes

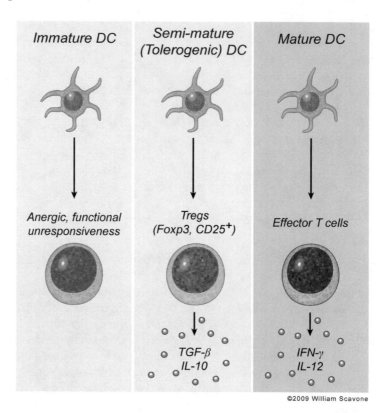

©2009 William Scavone

Figure 2.8 DC maturation: DCs are referred to as immature prior to binding and endocytosing antigen, as they are inactive and inefficient at stimulating T lymphocytes. Semi-mature DCs have demonstrated tolerogenic functions by skewing TH1/TH2 balance (producing IL-10 and TGFβ) as well as generating and interacting with regulatory T lymphocytes (CD4+CD25+FOXP3), to suppress autoimmunity. Mature DCs are immunogenic once antigens are encountered, endocytosed, and presented to T lymphocytes in an inflammatory microenvironment, resulting in effector functions (production of IFNγ and IL-2)

and other cells. They bind to their cognate receptors to induce a signaling cascade [5]. Cytokines function in both an autocrine and paracrine manner to induce a number of cellular responses. There are currently 35 interleukins (ILs) that have been cloned and characterized, tumor necrosis factor (TNF), chemokines, interferon-γ (IFNγ), and Type 1 Interferons α/β (T1IFNs). Many of the cytokines were found to be members of a family based on sequence similarity, sharing of subunits, sharing of receptors, or having cognate receptors that share subunits. For example, IL-2 is an important T-cell cytokine produced at high levels by naive CD4 T cells following antigen recognition. It serves as a growth and survival factor for T cells. IL-2 binds to its receptor, called the IL-2 receptor (IL-2R), which can consist of up to three chains; α, β, and c. The combination of receptor components determines the affinity of IL-2 to its receptor. On naive T cells, the α-chain, also known as CD25, is rapidly upregulated following antigen recognition, and in combination with the β and c chains forms a high-affinity receptor. The c chain, also called the IL-2R common c chain, is also a component of the IL-4, IL-7, and IL-15 receptors [5]. Monoclonal antibodies to cytokine receptors are being developed in order to suppress cytokine binding and proliferation of the cytokine production, leading to specific autoimmunity (i.e., Daclizumab, anti-CD25 (IL-2R)). There are a number of cytokine families that influence T-cell biology, and could be targeted in autoimmune disorders.

Endogenous T1IFN is a naturally occurring regulatory cytokine that is ubiquitously expressed except on red blood cells. Interferon (IFN) is pivotal for bridging the innate and adaptive immune response, as it is produced in response to viral stimuli by innate cells (T1IFN and IFNγ) as well as T lymphocytes (IFNγ) [15]. The key cell type that produces T1IFN is plasmacytoid dendritic cells (pDCs) [82]. pDCs are induced by toll-like receptors (TLR) on APCs. The pleiotropic effects of IFN include potent antiviral activity, antiproliferation, and immunomodulatory activities on the immune system [87]. T1IFN can stimulate the transcription of many genes primarily through the Janus kinase (JAK)-STAT pathway. In addition to gene induction, T1IFN can also inhibit the transcription of selected genes, although less is known about the mechanisms underlying IFN-b-mediated negative gene regulation [88]. Cells targeted by T1IFNs include, but are not limited to, DCs, lymphocytes, macrophages, astrocytes, and neurons. Type I IFNs are differentially involved with a number of autoimmune disorders [87], and therefore intriguing therapeutic targets.

Stem Cells

Stem cells have varying potential as therapeutic targets for neurologic autoimmune disorders. While highly controversial, embryonic stem cells are considered truly pluripotent and most versatile for regenerative medicine; adult stem cells also hold therapeutic potential. They are multipotent and far less controversial. Stem cells have common attributes that enable their self-renewal, survival, and maintenance of genomic integrity [89]. All tissues appear to have stem cells, and within each tissue type stem cells are located in a specialized vascular microenvironment called a "niche." Critical to the maintenance of the stem cell niche are microenvironmental cues and cell–cell interactions (cell adhesion molecules and integrins) that balance stem cell quiescence with proliferation, specification, and differentiation of progenitor cells [89, 90]. The microenvironment, a common theme in the homeostasis of immunity and health, plays a key role in the therapeutic potential of adult stem cells, whether endogenous or exogenous/transplanted.

Adult bone marrow contains at least three stem cell populations: hematopoietic stem cells (HSCs), mesenchymal stem/stromal cells (MSCs), and endothelial progenitor cells (EPCs) [89]. HSCs are rare amongst bone marrow cells, with a frequency of perhaps 1 in 10,000 or more [89]. Identification of HSCs is based upon the cell surface marker CD34+. Transdifferentiation/cell fusion [91, 92] is but one of many potentially therapeutic properties of adult stem cells, and possibly one of the most important [93, 94]. Other potential mechanisms include but are not limited to de-differentiation, transdetermination, true pluripotent stem cell behavior, and production of trophic factors [91]. The rationale behind autologous hematopoietic stem cell transplantation (HSCT) for MS, for example, is to induce new and self-tolerant lymphocytes (resetting the immune system) following chemotherapy-induced elimination of self-reactive lymphocytes [95]. Similar to malignancies response to HSCT, autoimmune diseases that respond to immunosuppressive therapy tend to respond to immunosuppressive conditioning followed by autologous HSCT rescue. Relapsing–remitting MS is an example of an inflammatory, immune responsive disease where an, autologous HSCT study showed positive results in the form of 100% progression-free survival after a mean follow-up of 3 years (as defined by "no deterioration in their Expanded Disability Status Scale") [95]. In contrast, traditional immune nonresponsive diseases such as primary progressive MS and late secondary progressive MS show little to no improvement following autologous HSCT [96]. Current research is ongoing to review the risk–benefit of autologous HSCT as well as the optimal conditioning regime (complete/partial/non-myeloablation) prior to autologous HSCT [95, 98].

MSCs have been studied in animal models, and following acute neurologic injury, migrate to the damaged brain [99]. MSCs can proliferate extensively in vitro, and differentiate under appropriate conditions into bone, cartilage, and other mesenchymal tissues, as well as multiple other cells including neuroectodermal cells [99, 101]. These results, albeit in animal models, suggest that human MSCs could provide an ideal cell source for repair of injured organs including the CNS. Studies with human MSCs have identified comprehensive immunomodulating properties [93]. Modulation of host immune responses due to low immunogenic properties [102, 103] and the ability to secrete neurotrophins, provides a microenvironment that induces neuronal cell survival and regeneration. Transplantation of MSCs, similar to HSCT, provide the most benefit in acute neurological injury and/or early inflammatory stages of disease. MSCs are rare and decline with age, so that alternative sources of MSCs may be integral for allogenic therapeutic application in the future, particularly MSCs isolated from human umbilical cord blood [104].

CNS stem cells have tri-lineage potential, capable of generating neurons, oligodendrocytes and astrocytes. During CNS development the neuroepithelial cells in the embryonic ventricular layer generate most of the neurons and glia (astrocytes and oligodendrocytes). A consensus view is that astrocytes are the main stem cell population, with small numbers of neural stem cells (NSCs) in other regions [89]. The niche for these NSCs has been identified as the subventricular zone (SVZ) lining the lateral ventricles, and the subgranular zone (SGZ) of the dentate gyrus of the hippocampus [105]. The neural stem cell niches define zones where stem cells are retained after embryonic development for the production of new cells of the nervous system. This continual supply of new neurons and glia then provides the postnatal and adult brain with an added capacity for cellular plasticity, neurogenesis, and gliogenesis that is restricted to the SVZ and SGZ within the brain [90]. In EAE, prolonged inflammation extensively alters the proliferative and migration of endogenous NSCs in vivo [106]. In animal models, research has demonstrated that transplanted NSCs migrate specifically to the injured CNS under the guidance of immune responsive cells, potentially directing targeted migration of stem cells toward the sites of inflammation/disease [107, 108]. Therapeutics aimed at facilitating endogenous or exogenous reparative processes will need to realize the timing of therapeutic potential, as it relates to stage and duration of disease process.

Remyelination represents one of the most compelling examples of adult multipotent progenitor cells contributing to the endogenous regeneration of the injured CNS [109]. This process has been noted to occur in the clinical disease MS [110], and the experimental disease EAE, revealing the impressive ability of the adult CNS to repair itself. The inconsistency of remyelination in MS, with loss of axonal integrity, makes enhancement of remyelination an important therapeutic objective. There is tremendous research in this area, looking to expand upon ways in which to improve specification, differentiation, translocation/mobilization, and function of endogenous NSCs and/or transplanted adult stem cells. The goal is to repair the degenerated or injured neuronal pathways [111, 112]. Autologous stem cell transplantation (HSC, MSC, NSC) may provide greater potential than just cell replacement. The concept of "therapeutic plasticity" refers to the capacity of stem cells to produce neuroprotection and immunomodulation in response to specific microenvironmental needs of different pathological conditions [108]. Pharmacological and cell-based restorative immunotherapies will need to demonstrate remodeling and enhancement of neurological function, while providing an acceptable risk–benefit ratio.

Conclusion

Bench and clinical research focused on autoimmunity have provided abundant details related to the pathogenesis of many neurological diseases, and greater understanding of the current and novel treatment approaches to regulate the immune system. Much remains in question. The immune microenvironment drives cellular response. In order to re-establish immune homeostasis and regain tolerance, it will require the concerted action of multiple cells types. If any one of the cell types are missing, peripheral tolerance will be avoided. The possibility of a single therapeutic agent, directed at a single target, resolving the complex interactions in disease pathogenesis may not be attainable. It may take multiple targets, treated simultaneously or serially, in order to restore the homeostatic balance needed for disease resolution. Restoration of the dysfunctional immune response will in all likelihood require careful dissection and manipulation rather than a sweeping ablative therapy that could be harmful. More bench and clinical research is needed to study other therapeutic targets such as, allogeneic HSCT, antimetabolites, toll-like receptors, statins, vitamin D and A (retinoic acid), commensal bacteria, continued genomic evaluation, and individualized treatments regimes.

References

1. Kasper L. Haque, Azizul., Haque, Sakhina DA Regulatory mechanisms of the immune system in multiple sclerosis. T regulatory cells: turned on to turn off. J Neurol. 2007;254 Suppl 1:110–4.
2. Duddy M et al. Distinct effector cytokine profiles of memory and naive human B cell subsets and implication in multiple sclerosis. J Immunol. 2007;178(10):6092–9.
3. Richman DP, Agius MA. Treatment principles in the management of autoimmune myasthenia gravis. Ann N Y Acad Sci. 2003;998:457–72.
4. Blanco P et al. Dendritic cells and cytokines in human inflammatory and autoimmune diseases. Cytokine Growth Factor Rev. 2008;19(1):41–52.
5. Dittel BN. CD4 T cells: balancing the coming and going of autoimmune-mediated inflammation in the CNS. Brain Behav Immun. 2008;22(4):421–30.

6. Costantino CM, Baecher-Allan C, Hafler DA. Multiple sclerosis and regulatory T cells. J Clin Immunol. 2008;28(6):697–706.

7. Kasper G et al. Matrix metalloprotease activity is an essential link between mechanical stimulus and mesenchymal stem cell behavior. Stem Cells. 2007;25(8):1985–94.

8. Chang X et al. Foxp3 controls autoreactive T cell activation through transcriptional regulation of early growth response genes and E3 ubiquitin ligase genes, independently of thymic selection. Clin Immunol. 2006;121(3):274–85.

9. Chang X et al. The Scurfy mutation of FoxP3 in the thymus stroma leads to defective thymopoiesis. J Exp Med. 2005;202(8):1141–51.

10. Sakaguchi S. Regulatory T cells: key controllers of immunologic self-tolerance. Cell. 2000;101(5):455–8.

11. Taylor A et al. Mechanisms of immune suppression by interleukin-10 and transforming growth factor-beta: the role of T regulatory cells. Immunology. 2006; 117(4):433–42.

12. Miyara M, Sakaguchi SD-M. Natural regulatory T cells: mechanisms of suppression. Trends Mol Med. 2007;13(3):108–16.

13. Reder AT et al. Low T8 antigen density on lymphocytes in active multiple sclerosis. Ann Neurol. 1984;16(2):242–9.

14. Sakaguchi S, Wing K, Miyara MD-N. Regulatory T cells – a brief history and perspective. Eur J Immunol. 2007;37 Suppl 1:S116–23.

15. Abbas AK, Lichtman A. Cellular and molecular immunology. 2nd ed. Philadelphia: Saunders Elsevier; 2006. p. 324.

16. Zhang C, Zhang J, et al. The regulatory effect of natural killer cells: do "NK-reg cells" exist? Cell Mol Immunol. 2006;3(4):241–54.

17. Li Z, Lim WK, et al. Cutting edge: in vivo blockade of human IL-2 receptor induces expansion of CD56(bright) regulatory NK cells in patients with active uveitis. J Immunol. 2005;174(9):5187–91.

18. Waldmann TA, Tagaya Y. The multifaceted regulation of interleukin-15 expression and the role of this cytokine in NK cell differentiation and host response to intracellular pathogens. Annu Rev Immunol. 1999;17:19–49.

19. Nowak M, Stein-Streilein J. Invariant NKT cells and tolerance. Int Rev Immunol. 2007;26(1–2):95–119.

20. Bendelac A, Savage PB, Teyton L. The biology of NKT cells. Annu Rev Immunol. 2007;25:297–336.

21. Yamaura A et al. Human invariant Valpha24+ natural killer T cells acquire regulatory functions by interacting with IL-10-treated dendritic cells. Blood. 2008;111(8):4254–63.

22. Godfrey DI, McCluskey J, Rossjohn J. CD1d antigen presentation: treats for NKT cells. Nat Immunol. 2005;6(8):754–6.

23. Burrows PD, Cooper MD. B-cell development in man. Curr Opin Immunol. 1993;5(2):201–6.

24. Tangye SG et al. BAFF, APRIL and human B cell disorders. Semin Immunol. 2006;18(5):305–17.

25. Uckun FM. Regulation of human B-cell ontogeny. Blood. 1990;76(10):1908–23.

26. Sun J, Lin Z, et al. BAFF-targeting therapy, a promising strategy for treating autoimmune diseases. Eur J Pharmacol. 2008;597(1–3):1–5.

27. Dalakas MC. B cells as therapeutic targets in autoimmune neurological disorders. Nat Clin Pract Neurol. 2008;4(10):557–67.

28. Schneider P et al. BAFF, a novel ligand of the tumor necrosis factor family, stimulates B cell growth. J Exp Med. 1999;189(11):1747–56.

29. Gross JA et al. TACI and BCMA are receptors for a TNF homologue implicated in B-cell autoimmune disease. Nature. 2000;404(6781):995–9.

30. Thompson JS et al. BAFF-R, a newly identified TNF receptor that specifically interacts with BAFF. Science. 2001;293(5537):2108–11.

31. Krumbholz M et al. BAFF is produced by astrocytes and up-regulated in multiple sclerosis lesions and primary central nervous system lymphoma. J Exp Med. 2005;201(2):195–200.
32. Nardelli B et al. Synthesis and release of B-lymphocyte stimulator from myeloid cells. Blood. 2001;97(1):198–204.
33. Ng LG et al. B cell-activating factor belonging to the TNF family (BAFF)-R is the principal BAFF receptor facilitating BAFF costimulation of circulating T and B cells. J Immunol. 2004;173(2):807–17.
34. Craxton A et al. Macrophage- and dendritic cell-dependent regulation of human B-cell proliferation requires the TNF family ligand BAFF. Blood. 2003;101(11): 4464–71.
35. Katsenelson N et al. Synthetic CpG oligodeoxynucleotides augment BAFF- and APRIL-mediated immunoglobulin secretion. Eur J Immunol. 2007;37(7):1785–95.
36. Meyer-Bahlburg A, Rawlings DG. B cell autonomous TLR signaling and autoimmunity. Autoimmun Rev. 2008;7(4):313–6.
37. Cheema GS et al. Elevated serum B lymphocyte stimulator levels in patients with systemic immune-based rheumatic diseases. Arthritis Rheum. 2001;44(6):1313–9.
38. Groom J et al. Association of BAFF/BLyS overexpression and altered B cell differentiation with Sjogren's syndrome. J Clin Invest. 2002;109(1):59–68.
39. Krumbholz M et al. Interferon-beta increases BAFF levels in multiple sclerosis: implications for B cell autoimmunity. Brain. 2008;131(Pt 6):1455–63.
40. Hamzaoui K et al. Serum BAFF levels and skin mRNA expression in patients with Behcet's disease. Clin Exp Rheumatol. 2008;26(4 Suppl 50):S64–71.
41. Thangarajh M et al. Expression of B-cell-activating factor of the TNF family (BAFF) and its receptors in multiple sclerosis. J Neuroimmunol. 2004;152(1–2):183–90.
42. Thien M et al. Excess BAFF rescues self-reactive B cells from peripheral deletion and allows them to enter forbidden follicular and marginal zone niches. Immunity. 2004;20(6):785–98.
43. Chen X, Jensen PE. The role of B lymphocytes as antigen-presenting cells. Arch Immunol Ther Exp (Warsz). 2008;56(2):77–83.
44. Hawker K. B-cell-targeted treatment for multiple sclerosis: mechanism of action and clinical data. Curr Opin Neurol. 2008;21 Suppl 1:S19–25.
45. Chan OT et al. A novel mouse with B cells but lacking serum antibody reveals an antibody-independent role for B cells in murine lupus. J Exp Med. 1999; 189(10):1639–48.
46. Lanzavecchia A. Receptor-mediated antigen uptake and its effect on antigen presentation to class II-restricted T lymphocytes. Annu Rev Immunol. 1990;8:773–93.
47. Lund FE et al. Regulatory roles for cytokine-producing B cells in infection and autoimmune disease. Curr Dir Autoimmun. 2005;8:25–54.
48. Pistoia V. Production of cytokines by human B cells in health and disease. Immunol Today. 1997;18(7):343–50.
49. Duddy ME, Alter A, Bar-Or A. Distinct profiles of human B cell effector cytokines: a role in immune regulation? J Immunol. 2004;172(6):3422–7.
50. Bancherau J et al. The CD40 antigen and its ligand. Annu Rev Immunol. 1994; 12:881–922.
51. Fillatreau S et al. B cells regulate autoimmunity by provision of IL-10. Nat Immunol. 2002;3(10):944–50.
52. Mizoguchi A et al. Chronic intestinal inflammatory condition generates IL-10-producing regulatory B cell subset characterized by CD1d upregulation. Immunity. 2002;16(2):219–30.
53. Mauri C et al. Prevention of arthritis by interleukin 10-producing B cells. J Exp Med. 2003;197(4):489–501.
54. Matsushita T et al. Regulatory B cells inhibit EAE initiation in mice while other B cells promote disease progression. J Clin Invest. 2008;118(10):3420–30.

55. Serafini B et al. Detection of ectopic B-cell follicles with germinal centers in the meninges of patients with secondary progressive multiple sclerosis. Brain Pathol. 2004;14(2):164–74.

56. Sims GP et al. Somatic hypermutation and selection of B cells in thymic germinal centers responding to acetylcholine receptor in myasthenia gravis. J Immunol. 2001;167(4):1935–44.

57. Roxanis I et al. Thymic myoid cells and germinal center formation in myasthenia gravis; possible roles in pathogenesis. J Neuroimmunol. 2002;125(1–2):185–97.

58. Aloisi F et al. Lymphoid chemokines in chronic neuroinflammation. J Neuroimmunol. 2008;198(1–2):106–12.

59. Magliozzi R et al. Meningeal B-cell follicles in secondary progressive multiple sclerosis associate with early onset of disease and severe cortical pathology. Brain. 2007;130(Pt 4):1089–104.

60. Engelhardt B, Ransohoff RM. The ins and outs of T-lymphocyte trafficking to the CNS: anatomical sites and molecular mechanisms. Trends Immunol. 2005;26(9):485–95.

61. Man S, Ubogu EE, Ransohoff RM. Inflammatory cell migration into the central nervous system: a few new twists on an old tale. Brain Pathol. 2007;17(2):243–50.

62. Allt G, Lawrenson JG. Is the pial microvessel a good model for blood-brain barrier studies? Brain Res Brain Res Rev. 1997;24(1):67–76.

63. Kivisakk P et al. Human cerebrospinal fluid central memory CD4+ T cells: evidence for trafficking through choroid plexus and meninges via P-selectin. Proc Natl Acad Sci USA. 2003;100(14):8389–94.

64. Provencio JJ et al. Comparison of ventricular and lumbar cerebrospinal fluid T cells in non-inflammatory neurological disorder (NIND) patients. J Neuroimmunol. 2005;163(1–2):179–84.

65. Weller RO et al. Lymphatic drainage of the brain and the pathophysiology of neurological disease. Acta Neuropathol. 2009;117(1):1–14.

66. Konat GW, Borysiewicz E, Fil D, James I. Peripheral challenge with double-stranded RNA elicits global up-regulation of cytokine gene expression in the brain. J Neurosci Res. 2009;87(6):1381–8.

67. Schenkel AR, Mamdouh Z. Locomotion of monocytes on endothelium is a critical step during extravasation. Nat Immunol. 2004;5(4):393–400.

68. Charo IF, Ransohoff RM. The many roles of chemokines and chemokine receptors in inflammation. N Engl J Med. 2006;354(6):610–21.

69. Cardona AE et al. Chemokines in and out of the central nervous system: much more than chemotaxis and inflammation. J Leukoc Biol. 2008;84(3):587–94.

70. Bazan JF et al. A new class of membrane-bound chemokine with a CX3C motif. Nature. 1997;385(6617):640–4.

71. Avolio C et al. Serum MMP-9/TIMP-1 and MMP-2/TIMP-2 ratios in multiple sclerosis: relationships with different magnetic resonance imaging measures of disease activity during IFN-beta-1a treatment. Mult Scler. 2005;11(4):441–6.

72. Takabe K et al. "Inside-out" signaling of sphingosine-1-phosphate: therapeutic targets. Pharmacol Rev. 2008;60(2):181–95.

73. Spiegel S, Milstien S. Sphingosine-1-phosphate: an enigmatic signalling lipid. Nat Rev Mol Cell Biol. 2003;4(5):397–407.

74. Cuvillier O et al. Suppression of ceramide-mediated programmed cell death by sphingosine-1-phosphate. Nature. 1996;381(6585):800–3.

75. Graler MH et al. The sphingosine 1-phosphate receptor S1P4 regulates cell shape and motility via coupling to Gi and G12/13. J Cell Biochem. 2003;89(3):507–19.

76. Wang W, Huang MC, Goetzl EJ. Type 1 sphingosine 1-phosphate G protein-coupled receptor (S1P1) mediation of enhanced IL-4 generation by CD4 T cells from S1P1 transgenic mice. J Immunol. 2007;178(8):4885–90.

77. Terai K et al. Edg-8 receptors are preferentially expressed in oligodendrocyte lineage cells of the rat CNS. Neuroscience. 2003;116(4):1053–62.
78. Allende ML et al. S1P1 receptor expression regulates emergence of NKT cells in peripheral tissues. FASEB J. 2008;22(1):307–15.
79. Shiow LR et al. CD69 acts downstream of interferon-alpha/beta to inhibit S1P1 and lymphocyte egress from lymphoid organs. Nature. 2006;440(7083):540–4.
80. Lande R et al. Plasmacytoid dendritic cells in multiple sclerosis: intracerebral recruitment and impaired maturation in response to interferon-beta. J Neuropathol Exp Neurol. 2008;67(5):388–401.
81. Wakkach A et al. Characterization of dendritic cells that induce tolerance and T regulatory 1 cell differentiation in vivo. Immunity. 2003;18(5):605–17.
82. Ito T et al. Plasmacytoid dendritic cells prime IL-10-producing T regulatory cells by inducible costimulator ligand. J Exp Med. 2007;204(1):105–15.
83. Meriggioli MN et al. Strategies for treating autoimmunity: novel insights from experimental myasthenia gravis. Ann N Y Acad Sci. 2008;1132:276–82.
84. Itano AA et al. Distinct dendritic cell populations sequentially present antigen to CD4 T cells and stimulate different aspects of cell-mediated immunity. Immunity. 2003;19(1):47–57.
85. Tarbell KV, Yamazaki S. The interactions of dendritic cells with antigen-specific, regulatory T cells that suppress autoimmunity. Semin Immunol. 2006;18(2): 93–102.
86. Groux H, Fournier N. Role of dendritic cells in the generation of regulatory T cells. Semin Immunol. 2004;16(2):99–106.
87. Javed A, Reder AT. Therapeutic role of beta-interferons in multiple sclerosis. Pharmacol Ther. 2006;110(1):35–56.
88. Zhao W et al. Stat2-dependent regulation of MHC class II expression. J Immunol. 2007;179(1):463–71.
89. Alison MR, Islam S. Attributes of adult stem cells. J Pathol. 2009;217(2):144–60.
90. Conover JC, Notti RQ. The neural stem cell niche. Cell Tissue Res. 2008;331(1): 211–24.
91. Rice CM, Scolding NJ. Adult stem cells-reprogramming neurological repair? Lancet. 2004;364(9429):193–9.
92. Singec I, Snyder EY. Inflammation as a matchmaker: revisiting cell fusion. Nat Cell Biol. 2008;10(5):503–5.
93. Whone AL, Scolding NJ. Mesenchymal stem cells and neurodegenerative disease. Clin Pharmacol Ther. 2009;85(1):19–20.
94. Korbling M, Estrov Z, Champlin R. Adult stem cells and tissue repair. Bone Marrow Transplant. 2003;32 Suppl 1:S23–4.
95. Burt RK et al. Autologous non-myeloablative haemopoietic stem cell transplantation in relapsing-remitting multiple sclerosis: a phase I/II study. Lancet Neurol. 2009;8(3):244–53.
96. Burt RK et al. Hematopoietic stem cell transplantation for progressive multiple sclerosis: failure of a total body irradiation-based conditioning regimen to prevent disease progression in patients with high disability scores. Blood. 2003; 102(7):2373–8.
97. Burt RK et al. The promise of hematopoietic stem cell transplantation for autoimmune diseases. Bone Marrow Transplant. 2003;31(7):521–4.
98. Freedman MS, Atkins HL. Suppressing immunity in advancing MS: too much too late, or too late for much? Neurology. 2004;62(2):168–9.
99. Li Y et al. Human marrow stromal cell therapy for stroke in rat: neurotrophins and functional recovery. Neurology. 2002;59(4):514–23.
100. Pittenger MF et al. Multilineage potential of adult human mesenchymal stem cells. Science. 1999;284(5411):143–7.
101. Zappia E et al. Mesenchymal stem cells ameliorate experimental autoimmune encephalomyelitis inducing T-cell anergy. Blood. 2005;106(5):1755–61.

102. Larghero J, Vija L, Lecourt S, Michel L, Verrecchia F, Farge D. Mesenchymal stem cells and immunomodulation: toward new immunosuppressive strategies for the treatment of autoimmune diseases? Rev Med Interne. 2009;30(3):287–99.

103. Bai L, Lennon DP, Eaton V, Maier K, Caplan AI, Miller SD, et al. Human bone marrow-derived mesenchymal stem cells induce Th2-polarized immune response and promote endogenous repair in animal models of multiple sclerosis. Glia. 2009;57(11):1192–203.

104. Wang M et al. The immunomodulatory activity of human umbilical cord blood-derived mesenchymal stem cells in vitro. Immunology. 2009;126(2):220–32.

105. Yadirgi G, Marino S. Adult neural stem cells and their role in brain pathology. J Pathol. 2009;217(2):242–53.

106. Pluchino S et al. Persistent inflammation alters the function of the endogenous brain stem cell compartment. Brain. 2008;131(Pt 10):2564–78.

107. Ben-Hur T et al. Transplanted multipotential neural precursor cells migrate into the inflamed white matter in response to experimental autoimmune encephalomy-elitis. Glia. 2003;41(1):73–80.

108. Pluchino S, Martino G. The therapeutic plasticity of neural stem/precursor cells in multiple sclerosis. J Neurol Sci. 2008;265(1–2):105–10.

109. Patrikios P et al. Remyelination is extensive in a subset of multiple sclerosis patients. Brain. 2006;129(Pt 12):3165–72.

110. Patani R et al. Remyelination can be extensive in multiple sclerosis despite a long disease course. Neuropathol Appl Neurobiol. 2007;33(3):277–87.

111. Franklin RJ, Kotter MR. The biology of CNS remyelination: the key to therapeutic advances. J Neurol. 2008;255 Suppl 1:19–25.

112. Kuhlmann T et al. Differentiation block of oligodendroglial progenitor cells as a cause for remyelination failure in chronic multiple sclerosis. Brain. 2008;131(Pt 7): 1749–58.

Part I

Multiple Sclerosis

MS: Pathology and Immunology

Patricia K. Coyle

Keywords: Plaques, Oligodendrocyte, Myelin, Microglia, Demyelination, Plasma cells

Introduction

The etiology of Multiple Sclerosis (MS) is unknown, but is believed to involve three factors (Table 3.1). The first is genetic vulnerability. Associated risk/susceptibility genes, protection genes, and disease severity genes are being identified at an increasing pace. Linked genes are not universal, and vary somewhat based on patient racial, ethnic, and geographic background. The second factor involves as yet unidentified environmental exposures, which probably occur at critical timepoints rather early in life. Both vitamin D deficiency and Epstein–Barr virus (EBV) infection have been implicated as important for development of MS. The final factor is the host immune system, which damages the central nervous system (CNS). MS is clearly an immune-mediated disease. It appears to be heterogeneous, however, with different pathways leading to disease expression [1]. Studies focused on pathology and immunology allow important insights into MS pathogenesis and pathophysiology. This chapter will review what has been learned from neuropathology, and current concepts on major immunologic disease factors.

Pathology

Since there are no good animal models for MS, neuropathologic studies are uniquely informative. Unfortunately biopsy and autopsy materials are limited, and subject to the criticism that they may not be representative of MS in general. Nevertheless, such studies have provided novel insights.

Abnormal pathology in MS is confined to the CNS. There are two major pathological processes. The first is focal inflammation leading to formation of macroscopic plaques, visualized initially as contrast-positive lesions on neuroimaging. This reflects major focal breach of the blood–brain barrier (BBB), and is a

From: *Clinical Neuroimmunology: Multiple Sclerosis and Related Disorders*, Current Clinical Neurology,
Edited by: S.A. Rizvi and P.K. Coyle, DOI 10.1007/978-1-60327-860-7_3,
© Springer Science+Business Media, LLC 2011

Table 3.1 Proposed etiologic factors in MS.

- Gene associations
    - HLA-DRB1*1501 (main susceptibility allele)
    - IL2RA, IL7R
    - TNFRSF1A (TNF receptor superfamily member 1A)
    - CD58, CD6, CD40, CD226
    - TYK2 (Tyrosine kinase 2)
    - IRF8
    - CLEC16A (C type lectin domain family 16 member A)
    - STAT3
    - EV15
    - CYP27B1
    - IL12A, MPHOSPH9/CDK2AP1, RGS1
- Environmental factors
    - Vitamin D deficiency (? prenatal)
    - Epstein–Barr virus (EBV) infection (? early childhood/symptomatic mononucleosis; high antibody levels to EBV nuclear antigen)
    - Tobacco smoking (particularly in context of high EBV antibodies)
- Immune system factors
    - CNS inflammation (both focal and diffuse)

Table 3.2 Pathologic changes in MS.

- Increased water content (edema)
- Endothelial cell injury
- Inflammation (lymphocytes, monocytes/macrophages, dendritic cells)
- Demyelination
- Axonal injury and loss
- Oligodendrocyte injury and loss
- Neuronal injury and loss
- Dendrites, synapses affected
- Microglial activation
- Astrocytosis
- Remyelination

hallmark of relapsing MS. The second pathologic process is neurodegeneration, with microscopic injury to axons and neurons and subsequent tissue volume loss. This is believed to be the neuropathologic substrate of progressive MS [2]. These two key pathologic processes, resulting in macroscopic and microscopic lesions, involve a spectrum of changes that can vary over time, as well as between patients (Table 3.2). It has been suggested that progression is age dependent, which might support neurodegeneration as a truly independent process from focal inflammation [3]. In this setting, transition to progressive MS might reflect critical loss of CNS reserve.

Macroscopic Injury

Multifocal lesions referred to as plaques occur in waves throughout the course of MS. They result from focal inflammation. About 80–85% of plaques are centered around small veins. Plaque pathology involves edema and inflammation early, variable degrees of myelin loss and axonal injury/loss, oligodendrocyte loss including via programmed cell death (apoptosis), myelin pallor or vacuolization, variable neuronal loss, normal or aberrant remyelination, microglial activation, and reactive astrocytosis. Early on there is infiltration of cells with marked BBB breakdown, identified by contrast enhancement on magnetic resonance imaging (MRI). This is followed by a local immune cascade, with proinflammatory cytokine and chemokine release, local cell activation, and injury to myelin, underlying axons, and oligodendrocytes. The edema and influx of serum components leads to nerve conduction block at nodes of Ranvier [4]. Over time cells clear, leaving a permanent area of damage surrounded by an astrocytic scar. These macroscopic lesions are visualized on MRI as hyperintense foci on T2/fluid attenuated inversion recovery (FLAIR) sequences. When there is marked tissue matrix damage, they will also appear as chronic hypointense black holes on T1 sequences.

Plaques form in preferential areas, including corpus callosum, periventricular white matter, optic nerves, cortical gray matter, juxtacortical white matter, brainstem/cerebellum, and spinal cord. They always seem to be close to blood or cerebrospinal fluid (CSF), raising the issue of diffusible humoral factors playing a role in their occurrence.

Microscopic Injury

MS CNS shows diffuse global injury. Much of the normal appearing brain, in between the macroscopic plaques, is microscopically abnormal [5]. Changes include BBB disturbances, low-grade (CD8+ T cell) inflammation, gliosis, microglial activation, axonal injury, and nerve fiber layer damage [6]. This has been documented using novel neuroimaging techniques such as magnetization transfer imaging, diffusion tensor imaging, and magnetic resonance spectroscopy, and confirmed with careful pathologic studies. Inflammatory cuffs are often seen in normal-appearing white matter. There is variable axonal injury, characterized by axonal spheroids and terminal swellings. Progressive MS patients in particular show both perivascular and parenchymal inflammatory infiltrates (see Progressive MS below). This microscopic injury is independent of macroscopic pathology.

Plaque Pathology

Formation of the MS lesion goes through stages with distinct differences. In an autopsy study of very early MS, the pathologic changes that preceded myelin phagocytosis involved marked loss of oligodendrocytes, often by apoptosis; marked microglial activation; myelin pallor without myelin loss; and virtually no systemic inflammatory cells [7]. The authors suggested these very early prephagocytic lesions, characterized by oligodendrocyte loss and microglial activation, preceded systemic inflammation. They interpreted this as most consistent with a primary in situ disturbance at the level of the oligodendrocyte and/or microglial cell, provoking a secondary systemic inflammation. This has important implications for the role of the systemic immune system in

MS, which will be discussed later. More recent reports suggest abnormalities in astrocyte foot processes may also be a very early lesion feature [8].

The next stage in very early lesions, still devoid of infiltrating B or T cells, is detection of macrophages ingesting myelin. Myelin phagocytosis represents an innate response of macrophages, and is not a CD4+ T-cell-mediated process [9]. Normal tissue surrounding these active lesions show microglial activation, except in very acute cases (when the duration is in days). Normal-appearing white matter also shows IgG-positive reactive astrocytes, and occasional IgG-positive oligodendrocytes and axons. Very early lesions show CD209+ dendritic cells in perivascular spaces within and surrounding new lesions, consistent with their being a major antigen-presenting cell (APC) in MS. Proliferating monocytes are present in the Virchow Robin spaces and adjacent tissues in very early lesions.

Subsequently CD4+ and CD8+ T cells are seen in perivascular spaces of parenchyma of recently demyelinated tissue, along with B cells and plasma cells and occasional regenerating oligodendrocytes. This has been interpreted as the start of an adaptive/acquired immune response, as opposed to the innate response of the very early lesion.

The tissue bordering active expanding lesions shows early loss of oligodendrocytes accompanied by activated microglia, with little inflammatory infiltrate. There is subsequent accumulation of activated T cells, B cells, and IgG-positive plasma cells, with some oligodendrocyte regeneration.

Early active lesions are marked by heavy infiltration of macrophages that phagocytize myelin fragments. Active plaques are defined by the presence of partially demyelinated axons with myelin-filled macrophages [10]. Male and female MS patients show no inflammation differences in T cells, CD8+ T cells, and macrophages in early MS lesions [11].

The dominant cell in active plaques is the myelin-laden macrophage, which originates largely from microglia with some participation of systemic infiltrating monocytes. They outnumber lymphocytes ten to one. With regard to T cells, clonally expanded CD8+ T cells markedly outnumber CD4+ T cells. B cells and plasma cells are limited. Immunoglobulin and complement products are found on the degenerating myelin sheaths, with variable loss of oligodendrocytes. This inflammatory infiltrate leads to upregulation of proinflammatory cytokines, such as interleukin-1 (IL-1) and IL-2; tumor necrosis factor (TNF); and interferon γ (IFNγ); and activation of endothelial cells, which will express stress proteins, MHC class II and adhesion molecules, and other factors.

Burnt out old plaques are marked by demyelination with little to no inflammation, and are surrounded by an astrocytic scar.

Autopsy Specimens

A recent study evaluated 67 MS autopsy brains compared to 28 control brains [12]. The MS cohort involved acute MS leading to death within 12 months (N=9); relapsing MS (N=5); secondary progressive MS (SPMS) (N=35); primary progressive MS (PPMS) (N=13); asymptomatic MS (N=4); and benign relapsing MS (N=1). A total of 1,148 lesions were evaluated: 378 were active, 222 were slowly expanding (an inactive center, surrounded by a rim of activated microglia and some macrophages at the lesion margin), and 548 were inactive (a sharp lesion border without macrophages, and no

microglial activation). Detailed quantitative analysis was performed on a subset of 228 lesions (85 active, 50 slowly expanding, 93 inactive). In addition, 139 normal-appearing white matter regions, 121 meninges, and 120 control areas were also analyzed from the MS brains.

Several important observations were made. The most marked inflammation was found in acute and relapsing MS brains. T cells were most marked in active lesions (which were most common in the acute and relapsing MS brains), followed by slowly expanding lesions (which were only found in progressive MS). Inactive lesions and normal-appearing white matter showed low T-cell numbers. T cells were virtually absent from cortex, but markedly present in meninges. Most of the lesional T cells were CD8+ as opposed to CD4+ cells. B cells showed a similar distribution pattern, but were tenfold fewer than T cells. They were predominantly found in perivascular cuffs or meninges; very few were within parenchyma. Macrophages (HLA-D+) were present in all active lesions, microglia were prominent in slowly expanding lesions, and a ramified microglia-like cell was present in inactive lesions. Plasma cells were mainly found in perivascular and meningeal connective tissue rather than lesions, parenchyma, cortex, or normal-appearing white matter. They were most common in progressive MS. Lymph node-like follicle structures were found only in 22% of the active progressive MS brains.

Acute axonal injury was most marked in active plaques, followed by slowly expanding lesions, inactive plaques, normal-appearing white matter, and cortex. Normal-appearing white matter from progressive MS showed greater axonal injury. Acute axonal injury correlated with inflammation in all MS subtypes, including progressive MS.

An intriguing observation was that in older MS brains (average age was 76 years), inflammation and axonal injury declined to levels consistent with age-matched controls. All lesions were inactive, suggesting the MS disease process burns out with age. There was active remyelination with evidence of shadow plaques. It could be speculated that clearance of activated microglia permitted resumption of remyelination. These patients could show concomitant vascular and Alzheimer pathology, however.

The authors concluded that progressive MS was associated with inflammation but did not show the degree of endothelial leakiness found in relapsing MS. There was differential cell distribution. T cells were seen in large perivascular cuffs, as well as in brain parenchyma. In contrast, B cells and especially plasma cells accumulated in connective tissue spaces (perivascular spaces and meninges). Plasma cells accumulated later than T and B cells, but persisted long after they had cleared.

The pathologic data supported a role for multiple cells (CD8+ T cells, B cells, plasma cells, macrophages, monocytes, microglia) in MS, in addition to CD4+ T cells.

Progressive MS

The neuropathology of progressive MS differs from relapsing MS. Although both contain focal inflammatory demyelinating lesions, with variable axonal injury and loss, progressive MS as noted above has been associated with a compartmentalized low-grade diffuse inflammatory process behind a relative intact BBB, slow expansion of white matter lesions, marked activated microglia, and extensive cortical demyelination. Most focal white matter lesions in progressive MS show slow expansion at the lesion edge, or are inactive [13]. The slowly expanding lesions show no oligodendrocyte precursors, and no active remyelination. They appear to reflect mitochondrial injury, and implicate an energy disturbance. The diffuse inflammation in progressive MS does not express apoptosis or proliferative markers. It is associated with marked neurodegeneration, with extensive axonal injury and microscopic changes. Such a process could be driven by local antigen exposure, or local cytokine production within the CNS microenvironment. There is diffuse injury to normal-appearing brain, along with marked gray matter demyelination within cerebral and cerebellar cortex. Fast axonal transport disturbances, resulting in neurodegeneration, correlate with inflammatory changes in T cells, B cells, and macrophages. Inflammatory lymphocytes predominate in perivascular cuffs. These T cells, B cells, and plasma cells are found largely in the meninges. Despite significant inflammation progressive MS patients show little to no contrast-enhancing lesion activity. This has been interpreted as progressive MS showing inflammation trapped behind a closed or repaired BBB.

In a recent study of brain and spinal cord of 34 SPMS patients and 13 PPMS patients, the SPMS patients showed larger brain plaques, greater demyelination and plaque inflammation, while PPMS showed greater remyelination with more remyelinated shadow plaques [14], Incomplete remyelination in spinal cord, but not in brain, correlated with greater disability.

Blood vessels in progressive patients may show thick perivascular infiltrates without leakiness [13]. Progressive patients also show ectopic lymphoid follicle-like structures, resembling secondary lymphoid tissue, in connective tissue compartments of the CNS. In a subset of secondary progressive MS these lymphoid follicles form within meninges where there is underlying inflammation and demyelination. They also form adjacent to large active subpial cortical lesions. The severity of meningeal inflammation and lymphoid follicles was said to correlate with extent of cortical lesion activity. However, in another study cortical demyelination did not correlate with meningeal inflammation [15]. It has been suggested that the chronically inflamed brain in progressive MS creates a local microenvironment favoring retention of inflammatory cells. In short, the neuropathology supports distinct mechanisms involved in progressive vs. relapsing MS [16].

MS Lesion Project

A consortium of neurologists and neuropathologists, funded to do research as the MS Lesion Project, have focused on examination of active MS lesions. In a series of publications based on autopsy or biopsy specimens, they described four discrete histopathologic patterns (Table 3.3) [17]. There was initial enthusiasm that these patterns formed a logical basis to define distinct MS subtypes. It was reported that all acute plaques in a given patient showed the same pattern, but that the pattern could differ between patients. It was also reported that only pattern II had a positive response to plasma exchange, indicating therapeutic implications for the classification system [18]. However, other investigators cannot confirm the Lesion Project findings [19]. Instead, it has been suggested that the patterns reflect temporal issues, with pattern III as the earliest lesion which later evolves into pattern I/II expression. This issue will need to be resolved in future studies.

Table 3.3 MS Lesion Project: proposed acute lesion pathology [160].

Pattern	Frequency	Features	Comment
I	15%	• Demyelination with abundant macrophages, some T cells • Oligodendrocyte survival with extensive remyelination • Sharp lesion borders	Macrophage-associated damage ? Myelin target
II	58%	• Demyelination as above, with immunoglobulin and complement deposition • Oligodendrocyte survival with extensive remyelination • Sharp lesion borders	Antibody, complement-associated damage ? Myelin target
III	26%	• Demyelination with limited inflammation • Oligodendrocyte loss (often by apoptosis), with no remyelination • Indistinct lesion borders	Distal oligodendrocyte gliopathy (? Ischemia) ? Oligodendrocyte target
IV	1%	• Demyelination with limited inflammation • Oligodendrocyte loss, with no remyelination • Indistinct lesion borders	Primary oligodendrocyte injury (? genetic) ? Oligodendrocyte target

Remyelination

Remyelination occurs in about 70–75% of MS plaques, and is associated with oligodendrocyte progenitor cell (OPC) recruitment. Chronic remyelinated lesions are referred to as shadow plaques. In the other 25–30% of lesions remyelination is absent and oligodendrocyte numbers are limited, suggesting a failure to recruit OPC cells [20]. Within a given macroscopic plaque, deeper sections can show signs of repair (remyelination, oligodendrocyte regeneration) even though the edges show continued destructive activity [21]. An important goal of current research efforts involves ways to enhance remyelination.

Axon Pathology

Acute axon injury including transection occurs in early MS, within both active and chronic plaques, as well as normal-appearing brain tissue and periplaque white matter [22–25]. Axon pathology correlates with degree of inflammation. Inflammatory intermediates reduce energy metabolism in demyelinated axons, perhaps by direct mitochondrial effects or by interfering with blood flow resulting in ischemia [4].

More specifically, CD8+ T-cell inflammation has been associated with axonal injury [26]. Although there is a symbiotic relationship between myelin and axon, axon changes can occur independent of demyelination [26].

In a recent study of MS spinal cord tissue, diffuse axonal loss correlated with density of both activated microglia and meningeal T cells [27].

With axon injury there is sodium influx, activation of calcium-dependent proteases, upregulation of voltage-gated calcium channels, and destruction of the axon cytoskeleton. Small axons (<2.5 mcm cross-sectional area) are preferentially lost within MS spinal cord and optic nerve [28, 29].

Cortical/Gray Matter Pathology

Although MS has been described as a demyelinating white matter disease, pathologic studies document marked gray matter involvement in deep nuclei as well as cortex. Thalamic neuronal loss in MS is estimated at 30–35% [30]. With regard to cortex, three types of lesions have been described. Type I lesions span cortex and white matter, Type II are completely intracortical, and Type III extend from the pial surface into the cortex, generally to cortical layer 3 or 4, and cover several gyri [31]. Although not visualized on conventional MRI, cortical lesions are common in MS. They are hypocellular compared to white matter plaques, and may not be associated with breakdown of the BBB. Although there are few inflammatory cells and no perivascular cuffs, activated microglia are plentiful. These lesions show loss of axons and neurons. As noted previously, progressive MS patients show more cortical pathology than relapsing patients.

Unusual MS Variants

Tumefactive MS refers to patients who present with an unusually large brain plaque, generally singular, with surrounding edema and mass effect. The lesion mimics a brain tumor or abscess, and may lead to urgent biopsy. In rare cases this is the presentation of MS. It can also occur in well-established MS. Neuroradiologic features involve size >2 cm and mass effect, with edema and/or ring enhancement [32]. The pathology shows active inflammation with myelin loss, reactive gliosis, myelin-laden macrophages, and relative axonal sparing.

Marburg variant MS refers to a clinically malignant severe disease expression, where patients go on to profound disability or even death within 1–2 years. Lesion pathology is more destructive [6]. There are many, often large, macroscopic lesions which may become confluent. Active lesions show massive macrophage infiltration, marked myelin loss, severe axon loss, and tissue necrosis. There may be deposition of immunoglobulin and complement activation in some cases. It has been suggested that Marburg variant is associated with increased (>80%) citrullinated myelin basic protein (MBP), a more immature and unstable form of this core CNS myelin component [33, 34].

Balo concentric sclerosis is an unusual demyelinating variant reported as more frequent in the Philippines and Asia. Cognitive features may be prominent. The striking pathology involves alternating rings of intact myelin, separated by demyelinated regions. Oligodendrocyte apoptosis along with selective loss of myelin-associated glycoprotein (MAG) has been noted in the demyelinated regions. In the MS Lesion Project, Balo cases were classified under Pattern III. The demyelinating pattern has been described as similar to what hypoxic injury might produce, with local expression of iNOS and upregulated expression of tissue preconditioning proteins at the lesion edge [6, 35, 36].

These lesions show defects in mitochondrial respiratory chain proteins [37]. Aquaporin 4 loss without complement or immunoglobulin deposition was extensive in both demyelinated and myelinated regions in four recent cases of Balo disease [38].

Myelinoclastic diffuse sclerosis (Schilder Disease) is a very rare predominantly pediatric disorder, characterized by one or two large (3×2 cm) cerebral inflammation demyelinating lesions [39].

Summary

Pathologic studies in MS have reinforced several key features, including the importance of abnormal inflammation, the presence of both macroscopic and microscopic pathology, extensive gray matter involvement, axonal and neuronal injury in addition to myelin and oligodendrocyte injury, and distinctive features for relapsing vs. progressive MS. More work is needed to clarify the role of initiating in situ pathology, and whether there are meaningful immunopathological subsets of MS.

Immunology

The conventional explanation for the immune disturbances that result in MS have focused on systemic autoreactive CD4+ T cells, sensitized to one or more CNS myelin components, along with proinflammatory cytokine production and a preferential T helper (Th)1 response. This is based on a key animal model discussed below. However, the immunology of MS is now appreciated to be much more complex. It is not even clear that MS is a true autoimmune disorder, since no critical autoantigen target (including any myelin component) has ever been identified. It is probably more accurate to describe MS as an immune-mediated disorder, with multiple immune system components and factors mediating the key pathologic changes of MS. It has even been suggested that changes in systemic immune factors (increase in innate immunity, including myeloid dendritic cells) contributes to development of SPMS, along with in situ CNS inflammation trapped behind a closed BBB [13, 40, 41].

Animal Models

The major animal model for MS is Experimental Allergic/Autoimmune Encephalomyelitis (EAE). This autoimmune CNS inflammatory demyelinating disease is produced in susceptible animal strains by immunizing with CNS whole myelin or myelin components such as myelin oligodendrocyte glycoprotein (MOG), MBP, and proteolipid protein. The immunization procedure requires potent adjuvants. Depending on the strain and immunization protocols, clinical expression can involve monophasic, relapsing, or progressive disease. In EAE both cellular (CD4+, CD8+ T cell) and humoral immune responses play a role. The most common model involves CD4+ Th1 cells initiating delayed type hypersensitivity responses to myelin antigens. Pathogenic CD4+ T cells adoptively transfer EAE, with the brunt of pathology seen in the spinal cord. Myelin-specific CD8+ T cells as well as Th17 cells can also induce EAE [42]. Recent studies suggest three forms of EAE, which can be driven by adoptive transfer of CD4+ Th1, Th17, or Th2/Th9 cells [43, 44]. In the EAE model inflammation first enters the subarachnoid space, and then the parenchyma. This may be similar to what happens in MS. Although MOG-induced EAE probably comes closest to looking like MS, no EAE model truly duplicates MS. EAE seems to be a truer model for Acute Disseminated Encephalomyelitis/Postinfectious Encephalomyelitis, which has an immunopathology distinct from MS [45].

The best infectious animal model for MS involves Theiler's Murine Encephalomyelitis virus (TMEV), a nonenveloped single-strand RNA picornavirus [42]. This causes an acute mild polioencephalomyelitis in mice, followed by a chronic inflammatory demyelinating spinal cord infection, with virus detectable in glial cells and macrophages. The chronic infection results in an immune-mediated myelopathy with features reminiscent of MS. However, it is relatively easy to document the persistent infection, whereas this has not been shown in MS. In brief, no animal model truly recapitulates MS.

MS Immunologic Scenarios

Several immunologic scenarios have been proposed for MS (Table 3.4). The first, and still the most popular (the so-called outside-in) hypothesis, involves proinflammatory CD4+ T cells, both Th1 and Th17, activated in the periphery by an unknown (likely antimicrobial) antigen. The triggering antigen presumably shares antigenic sequences with myelin or other CNS antigens. These proinflammatory cells attach to the CNS endothelium via adhesion molecules to cross the BBB. This is facilitated by release of proteolytic enzymes such as matrix metalloproteinases (MMPs). Once inside the CNS parenchyma molecular mimicry results in cross-reactivity, and the misdirected immune attack results in pathologic lesions. Instead of quickly exiting, the infiltrating cells see this shared antigen and are further activated locally to cause injury. This results in further leukocyte recruitment, inflammation, local cell activation, and damage to CNS tissue. There is evidence that immunity to myelin antigen targets can worsen MS. Altered peptide ligands (APL) are created as partial agonists or antagonists to the T-cell receptor of autoreactive lymphocytes. In a phase II trial of an APL to MBP 83-99, a subset of patients had marked worsening on MRI with clinical relapse, coincident with a marked expansion of MBP reactive T cells [46].

Table 3.4 MS immunologic scenarios.

- Environmental pathogen(s) or other factor leads to systemic immune response
    - This response cross-reacts with CNS/possibly myelin antigen
    - Sensitized systemic cells penetrate the CNS and result in primary tissue damage
- Intrinsic CNS abnormality (at level of oligodendrocyte, astrocyte, microglia, or neuron) leads to in situ disturbance
    - Secondary systemic immune cell penetration with secondary tissue damage
- Chronic cerebrospinal venous insufficiency
    - CNS venous stasis due to extra CNS venous stenoses
    - Hemosiderin/iron deposition around venules leads to local inflammation, perivenular damage

The second scenario (the inside-out hypothesis) is based on a primary in situ CNS abnormality which somehow provokes systemic immune cells to infiltrate, producing secondary inflammatory-mediated damage. This could reflect an abnormality of intrinsic CNS cells (oligodendrocytes, microglia, astrocytes, neurons) or their components (mitochondria, ion channels). The in situ disturbance could be a chronic CNS infection or metabolic defect. In this scenario, MS could be a neurodegenerative disorder, with demyelination a secondary issue [47].

A third recent scenario suggests MS is a vascular disorder, with CNS venous stasis leading to iron deposition, local inflammation, and secondary tissue damage [48]. Chronic cerebrospinal venous insufficiency (CCSVI) has been reported in a high rate of MS patients but not controls. Transcranial Doppler-ultrasound techniques find evidence for venous stasis and abnormal venous flow patterns within the CNS, associated with extraneural anatomic stenoses of major draining veins (particularly the internal jugular and azygous veins). This is discussed further below and in a separate chapter.

Since MS is most likely heterogeneous, it is quite possible that more than one scenario can cause MS. If this is the case, it would be important to define these distinct subsets.

Immune System Cells

T Cells

T cells have been a major focus in MS for years. Many still believe that MS represents a T-cell-mediated disease, with injury from autoreactive CD4+ Th1 cells. This certainly is true for most EAE models. Although the human immune system does not have true distinct Th1 and Th2 cells, CD4+ Th1-like cells do promote proinflammatory cytokines and enhance cellular immunity, while CD4+ Th2-like cells promote antagonistic regulatory cytokines and enhance humoral immunity. CD4+ T cells, depending on whether they are naïve or activated, can show abnormalities in number and/or function in MS patients vs. controls [49].

T regulatory (Treg) cells are immunosuppressive CD4+ T cells that express CD25 and Foxp3. They inhibit autoreactive effector cells [49]. CD4+ CD25+ T reg cells are implicated in development of autoimmune disorders. A number of studies have suggested that T reg number and function are abnormal in MS [50–52]. Transcription factor Foxp3 is the programmer for the suppressive function of T reg cells. Foxp3 mRNA and protein levels are reported as reduced in MS [53]. Recently CD8+ Treg cells were described, and found to be decreased in blood and CSF of MS patients who were in an acute attack [54].

CD4+ Th17 cells are distinct from Th1, Th2, and T reg cells, and have been associated with inflammation, autoimmunity, and response to extracellular pathogens [55]. Naïve T cells require exposure to transforming growth factor β (TGFβ) and either IL-6 or IL-21 to become Th17 cells, along with exposure to IL-23 produced by macrophages and dendritic cells [56]. IL-23 is a main driver. Th17 cells produce IL-17, which promotes inflammatory responses [52]. IL-17 messenger RNA is elevated in MS patients. These cells also produce IL-21 and IL-22. Th17 cells excel at infiltrating tissues to cause severe inflammation. They express the chemokine receptor CCR6 on their surface [50]. Th17 cells are clearly implicated in MS [57–59].

CD8+ T cells function as cytotoxic/regulatory cells. They are activated in the periphery, and then enter the CNS. They dramatically outnumber CD4+ T cells within MS lesions at all disease stages [54]. CD8+ T cells show the most profound and reproducible clonal and oligoclonal expansion [60], and memory CD8+ T cells are enriched in both blood and CSF of MS patients [61]. CD8+ T cells are associated with axonal injury in early MS [52]. They interact with autoreactive CD4+ T cells to suppress them. It has been suggested that CD8+ T cells are also reduced during MS relapses [53].

A small subpopulation of T cells have a T-cell receptor composed of γ/δ polypeptides, as opposed to the usual α/β polypeptides. They are mainly located in skin and mucosal tissues. These γ/δ T cells are involved in both innate and adaptive immune responses, and have been reported as clonally expanded in the CSF of early MS patients [62]. Another subset was associated with very aggressive MS [63]. They are increased in MS lesions, and may be involved in oligodendrocyte lysis [64]. γ/δ T cells in the EAE model control inflammatory cell migration into the CNS, promote apoptosis of encephalitogenic T cells, and play a key role in recovery. Their potential role in MS remains to be determined.

B Cells

B cells play a major role in MS (Table 3.5). B cells and plasma cells are present in the brain and CSF of MS patients [65]. There is clonal expansion and somatic mutation of B-cell receptor genes, consistent with an antigen-driven response [66, 67]. Healthy controls rarely show B cells in CSF. In contrast, MS patients show clonally expanded CSF memory B cells, centroblasts, and short lived plasmablasts as the predominant antibody-secreting cell in CSF [68]. Meningeal lymphoid follicles with germinal centers are detected in SPMS patient with younger age at MS onset, more severe disability, and more cortical demyelination [69]. It has been suggested that diffusion of antibodies or other soluble factors from the meningeal follicles to the cortex is responsible for enhanced gray matter lesions. EBV causes persistent infection of B cells, and this results in immunologic changes that might promote development of MS.

Table 3.5 Role for B cells in MS.

- B cells and plasma cells are present in CNS tissue
- Positive response to anti-CD20 monoclonal antibody
  - In relapsing MS
  - In younger, contrast+ MRI PPMS
- CSF oligoclonal bands, and intrathecal immunoglobulin production as diagnostic signatures
  - Some data suggests oligoclonal IgM, elevated IgG index may indicate poorer prognosis
- Lymphoid follicles in meninges of SPMS
- EBV persistently infects B cells

Oligoclonal IgG in CSF is a hallmark diagnostic signature in MS. The specificity of these band is not known, but they are not directed against myelin components and could represent a nonspecific polyantigenic exposure response [70]. Oligoclonal IgM (lipid specific) has been suggested to be a poor prognosis marker [71]. Although initial reports suggested anti-myelin antibodies to MBP and MOG might indicate more severe disease, these findings have not been confirmed [72–74]. Elevated IgG index, as a marker of intrathecal immunoglobulin production, is another less-specific CSF diagnostic marker.

Perhaps the most impressive data supporting a role for B cells in MS is the success of anti-CD20 monoclonal antibody therapy in relapsing MS, and specific subsets of PPMS [75, 76]. Because the benefits of therapy are seen within weeks, it suggests an effect on the B cells in their role as APCs or as T-cell regulators; the effect on humoral antibody response is delayed by months.

Plasma Cells

Plasma cells, along with B cells, also show clonal expansion in MS CSF [77]. Plasma cells show a distinct pattern from T and B cells. They accumulate in connective tissue spaces in the meninges and perivascular space [12]. They accumulate in MS CNS tissue later, but (unlike T and B cells) will persist. They are most marked in progressive MS. Clonally expanded plasma cells are the presumptive source of CSF oligoclonal bands and intrathecal immunoglobulin production [78].

Monocytes/Macrophages

Blood-borne monocytes/macrophages are known to be the major cell type in the perivascular infiltrates in MS. Monocytes also enhance T-cell migration across the BBB. Peripheral blood monocytes in MS were found to express higher levels of costimulatory molecule CD86, and to secrete higher levels of IL-6 and IL-12 [79]. Monocytes/macrophages along with microglia represent innate immunity. They are believed to play an important role in lesion pathogenesis and local tissue injury, phagocytic removal of debris, as well as repair processes [80].

Dendritic Cells

Dendritic cells are professional APCs which induce immunity and regulate tolerance. There are myeloid (CD11c+) and plasmacytoid (CD11c^{dim} CD123) types [81]. They are typically elevated in the blood, CSF, and lesions in MS [81, 82]. MS dendritic cells secrete higher levels of proinflammatory cytokines (IL-6, TNF, IL-23) than healthy controls, and show decreased expression of maturation markers [81]. There may be deficiencies in the maturation of dendritic cells in primary progressive MS [82, 83].

Natural Killer Cells

Natural killer (NK) cells, part of innate immunity, are cytotoxic to virus-infected cells and tumor cells; they also secrete cytokines [84]. These distinct functions coincide with two subsets, CD56 dim NK cells and CD56 bright NK cells. NK cells are found in MS lesions. NK cell abnormalities are described in MS, including certain subpopulations being increased during periods where patients are not actively relapsing [85, 86]. Other subpopulations are reduced in untreated MS, as well as first attack patients [84, 87]. A number of MS therapies (IFNβ, cyclophosphamide, natalizumab, daclizumab) increase NK cells [84, 88].

Invariant NK-T cells share properties of NK cells and T cells. These cells are reported as decreased in MS, and cell lines isolated from MS patients show higher secretion of IL-4 [50, 84].

Mast Cells

Mast cells are involved in allergic reactions, release histamine and cytokines, and interact with multiple immune system components [84]. Relatively limited studies have looked at mast cells in MS. They are detected in both plaques and normal-appearing white matter [89, 90]. Tryptase, a specific mast cell enzyme, is elevated in MS CSF [91].

Immune System Factors

Cytokines

The cytokine network is perturbed in MS, with Th1-mediated proinflammatory cytokines upregulated, and Th2-mediated anti-inflammatory regulatory cytokines downregulated. Several MS disease modifying therapies are believed to work in part through a Th1 to Th2 shift. The proinflammatory IFNγ cytokine has been reported to worsen MS [92], while IFNβ is used to treat MS. Blockade of another proinflammatory cytokine, TNFα, actually worsens MS [93, 94]. Progressive MS patients are reported to show greater IL-12 and IL-18 production by systemic immune cells [40, 95]. Targeted cytokine therapies continue to be developed for MS.

Chemokines

Chemokines are a family of small cytokines involved in chemo-attraction and cell migration. They are part of a network which also involves chemokine receptors. Chemokines control the selective CNS recruitment of inflammatory cells in MS [96]. In particular CCL5, CCL2, and CXCL10 are implicated in MS. CCL5 (Rantes) is upregulated at the edge of MS plaques to attract mononuclear cells [97]. CCL2 is expressed by local astrocytes to attract monocytes [98]. MS CSF shows elevated levels of CXCL10 and CCL5, which draws activated T cells [99]. Chemokines are another potential therapeutic target in MS.

Osteopontin

Osteopontin, early T lymphocyte activation-1, is a proinflammatory cytokine expressed by activated T cells, dendritic cells, and macrophages [43, 100]. It is a member of the small integrin-binding proteins, the SIBLING family [101]. It binds to α4β1 integrin, modulates TH1 and Th17 cytokines, and studies have reported elevated levels in the blood and CSF during relapses [102–104]. High expression of osteopontin has been found in MS brain lesions using cDNA microarray technology [105].

Adhesion Molecules

Cell adhesion molecules are located on the surface of cells, and mediate binding to other cells or to extracellular matrix via an adhesion process. This is important to cell penetration into the CNS in MS. Adhesion molecules involve four families (Immunoglobulin superfamily, integrins, cadherins, selectins). The endothelial cells within MS lesions express elevated levels of intercellular adhesion molecule (ICAM)-1 and vascular cell adhesion molecule (VCAM)-1 [96]. Activated immune cells express selectins and integrins such as lymphocyte function-associated antigen (LFA)-1 and very late antigen (VLA)-4 that bind to their ligand adhesion molecules on the endothelium. Anti-adhesion molecule therapy (such as Natalizumab, a monoclonal antibody directed against á4 integrin, a component of VLA-4) has been used successfully to treat MS.

Matrix Metalloproteinases

MMPs are part of a family of almost 40 endopeptidases, proteolytic enzymes that are involved in extracellular matrix and basement membrane degradation. These proteases include tissue inhibitors of matrix proteases (TIMPs), that downregulate MMPs. Activated immune cells secrete MMPs to help penetrate through the BBB basement membrane and extracellular matrix, to enter the CNS. Matrix proteinases may directly injure CSF cells, as well as activating membrane-bound proinflammatory cytokines, but may also promote CNS repair and regeneration. MMPs are implicated in BBB permeability and CNS inflammation in MS.

MMP-9 is elevated in the serum and CSF of MS, especially during relapses [106]. Elevated serum and CSF MMP-9 levels are reported to correlate with MS disease activity [107]. MMP-2 to TIMP-2 ratio is increased in the CSF and serum of relapsing MS, with evidence of intrathecal MMP-2 production [108]. Serum MMP-2 and MMP-2/TIMP-1 ratio is said to be elevated in progressive MS [109].

CNS Cells and Components

Microglia

Microglia are the resident CNS macrophages as well as immune cells. They act as APCs, produce cytokines, and are involved in phagocytosis. Activated microglia are noted in all MS patients, but are especially associated with the progressive subtypes.

Activated microglia and macrophages produce cytotoxic molecules including proinflammatory and cytotoxic cytokines, reactive oxygen and nitrogen intermediates, and proteolytic and lipolytic enzymes [80]. Microglia are likely to be an important component of the MS damage process, and are particularly involved in axonal injury [110]. It has been suggested that T cells in MS tissue may drive continued activation of microglia [111]. They may also be a repair-promoting component, since microglia can secrete neurotrophins (brain derived neurotrophic factor (BDNF), neurotrophin-3 (NT3), insulin growth factor (IGF-1)) and regulatory cytokines [84].

Oligodendrocytes and Myelination

Oligodendrocytes show variable degrees of loss in MS. They may be an early target, and can die by apoptosis prior to formation of demyelinating plaques [112]. Oligodendrocytes are especially vulnerable to oxidative stress because of their high metabolic rate, high ATP usage to synthesize myelin, large intracellular iron content, high hydrogen peroxide level, high levels of polyunsaturated fatty acid within the myelin, and low levels of antioxidants [113]. It has been suggested that intrinsic apoptosis due to oxidative stress is an important cause for oligodendrocyte loss in MS. Fas/CD95 is expressed on oligodendrocytes in chronic MS lesions; FasL expressed on microglia and inflammatory lymphocytes are likely to play a role in intrinsic oligodendrocyte apoptosis [113, 114].

Remyelination involves generating new mature oligodendrocytes [115]. Oligodendrocytes can be replaced by OPCs, a population of adult CNS stem/precursor cells widely placed within the adult CNS. They are present in white and gray matter at a density similar to microglia. They appear to be the main source of remyelination in MS, as opposed to surviving adult oligodendrocytes. Remyelination in MS is ultimately inadequate and fails. This is likely to represent in part non-disease-related factors (genetic and immune system background, sex, increasing age), as well as a failure of OPC differentiation and maturation [115–117].

Along with oligodendrocyte loss, MS involves extensive demyelination. Myelin is stripped and phagocytized by macrophages. The basis for myelin and oligodendrocyte injury is unknown and likely multifactorial (Table 3.6). There could even be intrinsic myelin instability.

MBP in MS shows a higher rate of citrullination/deimination (45%) compared to controls (15–20%) [112]. This is developmentally immature myelin, which is less compact and therefore destabilized. An unproven hypothesis is that unstable MBP is a primary factor leading to MS [34, 118, 119].

Table 3.6 Possible basis for myelin and oligodendrocyte injury in MS.

- Cell based
  - CD4+ T cells sensitized to myelin antigens
  - Antigen-specific cytotoxic CD8+ T cells
  - Astrocyte disturbance
- Immune system factors
  - Proinflammatory cytokines
  - Demyelinating antibodies
  - Complement cascade components
  - Bystander demyelination following infectious superantigen cell activation
- Hypoxic/ischemic stress
  - Reactive oxygen or nitrogen species
- CNS tissue infection
- Axonal dysregulation with 2° myelin loss
- Excitatory amino acids
  - Glutamate
- Proteolytic, lipolytic enzymes
- Fas antigen–ligand interactions

Astrocytes

Astrocytes are the most abundant CNS cell, and are involved in BBB function, glutamate metabolism, weak APC activity, extracellular potassium maintenance, and release of trophic factors for surrounding cells [120]. It is possible that MS could represent a primary disturbance of astrocytes, considering that another CNS inflammatory demyelinating disorder, Neuromyelitis Optica-Devic disease, is due to immune-mediated astrocyte destruction. MS patients show changes in sodium channels in reactive astrocytes. There is focal upregulation of the sodium channel Nav 1.5 within, as well as at the edge, of active and chronic MS lesions [121]. This upregulation is not seen in MS NAWM or control brain. It is also seen in astrocytes surrounding brain tumors and cerebrovascular accidents, suggesting it is a compensatory mechanism to CNS damage. Very active MS lesions show structural changes involving astrocytes [122]. A recent study reported decreased levels of creatine kinase B, localized to astrocytes, in the white matter of MS patients but not controls [123].

Neurons/Axons

Neurons, along with dendrites, axons, and nodes of Ranvier, are damaged and lost in MS [30, 124]. This is not just a sequelae of loss of trophic myelin, although demyelinated axons express increased sodium channels and deficits in ATP production, making them more vulnerable to physiologic stressors [125]. The increased expression of sodium channels on the demyelinated axon leads to excess sodium within the axons, requiring increased ATP to correct the sodium concentration. This increased energy demand, along with mitochondrial dysfunction, leads to axonal hypoxia [126]. This appreciation of ion channel changes has led to voltage-gated sodium channel blockade being proposed as a strategy to treat MS [127].

Acute axonal injury is prominent in active inflammatory plaques and correlates with inflammation (CD8+ T cells, macrophages, microglia) [12, 25]. Axonal injury does not require demyelination. Retinal nerve fiber layer, made up of unmyelinated axons, can be evaluated by optical coherence tomography, and shows deficits in MS [128]. Within cortical lesions, neuronal loss is estimated to be at least 20% of the total cell population [129].

The mechanism of axon damage is believed to be multifactorial, mediated by inflammatory cells and soluble factors, loss of trophic support from myelin and glia, wallerian degeneration, and antibodies. Autoantibodies directed against axo-glial gray matter antigens such as contactin 2, neurofilament light chain, and neurofascin are found in CSF and serum of MS patients [130]. Contactin 2 is a cell adhesion molecule expressed by neuronal subpopulations and juxtaparanodal axon/myelin [126, 131]. Neurofilaments are part of the axonal cytoskeleton. Elevated levels of the light and heavy subunits are reported in the CSF of progressive patients [132]. Neurofilament light protein is also elevated in CSF during acute relapses [133]. Increased CSF neurofilament levels may predict a worse prognosis [134]. Neurofascin is a cell adhesion molecule expressed by oligodendrocytes at the paranode [135, 136]. About 30% of MS patients show antibodies to neurofascin, an axonal component. This is much more common in progressive vs. relapsing MS, and seems to enhance axonal injury.

In addition, the neuronal 14-3-3 proteins are reported as elevated in the CSF of patients with more severe disability and disease progression [137]. Abnormally phosphorylated tau, with formation of insoluble tau, has been correlated with transition to secondary progressive MS, implicating tau as a neuronal damage mechanism [2].

Blood–Brain Barrier and Vascular System

The BBB involves multiple players that form a neurovascular unit: endothelia, perivascular astrocytes, pericytes, and neighboring CNS cells [138]. The BBB is disrupted in MS at two levels [139]. First, there is marked focal disruption characterized by contrast enhancement on neuroimaging, associated with focal edema and inflammation, which results in macroscopic plaque formation. This is characteristic of relapsing MS, but is also seen in progressive MS. Second, there is a much more subtle but diffuse BBB disturbance with abnormal permeability, tight junction disturbances, and changes in basement membrane and extracellular matrix [139–141]. This is present in normal appearing brain tissue, and not just the lesion areas. The BBB is also immunologically activated in MS, with upregulation and expression of surface markers as well as secretion of immune factors [138]. Although BBB abnormalities have been thought to be a secondary phenomenon in MS, it is not ruled out that they could reflect a primary disturbance.

Recent interest has focused on the venous system in MS. CCSVI refers to the concept that there is a venous drainage abnormality in MS, with longer venous outflow, increased mean transit time on MR perfusion, and opening of collaterals. This is detected through proposed ultra-sonography Doppler criteria, and in limited numbers has been associated with multiple stenoses in major extracranial venous drainage pathways. Preliminary reports have used percutaneous transluminal angioplasty, as well as stenting, to correct the vein defects. CCSVI has garnered huge interest, and is being addressed in multiple studies. Whether it is simply a risk factor for MS, or is responsible for actual damage, remains to be determined [41, 48, 143–146].

Excitotoxins

Glutamate is the major excitatory amino acid. Excess glutamate is capable of causing cell death. Glutamate-mediated exitotoxicity involves activation of ionotropic and metabotropic receptors, with calcium cytoplasmic accumulation leading to cell death. Glutamate is elevated within MS lesions and normal-appearing white matter, as well as CSF. This could be from activated immune cells, astrocytes, or axons [4]. AMPA, NMDA, and kainate receptors are all upregulated. Glutamate transporter expression is also altered [147]. Genetic variation is reported to play a role in glutamate levels [148]. Astrocytes, oligodendrocytes, and myelin all express glutamate receptors. They are all potential targets for exitotoxic damage.

Nitric Oxide

Nitric oxide (NO) is a free radical implicated as a damage mechanism in MS. It impairs the BBB [149]. Elevated levels of NO will modify function of ion channels, transporters, and glycolytic enzymes, resulting in axonal damage. Both NO and its derivative, peroxynitrite, inhibit mitochondria and the ability of the axon to generate ATP. A key enzyme involved in NO synthesis, NO synthase (iNOS) is upregulated in macrophages and reactive astrocytes in acute MS lesions [150]. NO activity in CSF rises during MS relapses [151–154].

Mitochondria

Mitochondria produce ATP, control calcium homeostasis, and play a role in apoptosis. They contain nonnuclear DNA which encodes subunits of the mitochondrial respiratory chain complexes. Mitochondrial abnormalities reported in MS include reduced respiratory chain complex activities, increase in neuron mitochondrial DNA copies, and evidence of oxidative damage to mitochondrial DNA [28, 37].

Mitochondria have been implicated in both conduction block and axonal injury, through calcium-mediated cytoskeletal changes as well as oxidative stress [28]. Mitochondria have been proposed as a therapeutic target in MS [155].

Neuotrophic Factors

Neurotrophic factors promote differentiation and survival of CNS cells and their components. They include brain-derived neurotropic factor, neurotrophin-3, and nerve growth factor. They are secreted by activated immune cells, and are the basis for the concept of neuroprotective autoimmunity. CNS inflammatory cells may help contain damage and boost repair and cell survival, by releasing these neurotrophic factors in MS brain and spinal cord [156–158].

Other Factors

Vitamin D

Vitamin D deficiency is a risk factor for MS. Vitamin D is obtained from synthesis in the skin (triggered by sunlight) and dietary intake. 25 Hydroxy vitamin D is the major circulating metabolite, and 1,25 dihydroxy vitamin D (calcitriol) is the biologically active metabolite. Biologic effects are mediated via the vitamin D receptor [159], a member of the steroid receptor superfamily. Vitamin D receptor is expressed by monocytes, APCs, and activated lympocytes. Vitamin D appears to shift immune responses to a more anti-inflammatory regulatory role, and enhances T reg function. It may play a role in immune modulation in MS, but this waits to be confirmed. The role of vitamin D in MS is the subject of ongoing research.

Conclusion

Recent studies on the immunology of MS have emphasized the likelihood that CNS damage is mediated by a number of immune and inflammatory factors beyond the CD4 Th1 cell. Key immunologic factors may differ based on subsets of MS patients, and different stages of the disease. A better appreciation of this immune system complexity is guiding therapeutic developments.

Novel targets are being proposed (ion channels, mitochondria, NO, glutamate) that may lead to improved outcomes. Personalized medicine may well see a more individualized approach, with therapeutic strategies determined by biomarkers obtained from genetic and immunologic studies on the individual patient.

References

1. Barnett MH, Parratt JDE, Pollard JD, et al. MS: Is it one disease? Int MS J. 2009;16:57–65.
2. Anderson JM, Hampton DW, Patani R, et al. Abnormally phosphorylated tau is associated with neuronal and axonal loss in experimental autoimmune encephalomyelitis and multiple sclerosis. Brain. 2008;131:1736–48.
3. Koch M, Mostert J, Heersema D, et al. Progression in multiple sclerosis: further evidence of an age dependent process. J Neurol Sci. 2007;255:35–41.
4. Trapp BD, Nave K-A. Multiple sclerosis: an immune or neurodegenerative disorder? Annu Rev Neurosci. 2008;31:247–69.
5. Kutzelnigg A, Lucchinetti CF, Stadelmann C, et al. Cortical demyelination and diffuse white matter injury in multiple sclerosis. Brain. 2005;128(pt 11):2705–12.
6. Hu W, Lucchinetti CF. the pathological spectrum of CNS inflammatory demyelinating diseases. Semin Immunopathol. 2009;31:439–53.
7. Barnett MH, Prineas JW. Relapsing and remitting multiple sclerosis: pathology of the newly forming lesion. Ann Neurol. 2004;55:458–68.
8. Parratt JDE, Prineas JW. Neuromyelitis optica: a demyelinating disease characterized by acute destruction and regeneration of perivascular astrocytes. Mult Scler. 2010;16:1156–72.
9. Henderson APD, Barnett MH, Parratt JDE, et al. Multiple sclerosis. Distribution of inflammatory cells in newly forming lesions. Ann Neurol. 2009;66:739–53.
10. Prineas JW, McDonald WI, Franklin RJM. Demyelinating diseases. In: Graham DI, Cantos PL, editors. Greenfield's neuropathology. 7th ed. London: Arnold; 2002. p. 471–550.
11. Kuhlmann T, Goldschmidt T, Antel J, et al. Gender differences in the histopathology of MS? J Neurol Sci. 2009;286:86–91.
12. Frischer JM, Bramow S, Dal-Bianco A, et al. The relation between inflammation and neurodegeneration in multiple sclerosis brains. Brain. 2009;132:1175–89.
13. Bradl M, Lassmann H. Progressive multiple sclerosis. Semin Immunopathol. 2009;31:455–65.
14. Bramow S, Frischer JM, Lassmann H, et al. Demyelination versus remyelination in progressive multiple sclerosis. Brain. 2010;133:2983–98.
15. Kooi EJ, Geurts JIG, van Horssen J, et al. Meningeal inflammation is not associated with cortical demyelination in chronic multiple sclerosis. J Neuropathol Exp Neurol. 2009;68:1021–8.
16. Lassmann H, Bruck W, Lucchinetti CF. The immunopathology of multiple sclerosis: an overview. Brain Pathol. 2007;17:210–8.
17. Lucchinetti C, Bruck W, Parisi J, et al. Heterogeneity of multiple sclerosis lesions: implications for the pathogenesis of demyelination. Ann Neurol. 2000;47:707–17.
18. Keegan M, Konig F, McClelland R, et al. Relation between humoral pathological changes in multiple sclerosis and response to therapeutic plasma exchange. Lancet. 2005;366:579–82.
19. Breij ECW, Brink BP, Veerhuis R, et al. Homogeneity of active demyelinating lesions in established multiple sclerosis. Ann Neurol. 2008;63:16–25.
20. Lucchinetti CF, Bruck W, Parisi J, et al. A quantitative analysis of oligodendrocytes in multiple sclerosis lesions: a study of 113 cases. Brain. 1999;122:2279–95.
21. Prineas JW, Barnard RO, Kwon EE, et al. Multiple sclerosis: remyelination of nascent lesions. Ann Neurol. 1993;33:137–51.
22. Ferguson B, Matyszak M, Esiri MM, et al. Axonal damage in acute multiple sclerosis lesions. Brain. 1997;120:393–9.

23. Trapp BD, Peterson J, Ransohoff RM, et al. Axonal transaction in the lesions of multiple sclerosis. N Engl J Med. 1998;338:278–85.
24. Evangelou N, Esiri MM, Smith S, et al. Quantitative pathological evidence for axonal loss in normal appearing white matter in multiple sclerosis. Ann Neurol. 2000;47:391–5.
25. Kuhlmann T, Lingfeld G, Bitsch A, et al. Acute axonal damage in multiple sclerosis is most extensive in early disease stages and decreases over time. Brain. 2002; 125:2202–12.
26. Bitsch A, Schuchart J, Bunkowski S, et al. Acute axonal injury in multiple sclerosis: correlation with demyelination and inflammation. Brain. 2000;123:1174–83.
27. Androdias G, Reynolds R, Chanal M, et al. Meningeal T cells associate with diffuse axonal loss in multiple sclerosis spinal cords. Ann Neurol. 2010;68:465–76.
28. Mahad D, Lassmann H, Turnbull D. Mitochondria and disease progression in multiple sclerosis. Neuropathol Appl Neurobiol. 2008;34:577–89.
29. Lassmann H. Axonal and neuronal pathology in multiple sclerosis: what have we learn from animal models. Exp Neurol. 2010;225:2–8.
30. Cifelli A, Arridge M, Jezzard P, et al. Thalamic neurodegeneration in multiple sclerosis. Ann Neurol. 2002;52:650–3.
31. Bo L, Vedeler CA, Nyland HI, et al. Subpial demyelination in the cerebral cortex of multiple sclerosis patients. J Neuropathol Exp Neurol. 2003;62:723–32.
32. Lucchinetti CF, Gavrilova RH, Metz I, et al. Clinical and radiographic spectrum of pathologically confirmed tumefactive multiple sclerosis. Brain. 2008;131: 1759–75.
33. Wood DD, Bilbao JM, O'Connors P, et al. Acute multiple sclerosis (Marburg type) is associated with developmentally immature myelin basic protein. Ann Neurol. 1996;40:18–24.
34. Harauz G, Musse AA. A tale of two citrullines – structural and functional aspects of myelin basic protein deamination in health and disease. Neurochem Res. 2007;32:137–58.
35. Yao DL, Webster H, Hudson LD, et al. Concentric sclerosis (Balo): morphometric and in situ hybridization study of lesions in six patients. Ann Neurol. 1994;35:18–30.
36. Stadelmann C, Ludwin SK, Tabira T, et al. Hypoxic preconditioning explains concentric lesions in Balo's type of multiple sclerosis. Brain. 2005;128:979–87.
37. Mahad D, Ziabreva I, Lassmann H, et al. Mitochondrial defects in acute multiple sclerosis lesions. Brain. 2008;131:1722–35.
38. Matsuoka T, Suzuki SO, Iwaki T, et al. Aquaporin-4 astrocytopathy in Balo's disease. Acta Neuropathol. 2010;120:651–60.
39. Bacigaluppi S, Polonara G, Zavanone ML, et al. Schilder's disease: non-invasive diagnosis? Neurol Sci. 2009;30:421–30.
40. Vaknin-Dembinsky A, Weiner HL. Relationship of immunologic abnormalities and disease stage in multiple sclerosis: implications for therapy. J Neurol Sci. 2007;259:90–4.
41. Meinl E, Krumbholz M, Derfuss T, et al. Compartmentalization of inflammation in the CNS: a major mechanism driving progressive multiple sclerosis. J Neurol Sci. 2008;274:42–4.
42. Sato F, Tanaka H, Hasanovic F, et al. Theiler's virus infection: pathophysiology of demyelination and neurodegeneration. Pathophysiology. 2010. doi:10.1010.
43. Steinman L. Shifting therapeutic attention in MS to osteopontin, type 1 and type 2 IFN. Eur J Immunol. 2009;39:2358–60.
44. Jager A, Dardalhon V, Sobel RA, et al. Th1, Th17, and Th9 effector cells induce experimental autoimmune encephalomyelitis with different pathological phenotypes. J Immunol. 2009;183:7169–77.
45. Wingerchuk DM, Lucchinetti CF. Comparative immunopathogenesis of acute disseminated encephalomyelitis, neuromyelitis optica and multiple sclerosis. Curr Opin Neurol. 2007;20:343–50.

46. Bielekova B, Goodwin B, Richert N, et al. Encephalitogenic potential of the myelin basic protein peptide in multiple sclerosis: results of a phase II clinical trial with an altered peptide ligand. Nat Med. 2000;6:1167–75.
47. Tsutsui S, Stys PK. Degeneration versus autoimmunity in multiple sclerosis. Ann Neurol. 2009;66:711–3.
48. Zivadinov R, Schirda C, Dwyer MG, et al. Chronic cerebrospinal venous insufficiency and iron deposition on susceptibility-weighted imaging in patients with multiple sclerosis: a pilot case-control study. Int Agiol. 2010;2:158–75.
49. Mikulkova Z, Praksova P, Stourac P, et al. Imbalance in T-cell and cytokine profiles in patients with relapsing-remitting multiple sclerosis. J Neurol Sci. 2010. doi:10.1016.
50. Batoulis H, Addicks K, Kuerten S. Emerging concepts in autoimmune encephalomyelitis beyond the CD4/Th1 paradigm. Ann Anat. 2010;192:179–93.
51. Vonken K, Hellings N, Hensen K, et al. Secondary progressive in contrast to relapsing-remitting multiple sclerosis patients show a normal CD4+CD25+ regulatory T-cell function and FoXP3 expression. J Neurosci Res. 2006;83:1432–46.
52. Bennett JL, Stuve O. Update on inflammation, neurodegeneration, and immunoregulation in multiple sclerosis: therapeutic implications. Clin Neuropharmacol. 2009;32:121–32.
53. Huan J, Cubertson N. Spencer l, et al. Decreased FOXP3 levels in multiple sclerosis patients. J Neurosci Res. 2005;81:45–52.
54. Correale J, Villa A. Role of CD8+ CD25+ Foxp3+ regulatory T cells in multiple sclerosis. Ann Neurol. 2010;67:625–38.
55. Harrington LE, Hatton RD, Mangan PR, et al. Interleukin 17-producing CD4+ effector T cells develop via a lineage distinct from the T helper type 1 and 2 lineages. Nat Immunol. 2005;6:1123–32.
56. Korn T. Pathophysiology of multiple sclerosis. J Neurol. 2008;255:2–6.
57. Lock C, Hermans G, Pedotti R, et al. Gene-microarray analysis of multiple sclerosis lesions yields new targets validated in autoimmune encephalomyelitis. Nat Med. 2002;8:500–8.
58. Tzartos JS, Friese MA, Craner MJ, et al. Interleukin-17 production in central nervous system-infiltrating T cells and glial cells is associated with active disease in multiple sclerosis. Am J Pathol. 2008;172:146–55.
59. Kebir H, Kreymborg K, Ifergan I, et al. Human T(H)17 lymphocytes promote blood-brain barrier disruption and central nervous system inflammation. Nat Med. 2007;13:1173–5.
60. Babbe H, Roers A, Waisman A, et al. Clonal expansions of CD8(+) T cells dominate the T cell infiltrate in active multiple sclerosis lesions as shown by micromanipulation and single cell polymerase chain reaction. J Exp Med. 2000;192:393–404.
61. Jacobsen M, Cepok S, Quak E, et al. Oligoclonal expansion of memory CD8+ T cells in cerebrospinal fluid from multiple sclerosis patients. Brain. 2002;125:538–50.
62. Shimonkevitz R, Colburn C, Burnham JA, et al. Clonal expansions of activated gamma/delta T cells in recent-onset multiple sclerosis. Proc Natl Acad Sci USA. 1993;90:923–7.
63. Chen Z, Freedman MS. Correlation of specialized CD16+ gammadelta cells with disease course and severity in multiple sclerosis. J Neuroimmunol. 2008;194:147–52.
64. Selmaj K, Brosnan CF, Raine CS. Colocalization of lymphocytes bearing gamma delta T-cell receptor and heat shock protein hsp65+ oligodendrocytes in multiple sclerosis. Proc Natl Acad Sci. 1991;88:6452–6.
65. Cepok S, Rosche B, Grummel V, et al. Short-lived plasma blasts are the main B cell effector subset during the course of multiple sclerosis. Brain. 2005;128:1667–76.

66. Harp C, Lee J, lambracht-Washignton D, et al. Cerebrospinal fluid B cells from multiple sclerosis patients are subject to normal germinal center selection. J Neuroimmunol. 2007;183:189–99.

67. Owens GP, Ritchie AM, Burgoon MP, et al. Single-cell repertoire analysis demonstrates that clonal expansion is a prominent feature of the B cell response in multiple sclerosis cerebrospinal fluid. J Immunol. 2003;171:2725–33.

68. Fraussen J, Vrolix K, Martinez-Martinez P, et al. B cell characterization and reactivity analysis in multiple sclerosis. Autoimmun Rev. 2009;8:654–8.

69. Magliozzi R, Howell O, Vora A, et al. Meningeal B-cell follicles in secondary progressive multiple sclerosis associate with early onset of disease and severe cortical pathology. Brain. 2007;130:1089–104.

70. Owens GP, Bennett JL, Lassmann H, et al. Antibodies produced by clonally expanded plasma cells in multiple sclerosis cerebrospinal fluid. Ann Neurol. 2009; 65:639–49.

71. Thangarajh M, Gomez-Rial J, Hedstrom AK, et al. Lipid-specific immunoglobulin M in CSF predicts adverse long-term outcome in multiple sclerosis. Mult Scler. 2008;14:1208–13.

72. Berger T, Rubner P, Schautzer F, et al. Antimyelin antibodies as a predictor of clinically definite multiple sclerosis after a first demyelinating event. N Engl J Med. 2003;349:139–45.

73. Kuhle J, Lindberg RL, Regeniter A, et al. Antimyelin antibodies in clinically isolated syndromes correlate with inflammation in MRI and CSF. J Neurol. 2007;254:160–8.

74. O'Connor KC, McLaughlin KA, De Jager PL, et al. Self-antigen tetramers discriminate between myelin autoantibodies to native or denatured protein. Nat med. 2007;13:211–7.

75. Hauser SI, Waubant F, Arnold Di, et al. B-cell depletion with rituximab in relapsing-remitting multiple slcerosis. N Engl J Med. 2008;358:676–88.

76. Hawker K, O'Connor P, Freedman MS, et al. Rituximab in patients with primary progressive Multiple Sclerosis. Ann Neurol. 2009;66:460–71.

77. Von Budingen HC, Harrer MD, Kuenzle S, et al. Clonally expanded plasma cells in the cerebrospinal fluid of MS patients produce myelin-specific antibodies. Eur J Immunol. 2008;38:2014–23.

78. Von Budingen HC, Gulati M, Kuenzle S, et al. Clonally expanded plasma cells in the cerebrospinal fluid of pateints with central nervous system autoimmune demyelination produce "oligoclonal bands". J Neuroimmunol. 2010;218: 134–9.

79. Kouwenhoven M, Teleshova N, Ozenci V, et al. Monocytes in multiple sclerosis: phenotype and cytokine profile. J Neuroimmunol. 2001;122:197–205.

80. Merson TD, Binder MD, Kilpatrick TJ. Role of cytokines as mediators and regulators of microglial activity in inflammatory demyelination of the CNS. Neuromolecular Med. 2010;12:99–132.

81. Comabella M, Montalban X, Munz C, et al. Targeting dendritic cells to treat multiple sclerosis. Nat Rev Neurol. 2010;6:499–507.

82. Zozulya AL, Clarkson BD, Ortler S, et al. The role of dendritic cells in CNS autoimmunity. J Mol Med. 2010;88:535–44.

83. Schwab N, Zozulya AL, Kieseier BC, et al. An imbalance of two functionally and phenotypically different subsets of plasmacytoid dendritic cells characterizes the dysfunctional immune regulation in multiple sclerosis. J Immunol. 2010;184: 5368–74.

84. Gandhi R, Laroni A, Weiner HL. Role of the innate immune system in the pathogenesis of multiple sclerosis. J Neuroimmunol. 2010;221:7–14.

85. O'Keefe J, Gately CM, Counihan T, et al. T-cells expressing natural killer (NK) receptors are altered in multiple sclerosis and responses to α-galactosylceramide are impaired. J Neurol Sci. 2008;275:22–8.

86. Sakuishi K, Miyake S, Yamamura T. Role of NK cells and invariant NKT cells in multiple sclerosis. Results Probl Cell Differ. 2010;51:127–47.

87. De Jager PL, Rossin E, Pyne S, et al. Cytometric profiling in multiple sclerosis uncovers patient population structure and a reduction of CD8 low cells. Brain. 2008;131:1701–11.

88. Putzki N, Baranwal MK, Tettenborn B, et al. Effects of natalizumab on circulating B cells, T regulatory cells and natural killer cells. Eur Neurol. 2010;63:311–7.

89. Olsson Y. Mast cells in plaques of multiple sclerosis. Acta Neurol Scand. 1974;50:611–8.

90. Toms R, Weiner HI, Johnson D. Identification of IgE-positive cells and mast cells in frozen sections of multiple sclerosis brains. J Neuroimmunol. 1990;30:169–77.

91. Rozniecki JJ, Hauser SL, Stein M, et al. Elevated mast cell tryptase in cerebrospinal fluid of multiple sclerosis patients. Ann Neurol. 1995;37:63–6.

92. Panitch HS, Hirsch RL, Schindler J, et al. Treatment of multiple sclerosis with gamma interferon: exacerbations associated with activation of the immune system. Neurology. 1987;27:1097–102.

93. Van Oosten BW, Barkhoff F, Truyen L, et al. Increased MRI activity and immune activation in two multiple sclerosis patients treated with the monoclonal anti tumor necrosis factor antibody cA2. Neurology. 1996;47:1531–4.

94. The Lenercept Multiple Sclerosis Study Group and the University of British Columbia MS/MRI Analysis Group. TNF neutralization in MS: results of a randomized, placebo-controlled multicenter study. Neurology. 1999;53:457–65.

95. Balashov KE, Smith DR, Khoury SJ, et al. Increased interleukin 12 production in progressive multiple sclerosis: induction by activated CD4+ T cells via CD40 ligand. Proc Natl Acad Sci USA. 1997;94:599.

96. Bar-Or A. The immunology of multiple sclerosis. Semin Neurol. 2008;28: 29–45.

97. Hvas J, McLean C, Justesen J, et al. Perivascular T cells express the pro-inflammatory chemokines. RANTES mRNA in multiple sclerosis lesions. Scand J Immunol. 1997;46:195–203.

98. Van Der Voorn P, Tekstra J, Beeden RH, et al. Expression of MCP-1 by reactive astrocytes in demyelinating multiple sclerosis lesions. Ann J Pathol. 1999; 154:45–51.

99. Szczucinski A, Losy J. CCL5, CXCL10 and CXCL11 chemokines in patients with active and stable relapsing-remitting multiple sclerosis. Neuroimmunomodulation. 2011;18:67–72.

100. Morimoto J, Kon S, Matsui Y, et al. Osteopontin; as a target molecule for the treatment of inflammatory diseases. Curr Drug Targets. 2010;11:494–505.

101. Bhat R, Steinman L. Innate and adaptive autoimmunity directed to the central nervous system. Neuron. 2009;64:123–32.

102. Vogt MH, Lopatinskaya L, Smits M, et al. Elevated osteopontin levels in active-remitting multiple sclerosis. Ann Neurol. 2003;53:819–22.

103. Comabella M et al. Plasma osteopontin levels in multiple sclerosis. J Neuroimmunol. 2005;158:231–9.

104. Chowdhury SA, Lin J, Sadiq SA. Specificity and correlation with disease activity of cerebrospinal fluid osteopontin levels in patients with multiple sclerosis. Arch Neurol. 2008;65:232–5.

105. Chabas D, Baranzini SE, Mitchell D, et al. The influence of the proinflammatory cytokine, osteopontin, on autoimmune demyelinating disease. Science. 2001;294:1731–5.

106. Leppert D, Ford J, Stabler G, et al. Matrix metalloproteinase-9 (gelatinase B) is selectively elevated in CSF during relapses and stable phases of multiple sclerosis. Brain. 1998;121:2327–34.

107. Fainardi E, Castellazzi M, Bellini T, et al. Cerebrospinal fluid and serum levels and intrathecal production of active matrix metalloproteinase-9 (MMP-9) as

markers of disease activity in patients with multiple sclerosis. Mult Scler. 2006; 12:294–301.

108. Fainardi E, Castellazzi M, Tamborino C, et al. Potential relevance of cerebrospinal fluid and serum levels and intrathecal synthesis of active matrix metalloproteinase-2 (MMP-2) as markers of disease remission in patients with multiple sclerosis. Mult Scler. 2009;15:547–54.

109. Benesova Y, Vasku A, Novotna H, et al. Matrix metalloproteinase-9 and matrix metalloproteinase-2 as biomarkers of various courses in multiple sclerosis. Mult Scler. 2009;15:316–22.

110. Howell OW, Rundle JL, Garg A, et al. Activated microglia mediate axoglial disruption that contributes to axonal injury in multiple sclerosis. J Neuropathol Exp Neurol. 2010;69:1017–33.

111. Friese MA, Fugger L. T cells and microglia as drivers of multiple sclerosis pathology. Brain. 2007;130:2755–7.

112. Artemiadis AK, Anagnostouli MC. Apoptosis of oligodendrocytes and post-translational modifications of myelin basic protein in multiple sclerosis: possible role for the early stages of multiple sclerosis. Eur Neurol. 2010;63:65–72.

113. Jana A, Pahan K. Sphingolipids in multiple sclerosis. Neuromolecular Med. 2010;12(4):351–61.

114. D'Souza SD, Bonetti B, Balasingman B, et al. Multiple sclerosis Fas signaling on oligodendrocyte cell death. J Exp Med. 1996;184:2361–70.

115. Franklin RJM, Ffrench-Constant C. Remyelination in the CNS: from biology to therapy. Nat Rev Neurosci. 2008;9:839–55.

116. Kuhlmann T, Miron V, Cuo Q, et al. Differentiation block of oligodendroglial progenitor cells as a cause for remyelination failure in chronic multiple sclerosis. Brain. 2008;131:1749–58.

117. Mi S, Miller RH, Tang W, et al. Promotion of central nervous system remyelination by induced differentiation of oligodendrocyte precursor cells. Ann Neurol. 2009;65:304–15.

118. Whitaker JN, Mitchell GW. A possible role for altered myelin basic protein in multiple sclerosis. Ann Neurol. 1996;40:3–4.

119. Moscarello MA, Mastronardi FG, Wood DD. The role of citrullinated proteins suggests a novel mechanism in the pathogenesis of multiple sclerosis. Neurochem Res. 2007;32:251–6.

120. Chastain EML, Duncan DS, Rodgers JM, et al. The role of antigen presenting cells in multiple sclerosis. Biochim Biophys Acta. 2010. doi:10.1016/J. BBADIS.2010.07.008.

121. Black JA, Newcombe J, Waxman SG. Astrocytes within multiple sclerosis lesions upregulate sodium channel Nav1.5. Brain. 2010;133:835–46.

122. Sharma R, Fischer MT, Bauer J, et al. Inflammation induced by innate immunity in the central nervous system leads to primary astrocyte dysfunction followed by demyelination. Acta Neuropathol. 2010;120:223–36.

123. Steen C, Wilczak N, Hoogduin JM, et al. Reduced creatine kinase B activity in multiple sclerosis normal appearing white matter. PLos One. 2010;5:e10811.

124. Pirko I, Lucchinetti CF, Sriram S, et al. Gray matter involvement in multiple sclerosis. Neurology. 2007;68:634–42.

125. Siffrin V, Vogt J, Radbruch H, et al. Multiple sclerosis – candidate mechanisms underlying CNS atrophy. Trends Neurosci. 2010;33:202–10.

126. Derfuss T, Linington C, Hohlfeld R. Axo-glial antigens as targets in multiple sclerosis: implications for axonal and grey matter injury. J Mol Med. 2010; 88:753–61.

127. Mantegazza M, Curia G, Biagini G, et al. Voltage-gated sodium channels as therapeutic targets in epilepsy and other neurological disorders. Lancet Neurol. 2010;9:413–24.

128. Henderson APD, Trip SA, Schlottmann PG, et al. An investigation of the retinal nerve fibre layer in progressive multiple sclerosis using optical coherence tomography. Brain. 2008;131:277–87.
129. Vercellino M, Plano F, Votta B, et al. Grey matter pathology in multiple sclerosis. J Neuropathol Exp Neurol. 2005;64:1101–7.
130. Meinl E, Derfuss T, Krumbholz M, et al. Humoral autoimmunity in multiple sclerosis. J Neurological Sci. 2010. doi:10.1016.
131. Derfuss T, Parikh K, Velhin S, et al. Contactin 2/TAG-1-directed autoimmunity is identified in multiple sclerosis patients and mediates gray matter pathology in animals. Proc Natl Acad Sci USA. 2009;106:8302–7.
132. Semra YK, Seidi OA, Sharief MK. Heightened intrathecal release of axonal cytoskeletal proteins in multiple sclerosis is associated with progressive disease and clinical disability. J Neuroimmunol. 2002;122:132–9.
133. Malmestrom C, Haghighi S, Rosengren L. Neurofilament light protein and flial fibrillary acidic protein as biological markers in MS. Neurology. 2003;61:1720–5.
134. Lim ET, Sellebjerg F, Jensen CV, et al. Acute axonal damage predicts clinical outcome in patients with multiple sclerosis. Mult Scler. 2005;11:532–6.
135. Mathey EK, Derfuss T, Storch MK, et al. Neurofascin as a novel target for autoantibody-mediated axonal injury. Exp Med. 2007;204:2363–72.
136. Pomicter AD, Shroff SM, Fuss B, et al. Novel forms of neurofascin 155 in the central nervous system: alterations in paranodal disruption models and multiple sclerosis. Brain. 2010;133:389–405.
137. Colucci M, Roccatagliata L, Capello E, et al. The 14-3-3 protein in multiple sclerosis: a marker of disease severity. Mult Scler. 2004;10:477–81.
138. Alvarez JI, Cayrol R, Prat A. Disruption of central nervous system barriers in multiple sclerosis. Biochim Biophys Acta. 2010. doi:10.1016.
139. Bennett J, Basivireddy J, Kollar A, et al. Blood-brain barrier disruption and enhanced vascular permeability in the multiple sclerosis model EAE. J Neuroimmunol. 2010. doi:10.1016.
140. Hochmeister S, Grundtner R, Bauer J, et al. Dysterlin is a new marker for leaky brain blood vessels in multiple sclerosis. J Neuropathol Exp Neurol. 2006;65:855–65.
141. Padden M, Leech S, Craig B, et al. Differences in expression of junctional adhesion molecule-A and beta-catenin in multiple sclerosis brain tissue: increasing evidence for the role of tight junction pathology. Acta Neuropathol. 2007;113:177–86.
142. Zamboni P, Galeotti R, Menegatti E, et al. Chronic cerebrospinal venous insufficiency in patients with multiple sclerosis. J Neurol Neurosurg Psychiatry. 2009;80:392–9.
143. Zamboni P, Galeotti R, Menegatti E, et al. A prospective open-label study of endovascular treatment of chronic cerebrospinal venous insufficiency. J Vasc Surg. 2009;50:1348–58.
144. Doepp F, Paul F, Valdueza JM, et al. No cerebrocervical venous congestion in patients with multiple sclerosis. Ann Neurol. 2010;68:173–83.
145. Hojnacki D, Zamboni P, Lopez-Soriano A, et al. Use of neck magnetic resonance venography, Doppler sonography and selective venography for diagnosis of chronic cerebrospinal venous insufficiency: a pilot study in multiple sclerosis patients and healthy controls. Int Angiol. 2010;29:127–39.
146. Khan O, Filippi M, Freedman MS, et al. Chronic cerebrospinal venous insufficiency and multiple sclerosis. Ann Neurol. 2010;67:286–90.
147. Centonze D, Muzio L, Rossi S, et al. The link between inflammation, synaptic transmission and neurodegeneration in multiple sclerosis. Cell Death Differ. 2010;17:1083–91.

148. Baranzini SE, Srinivasan R, Khankhanian P, et al. Genetic variation influences glutamate concentrations in brains of patients with multiple sclerosis. Brain. 2010;133:2603–11.
149. Thiel VE, Audus KL. Nitric oxide and blood-brain barrier integrity. Antioxid Redox Signal. 2001;3:273–8.
150. Oleszak EL, Zaczynska E, Bhattacharjee M, et al. Inducible nitric oxide synthase and nitrotyrosine are found in monocytes/macrophages and/or astrocytes in acute, but not in chronic, multiple slcerosis. Clin Diagn Lab Immunol. 1998;5:438–45.
151. Giovannoni G. Cerebrospinal fluid and serum nitric oxide metabolites in patients with multiple sclerosis. Mul Scler. 1998;4:27–30.
152. Brundin L, Morcos E, Olsson T, et al. Increased intrathecal nitric oxide formation in multiple sclerosis: cerebrospinal fluid nitrite as activity marker. Eur J Neurol. 1999;6:585–90.
153. Calabrese V, Scapagnini G, Ravagna A, et al. Nitric oxide synthase is present in the cerebrospinal fluid of patients with active multiple sclerosis and is associated with increases in cerebrospinal fluid protein nitrotyrosine and S-nitrosothiols and with changes in glutathione levels. J Neurosci Res. 2002;70:580–7.
154. Rejdak K, Eikelenboom MJ, Petzold A, et al. CSF nitric oxide metabolites are associated with activity and progression of multiple sclerosis. Neurology. 2004;63:1439–45.
155. Lassmann H. Pathophysiology of inflammation and tissue injury in multiple sclerosis: what are the targets for therapy. J Neurol Sci. 2010. doi:10.1016.
156. Linker R, Gold R, Luhder F. Function of neurotrophic factors beyond the nervous system: inflammation and autoimmune demyelination. Crit Rev Immunol. 2009;29:43–68.
157. De Santi L, Annunziata P, Setta E, et al. Brain-derived neurotrophic factor and TrkB receptor in experimental autoimmune cncephalomyelitis and multiple sclerosis. J Neurol Sci. 2009;287:17–26.
158. Urshansky N, Mausner-Fainberg K, Auriel E, et al. Dysregulated neurotrophin mRNA production by immune cells of patients with relapsing remitting multiple sclerosis. J Neurol Sci. 2010;295:31–7.
159. Smolders J, Damoiseaux J, Menheere P, et al. Vitamin D as an immune modulator in multiple sclerosis, a review. J Neuroimmunol. 2008;194:7–17.
160. Pittock SJ, Lucchinetti CF. The pathology of MS. New insights and potential clinical applications. Neurologist. 2007;13:45–56.

MS: Epidemiology and Genetics

Robert H. Gross and Philip L. De Jager

Keywords: Prevalence, Epstein–Barr, Omega3-fatty acids, Haplotype, Genetics

Introduction

Our understanding of multiple sclerosis (MS) has advanced rapidly over the past decade, but the inciting events of this chronic, disabling disease of the central nervous system remain elusive. Our working model is that environmental factors and stochastic events trigger MS in genetically susceptible individuals. Evidence for certain environmental factors is mounting, but the most exciting component of the MS susceptibility equation today lies in its genetic component as recent technological and analytic advances have allowed several polymorphisms to be discovered and validated in the last 2 years. How these genetic risk factors interact with putative environmental risk factors is one of the fascinating questions that we can now begin to explore in the hope of shedding light on the earliest events involved in the onset of MS.

Distribution of MS in Human Populations

MS affects about 350,000 people in the USA and about 1.1 million people throughout the world [1]. Most MS patients develop the disease between 20 and 40 years of age, with a preponderance of women being affected [1]. While the overall prevalence rate is generally cited as approximately 1 in 1,000 for populations of European ancestry, the lifetime risk in certain populations is as high as ~1 in 200 for women and slightly less for men [2, 3]. Indeed, MS is between 1.5 and 2.5 times more prevalent in women, and this skewed gender distribution may be rising over time [4, 5]. Much less is known about the prevalence of MS in non-European populations and admixed populations such as African-Americans. Nonetheless, the available evidence suggests that prevalence is reduced, particularly in populations of African and East Asian ancestry [4, 6].

From: *Clinical Neuroimmunology: Multiple Sclerosis and Related Disorders*, Current Clinical Neurology,
Edited by: S.A. Rizvi and P.K. Coyle, DOI 10.1007/978-1-60327-860-7_4,
© Springer Science+Business Media, LLC 2011

This difference in geographical distribution was noted early in the study of MS and is generally correct, and it is unlikely to be explained by issues such as access to medical care and lack of familiarity with a diagnosis of MS in areas of low prevalence. Overall, MS prevalence demonstrates a latitude gradient, with an increased prevalence in northern latitudes of Europe and North America and as in southern regions of Australia and New Zealand. However, there are notable exceptions to this general statement, with Sardinians having substantially higher rates of MS than other Italians and Parsis being more commonly affected than other ethnic groups in South Asia [7]. These observations and others reporting reduced prevalence rates among African-Americans regardless of geography [8, 9] suggest that the variable frequency of genetic susceptibility factors across human populations is likely to explain at least some of the geographical distribution of the disease.

There are a few observations that cannot be attributed to genetic factors. People who migrate to areas of greater MS prevalence tend to adopt the risk of their new homeland if they migrate in childhood, whereas those who migrate in later years retain the risk of their place of origin. Nor can genetics explain the differences in risk among those of common ancestry who migrate to areas of different MS prevalence [10]. It has also been argued that the recent decline in the latitude gradient and the relative increase in MS prevalence for white women in the USA and Canada must indicate exogenous factors, since genetic change does not occur over such a short period of time [2, 9, 11].

The much-quoted observation of change in risk depending on age at migration has been called into question. The cut-off for many years was assumed to be 15 years of age, but a study with a homogeneous Australian population demonstrated that when 15 years was used as the point of stratification, age of migration had no effect on MS susceptibility, suggesting that risk from migration must span a wider age range [12]. Overall, it is clear that neither genetic nor environmental risk factors are sufficient to independently explain the distribution of MS in different human populations; there is an active interplay between these two sets of risk factors.

Sunlight, Vitamin D, and MS

The search for environmental agents tied to latitude that might directly affect risk of MS has been difficult. Norman and colleagues studied a US veteran population and reported that air pollution index, concentrations of minerals in ground water, temperature measures, measures of annual rainfall and average humidity, and amount of annual solar radiation, when analyzed by multiple regression, did not influence MS risk independently from latitude [13]. That study notwithstanding, much of the research for a latitude correlate has centered on the amount and duration of sunlight [5, 14]. Studies measuring MS mortality as a function of occupation [15]; skin cancer rates in MS patients vs. sex-, age-, and location-matched controls [16]; and self-reported exposure to sunlight [17] all showed a protective role for sunlight. However, it should be noted that this evidence, while intriguing, might be misleading. The occupation and skin cancer-linkage studies that appear to show a relationship between less sunlight and MS risk may in fact reflect "reverse causation" – an epiphenomenon in which MS patients may preferentially avoid the sun as heat can exacerbate their symptoms, rather than sun exposure protecting against MS. Furthermore, case–control surveys can be confounded by recall bias if subjects with MS, aware of the posited relationship between sunlight and MS, over-report their exposure [18]. Nonetheless, increased sunlight exposure remains an attractive hypothesis that could contribute to the latitude gradient.

Exceptions to the latitude rule provide an important insight as to how sunlight might be acting to promote MS susceptibility. The first anomaly is the high prevalence of MS at low altitudes and the low MS rates at high altitudes in Switzerland [19]. The second is the high prevalence of MS inland and the lower MS prevalence along the coast in Norway [20, 21]. Both of these phenomena can be convincingly explained by examining the role of vitamin D in this pathway [22]. UV light is stronger at higher altitudes, encouraging endogenous production of vitamin D3, and coastal residents eat more vitamin D-rich fish oils than do inland residents. Epidemiological observations such as these are supported by experimental data showing that 1,25-dihydroxyvitamin D given exogenously prevents experimental autoimmune encephalomyelitis (EAE), the mouse model of MS [23, 24], while in vitamin D-deficient mice the onset of EAE is accelerated [25]. Clinical data also support a role for vitamin D: MS patients have been found to have low serum concentrations of 25-hydroxyvitamin D3 [25(OH)D] [26–28] and seasonal fluctuation of MS births and disease activity correlate with 25(OH)D seasonality [29–32].

Infectious Agents and MS

Given the geographical distribution of MS, the change in risk among migrants of different age, and the possible occurrence of MS epidemics [10, 33], the hypothesis that MS results from exposure to an infectious agent was proposed early and has been repeatedly explored. Certainly, the idea that a virus could infect many people but only cause pathological manifestations in a few was already evident from poliomyelitis and provided a possible model for MS. This model of a viral cause was conceptually supported by observations that several viruses were associated with demyelinating encephalomyelitis both in human patients and in experimental animals and that high concentrations of IgG (oligoclonal bands) are found in many patients with MS [34].

Two competing hypotheses have aimed to explain the relationship of microbes to MS. The prevalence hypothesis argues that MS comes about as a result of a pathogen that is more common in areas of high MS prevalence. Alternatively, the hygiene hypothesis states that a heavy burden of microbial or parasitic infections creates a persistent effect on the immune system early in childhood, conferring protection against MS (and other autoimmune diseases). The effect on the immune system may include a shift from pro-inflammatory helper T-cell (Th17) profile to a Th2 profile, such as that which is seen following helminthic infections and is associated with diminished inflammation in MS [4]. The hygiene hypothesis has generally been favored over the prevalence hypothesis in MS because it is better able to account for the latitude gradient, recent increases in prevalence (improved hygiene), and changing risk among migrants [35].

Over the years, various pathogens – such as human herpesvirus 6 (HHV6), Chlamydia pneumoniae and endogenous retroviruses – have been investigated for possible connection to MS but none have been definitively linked with the disease [36]. The pathogen with the most robust evidence to support it is the Epstein–Barr virus (EBV), the virus associated with infectious mononucleosis (IM), lymphoma, and nasopharyngeal carcinoma. The vast majority of adults have been infected with EBV. Interestingly, both IM and MS occur in adolescents and young adults and specifically target populations where EBV infection is known to occur at a later age (i.e., those with higher socioeconomic status and more education). IM also follows a similar latitude gradient to MS [37, 38]. Thus, late infection with EBV, marked by the appearance of IM, is associated with MS risk; conversely, early acquisition of EBV is seen in various parts of the world, like throughout Asia, where MS prevalence is low. MS risk was found to be associated with elevated levels of antibodies to the EBV nuclear antigen 1 (EBNA-1) many years prior to clinical manifestations of MS [39], with a secondary boost in anti-EBNA-1 titers (i.e., not from primary EBV infection) occurring at some point between ages 17 and 29 [40].

At this point, epidemiological and serological studies suggest a role for EBV in MS susceptibility, but how can the hygiene hypothesis and a putative role for EBV be reconciled? The hygiene hypothesis argues that a large burden of microbes in early childhood shifts the immunological profile toward protection from MS. EBV alone is unlikely to be sufficient to explain such a shift. However, it is known that children who are seronegative for EBV (presumably members of the high hygiene group) have a very low risk of MS as long as they are EBV-negative [35]. On the other hand, individuals who are infected and develop IM, have a relative risk of MS of 2.3 compared with those who never developed IM (95% CI, 1.7–3.0) [41]. The "EBV variant" of the hygiene hypothesis [35] argues that good hygiene is detrimental from the MS perspective only insofar as it causes one to be infected with EBV later in life and hence have a higher chance of developing MS.

Molecular evidence for the role of EBV in MS has extended these epidemiologic observations: Aloisi and colleagues have recently reported the presence of lymphoid follicles within the meninges of MS patients [42]. These structures were noted to contain many B cells and plasma cells with evidence of EBV infection. These results of technically challenging assays need to be validated and, if replicated, will offer a concrete link between EBV and MS-related neuropathology. The importance of B-cell dysregulation in MS has been suggested by the recent successful phase II trial of rituximab (an anti-CD20 monoclonal antibody) in patients with relapsing–remitting disease [43]. So, evaluating EBV further in this context is critical. In vitro studies have suggested that, because of amino acid sequence homologies between EBV proteins and myelin basic protein, immune responses directed against EBV antigen could cross-react with self-antigen. In a genetically susceptible host under the right circumstances, the threshold of such autoreactive reactions may be lower. For example, immune response to EBV may be modulated by vitamin D, and suboptimal levels could lead to the activation of autoreactive T cells [44]. Thus, while definitive evidence for a role of EBV or another microbial trigger remains elusive, it is likely that one or, more likely, several different infectious agents may play a role in the initiation of the inflammatory process in MS.

Smoking and MS

There is substantial evidence that smoking is a risk factor for multiple sclerosis [45]. Four longitudinal studies were undertaken in the 1990s and early 2000s, which, though varying in their definitions of smoking, all showed a relative risk of MS somewhere between 1.3 and 1.8 for smokers compared to subjects who had never smoked. The combined results from these four studies demonstrate a statistically significant association between a history of smoking and MS susceptibility ($P < 0.001$) [18]. One concern in the retrospective analyses done to date is that self-reported smoking status may not be very reliable, but Vollmer et al. recently showed that MS survey participants do reliably report their smoking status [46].

Smoking is also linked to transition to secondary progressive disease in MS [47], and it has been noted that smoking may promote acute exacerbations of MS [48]. Furthermore, it was shown by Di Pauli and colleagues that smoking is also a risk factor for early conversion to MS after an initial demyelinating event [49]. These results suggest that toxins in the environment may contribute to various steps in the MS disease process and that behavioral modifications may yield important dividends to patients, particularly if it is accomplished early in their course.

Diet, Neuro-Endocrine, and Other Factors

There is some evidence for the role of diet and hormones in MS risk; although, admittedly, it is not as robust as that for the aforementioned susceptibility factors. Given (1) the increased ratio of females to males affected with MS, (2) symptom onset in young adulthood and (3) the fact that women with MS appear to suffer somewhat fewer relapses in the second and third trimesters of pregnancy, sex hormones have been investigated for a possible role as modulators of MS risk. Progesterone appears to cause a switch from a Th1 to a Th2 immune response, while testosterone exerts anti-inflammatory and immunosuppressive effects in mouse models of autoimmunity [50]. The protection during pregnancy and the increased risk post-partum could be mediated by hormonal fluctuations of progesterone, estrogen, or other factors affected by pregnancy: for example, progesterone levels increase during gestation, reaching their peak during the third trimester, at which point evidence of protection from MS is the strongest, then plummet in the puerperium [51]. Further, it has been proposed that estradiol, the form of estrogen common in nonpregnant women, is deleterious with regard to MS, but that estriol, the predominant estrogen in pregnant women, is protective [52]. However, investigations of oral contraception use, parity, and age at first birth suggest that these beneficial effects from sex hormones are short-lived [18].

Researchers have also examined diet for a possible link to MS. Early epidemiological studies have suggested that diets high in saturated fats and low in polyunsaturated fats may increase risk; however, these are subject to recall bias [18]. As we have seen above, vitamin D deficiency has been implicated in MS pathogenesis, initially based in part on the observation that some populations whose geography would predispose them to the disease instead have a relatively low prevalence. However, not all studies of nutrients have been limited to this particular fat-soluble vitamin. Certain polyunsaturated fats like omega-3 fatty acids may in fact play a small role in reducing the severity of disease, according to results from several randomized control trials [53–55], but results remain inconclusive.

Integrating Environmental and Genetic Risk

With certain genetic factors now well established (such as the HLA DRB1*1501 haplotype) [56], specific hypotheses can be tested to see whether subjects with different levels of genetic susceptibility to MS respond differently to environmental exposures or whether certain environmental factors are dependent on a particular genetic architecture. Given that HLA DRB1 is a co-receptor for EBV entry and that the HLA DRB1*1501 allele may be able to present EBV antigen that may mimic self-antigen, assessing the interaction of these two strong risk factors is of great interest. A recent study suggests that these two risk factors are largely independent and may be multiplicative (Figure 4.1). Specifically, individuals who have both risk factors (the HLA DRB1*1501 allele and high levels of antibodies directed against the EBV protein EBNA1) have a ninefold increase in risk over individuals that have neither risk factor [57]. This observation requires validation in additional cohorts, but it suggests that diagnostic modeling may become practical as we further uncover the genetic architecture of MS. It is likely that environmental factors may have differential effects in different subsets of subjects with MS and that taking the genetic architecture of subjects into account will clarify the role of environmental susceptibility factors.

What about exposure to sunlight and vitamin D levels? Is their role similarly independent from genetic causes or can genetic predisposition account for their effect on MS risk? Researchers recently investigated the role of sun exposure using disease-discordant MZ twins. The avoidance of sunlight early in life seems to put people at risk for the future development of MS, independent of genetic susceptibility to MS [58]. Yet more evidence points in the direction of a complex interplay of genetic factors and vitamin D regulation: genetic variants in two candidate genes, vitamin D receptor and

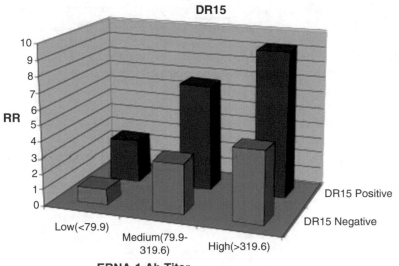

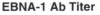

Figure 4.1 The synergistic effect of the HLA-DRB1*1501 and anti-EBNA1 antibody titer in conferring risk of MS. Relative risk increases independently with both the presence of the risk allele and with higher titers of antibody

1-alpha-hydroxylase (CYP27B1), were recently found to be associated with serum levels of 25 (OH)D [59]. Thus, diet, sun exposure, and genetics are all involved in vitamin D regulation. Since we know that serum levels of 25 (OH) D affect one's risk of MS, the exact degree to which diet and sunlight influence MS risk apart from genetics becomes more difficult to tease out without large sample sizes. Future epidemiological studies will benefit from knowledge of the genetic architecture of MS and will be better able to explore the independence, or interdependence, of genes and the environment.

Genetic Susceptibility in MS

This section will examine what is currently known about the genetics of MS. Unlike certain diseases, such as cystic fibrosis and sickle cell anemia, in which mutations in a single gene are wholly responsible for pathogenesis, MS is a genetically complex trait, with no simple Mendelian form described to date. That is to say, many different genetic loci with incomplete penetrance contribute to an individual's risk of developing MS. The evidence indicates that each of these genes probably only exert a modest influence [4]. For many years, the only chromosomal region or locus investigators known to be involved in MS was the Major Histocompatibility Complex (MHC). Then in 2007, the first genome-wide association scan (GWAS) was performed by the International Multiple Sclerosis Genetic Consortium (IMSGC), resulting in the identification of several new susceptibility loci [60]. This groundbreaking discovery was possible because of a combination of newly developed resources such as HapMap, a catalog of common genetic variation, technological advances, including novel high-throughput genotyping platforms, and more powerful statistical methodologies. Following this breakthrough, another GWAS study was performed, yielding a new set of candidate susceptibility loci that await replication [61]. A meta-analysis of three genome scans is currently underway, which will reveal more loci associated with MS susceptibility at genome-wide levels of significance. There are likely as many as 100 different genes suspected to be related to MS susceptibility. The risk alleles left to be discovered are likely of an effect size on the order of an odds ratio of 1.2 or smaller. In order to conduct a comprehensive scan to detect loci with such modest effect sizes, a much larger study is required, and the IMSGC has met this challenge by participating in the second generation of the Wellcome Trust Case Control Consortium which will generate genome-wide data on 11,000 MS patients, which will hopefully lead to the identification of nearly every susceptibility locus with an odds ratio of 1.2 or greater.

The Major Histocompatibility Complex

Human leukocyte antigen (HLA) genes, located within the MHC on chromosome 6p21, were first found to be associated with MS in 1972 [62]. Numerous linkage and association studies have since made this the most replicated finding in MS genetics [63]. In particular, the HLA-DRB1*1501 haplotype (also known by the HLA-DR2 and HLA-DR15 tissue types) has consistently demonstrated linkage and association with MS in different human populations [63]. However, other alleles within the MHC may separately confer MS risk. For example, Sardinians have a high concentration of HLA-DR3 and

HLA-DR4 [64, 65] , which may account for their high rates of MS, and HLA DR3 was found to be associated with susceptibility for MS in UK subjects [66]. Even within the MHC class I region, there may be alleles associated with MS: the best evidence for this was shown in a large population of MS subjects of European ancestry where HLA-Cw05 remained associated with MS susceptibility after subjects with HLA-DRB1 susceptibility alleles had been excluded [66]. However, additional Class I alleles such as HLA A2 may also have a role [67].

Because of strong linkage disequilibrium (LD, the co-occurrence of alleles at two or more loci more frequently than would be expected by chance) within the MHC, as well as the strong effect size (odds ratio [OR] = 2.7 for one copy of the allele) [68], it remains unclear where the true susceptibility factor resides or whether multiple linked alleles are required. In fact, it may be that DRB1*1501 is all one needs to inherit to have MHC-related increased MS susceptibility, with the other markers just incidentally linked to it. In a study of African-Americans with MS, Oksenberg and colleagues show not only that DRB1*0301 (HLA-DR3) and DRB1*1503 are associated with MS, but also that the DRB1*1501 allele confers MS risk independent of the tightly linked DQB1*0602 allele [69]. This pre-eminent role for HLA DRB1*1501 is also seen in rare individuals of European descent where these two alleles have been separated by recombination (De Jager, unpublished result). Further analysis of the African-American MS collection reveals that another HLA DRB1*1501 linked allele, DRB5*0101, is not a susceptibility factor but may influence disease severity [70]. While the linkage disequilibrium in the MHC and allelic heterogeneity at HLA DRB1 make it difficult to tease out the causal variant, it is clear that the HLA-DRB1*1501 allele is the strongest known MS susceptibility factor in the human genome and that the magnitude of its effect on MS susceptibility is unique for such a common allele.

Association-Based Mapping and Non-MHC Risk Alleles

The search for susceptibility loci in MS initially relied on linkage studies of families with multiple cases of MS, with limited success. This was consistent with theoretical discussions that highlighted the lack of statistical power of the linkage approach in discovering genetic variants of modest effect. Instead, an association-based approach such as a simple case–control design was put forward as the preferred method for gene discovery [71]. This realization led to the formation of the IMSGC, since an association study design requires very large sample sizes and very dense genotyping to be successful. However, one concern for the simple case–control study design is population stratification: unrecognized and irrelevant differences between cases and controls that produce spurious associations with MS susceptibility. It is for this reason that the IMSGC genome-wide association scan (GWAS) used transmission disequilibrium testing (TDT) as its primary analysis. TDT measures the number of times that a given allele present in the parent is passed on (transmitted) to an affected offspring; this family-based association study design, while more expensive, offered robustness to population stratification since the statistic is based on data from nuclear families and not disparate groups of affected and unaffected subjects [72, 73].

The 2007 GWAS was groundbreaking in two ways. First, by discovering novel associations with MS susceptibility using either the TDT method or a secondary case–control analysis with appropriate controls for stratification, it demonstrated that either method could be successfully applied in MS and other genetically complex diseases. The MS GWAS was one of the first such studies to be published, and therefore had an impact not only on the field of MS but also in the field of human genetics. Second, for the first time, a region outside of the MHC was discovered to be definitively associated with MS. The study identified several genetic variants associated with MS with high statistical significance. The top hit after the HLA-DRB1*1501 allele was rs12722489, in the region of the genes IL2RA and RBM17, which is referred to as the IL2RA locus. When analyzed with all the samples combined, it was found to have an odds ratio of 1.25 ($P=2.96\times10^{-8}$). This variant satisfied the requirement for significance at the genome level – the only one to do so officially in the study – when significance was set at $P<5\times10^{-8}$ to account for the statistical burden of testing polymorphisms genome-wide [74]. The next hit was rs2104286, also in the IL2RA and is in LD with the first SNP [75]. These associations were validated in subsequent studies [76, 77]. The IL2RA gene product IL2RA, also known as CD25, is expressed on the surface of regulatory T cells and also plays a role in another autoimmune disease, type 1 diabetes mellitus [78]. An intriguing observation is that daclizumab, a monoclonal antibody directed against CD25, is effective in treating patients with relapsing–remitting disease [79].

The SNP rs6897932, in the IL7R gene was just shy of genome-wide significance with a P value of 2.94×10^{-7}. However, candidate gene studies published in parallel with the GWAS confirm its role in susceptibility to MS [80, 81]. Looking further at the results, the 17 highest SNPs from the GWAS included variants in the regions of several other genes: KIAA0350/CLEC16A, RPL5, DBC1, CD58, ALK, FAM69A, ANKRD15, EVI5, KLRB1, CBLB, and PDE4B. Although none of these SNPs achieved a genome-wide level of significance in this study, subsequent data corroborated the association of several of these genetic loci with MS [82–86]. The CD58 locus is of interest given that there is evidence that the associated marker is also correlated with the level of CD58 RNA expression [86]. Similarly, the susceptible alleles at IL2RA are also associated with higher serum levels of soluble IL2RA [75]. Thus, we are beginning to have a handle on the functional consequences of some of these loci. However, among these 11 loci with suggestive evidence of association in the GWAS, the only locus to reach the threshold of genome-wide significance to date is KIAA0350/CLEC16A.

Two additional genome-wide scans have been published [61, 84], and KIF1B, a locus first identified in a Dutch genetically isolated population, appears to meet genome-wide levels of statistical significance. The most exciting lesson from these GWAS in MS is that the approach is successful and that we are only limited in our gene discovery efforts by the number of subjects that can be screened. How many subjects are needed? With the exception of HLA DRB1*1501 and its strong effect on disease risk, MS susceptibility alleles have modest effects on disease risk. Current estimates place odds ratios for these susceptibility alleles in the 0.75–1.25 range [60] (Figure 4.2). Thus, statistical modeling suggests that we should identify most susceptibility loci with an odds ratio of 1.2 or more once ~10,000 subjects have been scanned [71].

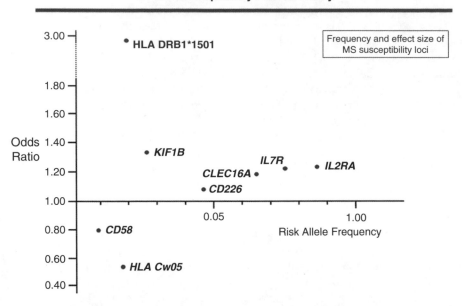

Figure 4.2 We have plotted the risk alleles that have been validated and have reached a genome-wide level of significance ($P=5\times10^{-8}$): HLA-DRB1*1501, CD226, CLEC16A, KIF1B, IL2RA, and IL7R. Also included are the alleles CD58 and HLA Cw05. The odds ratios and allele frequencies are based on those found in European populations

Influence of Genetics on Disease Course

As with the non-genetic risk factors for MS, it is important to determine whether those genetic variants that predispose an individual to develop MS also influence a patient's disease course. To date, there has been no validated evidence linking genetic loci with clinical endpoints, such as MRI lesions and expanded disability status score (EDSS). Some studies suggest an association between the HLA-DRB1*1501 haplotype and an earlier age of onset or certain MRI phenotypes, although this has yet to be demonstrated definitively [87–92]. It is entirely possible that a certain set of genes predisposes people to the disease, while a different set influences disease course.

High-density association scans of the genome can be used to detect associations with disease susceptibility, like the 2007 IMSGC GWAS, or they can also be used to look for associations with a different phenotype. This was the rationale behind a recent study to identify genes responsible for response to type I interferon therapy, whose results need to be validated [93]. The field of MS pharmacogenomics is still in the early stages of such studies given the need for precise, standardized outcome data in large numbers of subjects. While intriguing associations have been published, they remain preliminary and await replication. So far, alleles associated with susceptibility to MS have not demonstrated strong effects on the course of MS (De Jager PL, unpublished). Genotype–clinical phenotype correlations such as these may ultimately prove valuable in that they could be developed into biomarkers that can be used to predict disease course and response to therapy with the goal of providing more personalized medical care to MS patients.

Susceptibility to Other Inflammatory/Autoimmune Diseases

MS patients and their families tend to be affected by other autoimmune diseases more frequently than the general population [94, 95]. In the hopes of providing insights into common disease pathways, efforts have been made to identify susceptibility alleles shared among different autoimmune disorders. For example, like MS, the major susceptibility loci for Type 1 diabetes (T1DM), rheumatoid arthritis (RA), and autoimmune thyroid disease (AITD) are located in the MHC [96–98]. Additionally, the SNP rs6897932 (IL7R), found to be associated with MS in the IMSGC genome-wide scan, is also causally related to T1DM [99], and the IL2RA locus demonstrates a complex pattern of shared and discrete associations to MS, AITD [100], and T1DM [75].

Other genes have been linked to some autoimmune diseases but not to others. PTPN22 is located on chromosome 1p13 and encodes the lymphoid-specific tyrosine phosphatase LYP, involved in the suppression of T-cell activation. Evidence supports links between it and T1D [101, 102], RA [103], AITD [104], and SLE [105] but not MS [106]. A recent meta-analysis confirms the associations with these autoimmune diseases, but is unable to find similar ties between the polymorphism in question and other disorders with known autoimmune components, such as MS, IBD, psoriasis, Addison's disease, and Celiac disease [107]. STAT4, which encodes a transcription factor involved in the differentiation of Th1 and Th17 cells, is found to be linked to RA and SLE [108]. Ser307 allele of the CD226 gene, whose product is a transmembrane protein involved in adhesion and co-stimulation of T cells, predisposes to T1D, MS, and possibly AITD and RA [109]. Genes known to be involved in one autoimmune disorder are being tested to see whether they are also linked to another: it is in this way that CLEC16A and CD226 were found to be associated with MS at a genome-wide level of significance [85].

These data suggest that these and other genes – perhaps involved in basic immunological mechanisms like regulating the inflammatory response or promoting tolerance – increase susceptibility to autoimmune diseases through a shared mechanism whose clinical expression may be driven by other genetic and environmental factors. A representation of the type of clustering found with susceptibility loci to various autoimmune diseases can be seen in Figure 4.3. As these studies across inflammatory diseases are extended, it is likely that the majority of susceptibility loci will be shared between two or more diseases, with only a minority of loci being specific to a particular disease.

Conclusion

As we have seen, a variety of environmental and genetic factors have been implicated at various levels of statistical significance in the onset of MS. Sunlight exposure and vitamin D intake, infection with EBV, smoking, and other environmental risk factors have substantial epidemiological evidence supporting their role as MS risk factors. On the other hand, genetic association studies have already shown us convincingly that polymorphisms in the MHC and the CD226, CLEC16A, KIF1B, IL2RA, and IL7R loci predispose people to the disease. Fine gene mapping of MS patients will be required to determine which specific variant(s) is/are causal in each locus. The ability of genomewide scans to detect modest genetic associations has been a great boon for MS research,

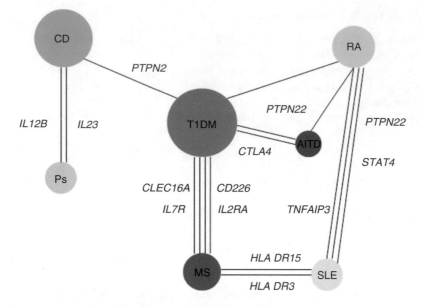

Figure 4.3 Shared susceptibility loci in autoimmune diseases. Each disease is connected to other diseases that share a locus of disease susceptibility at a genome-wide level of significance. The shared locus is listed next to the line that connects each disease pair. The diameter of each *colored circle* is proportional to the number of risk alleles discovered to date in each disease. *AITD* autoimmune thyroid disease, *CD* Crohn's disease, *MS* multiple sclerosis, *Ps* psoriasis, *RA* rheumatoid arthritis, *SLE* systemic lupus erythematosus, *T1DM* type 1 diabetes mellitus (figure produced from data collected by Drs. Chris Cotsapas and Mark Daly)

highlighting pathways to be pursued further. Soon, with the completion of the much larger GWAS planned by the IMSGC and the Wellcome Trust, we will have a nearly comprehensive map of common genetic variants that affect susceptibility to MS with an odds ratio of 1.2 or greater. There may be 50–100 loci that have this level of an effect on MS susceptibility. With a comprehensive map of the genetic architecture of MS in hand, we will be able to attack critical questions such as whether there are genetically distinct subgroups of patients within which particular alleles have a much greater effect or whether particular molecular pathways are preferentially targeted by genetic variants associated with MS susceptibility. The answers to these and many other questions will guide us in our dissection of disease pathways, in drug development, and in the design of clinical algorithms for diagnosis and possibly prognosis.

References

1. Hauser SL, Goodin DS. Multiple sclerosis and other demyelinating diseases. In: Kasper DL, Braunwald E, Hauser S, Longo D, Jameson LJ, Fauci AS, editors. Harrison's principles of internal medicine. 16th ed. New York: McGraw-Hill; 2004. p. 2461–71.
2. Hernán MA, Olek MJ, Ascherio A. Geographic variation of MS incidence in two prospective studies of US women. Neurology. 1999;53(8):1711–8.
3. Koch-Henriksen N, Hyllested K. Epidemiology of multiple sclerosis: incidence and prevalence rates in Denmark 1948–64 based on the Danish Multiple Sclerosis Registry. Acta Neurol Scand. 1988;78(5):369–80.

4. Compston A, Coles A. Multiple sclerosis. Lancet. 2008;372(9648):1502–17.

5. Ascherio A, Munger K. Epidemiology of multiple sclerosis: from risk factors to prevention. Semin Neurol. 2008;28(1):17–28. Review.

6. Smestad C, Sandvik L, Holmoy T, Harbo HF, Celius EG. Marked differences in prevalence of multiple sclerosis between ethnic groups in Oslo, Norway. J Neurol. 2008;255(1):49–55.

7. Rosati G. The prevalence of multiple sclerosis in the world: an update. Neurol Sci. 2001;22:117–39.

8. Kurtzke JF, Beebe GW, Norman Jr JE. Epidemiology of multiple sclerosis in US veterans. 1. Race, sex, and geographic distribution. Neurology. 1979;29:1228–35.

9. Wallin MT, Page WF, Kurtzke JF. Multiple sclerosis in US veterans of the Vietnam era and later military service: race, sex, geography. Ann Neurol. 2004;55(1): 65–71.

10. Gale CR, Martyn CN. Migrant studies in multiple sclerosis. Prog Neurobiol. 1995;47:425–48.

11. Orton SM, Herrera BM, Yee IM, et al. for the Canadian Collaborative Study Group. Sex ratio of multiple sclerosis in Canada: a longitudinal study. Lancet Neurol. 2006;5(11):932–6.

12. Hammond SR, English DR, McLeod JG. The age-range of risk of developing multiple sclerosis: evidence from a migrant population in Australia. Brain. 2000;123(5):968–74.

13. Norman Jr JE, Kurtzke JF, Beebe GW. Epidemiology of multiple sclerosis in U.S. veterans: 2. Latitude, climate, and the risk of multiple sclerosis. J Chronic Dis. 1983;36(8):551–9.

14. Hayes CE, Cantorna MT, DeLuca HF. Vitamin D and multiple sclerosis. Proc Soc Exp Biol Med. 1997;216:21–7.

15. Freedman DM, Dosemeci M, Alavanja MC. Mortality from multiple sclerosis and exposure to residential and occupational solar radiation: a case-control study based on death certificates. Occup Environ Med. 2000;57:418–21.

16. Goldacre MJ, Seagroatt V, Yeates D, Acheson ED. Skin cancer in people with multiple sclerosis: a record linkage study. J Epidemiol Community Health. 2004;58:142–4.

17. Van der Mei IA, Ponsonby AL, Dwyer T, et al. Past exposure to sun, skin phenotype and risk of multiple sclerosis: a case-control study. BMJ. 2003;327:316–21.

18. Ascherio A, Munger K. Environmental risk factors for multiple sclerosis. Part II. Noninfectious factors. Ann Neurol. 2007;61(6):504–13.

19. Kurtzke JF. On the fine structure of the distribution of multiple sclerosis. Acta Neurol Scand. 1967;43:257–82.

20. Swank RL, Lerstad O, Strom A, Backer J. Multiple sclerosis in rural Norway: its geographic and occupational incidence in relation to nutrition. N Engl J Med. 1952;246:722–8.

21. Westlund K. Distribution and mortality time trend of multiple sclerosis and some other diseases in Norway. Acta Neurol Scand. 1970;46:455–83.

22. Goldberg P. Multiple sclerosis: vitamin D and calcium as environmental determinants of prevalence (A viewpoint) part 1: sunlight, dietary factors and epidemiology. Int J Environ Stud. 1974;6:19–27.

23. Lemire JM, Archer DC. 1,25 dihydroxyvitamin D3 prevents the in vivo induction of murine experimental autoimmune encephalomyelitis. J Clin Invest. 1991;87:1103–7.

24. Pedersen LB, Nashold FE, Spach KM, Hayes CE. 1,25-dihydroxyvitamin D3 reverses experimental autoimmune encephalomyelitis by inhibiting chemokine synthesis and monocyte trafficking. J Neurosci Res. 2007;85(11):2480–90.

25. Cantorna MT, Hayes CE, DeLuca HF. 1,25-Dihydroxyvitamin D3 reversibly blocks the progression of relapsing encephalomyelitis, a model of multiple sclerosis. Proc Natl Acad Sci USA. 1996;93:7861–4.

26. Munger KL, Levin LI, Hollis BW, Howard NS, Ascherio A. Serum 25-hydroxyvitamin D levels and risk of multiple sclerosis. JAMA. 2006;296:2832–8.
27. Nieves J, Cosman F, Herbert J, Shen V, Lindsay R. High prevalence of vitamin D deficiency and reduced bone mass in multiple sclerosis. Neurology. 1994; 44:1687–92.
28. Ozgocmen S, Bulut S, Ilhan N, Gulkesen A, Ardicoglu O, Ozkan Y. Vitamin D deficiency and reduced bone mineral density in multiple sclerosis: effect of ambulatory status and functional capacity. J Bone Miner Metab. 2005;23:309–13.
29. Willer CJ, Dyment DA, Sadovnick AD, Rothwell PM, Murray TJ, Ebers GC. Timing of birth and risk of multiple sclerosis: population based study. BMJ. 2005; 330:120.
30. Sotgiu S, Pugliatti M, Sotgiu MA, et al. Seasonal fluctuations of multiple sclerosis births in Sardinia. J Neurol. 2006;253:38–44.
31. Embry AF, Snowdon LR, Vieth R. Vitamin D and seasonal fluctuations of gadolinium-enhancing magnetic resonance imaging lesions in multiple sclerosis. Ann Neurol. 2000;48:271–2.
32. Auer DP, Schumann EM, Kumpfel T, Gossl C, Trenkwalder C. Seasonal fluctuations of gadolinium-enhancing magnetic resonance imaging lesions in multiple sclerosis. Ann Neurol. 2000;47:276–7.
33. Kurtzke JF, Hyllested K. Multiple sclerosis in the Faroe Islands I. Clinical and epidemiological features. Ann Neurol. 1979;5(1):6–21.
34. Gilden DH. Infectious causes of multiple sclerosis. Lancet Neurol. 2005;4(3): 195–202.
35. Ascherio A, Munger K. Environmental risk factors for multiple sclerosis. Part I: the role of infection. Ann Neurol. 2007;61(4):288–99.
36. Giovannoni G, Cutter GR, Lunemann J, et al. Infectious causes of multiple sclerosis. Lancet Neurol. 2006;5:887–94.
37. Warner HB, Carb RI. Multiple sclerosis and Epstein-Barr virus. Lancet. 1981;2:1290.
38. Niederman JC, Evans AS. Epstein-Barr virus. In: Evans AS, Kaslow RA, editors. Epidemiology and control. 4th ed. New York: Plenum; 1997. p. 253–83.
39. Levin LI, Munger KL, Rubertone MV, et al. Multiple sclerosis and Epstein-Barr virus. JAMA. 2003;289:1533–6.
40. Levin LI, Munger KL, Rubertone MV, et al. Temporal relationship between elevation of Epstein Barr virus antibody titers and initial onset of neurological symptoms in multiple sclerosis. JAMA. 2005;293:2496–500.
41. Thacker EL, Mirzaei F, Ascherio A. Infectious mononucleosis and risk for multiple sclerosis: a meta-analysis. Ann Neurol. 2006;59(3):499–503.
42. Serafini B, Rosicarelli B, Franciotta D, et al. Dysregulated Epstein-Barr virus infection in the multiple sclerosis brain. J Exp Med. 2007;204(12):2899–912.
43. Hauser SL, Waubant E, Arnold DL, et al. B-cell depletion with rituximab in relapsing-remitting multiple sclerosis. N Engl J Med. 2008;358(7):676–88.
44. Holmoy T, Vitamin D. modulates the immune response to Epstein-Barr virus: synergistic effect of risk factors in multiple sclerosis. Med Hypotheses. 2008; 70(1):66–9.
45. Riise T, Nortvedt MW, Ascherio A. Smoking is a risk factor for multiple sclerosis. Neurology. 2003;61:1122–4.
46. Marrie RA, Cutter G, Tyry T, Campagnolo D, Vollmer T. Smoking status over two years in patients with multiple sclerosis. Neuroepidemiology. 2008;32(1):72–9.
47. Hernán MA, Jick SS, Logroscino G, Olek MJ, Ascherio A, Jick H. Cigarette smoking and the progression of multiple sclerosis. Brain. 2005;128:1461–5.
48. Courville CB, Maschmeyer JE, DeLay CP. Effects of smoking on the acute exacerbations of multiple sclerosis. Bull Los Angeles Neurol Soc. 1964;29:1–6.
49. Di Pauli F, Reindl M, Ehling R, et al. Smoking is an early risk factor for conversion to clinically definite multiple sclerosis. Mult Scler. 2008;14:1026–30.

50. Whitacre CC, Reingold SC, O'Loony PA. A gender gap in autoimmunity. Science. 1999;283:1277–8.
51. Whitacre CC. Sex differences in autoimmune disease. Nat Immunol. 2001;2: 777–80.
52. Tanzer J. Estrogen effect in multiple sclerosis more nuanced than described. Ann Neurol. 2008;63(2):263. Letter.
53. Dworkin RH, Bates D, Millar JHD, Paty DW. Linoleic acid and multiple sclerosis: a reanalysis of three double-blind trials. Neurology. 1984;34:1441–5.
54. Bates D, Cartlidge NE, French JM, et al. A double-blind controlled trial of long chain n-3 polyunsaturated fatty acids in the treatment of multiple sclerosis. J Neurol Neurosurg Psychiatry. 1989;52:18–22.
55. Weinstock-Guttman B, Baier M, Park Y, et al. Low fat dietary intervention with omega-3 fatty acid supplementation in multiple sclerosis patients. Prostaglandins Leukot Essent Fatty Acids. 2005;73:397–404.
56. Oksenberg JR, Baranzini SE, Sawcer S, Hauser SL. The genetics of multiple sclerosis: SNPs to pathways to pathogenesis. Nat Rev Genet. 2008;9(7):516–26.
57. De Jager PL, Simon KC, Munger KL, Rioux JD, Hafler DA, Ascherio A. Integrating risk factors: HLA-DRB1*1501 and Epstein-Barr virus in multiple sclerosis. Neurology. 2008;70(13 Pt 2):1113–8.
58. Islam T, Gauderman WJ, Cozen W, Mack TM. Childhood sun exposure influences risk of multiple sclerosis in monozygotic twins. Neurology. 2007;69(4): 381–8.
59. Orton SM, Morris AP, Herrera BM, et al. Evidence for genetic regulation of vitamin D status in twins with multiple sclerosis. Am J Clin Nutr. 2008;88(2):441–7.
60. Hafler DA, Compston A, Sawcer S. for the International Multiple Sclerosis Genetics Consortium. Risk alleles for multiple sclerosis identified by a genome-wide study. N Engl J Med. 2007;357:851–62.
61. Baranzini SE, Wang J, Gibson RA, et al. Genome-wide association analysis of susceptibility and clinical phenotype in multiple sclerosis. Hum Mol Genet. 2009;18(4):767–78.
62. Jersild C, Svejgaard A, Fog T. HL-A antigens and multiple sclerosis. Lancet. 1972;1: 1240–1.
63. Fernando MM, Stevens CR, Walsh EC, et al. Defining the role of the MHC in autoimmunity: a review and pooled analysis. PLoS Genet. 2008;4(4):e1000024. Review.
64. Marrosu MG, Murru MR, Costa G, et al. Multiple sclerosis in Sardinia is associated and in linkage disequilibrium with HLA-DR3 and HLA-DR4 alleles. Am J Hum Genet. 1997;61:454–7.
65. Marrosu MG, Murru MR, Costa G, Murru R, Muntoni F, Cucca F. DRB1-DQA1-DQB1 loci and multiple sclerosis predisposition in the Sardinian population. Hum Mol Genet. 1998;7:1235–7.
66. Yeo TW, De Jager PL, Gregory SG, et al. A second major histocompatibility complex susceptibility locus for multiple sclerosis. Ann Neurol. 2007;61(3):228–36.
67. Fogdell-Hahn A, Ligers A, Gronning M, Hillert J, Olerup O. Multiple sclerosis: a modifying influence of HLA class I genes in an HLA class II associated autoimmune disease. Tissue Antigens. 2000;55(2):140–8.
68. Barcellos LF, Oksenberg JR, Begovich AB, et al. HLA-DR2 dose effect on susceptibility to multiple sclerosis and influence on disease course. Am J Hum Genet. 2003;72:710–6.
69. Oksenberg JR, Barcellos LF, Cree BA, et al. Mapping multiple sclerosis susceptibility to the HLA-DR locus in African-Americans. Am J Hum Genet. 2004;74(1):160–7.
70. Caillier SJ, Briggs F, Cree BA, et al. Uncoupling the roles of HLA-DRB1 and HLA-DRB5 genes in multiple sclerosis. J Immunol. 2008;181(8):5473–80.

71. Risch N, Merikangas K. The future of genetic studies of complex human diseases. Science. 1996;273(5281):1516–7.
72. Spielman RS, McGinnis RE, Ewens WJ. Transmission test for linkage disequilibrium: the insulin gene region and insulin-dependent diabetes mellitus (IDDM). Am J Hum Genet. 1993;52(3):506–16.
73. Spielman RS, Ewens WJ. The TDT and other family-based tests for linkage disequilibrium and association. Am J Hum Genet. 1996;59(5):983–9.
74. Pe'er I, Yelensky R, Altshuler D, Daly MJ. Estimation of the multiple testing burden for genomewide association studies of nearly all common variants. Genet Epidemiol. 2008;32(4):381–5.
75. Maier LM, Lowe CE, Cooper J, et al. IL2RA genetic heterogeneity in multiple sclerosis and type 1 diabetes susceptibility and soluble interleukin-2 receptor production. PLoS Genet. 2009;5(1):e1000322.
76. Weber F, Fontaine B, Cournu-Rebeix I, et al. IL2RA and IL7RA genes confer susceptibility for multiple sclerosis in two independent European populations. Genes Immun. 2008;9:259–63.
77. Ramagopalan SV, Anderson C, Sadovnick AD, Ebers GC. Genomewide study of multiple sclerosis. N Engl J Med. 2007;357:2199–201 (correspondence).
78. Lowe CE, Cooper JD, Brusko T, et al. Large-scale genetic fine mapping and genotype-phenotype associations implicate polymorphism in the IL2RA region in type 1 diabetes. Nat Genet. 2007;39(9):1074–82.
79. Schippling DS, Martin R. Spotlight on anti-CD25: daclizumab in MS. Int MS J. 2008;15(3):94–8.
80. Gregory SG, Schmidt S, Seth P, et al. Interleukin 7 receptor alpha chain (IL7R) shows allelic and functional association with multiple sclerosis. Nat Genet. 2007;39:1083–91.
81. Lundmark F, Duvefelt K, Iacobaeus E, et al. Variation in interleukin 7 receptor alpha chain (IL7R) influences risk of multiple sclerosis. Nat Genet. 2007;39:1108–13.
82. Hoppenbrouwers IA, Aulchenko YS, Ebers GC, et al. EVI5 is a risk gene for multiple sclerosis. Genes Immun. 2008;9:334–7.
83. Rubio JP, Stankovich J, Field J, et al. Replication of KIAA0350, IL2RA, RPL5, and CD58 as multiple sclerosis susceptibility genes in Australians. Genes Immun. 2008;9(7):624–30.
84. Aulchenko YS, Hoppenbrouwers IA, Ramagopalan SV, et al. Genetic variation in the KIF1B locus influences susceptibility to multiple sclerosis. Nat Genet. 2008;40(12):1402–3.
85. International Multiple Sclerosis Genetics Consortium (IMSGC). The expanding genetic overlap between multiple sclerosis and type I diabetes. Genes Immun. 2009;10:11.
86. De Jager PL, Baecher-Allan C, Maier LM, et al. The role of the CD58 locus in multiple sclerosis. Proc Natl Acad Sci USA. 2009;106(13):5264–9.
87. Smestad C, Brynedal B, Jonasdottir G, et al. The impact of HLA-A and –DRB1 on age at onset, disease course, and severity in Scandinavian multiple sclerosis patients. Eur J Neurol. 2007;14:835–40.
88. Weatherby SJ, Thomson W, Pepper L, et al. HLA-DRB1 and disease outcome in multiple sclerosis. J Neurol. 2001;248:304–10.
89. Weinshenker BG, Santrach P, Bissonet AS, et al. Major histocompatibility complex class II alleles and the course and outcome of MS: a population-based study. Neurology. 1998;51:742–7.
90. Hensiek AE, Sawcer SJ, Feakes R, et al. HLA-DR 15 is associated with female sex and younger age at diagnosis in multiple sclerosis. J Neurol Neurosurg Psychiatry. 2002;72:184–7.
91. Barcellos LF, Sawcer S, Ramsay PP, et al. Heterogeneity at the HLA-DRB1 locus and risk for multiple sclerosis. Hum Mol Genet. 2006;15(18):2813–24.

92. Okuda DT, Srinivasan R, Oksenberg JR, et al. Genotype-Phenotype correlations in multiple sclerosis: HLA genes influence disease severity inferred by 1HMR spectroscopy and MRI measures. Brain. 2009;132(Pt 1):250–9.

93. Byun E, Caillier SJ, Montalban X, et al. Genome-wide pharmacogenomic analysis of the response to interferon beta therapy in multiple sclerosis. Arch Neurol. 2008;65(3):337–44.

94. Barcellos LF, Kamdar BB, Ramsay PP, et al. Clustering of autoimmune diseases in families with a high-risk for multiple sclerosis: a descriptive study. Lancet Neurol. 2006;5:924–31.

95. Broadley SA, Deans J, Sawcer SJ, Clayton D, Compston DA. Autoimmune disease in first-degree relatives of patients with multiple sclerosis. A UK survey. Brain. 2000;123(6):1102–11.

96. Todd JA, Bell JI, McDevitt HO. HLA-DQ beta gene contributes to susceptibility and resistance to insulin-dependent diabetes mellitus. Nature. 1987;329:599–604.

97. Stastny P. Association of the B-cell alloantigen DRw4 with rheumatoid arthritis. N Engl J Med. 1978;298:869–71.

98. Simmonds MJ, Howson JM, Heward JM, et al. A novel and major association of HLA-C in Graves' disease that eclipses the classical HLA-DRB1 effect. Hum Mol Genet. 2007;16:2149–53.

99. Todd JA, Walker NM, Cooper JD, et al. Robust associations of four new chromosome regions from genome-wide analyses of type 1 diabetes. Nat Genet. 2007;39(7):857–64.

100. Brand OJ, Lowe CE, Heward JM, et al. Association of the interleukin-2 receptor alpha (IL-2Ralpha)/CD25 gene region with Graves' disease using a multilocus test and tag SNPs. Clin Endocrinol (Oxf). 2007;66:508–12.

101. Gregersen PK, Lee HS, Batliwalla F, Begovich AB. PTPN22: setting thresholds for autoimmunity. Semin Immunol. 2006;18(4):214–23.

102. Bottini N, Musumeci L, Alonso A, et al. A functional variant of lymphoid tyrosine phosphatase is associated with type I diabetes. Nat Genet. 2004;36:337–8.

103. Michou L, Lasbleiz S, Rat AC, et al. Linkage proof for PTPN22, a rheumatoid arthritis susceptibility gene and a human autoimmunity gene. Proc Natl Acad Sci USA. 2007;104(5):1649–54.

104. Velaga MR, Wilson V, Jennings CE, et al. The codon 620 tryptophan allele of the lymphoid tyrosine phosphatase (LYP) gene is a major determinant of Graves' disease. J Clin Endocrinol Metab. 2004;89:5862–5.

105. Wu H, Cantor RM, Graham DS, et al. Association analysis of the R620W polymorphism of protein tyrosine phosphatase PTPN22 in systemic lupus erythematosus patients with autoimmune thyroid disease. Arthritis Rheum. 2005;52:2396–402.

106. De Jager PL, Sawcer S, Waliszewska A, et al. Evaluating the role of the 620W allele of protein tyrosine phosphatase PTPN22 in Crohn's disease and multiple sclerosis. Eur J Hum Genet. 2006;14(3):317–21.

107. Lee YH, Rho YH, Choi SJ, et al. The PTPN22 C1858T functional polymorphism and autoimmune diseases – a meta-analysis. Rheumatology (Oxford). 2007;46(1):49–56.

108. Remmers EF, Plenge RM, Lee AT, et al. STAT4 and the risk of rheumatoid arthritis and systemic lupus erythematosus. N Engl J Med. 2007;357:977–86.

109. Hafler JP, Maier LM, Cooper JD, et al. CD226 Gly307Ser association with multiple autoimmune diseases. Genes Immun. 2008;10:5–10.

MS: Clinical Features, Symptom Management, and Diagnosis

James M. Stankiewicz and Guy J. Buckle

Keywords: Symptoms, Fatigue, Spasticity, Hyper reflexia, Tremor, Neuritis

Introduction

Given its potential for diffuse dissemination throughout virtually every portion of the central nervous system (optic nerves, brain, and spinal cord), it is perhaps not surprising that a broad array of symptoms may be reported by patients with Multiple Sclerosis (MS). Nonetheless, the majority of patients with MS will at some point present with a stereotyped constellation of symptoms and signs constituting a first clinical "attack" of demyelination, often referred to as a Clinically Isolated Syndrome (CIS). CIS typically comprises unilateral optic neuritis, partial transverse myelitis, or a brainstem–cerebellar syndrome (see below). The majority of patients presenting with CIS will also have characteristic lesions on brain MRI not accounting for their clinical presentation and indicative of prior asymptomatic episodes of inflammatory demyelination. These patients should be managed based on their risk of having a second attack and thus converting to Relapsing–Remitting MS (RRMS), also termed Clinically Definite MS (CDMS). In the Optic Neuritis Treatment Trial (ONTT) [1], the cumulative probability of developing MS by 15 years after onset of optic neuritis was 50% (95% confidence interval, 44–56%) and strongly related to presence of lesions on the baseline non-contrast-enhanced brain (MRI). Twenty-five percent of patients with no lesions on baseline brain MRI developed MS during follow-up compared with 72% of patients with one or more lesions. In longitudinal studies of a separate cohort of CIS patients, 83% (45/54) of patients with CIS who had abnormal results on brain MRI at baseline developed CDMS after a 10-year follow-up period and baseline lesion number and lesion volume increase over the first 5 years predicted the extent of clinical disability measured by the Expanded Disability Status Scale (EDSS) at the 14-year follow-up examination [2, 3]. These findings underscore the prognostic value of MRI early in MS. Using modern imaging criteria, it is now also possible to make a diagnosis of MS prior to a second clinical attack by

From: *Clinical Neuroimmunology: Multiple Sclerosis and Related Disorders*, Current Clinical Neurology,
Edited by: S.A. Rizvi and P.K. Coyle, DOI 10.1007/978-1-60327-860-7_5,
© Springer Science+Business Media, LLC 2011

demonstrating new asymptomatic lesions on MRI (i.e., dissemination in time), and most disease-modifying therapies (DMTs) are utilized in both RRMS and CIS with characteristic abnormal MRI findings. In this chapter, we will discuss the signs and symptoms experienced by MS patients as well as the diagnosis and differential diagnosis of MS.

Signs and Symptoms

No single symptom or sign is pathognomonic for MS, although in younger age groups, the typical symptoms and signs of CIS should always prompt an investigation into demyelinating disease. These include (1) optic neuritis, typically subacute monocular visual loss with pain on eye movement, red desaturation and relative afferent pupillary defect (RAPD); (2) partial transverse myelitis, typically unilateral or bilateral ascending sensory disturbances and paresthesiae, often with L'Hermitte phenomenon, and with posterior column sensory loss and varying degrees of paraparesis and hyperreflexia; or (3) brainstem–cerebellar syndromes, typically combinations of diplopia, dysarthria, weakness, and incoordination with unilateral or bilateral internuclear opthalmoparesis (INO) and varying degrees of ataxic hemiparesis.

Conversely, some symptoms (e.g., fatigue, overactive bladder) while nonspecific, occur with such frequency in MS that their conspicuous absence may warn the practitioner that other diagnoses should at least be more carefully considered. There is as yet no specific biomarker for MS (MRI comes closest), and diagnosis is ultimately based on clinical presentation and elimination of other possible etiologies/explanations (MS mimickers), so that MS is ultimately a "diagnosis of exclusion." In practice, however, MS is relatively common in the young adult population, alternative etiologies for the typical CIS presentations are comparatively rare, especially when they are accompanied by MRI findings typical for demyelination, and the majority of CIS cases will evolve into CDMS over time.

Cranial Nerves

Though any cranial nerve can be involved in MS, certain characteristic syndromes are so common in MS that they should always prompt a workup for demyelinating disease.

Optic Neuritis

Optic nerve involvement typically presents as a subacute but often rapidly progressive loss of visual acuity; as well as pain on eye movement and color (especially red) desaturation. Nadir is generally reached within hours or days, not minutes or weeks. Pain with eye movement occurred in 92% of patients in the optic neuritis treatment trial and is thought to result from stretching of the dural sheath around an inflamed optic nerve. Acutely, fundoscopic examination is normal in two-third of cases. A relative afferent pupillary defect (RAPD) can often be detected in the acute or subacute setting with the (Marcus-Gunn) swinging flashlight test and is estimated to be present chronically in 50% of MS patients that have experienced an episode of optic neuritis [4]. Almost all patients in the ONTT had improvement in visual acuity in 1 month, and at 15-year follow-up 72% of patients had at least 20/20 vision in the affected eye, though even patients improving to 20/20 acuity can note blurred or "washed-out" vision [5]. Visual Evoked Potentials (VEPs) classically show an increased P100 latency in the affected eye with preserved waveform, though amplitude can be slightly diminished. Central scotomata are common, and peripheral visual loss occurs far less frequently. Uhthoff's phenomenon classically denotes enlargement of a central scotoma or "blind spot" with exercise, although the term has been generalized to denote the return of nearly any prior MS symptom upon even a mild elevation of core body temperature.

Eye Movement Abnormalities

Complex cerebral, cerebellar, and brainstem circuitry mediates coordination of eye movements through some of the most heavily myelinated and rapidly conducting tracts of the CNS. The most common finding in MS is breakdown of smooth pursuit movements, which is frequently found in the absence of any overt symptoms. This is believed to be due to damage to cerebellar and descending supranuclear fibers and may implicate a second site of involvement of the CNS in patients presenting with an attack not involving these connections clinically. Up-beating vertical nystagmus is uncommon but often attributable to a lesion of the rostral interstitial medial longitudinal fasciculus (riMLF). Down-beating vertical nystagmus classically localizes to the cervicomedullary junction and can be caused by MS, but it can also occur with a Chiari malformation or paraneoplastic cerebellar degeneration, two conditions which may occasionally mimic MS. Internuclear ophthalmoplegia (INO) results from damage to the medial longitudinal fasciculus (MLF), located in the dorsal pons/midbrain, which leads to poor integration between the oculomotor and abducens cranial nerve nuclei and consequent failure of binocular fusion. This is classically manifested as diplopia, although blurring, jumping, or shadowing of images may be described. Though classically the affected side experiences an inability to adduct past the midline, with nystagmus in the contralateral abducting eye, in practice it is more common to observe slowed adduction rather than paralysis, and in its mildest form (*forme fruste*) only a subtle nystagmus of the abducting eye may be present. Convergence is preserved, indicating intact third nerve nuclei rostrally. In a survey of 100 patients, Muri and Meienberg [6] reported a unilateral INO in 20 patients, bilateral in 14. Bilateral INO is nearly pathognomonic for MS, and longstanding cases may develop "wall-eyed," bilateral INO (WEBINO) secondary to complete failure of adduction and resulting bilateral exotropia. Complete gaze palsy on one side and an INO on gaze to the opposite side constitutes the "one-and-a-half" syndrome, resulting from a lesion that damages either the paramedian pontine reticular formation (PPRF) or abducens nucleus (or both), together with the MLF on the same side. Individual palsies of cranial nerves III, IV, and VI are relatively uncommon. Other rarer eye movement abnormalities have been described.

Other Cranial Nerves

The olfactory nerve may be involved in up to 40% of patients [7] but is infrequently tested. Trigeminal involvement is common, and, when it occurs, generally involves the second and/or third divisions and is often painful, i.e., trigeminal neuralgia (TGN). When facial palsy occurs it is usually subtle, and upper vs. lower motor neuron involvement can be difficult to distinguish at the bedside in the absence of other brainstem or cerebellar findings. A "lower motor neuron" CN VII palsy can occasionally be seen from a CNS lesion involving the nerve root exit zone, although more commonly, frontalis and orbicularis oculi muscles are spared in MS. Often isolated cranial nerve palsies are not always reflected on MRI and may be more sensitively identified with electrophysiologic testing [8] although in practice this is rarely done, and clinical examination remains the most relevant and practical means of evaluation.

The vestibular-cochlear system is often involved in MS, and subtle forms of vertigo are frequent complaints. Patients often have concomitant spasticity and posterior column loss and frequently complain of difficulty with balance, station, and gait. They may describe a sensation of being suddenly "pushed" or "shoved," as if by an unseen force, and have particular difficulty on descending stairs. Lesions of the brainstem and cerebellum can cause patients to become frankly vertiginous, even to the point of nausea and vomiting acutely, but benign positional vertigo occurs in MS patient as well [9]. Though usually a low grade and frequently persistent symptom, vertigo can sometimes be intermittent and intense, simulating a labyrinthitis. Hearing loss can be an MS-related symptom, though it rarely occurs in isolation. Demyelinating lesions responsible for hearing loss are typically unilateral and also frequently cause vertigo and tinnitus on the affected side. Isolated retrocochlear hearing loss seen in an MS-like presentation with monocular visual loss and nonspecific T2 signal abnormalities on brain MRI should arouse suspicion for Susac syndrome. Spastic dysarthria occurs in patients with prominent motor involvement while "scanning speech" occurs classically with cerebellar dysfunction. Isolated tongue or palatal weakness is an uncommon manifestation, and difficulty swallowing is typically due to a failure of coordination of motor control and is generally seen only as an end-stage complication in the tetraplegic and otherwise severely disabled patient.

Weakness, Hyper-reflexia, and Spasticity

Weakness is extremely common in MS and generally results from involvement of the spinal cord or brainstem, although capsular and even hemispheric syndromes occur on occasion, especially with "tumefactive" presentations. Weakness and spasticity often increase over time, especially in progressive forms of MS, and tend to parallel the degree of spinal cord involvement. Isolated limb weakness is comparatively rare but can occur in presentations of primary progressive MS. Atrophy can occur as a result of deconditioning, but is not a common finding in early MS. Fasciculations in the setting of progressive motor weakness should of course always prompt a workup for motor neuron disease.

Brisk reflexes alone are not clearly pathologic and can be seen in young adults and anxious patients. Clinical experience suggests that evidence of reflex spread, sustained clonus, or upgoing toes relates better to evidence of CNS damage. The degree of hyperreflexia seen in MS is often severe and frequently parallels that seen in other forms of spinal cord injury. Absence of lower extremity reflexes in the setting of upgoing toes, progressive weakness, sensory loss and other signs of myelopathy should prompt consideration of subacute combined degeneration of the spinal cord from vitamin B12 deficiency, hereditary ataxias, and a variety of other conditions which may mimic progressive forms of MS.

Spasticity occurs in up to 75% of MS patients [10]. Patients frequently complain of pain, stiffness, and incoordination in the lower extremities on first rising in the morning or after prolonged periods of inactivity, such as long car rides or airplane flights. Symptoms of spasticity improve with stretching, exercise or ambulation, in contrast to weakness, which typically worsens with prolonged ambulation, although frequently the two occur together as a consequence of spinal cord involvement. Spasticity can impair gait and lead to increased disability early on, while treatment of spasticity may unmask muscle weakness in more disabled patients, because involuntary spastic muscle contraction of the quadriceps can compensate for decreased strength in the lower extremities and is often relied upon for short-distance ambulation and transfers, especially in secondary progressive patients. Spasticity is the functional consequence of damage to the corticospinal, vestibulospinal, or reticulospinal tracts and frequently coexists with autonomic dysfunction of the bladder. Bladder and bowel abnormalities, such as urinary tract infections and constipation, can increase weakness and/or spasticity, even in the absence of detectable fever, by poorly understood mechanisms. Medication options for treatment of spasticity include "muscle relaxants" such as baclofen and tizanidine, which have comparable efficacy, but differ in their side-effect profiles. Baclofen stimulates gamma-aminobutyric acid (GABA) receptors and can cause lightheadedness, dry mouth, and drowsiness. Abrupt withdrawal of baclofen at high doses can precipitate seizures. Tizanidine is an adrenergic receptor agonist. It tends to be more sedating than Baclofen and can also precipitate hypotension, dry mouth, constipation, and asthenia. Benzodiazepines such as diazepam and clonazepam work well for spasticity but are sedating and have potential for dependence and withdrawal phenomena. Injectable botulinum toxin also can help treat MS-related spasticity, especially in small muscles of the upper extremity. Larger doses required for the quadriceps and other large lower extremity muscles frequently lead to neutralizing antibody formation. Intrathecal baclofen (ITB) pump implantation, once considered a "last resort" for wheelchair bound patients with painful lower extremity spasticity, is now relatively commonplace and is increasingly initiated in ambulatory patients with moderate to severe painful lower extremity spasticity that are unable to tolerate the side effects of the oral medications.

Incoordination and Tremor

Up to 50% of MS patients may have various forms of tremor [11, 12] and in some cases this may be the most disabling feature of their disease. From 100 randomly chosen patients at an MS clinic Alusi et al. detected tremor in 58% of patients. The upper extremity was most frequently involved (56%) and action tremor was most frequently detected. Upper extremity intention or "target seeking" cerebellar tremor is typical and can be severely disabling; resting tremor is comparatively rare, although titubation and truncal instability are relatively common in severely disabled patients. Many MS patients with advanced disease walk with a wide-based gait, and often there is an ataxic component to their disability in combination with spasticity and posterior column sensory loss. Imbalance with feet together and eyes open suggests potential cerebellar involvement, in contrast to Romberg's test, which classically invokes posterior column sensory loss. MS-related tremor can be notoriously difficult to treat. Small controlled trials suggest that some therapeutic benefit might be achieved with propranolol, ethanol, isoniazid, carbamazepine, ondansetron, or dolasetron [13]. Remeron, primidone, diazepam, and clonazepam are sometimes helpful but are all sedating. Severe cases are sometimes treated by implantation of a deep brain stimulator. In the three studies on thalamic DBS with longer than 1-year follow-up, 69–100% of the patients experienced reduced tremor [13], although in our experience results are less impressive, especially in severe cases.

Sensory Loss

Patients with MS frequently have involvement of the posterior columns, and sensory complaints are common. Impairment of vibratory sensation in the lower extremities is especially common, even in the absence of sensory complaints or other motor or sensory findings, and should always be tested. Proprioceptive loss occurs later and is unusual without concomitant weakness. Spinothalamic tract involvement is less common, and pain and temperature loss may be relative rather than absolute, so that patients report a dulling of pinprick rather than an absence. Patients with acute spinal cord attacks can exhibit a clear sensory level to pain and temperature, though the posterior columns are typically also involved, and a true Brown–Sequard syndrome is rare. Paresthesias are common in MS and often persist after relapses with sensory disturbance.

Ambulatory Difficulties

Gait abnormalities and slowed walking are common in MS. Multiple factors can impinge on an MS patient's ability to walk including cerebellar or vestibular dysfunction, weakness, spasticity, and sensory loss. Walking time also tends to slow as the disease progressed. Dalfampridine (Ampyra) has been approved by the FDA based on trials documenting improvement in walking in about a third of patients [14, 15]. It is a sustained released preparation of a long time available compounded medication, 4AP, which blocks potassium channels, serving to speed conduction along damaged demyelinated axons. It is possible that through its mechanism of action dalfampridine may have other beneficial effects in MS, though this has not yet been well studied. Compounded 4AP was associated with increased risk of seizure though in trials seizure was no more frequently reported in the dalfampridine group than placebo. It is important, however, to highlight that patients with prior seizures were excluded from the trials and it is considered a contraindication to drug use. Side-effect profile otherwise was benign.

Subjective or "Invisible" Symptoms of MS

Fatigue
Point estimates indicate that fatigue is present in over 75% of MS patients [16] and is commonly present even in those with low T2 lesion load on brain MRI and little motor impairment or other disability. Many patients will complain of episodes of severe fatigue unrelated to effort. Though many affected patients typically awake reasonably well rested, they describe, "hitting a wall" in the early afternoon, suggesting an effect related to MS itself rather than poor

quality of sleep. Fatigue is frequently seen in otherwise normal-appearing, nondisabled patients with MS, but the possibility of depression or metabolic abnormalities such as anemia or hypothyroidism should also be considered in patients with this frequent complaint. The underlying explanation for MS-related fatigue has yet to be determined.

Pharmacologic intervention for fatigue includes amantadine, modafinil, and amphetamines. Extensive clinical experience confirms that modafinil is effective, well tolerated, nonhabit-forming, and works well in most patients, although placebo controlled trials differ in terms of efficacy results [17, 18] Support for the use of amantadine is largely anecdotal, although it is generally safe and may provide benefit in some patients for largely unknown reasons. Amphetamines are effective but are generally considered a last resort secondary to their potential for long-term dependence, addiction, and withdrawal. The active enantiomer of modafinil (Armodafinil) has recently been released and has a longer half-life than the parent compound, although there are no controlled clinical trials to date in MS.

Depression

Lifetime prevalence rates of depression in MS range from 25 to 50% [19]. A study comparing patients with MS to patients who had similar levels of disability resulting from peripheral nervous system disorders found that depression was more common in the MS group, suggesting that depression in MS is likely related to the direct pathophysiologic effects of the disease on the brain [20]. Compared with nondepressed MS patients, patients with major depression had a greater T2-weighted lesion volume and less gray matter volume [21]. Interferon treatment in the past has been implicated as having the potential to exacerbate underlying depression, but recent studies suggest that interferon likely does not increase risk of depression [22, 23].

Standard anti-depressant medications are generally effective in MS, although use of selective serotonin reuptake inhibitors (SSRIs) may be limited by sexual side effects, especially in patients with spinal cord involvement. Tricyclic anti-depressants can be limited by anti-cholinergic side effects at high doses, although low doses at bedtime often help with chronic pain, overactive bladder, and sleep disturbances in addition to mood. Many practitioners prefer atypical agents such as bupropion as first line, because of its relative lack of sedative and sexual side effects, although increased seizure risk should be kept in mind, especially in patients on interferons, which may also reduce seizure threshold.

Cognitive Dysfunction

Estimates are that nearly half of MS patients suffer some level of cognitive impairment [24]. Problems with executive function, attention, and ability to organize and maintain multiple simultaneous trains of thought (multitasking) typically occur before demonstrable memory deficits. If memory is impaired, working memory is most often affected before remote recall. Language abilities are sometimes affected in terms of word-finding difficulties, but aphasia, apraxia, visuospatial deficits, and other cortical syndromes are relatively rare. Studies have demonstrated that patients early in the disease course, who may not manifest significant physical disability, still exhibit cognitive impairment [25].

Patients with cognitive difficulty can have social functional impairment and are more likely to be disabled or unemployed [26]. Fatigue and depression are common intercurrent morbidities in MS, and, although quality of life frequently suffers over dementia is rare [27]. Patients with greater MRI disease burden tend to have more cognitive impairment, as do patients with brain volume loss, especially gray matter atrophy [28, 29]. Donepezil has been tested in a small group of cognitively impaired MS patients with some success and larger trials are currently ongoing [30].

Pain

Though a survey found that the percentage of MS patients reporting pain (80%) was not substantively different than a normal population (75%), MS patients experience pain of greater intensity, more frequently require medication for pain relief, and suffer greater impairment of quality of life from pain [31]. Several pain syndromes are highly suggestive of demyelinating disease, especially in younger age groups and when accompanied by focal neurologic signs and symptoms. Perhaps the most common pain phenomenon in MS is Lhermitte's sign, a sudden, brief and reproducible sensation of tingling, vibration or electrical shock-like sensations that spread down the spine, into the extremities, or throughout the body on flexion of the neck, generally indicative of posterior column involvement in the cervical spine. Two prospective studies estimate prevalence of Lhermitte's sign at nearly 40% patients [32, 33] while estimates of incidence range are lower (9–13%) [32, 34]. Although a strong association between Lhermitte's sign and intra medullary cervical spinal cord abnormalities on MRI has been demonstrated [35], it is not specific to demyelinating disease, and other conditions such as subacute combined degeneration of the cord, neck trauma, radiation myelitis, or herniated cervical disc can cause it. Another common pain syndrome seen in MS is trigeminal neuralgia (TGN). It typically manifests as a unilateral intermittent lancinating pain in the second or third division of the Trigeminal nerve felt in the cheek, teeth, or gums. Pain can be quite severe and is frequently precipitated by "triggers" such as brushing the teeth or hot or cold beverages. TGN can be notoriously difficult to treat. First-line agents include anticonvulsants such as carbamazepine and gabapentin, although opiates are frequently needed for severe attacks. Surgical rhizotomy or radiofrequency ablation of the Gasserion ganglion may be required in refractory cases.

"Tonic spasms" can also occur with MS and are typified by sudden brief (generally less than 1 min) involuntary contractions of an extremity, which may be mistaken for simple partial or partial-onset seizures, except that they are usually painful and do not result in loss of consciousness. They can be frequent throughout the day and disabling, although they generally respond to carbamazepine or benzodiazepines. They are most often associated with spinal cord lesions, often near a root exit zone, and are thought to be caused by ephaptic transmission of nerve impulses.

Bladder, Bowel, and Sexual Dysfunction

A recent study by Marrie et al. of nearly 10,000 MS patients found that 80% of patients reported either bowel or bladder symptoms [36]. Urinary tract infections were reported in 64% of patients within 6 months of survey, which was roughly six times higher than observed in the general female population. Symptoms reported as "greatly bothersome" included urinary frequency (16.5%), urgency (17.0%), urge incontinence (8.4%), difficulty with bladder emptying (12.5%), and nocturia (20.9%). Patients were at greater risk for urologic dysfunction if they were female, had a longer disease duration, or higher degree of disability. Clinically, it is commonly observed that patients with lower extremity weakness and spasticity are more likely to have autonomic nervous system involvement as well. Nocturia can be a significant cause of sleep disturbance and can result in falls. The pons contains a micturation center which coordinates uretheral sphincter relaxation and bladder detrusor contraction via a complex network of sympathetic and parasympathetic fibers arising from multiple levels throughout the thoracic and lumbar spinal cord. An MRI study showed that detrusor hyporeflexia occurred more frequently with pontine involvement and detrusor-sphincter dyssynergia (a lack of coordination between bladder and external urethral sphincter) more commonly with spinal cord lesions [37]. Patients with detrusor hyperactivity often respond well to anticholinergics such as oxybutynin and tolterodine. Detrusor-sphincter dyssynergia may respond to a combination of anticholinergics and adrenergic antagonists or may require self-catheterization. Urinary retention frequently does not respond to pharmacologic treatment and requires self-catheterization, though adrenergic antagonists (i.e., tamsulosin, terazosin, doxazosin) can be trialed. Intra-detrusor botulinum neurotoxin injections have been shown to decrease incontinence, urinary urgency, and nocturia and to improve quality of life [38]. Urologic referral should be initiated for recurrent UTIs, uncontrolled incontinence, or persistent urinary retention with elevated post-void residuals.

In a patient population with urologic issues and clinical evidence of spinal cord disease only 25% of patients reported normal bowel function; 36% of patients had constipation, and 30% reported one episode of fecal incontinence in the past 3 months [39]. Similar numbers were reported in an earlier study by Hinds et al. in an unselected MS population [40]. The underlying causes of MS-related bowel dysfunction are unclear. Bowel issues are important to address because they can cause embarrassment, predispose to infection, and worsen spasticity. Anticholinergics taken for bladder dysfunction and muscle relaxants such as baclofen can worsen constipation. Copious fluid intake, fiber, and docusate may help keep bowels regular. If these are ineffective laxatives can be considered. In severely disabled and immobile patients with MS, abdominal pain resulting from abnormal colonic motility can occur, and manual disimpaction may be necessary.

Sexual dysfunction is common in MS. A recent survey of 56 Norwegian MS patients 2–5 years after diagnosis found that 50% of males and 14% of females were not satisfied with their sexual functioning [41]. Men most often complained of difficulty achieving or maintaining an erection, while women most often complained of difficulty having an orgasm. It is always important to review all patient medications when addressing sexual dysfunction, because some medications frequently used in MS, such as SSRIs, can cause impairment in sexual functioning. Mixed results have been achieved with sildenafil citrate in both men and women in clinical trials, although in practice erectile dysfunction often responds to this or similar agents [42–44].

Seizures

Seizure prevalence is increased slightly in MS (approx. 2%) relative to the general population (0.5–1%) [45]. Two-thirds of seizures in MS are generalized. Simple partial seizures are more common than partial complex seizures, the reverse of what is expected in the general population. To date no studies evaluating specific anti-epileptic medication efficacy in MS have been performed, although in practice seizure disorders in MS generally respond to conventional anticonvulsants and are rarely intractable. Cortical and juxtacortical lesions are increasingly recognized in MS and are typically not well visualized on conventional MRI sequences. New onset partial and/or secondarily generalized seizures may occasionally herald a new juxtacortical enhancing brain lesion, which may respond to steroid treatment acutely. Interferons have the potential to lower seizure threshold and should be used cautiously in patients with a preexisting seizure disorder, though in practice this is not necessarily an absolute contraindication.

Sleep Difficulties

A higher prevalence of sleep disturbance is observed in MS patients than in the general population, and women may be more frequently affected [46]. Risk of developing restless legs syndrome is increased fivefold in MS patients (prevalence of 19% vs. 4% for controls). Risk factors for development of RLS include older age, longer disease duration, and increased disability [47].

Other Symptoms

Patients may suffer from other paroxysmal symptoms such as intermittent dysarthria, ataxia, tonic spasms, itching, transient akinesia, and radicular thoracic sensations of pain or tightness (so-called MS hug), or other radicular-type pain in an extremity. Some of these symptoms are covered in the section on pain. Anticonvulsants such as carbamazepine and gabapentin often are helpful to decrease the frequency and severity of these spells.

Diagnosis of Multiple Sclerosis

The majority of MS cases can be diagnosed by clinical or clinical and imaging parameters alone, provided these are properly applied and that other causes of CNS inflammatory white matter disease (so-called MS mimickers) are ruled out, usually by history, appropriate blood tests, and occasionally by CSF analysis. A CSF analysis which is positive for markers of abnormal intrathecal immunoglobulin synthesis (increased IgG index, synthesis rate, and/or oligoclonal bands) can be useful in unusual presentations of MS with uncharacteristic features on MRI, as well as in primary progressive MS, where imaging may be negative, especially early in the disease course. Frequently, however, the CSF is negative for these markers, especially early in the disease course, and provides no supportive evidence in either direction. Visual evoked potential (VEP) recordings are usually unnecessary in the setting of acute optic neuritis but can be useful in documenting a prior episode of retrobulbar neuritis when they show a unilaterally prolonged P100 latency with preserved wave form; beyond this, further evoked potential (EP) studies are not often helpful or reliable.

Diagnostic Criteria

Initial criteria used to diagnose Multiple Sclerosis (MS) were based on clinical features alone and required demonstration of CNS lesions disseminated in space and time by objective abnormalities on the neurological examination, as well as the elimination of alternative diagnoses which might present with a similar clinical picture, ultimately rendering MS a diagnosis of exclusion, as is still the case today. In 1983, the "Poser Criteria" [48] were proposed, which used para-clinical findings (neuroimaging, evoked potentials, and spinal fluid analysis) to supplement clinical evidence for the diagnosis in situations where strict clinical criteria were not met. An international panel chaired by W. Ian McDonald met in July 2000 to review preexisting criteria for the diagnosis of MS and to incor-porate modern imaging techniques into a diagnostic scheme that would allow the physician to satisfy a requirement for dissemination of lesions in time and/ or space without having to wait for a second clinical manifestation of disease, as had previously been the norm [49]. The resulting "McDonald Criteria" may appear cumbersome at first, but, if properly applied, show a sensitivity of 83%, specificity of 83%, negative predictive value of 89%, and accuracy of 83% for clinically definite MS at 3 years in patients initially presenting with a clinically isolated syndrome (CIS) suggestive of demyelinating disease [50]. These crite-ria were revised in 2005 in order to further simplify the possibility of making a definitive diagnosis of MS after either a monosymptomatic presentation or a progressive course from the outset (primary progressive MS) [51]. Nearly all subsequent clinical trials in RRMS have relied on the McDonald criteria for inclusion. Since initiation of treatment at the time of CIS in patients with abnormal MRI findings has been shown to delay the onset of a second clinical attack, i.e., clinically definite MS (CDMS), most MS specialists now advocate early treatment, at the time of CIS, if the baseline MRI shows at least two characteristic lesions indicative of prior asymptomatic demyelination. Earlier recognition allows for treatment to at least be considered after a first clinical episode and to tailor the follow-up approach with the patient. It should also be re-emphasized that the McDonald criteria do not absolutely require an MRI in order to diagnose MS. Two or more attacks with objective clinical evidence of two or more CNS lesions will suffice. In contradistinction, the criteria also do not provide for a diagnosis of MS based on imaging alone. At least one attack with objective clinical evidence of a CNS lesion on examination (CIS) is required before paraclinical data (chiefly MRI) come into play. Furthermore, it cannot be overemphasized that there must be no better explanation for any clinical or paraclinical abnormalities in order for the diagnosis to be secure, i.e., "MS mimickers" must be ruled out.

To simplify the McDonald criteria (Table 5.1) we can apply them to five common clinical scenarios:

1. *Two clinical attacks and two objective lesions on neurologic examination*:
   Here no further paraclinical testing is technically needed, and a diagnosis of relapsing–remitting MS (RRMS) can be made anywhere in the world without the benefit of MRI or other paraclinical testing, provided other

Table 5.1 2001 McDonald diagnostic criteria.

Clinical presentation	Additional data needed for MS diagnosis
Two or more attacks; objective clinical evidence of two or more lesions	None[a]
Two or more attacks; objective clinical evidence of one lesion	Dissemination in space, demonstrated by MRI[b] *or* two or more MRI-detected lesions consistent with MS plus positive CSF[c] *or* await further clinical attack implicating a different site
One attack; objective clinical evidence of two or more lesions	Dissemination in time, demonstrated by MRI[d] *or* second clinical attack
One attack; objective clinical evidence of one lesion (monosymptomatic presentation; clinically isolated syndrome)	Dissemination in space, demonstrated by MRI[b] *or* two or more MRI-detected lesions consistent with MS plus positive CSF[c] *and* dissemination in time, demonstrated by MRI[d] *or* second clinical attack
Insidious neurological progression suggestive of MS	Positive CSF[c] *and* dissemination in space, demonstrated by (1) nine or more T2 lesions in brain *or* (2) two or more lesions in spinal cord, *or* (3) 4–8 brain plus 1 spinal cord lesion *or* abnormal VEP[e] associated with 4–8 brain lesions, or with fewer than four brain lesions plus one spinal cord lesion demonstrated by MRI *and* dissemination in time, demonstrated by MRI[d] *or* continued progression for 1 year

If criteria indicated are fulfilled, the diagnosis is multiple sclerosis (MS); if the criteria are not completely met, the diagnosis is "possible MS"; if the criteria are fully explored and not met, the diagnosis is "not MS".

From McDonald WI, Compston A, Edan G, et al. Recommended diagnostic criteria for multiple sclerosis: guidelines from the International Panel on the diagnosis of multiple sclerosis. Ann Neurol. 2001;50:121–7. With permission.

[a] No additional tests are required; however, if tests [magnetic resonance imaging (MRI), cerebral spinal fluid (CSF)] are undertaken and are *negative,* extreme caution should be taken before making a diagnosis of MS. Alternative diagnoses must be considered. There must be no better explanation for the clinical picture.

[b] MRI demonstration of space dissemination must fulfill the criteria listed in Table 5.2.

[c] Positive CSF determined by oligoclonal bands detected by established methods (preferably isoelectric focusing) different from any such bands in serum or by a raised IgG index.

[d] MRI demonstration of time dissemination must fulfill the criteria listed in Table 5.2.

[e] Abnormal visual evoked potential of the type seen in MS (delay with a well-preserved wave form).

diagnostic possibilities have been ruled out, i.e., there is "no better explanation" for the findings.

2. *Two clinical attacks and only one objective lesion on neurologic examination*: Here the diagnosis can be made either by waiting for an additional attack, or by demonstrating dissemination in space by paraclinical testing. The requirement for dissemination in space can be demonstrated by documenting two or more characteristic demyelinating lesions on MRI plus a positive cerebrospinal fluid (CSF) exam, or by MRI alone provided at least three of the criteria summarized in Table 5.2 are met.

Table 5.2 Magnetic resonance imaging criteria for brain abnormality.

Three of four of the following
1. One gadolinium-enhancing lesion or nine T2-hyperintense lesions if there is no gadolinium-enhancing lesion
2. At least one infratentorial lesion
3. At least one juxtacortical lesion
4. At least three periventricular lesions

Note: One spinal cord lesion can be substituted for one brain lesion.
From McDonald WI, Compston A, Edan G, et al. Recommended diagnostic criteria for multiple sclerosis: guidelines from the International Panel on the diagnosis of multiple sclerosis. Ann Neurol. 2001;50:121–7. With permission.

3. *One clinical attack and two or more objective lesions on neurologic examination*: In this case, the criterion for dissemination in space was fulfilled by the neurological exam and the criterion for dissemination in time can be demonstrated by either waiting for a second attack, or by at the demonstration of a new lesion on an MRI scan done at least 3 months out from the initial clinical event. The choice of a 3-month interval is arbitrary, but it reduces the risk of misdiagnosing MS in cases of acute disseminated encephalomyelitis with a stuttering onset.

4. *One clinical attack and one objective lesion on neurologic examination*: The monosymptomatic presentation or so-called clinically isolated syndrome (CIS) is currently the focus of many clinical trials of the disease-modifying therapies (DMT). CIS generally comprises optic neuritis, partial transverse myelitis, and brainstem–cerebellar syndromes, although a capsular or large hemispheric lesion may occasionally present in this fashion. Here the criterion for dissemination in space can again be satisfied by documenting nine additional clinically silent lesions by MRI (Table 5.2) or, if that is lacking, at least two brain lesions consistent with MS plus a positive CSF exam. The criterion for dissemination in time is then satisfied either by a second clinical attack or by documenting additional new lesions on a follow-up MRI done at some point after the initial evaluation.

5. *Insidious neurological progression from the outset or primary progressive MS (PPMS)*: Here it is difficult to prove dissemination in time or space and the MRI may not show characteristic demyelinating lesions, especially early in the disease course, so in order to diagnose PPMS alternative criteria must be met (Table 5.1).

In each case, if criteria indicated are fulfilled, the diagnosis is multiple sclerosis; if the criteria are not completely met, the diagnosis is "possible MS"; if the criteria are fully explored and not met, the diagnosis is "not MS."

In 2006, new MRI criteria were proposed by Swanton et al. to diagnose MS in patients who present with CIS, in which dissemination in space requires only one or more T2 lesion(s) in at least two of four locations (juxtacortical, periventricular, infratentorial, and spinal cord), and dissemination in time requires only a new T2 lesion on a follow-up scan done at any point after the baseline MRI [52]. When all three criteria were applied in a large cohort of CIS patients to assess their performance, it was found that

Table 5.3 Comparison of MRI Criteria for Dissemination in Space (DIS) and Dissemination in Time (DIT).

	DIS[a]	DIT
McDonald 2001	≥3 of the following: 9 T2 lesions or 1 Gd-enhancing lesion; ≥3 periventricular lesions; ≥1 juxtacortical lesion; ≥1 posterior fossa lesion 1 spinal cord lesion can replace 1 brain lesion	A Gd-enhancing lesion ≥3 months after CIS onset A new T2 lesion with reference to a previous scan ≥3 months after CIS onset
McDonald 2005	≥3 of the following: 9 T2 lesions or 1 Gd-enhancing lesion; ≥3 periventricular lesions; ≥1 juxtacortical lesion; ≥1 posterior fossa lesion or spinal cord lesion A spinal cord lesion can replace an infratentorial lesion Any number of spinal cord lesions can be included in total lesion count	A Gd-enhancing lesion ≥3 months after CIS onset A new T2 lesion with reference to a baseline scan obtained ≥30 days after CIS onset
New criteria	≥1 lesion in each of ≥2 characteristic locations: periventricular, juxtacortical, posterior fossa, spinal cord All lesions in symptomatic region excluded in brainstem and spinal cord syndromes	A new T2 lesion on follow-up MRI irrespective of timing of baseline scan

CIS clinically isolated syndrome, *Gd* gadolinium.

[a] On baseline or follow-up MRI. The McDonald 2001 and 2005 DIS criteria also include the presence of two or more T2 lesions plus cerebrospinal fluid oligoclonal bands. Because cerebrospinal fluid was not examined systematically in the Magnims cohort, only the MRI criteria for DIS were used in this study. From Swanton JK, Rovira A, Tintore M, et al. MRI criteria for multiple sclerosis in patients presenting with clinically isolated syndromes: a multicentre retrospective study. Lancet Neurol. 2007;6:677–86, with permission.

the specificity of all criteria for predicting conversion to clinically definite MS (CDMS) was high (2001 McDonald, 91%; 2005 McDonald, 88%; new criteria, 87%), but the sensitivity of the new criteria and the 2005 revised McDonald criteria were higher (72% and 60%, respectively) than the original 2001 McDonald criteria (47%). The newly proposed (Swanton) criteria have not yet been accepted as the gold standard for diagnosis or inclusion in clinical trials, but in practice are much simpler to use than the McDonald criteria (Table 5.3).

A common obfuscation in the application of the McDonald criteria seems to arise from the dual meaning of the word "lesion." In the context of the initial clinical presentation, "lesion" refers to a demonstrable clinical abnormality of the CNS on neurological examination and not to an area of signal abnormality on MRI. Unfortunately (but perhaps unavoidably), "lesion" is also commonly used to define an area of signal abnormality seen on MRI. In our experience the most common difficulty, however, arises from the failure to differentiate MRI lesions that are typical for MS from those that are "nonspecific" and are frequently noted as incidental findings on routine imaging of patients with headache, vertigo, and a variety of other common conditions. While the McDonald criteria, address to some extent the issues of lesion size (>3 mm), number (≥9 T2 hyperintense lesions if no Gad+ lesion is present), and location (infratentorial, juxtacortical, periventricular, spinal cord) in satisfying a requirement for dissemination in space, the issue of lesion morphology (rounded, ovoid, etc.) is not well-addressed in any of the criteria. Also, while the criteria fairly carefully spell out what is needed to satisfy a requirement for dissemination in time, they do not specifically address the issue of follow-up of CIS with a normal initial brain MRI. Nor do they address the increasingly common scenario of the asymptomatic patient, with no prior history of a demyelinating episode, but who has incidental MRI findings characteristic of prior areas of demyelination on a scan which was done for other reasons (headache, vertigo, trauma, etc.), or so-called Radiographically Isolated Syndrome (RIS).

Differential Diagnosis

A key element in the diagnosis of MS is the exclusion of other possible disease entities. Distinguishing an MS presentation from that of another neurologic disease can at times be challenging, due to lack of homogeneity in clinical presentation and absence of a definitive paraclinical confirmatory test. Overlap between MS and other diseases that may have similar presentations and can also be difficult to diagnose (e.g., SLE, neurosarcoidosis, etc.) further compounds the problem. For this reason, an awareness of neurologic diseases that are MS "look alikes" or "mimics" is important. While parsimony of diagnosis (Ockham's razor) is desirable heuristically, a single diagnosis is not infrequently elusive, and patients may indeed have an overlapping presentation of various neurologic and/or autoimmune phenomena.

A consensus panel recently convened and identified common "red flags" that can alert the neurologist to a potential alternate diagnosis [53] (Table 5.4). Since other autoimmune disorders are covered in greater detail elsewhere in this book, we will limit ourselves to some more general comments. The first is that different MS subtypes overlap with alternate potential differential diagnoses. For example, because amyotrophic lateral sclerosis (ALS) is a progressive disease of motor neurons, it would be difficult to confuse with CIS or relapsing forms of MS. On the other hand, primary progressive MS and ALS could be, and are, more readily confused. Symptoms and signs attributable to relapsing MS can also be seen in other autoimmune, vasculitic, infectious, metabolic, and paraneoplastic presentations, while infectious, metabolic, and structural entities most commonly overlap with a more progressive MS phenotype. Table 5.4 lists diseases more commonly mistaken for MS with some basic differential diagnosis points.

Table 5.4

Disease	Symptoms/exam	Paraclinical
Diseases which may mimic relapsing presentations of MS		
Neurosarcoidosis	Cranial neuropathy (80%), headaches (27%), visual failure (27%), ataxia (20%), vomiting (23%), seizures (17%)	Serum ACE+(29%) [55]
		CSF OCB+(27%)
		CSF ACE (55–94%)
	Note: 10% no evidence of systemic sarcoidosis [54]	MRI leptomeningeal enhancement (36%) [56]
		Abnormal CXR (48%)
		Gallium scanning+(67%)
Behcet disease	Brainstem involvement (51%), hemiparesis (60%), behavioral changes (54%), arthritis (33%), thrombophlebitis (33%), oral ulcerations (100%), genital ulcerations (94%)	CSF OCB not typically seen
		CSF pleocytosis (approx. 50%)
		MRI abnormal about 2/3 patients, no specific feature
	Note: Rare without evidence of ulcerations [57]	
Systemic Lupus Erythematosis (SLE)	Neuropsychiatric (60%)	Serum ANA+(59%)
	Malar rash, photosensitivity, arthritis	Double-stranded DNA+(28%)
	Visual loss frequently severe and painless if occurs	Antiphospholipid antibody (33%) [58]
		CSF OCB (approx. 50%)
		MRI can look MS-like or stroke-like
Antiphospholipid antibody syndrome	Hx of thrombosis, miscarriages, livedo reticularis, thrombocytopenia, transverse myelitis [59]	Antiphospholipid antibodies frequently+in active disease
		MRI spinal cord involvement usually >2 vertebral levels, typically thoracic
Sjogren syndrome	Peripheral nervous system involvement (62%), multiple mononeuropathies (9%), seizures (9%), cranial nerves (20%)	CSF OCB (30%)
		VEP abnl (61%)
		Anti-Ro/anti-La+(21%)
	Sicca sx (53%) [60]	ANA+(54%)
		MRI WM lesions (70%)
Lyme disease	Aseptic meningitis, radicular pain, cranial neuropathy (VII), tic bite	CSF OCB, pleocytosis frequently present
		MRI WM lesion common
		Lyme testing very sensitive [61]
Vasculitis	Peripheral neuropathies, mononeuritis-multiplex, oculomotor palsies, seizures, encephalopathy	CSF leukocytosis
		MRI stroke, hemorrhage, or meningeal enhancement, or multiple punctuate enhancing lesions
	Fatigue, fever, night sweats, headaches, oligoarthropathy	Gold standard for dx: brain biopsy [62]
Cerebral Autosomal Dominant Arteriopathy with Subcortical Infarcts and Leukoencephalopathy (CADASIL)	Headache, stroke-like episodes	CSF OCB rarely present
	FH stroke common	MRI diffuse extensive WM changes with anterior temporal and external capsule involvement
		NOTCH 3 gene present

(continued)

Table 5.4 (continued)

Disease	Symptoms/exam	Paraclinical
Leber Hereditary Optic Neuropathy (LHON)	Consider with recurrent optic neuritis	Point mutation in mitochondrial DNA
	Vision loss most commonly painless, progressive, and binocular	
	Affects men only	
Diseases which may mimic progressive presentations of MS		
Vitamin B12 deficiency	Peripheral neuropathy, myelopathy	Macrocytic anemia
	Cognitive impairment (25%)	B12 or methylmalonic acid low
	Bilateral+Babinski, ankle jerks lost [63]	
Copper deficiency	Gait difficulty, myelopathy, lower extremity paresthesias, bilateral+Babinski, ankle jerks lost	Anemia frequent, ceruloplasmin, or copper levels low
		MRI can show brain or spinal cord involvement
Paraneoplastic syndromes	Gait unsteadiness, dysarthria, diplopia, dysphagia, weight loss, pruritis, fevers	CSF lymphocytic pleocytosis, elevated protein, OCB
		MRI can show late cerebellar atrophy
		Anti-Yo, anti-HU, anti-Tr most frequently associated [64]
HTLV-1 myelopathy/ tropical spastic paraparesis	Chronically progressive myelopathy	CSF OCB typically present
		MRI spinal cord lesions, brain can have white matter lesions
		Thoracic cord atrophy common
		HTLV-1 antibodies found in both serum and CSF
Whipple disease	Cognitive changes	OCB can be present
	Supranuclear gaze palsies	MRI can look MS-like
	Neuro. symptoms rare before systemic (arthralgia, wt. loss, diarrhea, fever)	PCR+*t. whipplei*
	Oculomasticatory myorhythmia (20%) [65]	
Spinocerebellar Ataxias (SCA)	Primarily disequilibrium, incoordination	CSF OCB likely negative
		MRI atrophy of cerebellum, brainstem but T2/FLAIR changes unlikely
		Genetic testing available
Friedrich ataxia	Ataxia, weakness later, skeletal abnormalities, diabetes common, diminished reflexes, toes up-going [66]	CSF OCB can be present
		MRI at time gray and white matter involvement
		Genetic testing available (trinucleotide repeat)
Amyotrophic Lateral Sclerosis (ALS)	No sensory involvement	EMG/NCS confirmatory in advanced disease
	Upper and lower motor neuron	
	Fasciculations	
	Bulbar symptoms	
Primary Lateral Sclerosis (PLS)	Similar to ALS, no lower motor neuron involvement	EMG/NCS confirmatory in advanced disease

(continued)

Table 5.4 (continued)

Disease	Symptoms/exam	Paraclinical
Celiac sprue	Progressive spinal and cerebellar decline Myoclonus, peripheral neuropathy, encephalopathy and seizures can occur	MRI can look MS-like [67] Antigliadin antibodies nonspecific, duodenal biopsy recommended
Leukodystrophies	In adults can look like progressive myelopathy Adrenoleukodystophy (ALD): Addisonian features, bronzing of skin, abdominal pain, family history. Metachromatic leukodystrophy (MLD): progressive myelopathy	OCB absent ALD-serum very long chain fatty acids MLD-serum arylsulfatase A deficiency MRI ALD: WM involvement can occur [68] MRI MLD: WM involvement, sparing of "U" fibers [69]

Hx history, *sx* symptoms, *FH* family history, *wt* weight, ALS+amyotrophic lateral sclerosis, *ACE* angiotensin converting enzyme, *OCB* oligoclonal bands, *CXR* chest x-ray, *ANA* antinuclear antibodies, *VEP* visual evoked potential, *WM* white matter, *CSF* cerebrospinal fluid, *dx* diagnosis, EMG/NCS electromyogram/nerve conduction studies, *PCR* polymerase chain reaction.

Conclusion

MS can present with a wide variety of symptoms and signs, and there remains no substitute for clinical judgment. One must remain alert to alternate possible diagnoses, both at the initial visit and in follow-up. MRI is a remarkably sensitive paraclinical test that can be repeatedly used to demonstrate both the acute and chronic changes in CNS signal characteristics that are typically seen in MS. As such, it is used increasingly as both a diagnostic tool to establish dissemination in time and space, a prognostic tool at the time of CIS, and as a tool to monitor disease activity and the effectiveness of treatments. Ultimately, conventional (proton) MRI is not specific to any disease process and can be misleading if not interpreted in the proper clinical context. The typical "laundry list" differential generated by the radiologist in response to common nonspecific T2 signal changes in the white matter is daily proof of this and is almost never helpful. For this reason, it is the obligation of the diagnosing and treating neurologist to consider all clinical data and personally review the MRI scans. Neither do conventional measures of disease burden or activity, such as T2 lesion number or volume, or Gadolinium enhancement correlate particularly well with symptoms or disability on cross-sectional studies, much less at the office visit. One should not be drawn into the type of simple structure/function explanation that characterizes other CNS lesions. Surprising numbers of MS lesions may be found in supposedly "eloquent" areas of the CNS, including the brainstem and spinal cord, without any corresponding symptoms or signs on examination. One must incorporate the MRI into an overall picture of the patient that also includes clinical measures of disease activity, such as relapse rate, disability progression, and cognitive and psychosocial parameters when deciding when to initiate or change treatment. Longitudinal studies and improving MRI techniques are beyond the scope of this chapter and are addressed in a separate chapter. These will undoubtedly shed new light on the disease process, but will also raise new questions, as increased sensitivity shows us pathologic processes in what we even now tentatively deem the "normal-appearing" brain tissue.

References

1. Optic Neuritis Study Group. Visual function 15 years after optic neuritis: a final follow-up report from the Optic Neuritis Treatment Trial. Ophthalmology. 2008; 115:1079–82.
2. O'Riordan JI, Thompson AJ, Kingsley DPE, et al. The prognostic value of brain MRI in clinically isolated syndromes of the CNS: a 10-year follow-up. Brain. 1998;121:495–503.
3. Brex PA, Ciccarelli O, O'Riordan JI, Sailer M, Thompson AJ, Miller DH. A longitudinal study of abnormalities on MRI and disability from multiple sclerosis. N Engl J Med. 2002;346:158–64.
4. Honan WP, Heron JR, Foster DH, Edgar GK, Scase MO, Collins MF. Visual loss in multiple sclerosis and its relation to previous optic neuritis, disease duration and clinical classification. Brain. 1990;113:975–87.
5. Cole SR, Beck RW, Moke PS, Gal RL, Long DT. The National Eye Institute Visual Function Questionnaire: experience of the ONTT. Optic Neuritis Treatment Trial. Invest Ophthalmol Vis Sci. 2000;41:1017–21.
6. Müri RM, Meienberg O. The clinical spectrum of internuclear ophthalmoplegia in multiple sclerosis. Arch Neurol. 1985;42:851–5.
7. Zorzon M, Ukmar M, Bragadin LM, et al. Olfactory dysfunction and extent of white matter abnormalities in multiple sclerosis: a clinical and MR study. Mult Scler. 2000;6:386–90.
8. Thömke F, Lensch E, Ringel K, Hopf HC. Isolated cranial nerve palsies in multiple sclerosis. J Neurol Neurosurg Psychiatry. 1997;63:682–5.
9. Frohman EM, Zhang H, Dewey RB, Hawker KS, Racke MK, Frohman TC. Vertigo in MS: utility of positional and particle repositioning maneuvers. Neurology. 2000;55:1566–9.
10. Paisley S, Beard S, Hunn A, Wight J. Clinical effectiveness of oral treatments for spasticity in multiple sclerosis: a systematic review. Mult Scler. 2002;8: 319–29.
11. Alusi SH, Worthington J, Glickman S, Bain PG. A study of tremor in multiple sclerosis. Brain. 2001;124:720–30.
12. Pittock SJ, McClelland RL, Mayr WT, Rodriguez M, Matsumoto JY. Prevalence of tremor in multiple sclerosis and associated disability in the Olmsted County population. Mov Disord. 2004;19:1482–5.
13. Koch M, Mostert J, Heersema D, De Keyser J. Tremor in multiple sclerosis. J Neurol. 2007;254:133–45.
14. Goodman AD, Brown TR, Krupp LB, et al. Fampridine MS-F203 Investigators. Sustained-release oral fampridine in multiple sclerosis: a randomised, double-blind, controlled trial. Lancet. 2009;373:732–8.
15. Goodman AD, Brown TR, Cohen JA, et al. Fampridine MS-F202 Study Group. Dose comparison trial of sustained-release fampridine in multiple sclerosis. Neurology. 2008;71:1134–41.
16. Iriarte J, Subirá ML, Castro P. Modalities of fatigue in multiple sclerosis: correlation with clinical and biological factors. Mult Scler. 2000;6:124–30.
17. Rammohan KW, Rosenberg JH, Lynn DJ, Blumenfeld AM, Pollak CP, Nagaraja HN. Efficacy and safety of modafinil (Provigil) for the treatment of fatigue in multiple sclerosis: a two centre phase 2 study. J Neurol Neurosurg Psychiatry. 2002;72:179–83.
18. Stankoff B, Waubant E, Confavreux C, et al. Modafinil for fatigue in MS: a randomized placebo-controlled double-blind study. Neurology. 2005;64:1139–43.
19. Minden SL, Schiffer RB. Affective disorders in multiple sclerosis. Review and recommendations for clinical research. Arch Neurol. 1990;47:98–104.
20. Schiffer RB, Babigian HM. Behavioral disorders in multiple sclerosis, temporal lobe epilepsy, and amyotrophic lateral sclerosis. An epidemiologic study. Arch Neurol. 1984;41:1067–9.

21. Feinstein A, Roy P, Lobaugh N, Feinstein K, O'Connor P, Black S. Structural brain abnormalities in multiple sclerosis patients with major depression. Neurology. 2004;62:586–90.
22. Feinstein A. Multiple sclerosis, disease modifying treatments and depression: a critical methodological review. Mult Scler. 2000;6:343–8.
23. Patten SB, Fridhandler S, Beck CA, Metz LM. Depressive symptoms in a treated multiple sclerosis cohort. Mult Scler. 2003;9:616–20.
24. Rao SM, Leo GJ, Bernardin L, Unverzagt F. Cognitive dysfunction in multiple sclerosis. I. Frequency, patterns, and prediction. Neurology. 1991;41:685–91.
25. Glanz BI, Holland CM, Gauthier SA, et al. Cognitive dysfunction in patients with clinically isolated syndromes or newly diagnosed multiple sclerosis. Mult Scler. 2007;13:1004–10.
26. Rao SM, Leo GJ, Ellington L, Nauertz T, Bernardin L, Unverzagt F. Cognitive dysfunction in multiple sclerosis. II. Impact on employment and social functioning. Neurology. 1991;41:692–6.
27. Benito-León J, Morales JM, Rivera-Navarro J. Health-related quality of life and its relationship to cognitive and emotional functioning in multiple sclerosis patients. Eur J Neurol. 2002;9:497–502.
28. Rovaris M, Comi G, Filippi M. MRI markers of destructive pathology in multiple sclerosis-related cognitive dysfunction. J Neurol Sci. 2006;245:111–6.
29. Pirko I, Lucchinetti CF, Sriram S, Bakshi R. Gray matter involvement in multiple sclerosis. Neurology. 2007;68:634–42.
30. Krupp LB, Christodoulou C, Melville P, Scherl WF, MacAllister WS, Elkins LE. Donepezil improved memory in multiple sclerosis in a randomized clinical trial. Neurology. 2004;63:1579–85.
31. Svendsen KB, Jensen TS, Overvad K, Hansen HJ, Koch-Henriksen N, Bach FW. Pain in patients with multiple sclerosis: a population-based study. Arch Neurol. 2003;60:1089–94.
32. Al-Araji AH, Oger J. Reappraisal of Lhermitte's sign in multiple sclerosis. Mult Scler. 2005;11:398–402.
33. Kanchandani R, Howe JG. Lhermitte's sign in multiple sclerosis: a clinical survey and review of the literature. J Neurol Neurosurg Psychiatry. 1982;45:308–12.
34. Solaro C, Brichetto G, Amato MP, et al. The prevalence of pain in multiple sclerosis: a multicenter cross-sectional study. Neurology. 2004;63:919–21.
35. Gutrecht JA, Zamani AA, Slagado ED. Anatomic-radiologic basis of Lhermitte's sign in multiple sclerosis. Arch Neurol. 1993;50:849–51.
36. Marrie RA, Cutter G, Tyry T, Vollmer T, Campagnolo D. Disparities in the management of multiple sclerosis-related bladder symptoms. Neurology. 2007;68:1971–8.
37. Araki I, Matsui M, Ozawa K, Takeda M, Kuno S. Relationship of bladder dysfunction to lesion site in multiple sclerosis. J Urol. 2003;169:1384–7.
38. Kalsi V, Gonzales G, Popat R, et al. Botulinum injections for the treatment of bladder symptoms of multiple sclerosis. Ann Neurol. 2007;62:452–7.
39. Chia YW, Fowler CJ, Kamm MA, Henry MM, Lemieux MC, Swash M. Prevalence of bowel dysfunction in patients with multiple sclerosis and bladder dysfunction. J Neurol. 1995;242:105–8.
40. Hinds JP, Eidelman BH, Wald A. Prevalence of bowel dysfunction in multiple sclerosis. A population survey. Gastroenterology. 1990;98:1538–42.
41. Nortvedt MW, Riise T, Frugård J, et al. Prevalence of bladder, bowel and sexual problems among multiple sclerosis patients two to five years after diagnosis. Mult Scler. 2007;13:106–1012.
42. Safarinejad MR. Evaluation of the safety and efficacy of sildenafil citrate for erectile dysfunction in men with multiple sclerosis: a double-blind, placebo controlled, randomized study. J Urol. 2009;181:252–8.

43. Fowler CJ, Miller JR, Sharief MK, Hussain IF, Stecher VJ, Sweeney M. A double blind, randomised study of sildenafil citrate for erectile dysfunction in men with multiple sclerosis. J Neurol Neurosurg Psychiatry. 2005;76:700–5.

44. Dasgupta R, Wiseman OJ, Kanabar G, Fowler CJ, Mikol DD. Efficacy of sildenafil in the treatment of female sexual dysfunction due to multiple sclerosis. J Urol. 2004;171:1189–93.

45. Koch M, Uyttenboogaart M, Polman S, De Keyser J. Seizures in multiple sclerosis. Epilepsia. 2008;49:948–53.

46. Bamer AM, Johnson KL, Amtmann D, Kraft GH. Prevalence of sleep problems in individuals with multiple sclerosis. Mult Scler. 2008;14:1127–30.

47. Italian REMS Study Group. Multicenter case-control study on restless legs syndrome in multiple sclerosis: the REMS study. Sleep. 2008;31:944–52.

48. Poser CM, Paty DW, Scheinberg L, et al. New diagnostic criteria for multiple sclerosis: guidelines for research protocols. Ann Neurol. 1983;13:227–30.

49. McDonald WI, Compston A, Edan G, et al. Recommended diagnostic criteria for multiple sclerosis: guidelines from the International Panel on the Diagnosis of Multiple Sclerosis. Ann Neurol. 2001;50:121–7.

50. Dalton CM, Brex PA, Miszkiel KA, et al. Application of the new McDonald criteria to patients with clinically isolated syndrome suggestive of multiple sclerosis. Ann Neurol. 2002;52:47–53.

51. Polman CH, Reingold SC, Edan G, et al. Diagnostic criteria for multiple sclerosis: 2005 revisions to the "McDonald Criteria". Ann Neurol. 2005;58:840–6.

52. Swanton JK, Rovira A, Tintore M, et al. MRI criteria for multiple sclerosis in patients presenting with clinically isolated syndromes: a multicentre retrospective study. Lancet Neurol. 2007;6:677–86.

53. Miller DH, Weinshenker BG, Filippi M, et al. Differential diagnosis of suspected multiple sclerosis: a consensus approach. Mult Scler. 2008;14:1157–74.

54. Joseph FG, Scolding NJ. Neurosarcoidosis: a study of 30 new cases. J Neurol Neurosurg Psychiatry. 2009;80:297–304.

55. Marangoni S, Argentiero V, Tavolato B. Neurosarcoidosis. Clinical description of 7 cases with a proposal for a new diagnostic strategy. J Neurol. 2006;253:488–95.

56. Pickuth D, Heywang-Köbrunner SH. Neurosarcoidosis: evaluation with MRI. J Neuroradiol. 2000;27:185–8.

57. Akman-Demir G, Serdaroglu P, Tasçi B. Clinical patterns of neurological involvement in Behçet's disease: evaluation of 200 patients. The Neuro-Behçet Study Group. Brain. 1999;122:2171–82.

58. Roussel V, Yi F, Jauberteau MO, Couderq C, et al. Prevalence and clinical significance of anti-phospholipid antibodies in multiple sclerosis: a study of 89 patients. J Autoimmun. 2000;14:259–65.

59. Kovacs B, Lafferty TL, Brent LH, DeHoratius RJ. Transverse myelopathy in systemic lupus erythematosus: an analysis of 14 cases and review of the literature. Ann Rheum Dis. 2000;59:120–4.

60. Delalande S, de Seze J, Fauchais AL, et al. Neurologic manifestations in primary Sjögren syndrome: a study of 82 patients. Medicine (Baltimore). 2004;83:280–91.

61. Steere AC, McHugh G, Damle N, Sikand VK. Prospective study of serologic tests for lyme disease. Clin Infect Dis. 2008;47:188–95.

62. Stone JH, Pomper MG, Roubenoff R, Miller TJ, Hellmann DB. Sensitivities of noninvasive tests for central nervous system vasculitis: a comparison of lumbar puncture, computed tomography, and magnetic resonance imaging. J Rheumatol. 1994;21:1277–82.

63. Shorvon SD, Carney MW, Chanarin I, Reynolds EH. The neuropsychiatry of megaloblastic anaemia. Br Med J. 1980;281:1036–8.

64. Dalmau J, Rosenfeld MR. Paraneoplastic syndromes of the CNS. Lancet Neurol. 2008;7:327–40.

65. Louis ED, Lynch T, Kaufmann P, Fahn S, Odel J. Diagnostic guidelines in central nervous system Whipple's disease. Ann Neurol. 1996;40:561–8.
66. Harding AE, Sweeney MG, Miller DH, et al. Occurrence of a multiple sclerosis-like illness in women who have a Leber's hereditary optic neuropathy mitochondrial DNA mutation. Brain. 1992;115:979–89.
67. Ghezzi A, Filippi M, Falini A, Zaffaroni M. Cerebral involvement in celiac disease: a serial MRI study in a patient with brainstem and cerebellar symptoms. Neurology. 1997;49:1447–50.
68. Eichler F, Mahmood A, Loes D, et al. Magnetic resonance imaging detection of lesion progression in adult patients with X-linked adrenoleukodystrophy. Arch Neurol. 2007;64:659–64.
69. Rauschka H, Colsch B, Baumann N, et al. Late-onset metachromatic leukodystrophy: genotype strongly influences phenotype. Neurology. 2006;67:859–86.

Advances in Magnetic Resonance Imaging of Multiple Sclerosis

Robert Zivadinov

Keywords: Multiple sclerosis, Magnetic resonance imaging, Conventional MRI techniques, Non-conventional MRI techniques, Gray matter, White matter

Introduction

Magnetic resonance imaging (MRI) is the most important paraclinical measure for assessing and monitoring the pathologic changes implicated in the onset and progression of multiple sclerosis (MS). Conventional MRI sequences, such as T1-weighted gadolinium (Gd)-enhanced and spin-echo T2-weighted imaging, provide an incomplete picture of the degree of inflammation and underlying neurodegenerative changes in this disease. Two- and three-dimensional fluid-attenuated inversion recovery and double-inversion recovery sequences allow better identification of cortical, periventricular, and infratentorial lesions. High field strength MRI has the potential to detect more cortical and deep gray matter lesions, but the detection of subpial cortical lesions in MS remains challenging. Unenhanced T1-weighted imaging can reveal hypointense black holes, a measure of chronic neurodegeneration. Magnetization transfer imaging (MTI) is increasingly used to characterize the evolution of MS lesions and normally appearing brain tissue, and evidence suggests that the dynamics of magnetization transfer changes correlate with the extent of demyelination and remyelination. Magnetic resonance spectroscopy, which provides details on tissue biochemistry, metabolism, and function, also has the capacity to reveal neuroprotective mechanisms. By measuring the motion of water, diffusion imaging can provide information about the orientation, size, and geometry of tissue damage in white and gray matters. Iron imaging-related techniques such as susceptibility-weighted imaging (SWI) have enormous potential for identifying iron-related pathology in MS. These advanced non-conventional MRI techniques relate better to clinical impairment, disease progression, and accumulation of disability and have the potential to detect neuroprotective effects of treatment.

From: *Clinical Neuroimmunology: Multiple Sclerosis and Related Disorders*, Current Clinical Neurology,
Edited by: S.A. Rizvi and P.K. Coyle, DOI 10.1007/978-1-60327-860-7_6,
© Springer Science+Business Media, LLC 2011

Conventional MRI Imaging and Clinical Status on MS

The presence and accumulation of T2-weighted and gadolinium (Gd)-enhancing T1-weighted lesions have represented the MRI gold standard for making a diagnosis and evaluating long-term prognosis in MS. These measures have also been used for a long time as principal MRI outcomes in clinical trials. One of the principal limitations of these techniques is that they incompletely reveal the pathophysiologic process in this disease. At least 20 clinical trials have demonstrated very pronounced inhibition of these inflammatory MRI measures without concurrent clinical benefit over the long term. A meta-analysis study [1] analyzed data from five natural history studies and the placebo groups from four clinical trials included a total of 307 patients. A moderate correlation was found between the mean cumulative number of Gd-enhancing lesions (Figure 6.1) observed during the first 6 months and relapse rate during the first year. Nevertheless, little correlation was observed between the number of these lesions at baseline or over the first 6 months and progression of disability, as measured by change in the expanded disability status scale (EDSS) score at 1 or 2 years. Therefore, Gd-enhancing lesions are very good short-term (6–12 months) predictors of clinical activity but not of long-term development of disability [2].

The apparent mismatch between conventional MRI imaging and clinical status can be explained by several possibilities. It is difficult to distinguish between demyelinated and remyelinated lesions using standard proton transfer MRI [3]. Demyelinated lesions appear as hyperintense loci on T2-weighted images (WI) (Figure 6.2) and hypointense loci on T1-WI (Figure 6.3), and the same is true for partially remyelinated lesions. Fully remyelinated lesions have the same general appearance on T2-WI, whereas on T1-WI the signal may be weaker and they usually appear as shadow plaques [4]. T1-WI was shown to reflect remyelination better than did T2-WI in a systematic comparison between MRI and histopathologic evaluation of myelination status in lesions

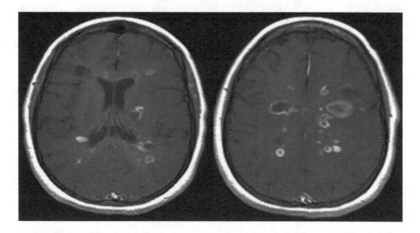

Figure 6.1 Enhancing lesions typical of MS on axial T1-WI postcontrast scans after gadolinium injection (0.1 mmol/kg). Two types of enhancing lesions are present in a 35-year-old female with RRMS with significant residual deficit and disability: homogenous lesions (hyperintense on T1-WI) and open-ring lesions (with central hypointense and external hyperintense rim)

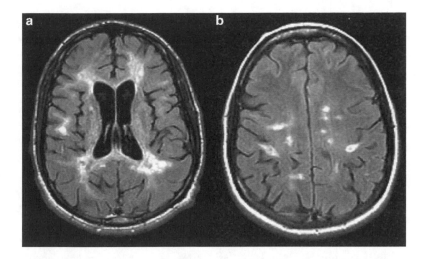

Figure 6.2 Representative axial FLAIR image shows widespread white matter lesions in the periventricular region (**a**). Supratentorial periventricular lesions are especially well visualized by FLAIR imaging compared with T2-WI where cerebrospinal fluid may mask the visualization of these lesions (**a**). White matter lesions may also be seen at the cortical level (**b**). Three different types of cortical lesions are found in patients with MS: (1) juxtacortical lesions (Type I); (**b**) located on the border between GM and WM; (2) intracortical lesions (Type II) (b); and (3) subpial cortical lesions (Type III), a class of GM lesion recently identified using new myelin basic protein-based pathologic staining methods

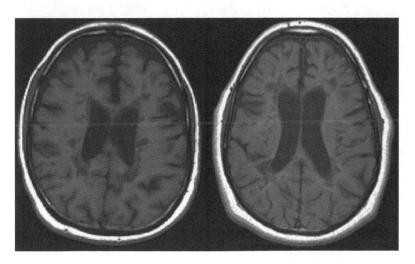

Figure 6.3 Axial T1-WI in a 43-year-old female with RRMS and EDSS score of 5.5. On T1-WI, multiple lesions are hypointense or appear as "black holes"

that were detected in 36 autopsy samples [5], with those lesions that were slightly hypointense or mostly isointense being most likely to be remyelinated and the strongly hypointense lesions being most likely to be demyelinated [3]. It is known that spontaneous remyelination does occur in MS lesions, but its extent within the global MS population is presently unknown [3]. A pathologic study explored the incidence and distribution of completely or partially remyelinated lesions in 51 autopsies of patients with different clinical courses and disease durations [6]. The authors showed that the extent of remyelination varied between MS patients; in 20% of the patients remyelination may be extensive, involving 60–96% of the global lesion area. These findings suggest that the hyperintense lesions observed on T2-WI in MS could be remyelinated to varying degrees and that the level of remyelination might be influenced by age, disease duration, and disease type.

A number of studies have followed patients over time with serial MRI scans, and these have allowed the evolution of individual lesion appearance over time to be mapped [7–10]. Approximately 98% of the lesions first appear on T1-WI as bright Gd-enhancing spots, which represent acute inflammatory lesions where the blood–brain barrier (BBB) has broken down locally [4]. On T2-WI, these lesions may or may not appear concomitantly hyperintense. A small part of these lesions (~5%) will disappear completely and no longer be visible on either T1-WI or T2-WI. They correspond to those lesions that achieve complete remyelination with no residual inflammation or edema. Enhancement duration is short (around 3–6 weeks) [7], and after 4–6 weeks, most lesions do not enhance. These lesions thus disappear from T1-WI, but remain visible in most cases as hyperintense areas on T2-WI. From a histologic point of view, these lesions are characterized by limited inflammatory activity, but are heterogeneous in terms of remyelination status, ranging from extensively demyelinated to fully remyelinated lesions [5, 6]. Approximately two-thirds of lesions remain visible on T1-WI as hypointense areas after Gd-enhancement is lost 1 or 2 months after their first appearance. These lesions, called "acute black holes," may evolve over the following months into demyelinated or partially/completely remyelinated lesions invisible on T1-WI. This process presumably corresponds to acute phase remyelination. Approximately one-third of these acute black holes persist on T1-WI as hypointense areas. These T1 chronic black holes are characterized histopathologically by extensive axonal loss and gliosis and their density is associated with the degree of chronic neurologic impairment [11]. Prevention of evolution of initially Gd-enhancing lesions into T1 chronic black holes may thus be considered as a key treatment objective [12–14].

Different pathologic lesion states may give rise to a similar appearance on conventional MRI imaging and, conversely, lesions with similar myelination status may take different forms on MRI images. This suggests that lesion appearance on conventional MRI images may not be specific in terms of underlying pathology, and probably accounts in part for the mismatch between these MRI measures and clinical outcome.

The conventional MRI techniques are also not sensitive enough, as they cannot detect pathology in gray matter (GM) or diffuse damage in "normally appearing" (NA) white matter (WM), which we now know to be very important for long-term outcome, notably for the accumulation of irreversible neurologic impairment [3, 15].

Clinical-MRI mismatch may also be related to the fact that not all lesions are equivalent in terms of their functional impact. Lesions, even a small number, in strategic areas in the brain may lead to very significant disability, whereas widespread lesion activity in nonstrategic areas may be clinically silent. Lesions in the spinal cord may cause disability related to walking ability [4].

The central nervous system (CNS) is plastic. Some patients may develop compensatory mechanisms through the use of alternative neural circuits to execute functions initially assured by pathways damaged by the lesion [16]. Remyelination or neuroprotective immunity may allow function to be restored without this being visible on conventional MRI. Not all patients seem to be able to compensate for lesion damage to the same extent and understanding why this is so represents an important clinical challenge. One factor that appears to influence compensatory capacity is age, with younger patients being able to compensate better.

Classic measures of total T2 lesion burden do not take into account dynamic changes within individual lesions. These changes can be investigated now using voxel-wise dynamic lesion change mapping [17] and subtraction techniques [18], in which the state of the lesion is compared on a voxel-by-voxel basis on serial MRI scans.

Strategies Proposed to Overcome the Limits of Conventional MRI

Several strategies have been proposed to overcome the limitations of conventional MRI scanning for better visualization of the global pathology in MS. One is related to the development of more advanced conventional sequences and application of newer contrast agents that are able to detect, in real time on the scanner, pathology that is currently invisible with standard conventional sequences. Newer imaging hardware strategies (such as high field strength scanners) (Figure 6.4) may increase the sensitivity of conventional scanning paradigms for the detection of invisible pathology. Finally, currently available non-conventional techniques using fully automated postimaging voxel-wise techniques can be applied in real time to help visualize or quantify this indirect damage in the CNS.

Advanced Conventional Sequences and New Contrast Agents

Of all advanced conventional sequences, two are particularly promising, namely three-dimensional fluid-attenuated inversion recovery (3D FLAIR) and double-inversion recovery (DIR). Newer contrast techniques continue to emerge.

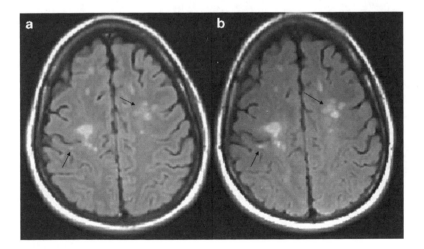

Figure 6.4 Evaluation of T2 hyperintense lesions in patients with RRMS on FLAIR images. 1.5T Scanner (**a**) shows less T2 lesions than 3T (**b**) (*arrows*)

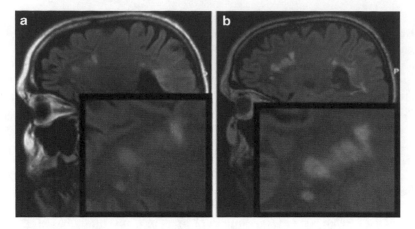

Figure 6.5 Data are reproduced with permission from Bink et al. [20] Comparison of 2D-FLAIR (**a**) vs. 3D-FLAIR (**b**). 3D-FLAIR shows significantly better delineation of the frontal lesions compared with 2D-FLAIR

Three-Dimensional Fluid-Attenuated Inversion Recovery

One limitation of 3D FLAIR involves distinguishing the anatomical border between juxtacortical, mixed WM and GM, and intracortical tissue and accounting for partial volume effect [19]. A comparison study of conventional 2D FLAIR and single-slab 3D FLAIR sequences in detecting lesions in eight patients with MS showed that the 3D FLAIR sequence detected 1.7 times the number of lesions visible on the 2D sequence (Figure 6.5) [20]. The difference was particularly striking for infratentorial lesions. This increased performance is likely to lead, over the next few years, to the substitution of 2D FLAIR with 3D FLAIR both as a research tool and in routine clinical practice.

Double-Inversion Recovery

Three-dimensional DIR overcomes this limitation by allowing the combination of two different inversion pulses that lead to the suppression of two tissue types, such as cerebrospinal fluid and WM, resulting in visualized images showing superior delineation of GM (Figure 6.6). A prospective clinical study compared visualization of intracortical lesions using 3D DIR, 3D FLAIR, and T2-WI spin-echo MRI in patients with MS ($n=10$) and age-matched healthy controls ($n=11$) [19]. No difference was observed in the total number of lesions visualized with 3D DIR or 3D FLAIR; however, 3D DIR detected 21% more lesions than T2-WI spin-echo. Furthermore, 3D DIR depicted significantly more intracortical lesions than 3D FLAIR or T2-WI spin-echo (152% and 538%, respectively). Another prospective study also demonstrated the greater sensitivity of 3D DIR in detecting cortical lesions in patients with CIS ($n=17$) or with a definite diagnosis of MS ($n=9$) compared with 3D FLAIR ($p=0.04$) and T2-WI spin-echo ($p=0.01$) [21]. Despite the improvement in lesion detection with 3D MRI, relatively long acquisition times of these multi-slab 3D imaging techniques have hampered their introduction into a clinical setting. Recently, single-slab 3D methods have shown reduced acquisition times and fewer flow artifacts [22]. The performance of single-slab 3D DIR

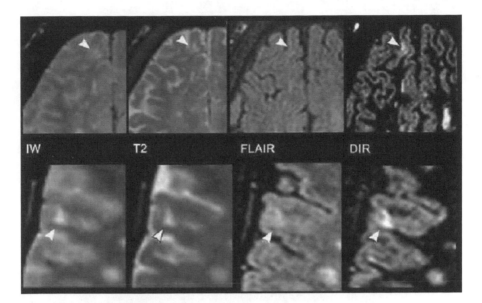

Figure 6.6 Data are reproduced with permission from Geurts et al. [19]. Cortical lesions detected in patients with MS using three different conventional MRI sequences. *T2-SE* T2-weighted spin-echo, *3D-FLAIR* three-dimensional fluid-attenuated inversion recovery, *3D-DIR* three-dimensional double-inversion recovery. *Top row*: lesion (*arrow*) in the cortical gray matter, with a possible juxtacortical component; the intracortical lesion is particularly poorly visible on intermediate-and T2-weighted images, as well as on the FLAIR image, whereas it is depicted clearly on the DIR image. *Bottom row* (different patient): DIR image shows very good delineation of the intracortical lesion (*arrow*), which may be mistaken for a juxtacortical lesion or a partial volume artifact on the T2-weighted image and may even be missed on the FLAIR image. No contrast agent was used

has been compared with 2D T2-WI spin-echo imaging in detecting MS brain lesions [22]. Single-slab 3D MRI allowed an improved detection of both GM and WM lesions compared with 2D T2-WI spin-echo imaging. In addition, DIR can increase the detection of cortical lesions over a short-term period compared with conventional MRI sequences [23]. Brain imaging using 3D DIR provides possibly the highest overall sensitivity in detecting MS lesions compared with other traditional and advanced MRI measures, a characteristic that emphasizes its potential utility in clinical trials evaluating the efficacy of disease-modifying treatments in patients with MS.

High-Resolution Microautoradiography

Inflammatory lesions observed in patients with MS are characterized by the activation of microglia and infiltration of lymphocytes and macrophages across the BBB. Preclinical studies of the experimental autoimmune encephalomyelitis rat model of MS detected intracellular phagocytosis occurring in inflammatory lesions by imaging with ultra-small particle iron oxide (USPIO), a new contrast agent that accumulates in phagocytic cells. One prospective, open-label, phase 2 imaging study investigated macrophage infiltration into the CNS in patients with clinically diagnosed RRMS [24]. Ten patients experiencing an acute relapse of MS were injected with intravenous USPIO 2.6 mg Fe/kg. Gadolinium enhancement, a marker of increased BBB permeability, was also evaluated in the same patients. Twenty-four hours following injection, 33 USPIO-enhanced lesions were observed on T1-WI images in nine of ten patients, and 55 Gd-enhanced lesions were visualized in seven of ten patients. Additionally, findings were similar in four patients receiving long-term treatment with IFN-beta or immunosuppressive therapy (13 USPIO lesions and 25 Gd lesions) compared with six untreated patients (20 USPIO lesions and 30 Gd lesions). In a phase 2 clinical study of 19 patients with RRMS, lesion enhancement with the novel USPIO nanoparticle SHU555C occurred more frequently and remained visible for a longer period of time compared with Gd-lesion enhancement [25]. Overall, the application of MRI using USPIO permitted visualization of different inflammatory aspects of CNS lesions and provided evidence that infiltration of macrophages and other inflammatory cells can be evaluated either with or without increased permeability of the BBB. High-resolution microautoradiography using USPIO is an important new imaging tool that may accurately predict the progression of MS. However, longitudinal studies are needed to further investigate the pathologic processes occurring within USPIO-enhanced lesions in patients with relapsing and progressive forms of MS and their relation to disease-modifying treatments.

High Field Strength MRI

High Field Strength MRI and Diagnosis

Another way to increase the sensitivity of conventional MRI sequences for the detection of inflammatory pathology in patients with MS is to use high field strength (Figure 6.4). In this respect, 3T scanners are being used increasingly for visualizing inflammatory pathology. Use of a 3T scanner allows the detection of around 20–50% more Gd-enhancing and T2 lesions compared with a 1.5T scanner [26–28].

The utility of high field strength scanning is still limited in MS patients who are diagnosed, treated, and stable. In patients presenting with a CIS suggestive of MS high strength MRI can provide vital supplementary information for confirming the diagnosis of MS. The improved image acquisition provided by high field strength MRI stands to benefit clinical trials assessing neuronal tissue damage and the efficacy of disease-modifying treatments in patients with MS. In this regard, a prospective, comparative clinical study employed 1.5 and 3T imaging to evaluate 40 patients with CIS to determine whether MR field strength affected classification of patients [29]. The authors reported that 11 of 40 patients (28%) met MRI diagnostic criteria with 3T imaging. However, although high field MRI shows a higher detection rate of inflammatory brain lesion in CIS and MS patients with an influence according to MRI criteria, this influence does not lead to an earlier diagnosis of lesion dissemination in time and therefore definite MS [30].

High Field Strength MRI and Detection of Type III Cortical Lesions

High- and ultra-high field MRI protocols do not contribute to the detection of lesions in GM in general and in the cortex in particular (Type III lesions) – that are now known to be widespread in subpial regions [31] – and possibly critical for the development of irreversible disability. GM lesions are also thought to represent the major type of pathology in progressive MS. The reason why cortical lesions are so difficult to detect using conventional MRI may relate to the fact that they are only weakly infiltrated by T cells, and thus associated with little inflammation and edema, so that the water content of the lesion, which is the source of the MRI signal, is relatively normal. Recent studies suggest

B cell-related pathophysiology of those lesions, although such a hypothesis is under intensive investigation [32]. The use of high field strength imaging provides only modest gains in the ability to identify Type III lesions, although the newer WM suppression inversion recovery techniques do improve the ability to detect Type I and Type II cortical lesions. Only one ultra-high field MRI study [33] has partially succeeded in demonstrating cortical pathology convincingly, and this in postmortem brain tissue. It required the use of an 8T scanner and very long scanning times, which are clearly unfeasible for routine monitoring or diagnosis of patients with MS.

It has been found that the extensive subpial demyelination is not associated with a significant increase in the area of focal and diffuse WM pathologic changes as assessed by histochemistry or by MRI findings in a recent study performed on samples from six patients with different degrees of cortical involvement [34]. This study demonstrated that those patients with principally GM lesions displayed few lesions in WM visible on T2-WI. Conversely, those patients who displayed a high T2 lesion burden in WM did not show prominent GM pathology. The only characteristic of the patients with GM lesions was that all presented severe cognitive problems. This may suggest that GM demyelination in MS occurs largely independent of WM pathologic changes, and that there are no major differences in the extent of WM pathologic features on MRI that may be used to distinguish patients with extensive subpial demyelination in clinical practice.

MRI Methods for Measuring Neuronal Damage and Repair

Above discussed MRI methods can effectively detect inflammatory damage to WM, although they do not permit us to visualize the processes of neuronal injury and repair that are the critical determinants of long-term clinical outcome in MS. A number of non-conventional MRI methods have been developed to allow these processes to be detected.

Brain Atrophy Measurements

Brain atrophy is the most accepted imaging biomarker of neurodegeneration and progression of disability in MS [35]. It should be noted that the terms "brain atrophy" and "brain volume (BV) loss" are not clearly distinct in the MS literature. Measured changes in BV in MS can be caused by two mechanisms [36]. First, changes in the degree of brain edema are associated with inflammation. Second, these changes may be caused by actual tissue loss (including loss of oligodendrocytes, myelin, axons, and possibly also astrocytes) or increases in BV could be due to tissue regeneration (such as remyelination). Focal edema in new lesions may mask reductions in BV caused by true atrophy, especially in those WM areas where inflammation is most pronounced. Massive cortical demyelination and diffuse axonal loss in the NAWM contributing to the loss of BV are present in the later stages of MS [31].

Dynamic changes in BV in MS can be considered a composite of volume-gaining and volume-losing processes that are influenced by the extent of inflammatory, neurodegenerative, and remyelinating processes, potency of anti-inflammatory therapy, and its neuroprotective effects. One problem with every anti-inflammatory drug used in patients with MS is that each of them decreases whole BV more rapidly in the treated vs. the placebo group

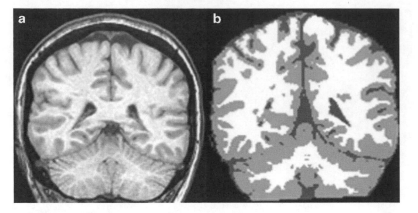

Figure 6.7 Representative images of brain segmentation with SIENAX in patient with RRMS. The 3D-T1 image is used for tissue segmentation (**a**). Three tissue class image is presented showing cerebrospinal fluid (*slightly gray*), neocortical gray matter (*dark gray*), and white matter (*mid gray*) (**b**)

due to reduced inflammation in the first couple of months of treatment [36]. The result is that none of the disease-modifying treatments shows efficacy in preventing BV loss when the treatment vs. the placebo group are compared in the first year, with any beneficial effect only becoming evident in the second year and beyond. This accelerated treatment-related BV reduction was named pseudoatrophy [36]. At this point, it is not clear whether pseudoatrophy is inseparable from true BV decline or represents only accelerated water loss (fluid shifts) with no associated loss of cell structures. Also, it has not yet been elucidated whether this is a temporary phenomenon.

CNS atrophy is a moderate but significant predictor of neurologic impairment that is independent of the effect of conventional MRI lesions [37, 38]. The relationship between spinal cord atrophy and disability is strong [39]. Evidence of brain atrophy can be found from the earliest stages of disease [35, 40, 41]. Total and regional brain volumes are further decreased in patients with a confirmed diagnosis of MS, particularly in those in advanced stages of the disease [42–44]. In the latter, the decrease of thalamic and putamen volumes is pronounced [45, 46]. The loss of deep GM volumes is accompanied by a striking increase in the volume of the lateral ventricles [47]. Cortical atrophy is less prominent than atrophy of the deep GM. Such findings indicate that selective regional atrophy is occurring in periventricular, deep GM, and cortical regions. Recent cross-sectional [48, 49] and longitudinal [50, 51] studies evaluated the evolution of atrophy in different tissue compartments. Findings from these studies suggest that the disease process in MS is not limited only to WM, but that GM atrophy develops at a much faster rate than WM atrophy, and that inclusion of GM atrophy in the assessment of patients with MS may further improve the usefulness of MRI measurements (Figure 6.7). The degree of correlation of GM and WM atrophy with neurological impairment is under intensive investigation.

Magnetization Transfer Imaging

Magnetization transfer imaging (MTI) contrast is obtained by applying a radiofrequency only to the proton magnetization of the macromolecules based on the interaction and exchange of protons unbound in free water with those

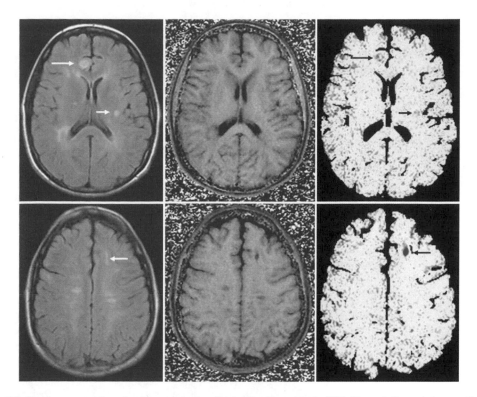

Figure 6.8 Data are reproduced with permission from Zivadinov et al. [72]. From left to right are displayed FLAIR image, MTR map, and raw voxel-wise dynamic MTR map. The raw voxel-wise MTR map shows areas of MTR stability (*yellow*) decrease of MTR (*red*) and increase in MTR (*green*) associated with lesions and normal appearing brain tissue in a patient with multiple sclerosis over 1 year. *Upper row*: Note the two T2 lesions (*arrows*) corresponding to the *green areas* (increase of MTR) on the voxel-vise MTR map (*arrows*) over the follow-up possibly reflecting remyelination. *Lower row*: Note the T2 lesion (*arrow*) corresponding to the *red area* (decrease of MTR) on the voxel-wise MTR map (*arrow*) over the follow-up possibly reflecting demyelination. *Upper and lower rows*: Note the high number of *red* and *green voxels* widespread in the brain reflecting possible demyelinating and remyelinating processes

bound with macromolecules. Although MTR decreases are not specific to any of the various MS pathologic substrates, MTI allows the detection of diffuse demyelination in lesions and normal appearing (NA) brain tissue (NABT). Demyelination is visualized as a reduced proton exchange, or a decrease in the magnetization transfer ratio (MTR), whereas an elevated proton exchange, or increased MTR, is evidence of possible remyelination or resolution of edema. MTI is probably the best adapted technique to measure the extent of remyelination in patients with MS [52–54]. A voxel-by-voxel comparison of MTR changes in serial MRI scans allows demyelination and remyelination to be captured on a dynamic basis (Figure 6.8) [55–58]. Different lesions can thus be characterized as predominantly demyelinating or remyelinating and, even within the same lesion, heterogeneity in myelination status over time can be observed. A histopathologic-MRI correlation study analyzed the evolution of MTR in individual voxels of an acute, Gd-enhancing lesion that was available for a pathology examination [57]. Over 6.5 months following enhancement, MTR was low and stable in the lesion center and MTR increased at the lesion border with NA white matter (NAWM). Histopathologic analysis confirmed a demyelinated lesion center with diffuse presence of macrophages/microglia and marked loss of oligodendrocytes and a partially remyelinated lesion border with diffuse presence of macrophages/microglia and relatively more oligodendrocytes compared with the lesion center. These findings support the validity and sensitivity of voxel-wise-based MTR image processing for monitoring demyelination and remyelination in vivo.

We recently introduced a threshold-free cluster enhancement (TFCE) technique in combination with a Monte Carlo estimation approach. TFCE is first applied to enhance individual voxels based on their level of local cluster support, and then Monte Carlo estimation is performed to allow meaningful statistical interpretation of the resulting TFCE values [58]. We validated this technique in three complementary ways: healthy control scan–rescan analysis, analysis of a "gold standard" simulated dataset, and analysis of a group of MS patients and healthy volunteers with 1-year longitudinal MRI scans. Scan–rescan analysis demonstrated a very low false-positive rate (1.44 mL increasing and 1.48 mL decreasing at the optimal detection threshold). Simulated dataset analysis yielded an area under receiver-operating characteristic curve of 0.942 (compared with 0.801 for a more conventional voxel-wise thresholding analysis). Finally, analysis of the real subject population showed highly significant differences ($p < 0.001$) in volume of decreasing MTR between patients and controls. The proposed method provides a valuable means for quantifying MS-related tissue changes, particularly demyelination and remyelination, in vivo and without the use of highly complex or experimental MRI acquisition techniques. It improves on the sensitivity of other approaches and may increase the statistical power of studies investigating the effects of therapy on MRI outcomes in MS.

Magnetic Resonance Spectroscopy

A magnetic resonance spectroscopy (MRS) signal does not derive from protons in water, but from protons in organic molecules contained in living tissue. This distinguishes MRS from the other MRI techniques discussed above. The most relevant metabolites of the brain are creatine (Cr), N-acetylaspartate (NAA), choline, glutamate, or myo-inositol (Figure 6.9). Increases in lactate, choline, and lipids reflect evidence of inflammation and demyelination. Cr is present in both neurons and glial cells, and Cr changes can be indicative of neuroaxonal injury (which is likely associated with decreases in both NAA and Cr signals), oligodendroglial disturbance (which is likely associated with decreases in Cr signals), and astrocytic proliferation (which is likely associated with increases in Cr signals). Of particular interest in MS is measuring the signal from NAA, since this metabolite is specifically localized in the neuronal compartment [59]. Decreases in the relative size of the NAA signal can thus be used to measure neuronal loss. Decrease in the NAA/Cr ratio was strongly correlated with disability, both in cross-sectional and longitudinal studies [60].

Diffusion-Weighted and Tensor Imaging

Diffusion imaging, which includes diffusion-weighted imaging (DWI) and diffusion tensor imaging (DTI), measures random translational motion of molecules in a fluid system to ascertain information about the orientation, size, and geometry of tissue damage occurring in NABT [61]. Because processes

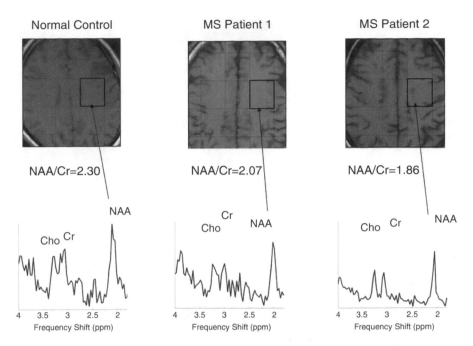

Figure 6.9 Magnetic resonance spectroscopy imaging in normal control (*left*), and MS patients (*middle and right images*). LC model was used to estimate the value of the spectra. The *N*-acetyl-aspartate to creatine ratio (NAA/Cr) is the highest in the normal appearing white matter (NAWM) of normal control (*left*), lower in the NAWM of the MS patients (*middle*), and the lowest in T1 hypointense lesion of the MS patient (*right*)

of demyelination and remyelination alter brain tissue geometry and increase water diffusivity, an increasing number of clinical studies have assessed characteristics of neurologic damage in MS patients with DWI and DTI [62, 63]. Results from these studies confirm that DWI is a highly sensitive marker of subtle damage occurring within the NAWM and has the ability to detect short-term changes in the NAGM, which may accurately predict cumulative physical disability in patients with MS [61]. Alternatively, DTI provides quantitative information regarding structural characteristics of neuronal tissue, and studies of DTI measures have reported the detection of neuronal tissue damage in T1-WI and T2-WI lesions, in the tissue adjacent to these lesions, and in the remote NAWM and NAGM [63]. Overall, the specific information provided by both DWI and DTI measures with regard to tissue abnormalities of the NAWM could provide a more accurate evaluation of disease-modifying treatments for patients with MS.

Functional MRI

Functional MRI is an emerging technique that assesses changes in brain activation occurring as the result of altered deoxygenated hemoglobin concentrations, providing noninvasive spatial localization of brain function [16]. Functional imaging studies have evaluated the relationship between cortical adaptive changes and clinical symptoms in patients with MS, based on the rationale that substantial alterations in neuronal tissue (e.g., axonal injury

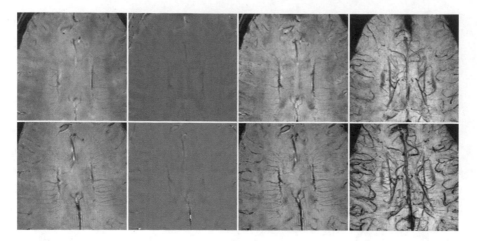

Figure 6.10 Susceptibility-weighted imaging (SWI) in a 45-year-old SPMS patient. The *upper row* represents images with single-dose of gadolinium (0.1 mmol/kg), whereas the *lower row* shows the SWI images with triple dose of gadolinium (0.3 mmol/kg). From the left to the right are represented: magnitude image, high pass filtered phase image, SWI image, and minimum intensity projection (minIP). The SWI images are showing focal areas of hypointensity representing iron deposition (please note advantages of single vs. triple dose in visualization of these hypointensities). The minIP images are used to reconstruct the vein architecture in the brain (please note advantages of single vs. triple dose in visualization of the veins)

and neurodegeneration) occur in the earliest stages of MS pathology [64, 65]. One small clinical study ($n = 21$) identified the activation of the medial prefrontal cortex as a mechanism of cortical plasticity in MS patients with functional impairment [65]. Additionally, the progressive decrease in functional MRI cortical activation in combination with movement recovery demonstrated that cortical reorganization of the motor cortex appears to accompany remission of MS symptoms. Controlled, clinical trials demonstrating the utility of functional imaging in MS are limited, and longitudinal clinical studies designed to evaluate the effects of disease-modifying treatments on cortical plasticity are needed to better understand the role of functional brain changes in symptom progression and remission in patients with MS.

Susceptibility-Weighted Imaging

Susceptibility-weighted imaging (SWI) is a new neuroimaging technique, which uses tissue magnetic susceptibility differences to generate a unique contrast, different from that of spin density, T1, T2, and T2* [66, 67]. SWI consists of using both magnitude and phase images from a high-resolution, three-dimensional fully velocity-compensated gradient echo sequence (Figure 6.10). Phase mask is created from the MR phase images, and multiplying these with the magnitude images increase the conspicuousness of the smaller veins and other sources of susceptibility effects, which is depicted using minimal intensity projection (minIP) (Figure 6.10). The phase images are useful in differentiating between diamagnetic and paramagnetic susceptibility effects of calcium and blood, respectively. This unique MR sequence will help in detecting occult low flow vascular lesions, calcification and cerebral microbleed in various pathologic conditions and aids in characterizing tumors and degenerative diseases of the brain. This sequence can also be used for prominent display of normal brain structures. Using phase as an iron marker may be useful for studying absorption of iron in diseases such as Parkinson's, Huntington's, neurodegeneration with brain iron accumulation, Alzheimer's, and MS and other iron-related diseases.

The use of SWI in MS has gained increasing attention in the last couple of years. Although, the use of SWI in MS is in its infancy, the detection of vein abnormalities, and areas of iron deposition in the brain are two main topics of interest. Ge et al. [68] demonstrated markedly enhanced detection of unique microvascular involvement associated with most of the visualized MS lesions with abnormal signals on and around the venous wall on 7-T compared with 3-T MRI. These findings, which have never been seen on conventional fields of MRI, allowed for direct evidence of vascular pathogenesis in MS in vivo and have important implications for monitoring lesion activity and therapeutic response. Hammond et al. [69] studied seven patients with MS and observed small phase-shifted plaques in the region of the deep medullary veins; this observation supports the contention that the disease progresses along the vasculature. They found that a subset of MS plaques showed contrast uptake only at the peripheral margin of the lesion in the phase images. More recently, Haacke et al. [70] completed a study of 27 patients with MS by using SWI-filtered phase images. They found that there is a negative correlation of iron with T2 hyperintensity. The higher the iron content, the less visible the lesions seem to be in T2-weighted images.

This may suggest that significant damage to the tissue occurs following chronic inflammation, such that the tissue no longer shows signs of inflammation. They also noted that there were marked hypointense rings around some lesions, lesions with uniform iron content, and regions with central iron but no rings. On occasion, lesions were also seen in the GM as well. Overall, in that particular study, using SWI permitted a more accurate measurement of the extent of MS and increased the number of lesions detected by 50% [71].

Conclusion

The various MRI techniques that have been developed over the last two decades differ in their utility for predicting clinical status in MS. In this respect, Gd-enhancing T1- and T2 lesions have only limited value due to their poor sensitivity and specificity for the underlying pathophysiological process. Use of high field imaging protocols, advanced conventional sequences and fully automated non-conventional techniques may increase sensitivity in detecting lesions and help identify pathology invisible on 1.5 and 3T protocols [72]. Characterizing the pathology visualized with these new protocols is an important goal of current MRI research. Evaluation of T1 black holes, atrophy measures, MRS, MTI, SWI, and diffusivity outcomes is more useful in predicting neurologic impairment. These different MRI techniques can be used to evaluate the effects of disease-modifying therapy.

References

1. Kappos L, Moeri D, Radue EW, Schoetzau A, Schweikert K, Barkhof F, et al. Predictive value of gadolinium-enhanced magnetic resonance imaging for relapse rate and changes in disability or impairment in multiple sclerosis: a meta-analysis. Gadolinium MRI Meta-analysis Group. Lancet. 1999;353(9157):964–9.

2. Zivadinov R, Leist TP. Clinical-magnetic resonance imaging correlations in multiple sclerosis. J Neuroimaging. 2005;15(4 Suppl):10S–21.
3. Zivadinov R. Can imaging techniques measure neuroprotection and remyelination in multiple sclerosis? Neurology. 2007;68(3):S72–82.
4. Zivadinov R, Hussein S, Stosic M, Durfee J, Cox JL, Cookfair DL, et al. Glatiramer acetate recovers microscopic tissue damage in patients with multiple sclerosis. A case-control diffusion imaging study. Pathophysiology. 2011;18:61–8.
5. Barkhof F, Bruck W, De Groot CJ, Bergers E, Hulshof S, Geurts J, et al. Remyelinated lesions in multiple sclerosis: magnetic resonance image appearance. Arch Neurol. 2003;60(8):1073–81.
6. Patrikios P, Stadelmann C, Kutzelnigg A, Rauschka H, Schmidbauer M, Laursen H, et al. Remyelination is extensive in a subset of multiple sclerosis patients. Brain. 2006;129(Pt 12):3165–72.
7. Cotton F, Weiner HL, Jolesz FA, Guttmann CR. MRI contrast uptake in new lesions in relapsing-remitting MS followed at weekly intervals. Neurology. 2003;60(4):640–6.
8. Rovira A, Alonso J, Cucurella G, Nos C, Tintore M, Pedraza S, et al. Evolution of multiple sclerosis lesions on serial contrast-enhanced T1-weighted and magnetization-transfer MR images. AJNR Am J Neuroradiol. 1999;20(10):1939–45.
9. van Waesberghe JH, van Walderveen MA, Castelijns JA, Scheltens P, Lycklama a Nijeholt GJ, Polman CH, et al. Patterns of lesion development in multiple sclerosis: longitudinal observations with T1-weighted spin-echo and magnetization transfer MR. AJNR Am J Neuroradiol. 1998;19(4):675–83.
10. Guttmann CR, Ahn SS, Hsu L, Kikinis R, Jolesz FA. The evolution of multiple sclerosis lesions on serial MR. AJNR Am J Neuroradiol. 1995;16(7):1481–91.
11. Bagnato F, Jeffries N, Richert ND, Stone RD, Ohayon JM, McFarland HF, et al. Evolution of T1 black holes in patients with multiple sclerosis imaged monthly for 4 years. Brain. 2003;126(Pt 8):1782–9.
12. Dalton CM, Miszkiel KA, Barker GJ, MacManus DG, Pepple TI, Panzara M, et al. Effect of natalizumab on conversion of gadolinium enhancing lesions to T1 hypointense lesions in relapsing multiple sclerosis. J Neurol. 2004;251(4):407–13.
13. Filippi M, Rovaris M, Rocca MA, Sormani MP, Wolinsky JS, Comi G. Glatiramer acetate reduces the proportion of new MS lesions evolving into "black holes". Neurology. 2001;57(4):731–3.
14. Bagnato F, Gupta S, Richert ND, Stone RD, Ohayon JM, Frank JA, et al. Effects of interferon beta-1b on black holes in multiple sclerosis over a 6-year period with monthly evaluations. Arch Neurol. 2005;62(11):1684–8.
15. Dwyer MG, Abdelrahman N, Weinstock-Guttman B, Srinivasaraghavan B, Prakash R, Hussein S, et al. Quantitative analysis of lesion load progression in advanced multiple sclerosis. Mult Scler. 2005;11 Suppl 1:68. S14.
16. Rocca MA, Filippi M. Functional MRI in multiple sclerosis. J Neuroimaging. 2007;17 Suppl 1:36S–41.
17. Zivadinov R, Fritz D, Hani N, Nussenbaum F, Weinstock-Guttman B, Durfee J, Abdelrahman N, Hussein N, De Brujin M, Cox JL, Dwyer MG. Voxel-wise dynamic classification of new, stable, resolving and atrophied T2 hyperintense lesion volumes in patients with multiple sclerosis. A 2-year longitudinal study. Mult Scler. 2007;13(Suppl 2):P605:S182.
18. Moraal B, Meier DS, Poppe PA, Geurts JJ, Vrenken H, Jonker WM, et al. Subtraction MR images in a multiple sclerosis multicenter clinical trial setting. Radiology. 2009;250(2):506–14.
19. Geurts JJ, Pouwels PJ, Uitdehaag BM, Polman CH, Barkhof F, Castelijns JA. Intracortical lesions in multiple sclerosis: improved detection with 3D double inversion-recovery MR imaging. Radiology. 2005;236(1):254–60.

20. Bink A, Schmitt M, Gaa J, Mugler 3rd JP, Lanfermann H, Zanella FE. Detection of lesions in multiple sclerosis by 2D FLAIR and single-slab 3D FLAIR sequences at 3.0 T: initial results. Eur Radiol. 2006;16(5):1104–10.
21. Wattjes MP, Lutterbey GG, Gieseke J, Traber F, Klotz L, Schmidt S, et al. Double inversion recovery brain imaging at 3T: diagnostic value in the detection of multiple sclerosis lesions. AJNR Am J Neuroradiol. 2007;28(1):54–9.
22. Moraal B, Roosendaal SD, Pouwels PJ, Vrenken H, van Schijndel RA, Meier DS, et al. Multi-contrast, isotropic, single-slab 3D MR imaging in multiple sclerosis. Eur Radiol. 2008;18(10):2311–20.
23. Calabrese M, Filippi M, Rovaris M, Mattisi I, Bernardi V, Atzori M, et al. Morphology and evolution of cortical lesions in multiple sclerosis. A longitudinal MRI study. Neuroimage. 2008;42(4):1324–8.
24. Dousset V, Brochet B, Deloire MS, Lagoarde L, Barroso B, Caille JM, et al. MR imaging of relapsing multiple sclerosis patients using ultra-small-particle iron oxide and compared with gadolinium. AJNR Am J Neuroradiol. 2006;27(5):1000–5.
25. Vellinga MM, Oude Engberink RD, Seewann A, Pouwels PJ, Wattjes MP, van der Pol SM, et al. Pluriformity of inflammation in multiple sclerosis shown by ultra-small iron oxide particle enhancement. Brain. 2008;131(Pt 3):800–7.
26. Erskine MK, Cook LL, Riddle KE, Mitchell JR, Karlik SJ. Resolution-dependent estimates of multiple sclerosis lesion loads. Can J Neurol Sci. 2005;32(2):205–12.
27. Sicotte NL, Voskuhl RR, Bouvier S, Klutch R, Cohen MS, Mazziotta JC. Comparison of multiple sclerosis lesions at 1.5 and 3.0 Tesla. Invest Radiol. 2003;38(7):423–7.
28. DiPerri C, Dwyer M, Wack D, Cox JL, Hashmi K, Saluste E, et al. Lesion characteristics at 1.5 and 3 Tesla in multiple sclerosis patients and healthy controls: a morphological and topological quantitative comparison study. Mult Scler. 2008;14(Supp 1):S102.
29. Wattjes MP, Harzheim M, Kuhl CK, Gieseke J, Schmidt S, Klotz L, et al. Does high-field MR imaging have an influence on the classification of patients with clinically isolated syndromes according to current diagnostic mr imaging criteria for multiple sclerosis? AJNR Am J Neuroradiol. 2006;27(8):1794–8.
30. Wattjes MP, Harzheim M, Lutterbey GG, Hojati F, Simon B, Schmidt S, et al. Does high field MRI allow an earlier diagnosis of multiple sclerosis? J Neurol. 2008;255(8):1159–63.
31. Kutzelnigg A, Lucchinetti CF, Stadelmann C, Bruck W, Rauschka H, Bergmann M, et al. Cortical demyclination and diffuse white matter injury in multiple sclerosis. Brain. 2005;128(Pt 11):2705–12.
32. Magliozzi R, Howell O, Vora A, Serafini B, Nicholas R, Puopolo M, et al. Meningeal B-cell follicles in secondary progressive multiple sclerosis associate with early onset of disease and severe cortical pathology. Brain. 2007;130(Pt 4):1089–104.
33. Kangarlu A, Bourekas EC, Ray-Chaudhury A, Rammohan KW. Cerebral cortical lesions in multiple sclerosis detected by MR imaging at 8 Tesla. AJNR Am J Neuroradiol. 2007;28(2):262–6.
34. Bo L, Geurts JJ, van der Valk P, Polman C, Barkhof F. Lack of correlation between cortical demyelination and white matter pathologic changes in multiple sclerosis. Arch Neurol. 2007;64(1):76–80.
35. Zivadinov R, Bakshi R. Role of MRI in multiple sclerosis II: brain and spinal cord atrophy. Front Biosci. 2004;9:647–64.
36. Zivadinov R, Reder A, Filippi M, Minagar A, Stüve O, Lassmann H, et al. Mechanisms of action of disease-modifying agents and brain volume changes in multiple sclerosis. Neurology. 2008;71:136–44.
37. Zivadinov R, Bakshi R. Central nervous system atrophy and clinical status in multiple sclerosis. J Neuroimaging. 2004;14(3 Suppl):S27–35.

38. Anderson VM, Fox NC, Miller DH. Magnetic resonance imaging measures of brain atrophy in multiple sclerosis. J Magn Reson Imaging. 2006;23(5):605–18.
39. Evangelou N, DeLuca GC, Owens T, Esiri MM. Pathological study of spinal cord atrophy in multiple sclerosis suggests limited role of local lesions. Brain. 2005;128(Pt 1):29–34.
40. Dalton CM, Brex PA, Jenkins R, Fox NC, Miszkiel KA, Crum WR, et al. Progressive ventricular enlargement in patients with clinically isolated syndromes is associated with the early development of multiple sclerosis. J Neurol Neurosurg Psychiatry. 2002;73(2):141–7.
41. Dalton CM, Chard DT, Davies GR, Miszkiel KA, Altmann DR, Fernando K, et al. Early development of multiple sclerosis is associated with progressive grey matter atrophy in patients presenting with clinically isolated syndromes. Brain. 2004;127(Pt 5):1101–7.
42. Pagani E, Rocca MA, Gallo A, Rovaris M, Martinelli V, Comi G, et al. Regional brain atrophy evolves differently in patients with multiple sclerosis according to clinical phenotype. AJNR Am J Neuroradiol. 2005;26(2):341–6.
43. Carone DA, Benedict RH, Dwyer MG, Cookfair DL, Srinivasaraghavan B, Tjoa CW, et al. Semi-automatic brain region extraction (SABRE) reveals superior cortical and deep gray matter atrophy in MS. Neuroimage. 2006;29(2):505–14.
44. Chen JT, Narayanan S, Collins DL, Smith SM, Matthews PM, Arnold DL. Relating neocortical pathology to disability progression in multiple sclerosis using MRI. Neuroimage. 2004;23(3):1168–75.
45. Cifelli A, Arridge M, Jezzard P, Esiri MM, Palace J, Matthews PM. Thalamic neurodegeneration in multiple sclerosis. Ann Neurol. 2002;52(5):650–3.
46. Houtchens MK, Benedict RH, Killiany R, Sharma J, Jaisani Z, Singh B, et al. Thalamic atrophy and cognition in multiple sclerosis. Neurology. 2007;69(12):1213–23.
47. Horakova D, Cox JL, Havrdova E, Hussein S, Dolezal O, Cookfair D, et al. Evolution of different MRI measures in patients with active relapsing-remitting multiple sclerosis over 2 and 5 years: a case-control study. J Neurol Neurosurg Psychiatry. 2008;79(4):407–14.
48. Chard DT, Griffin CM, Parker GJ, Kapoor R, Thompson AJ, Miller DH. Brain atrophy in clinically early relapsing-remitting multiple sclerosis. Brain. 2002;125(Pt 2): 327–37.
49. Sanfilipo MP, Benedict RH, Sharma J, Weinstock-Guttman B, Bakshi R. The relationship between whole brain volume and disability in multiple sclerosis: a comparison of normalized gray vs. white matter with misclassification correction. Neuroimage. 2005;26(4):1068–77.
50. Fisher E, Lee JC, Nakamura K, Rudick RA. Gray matter atrophy in multiple sclerosis: a longitudinal study. Ann Neurol. 2008;64(3):255–65.
51. Fisniku LK, Chard DT, Jackson JS, Anderson VM, Altmann DR, Miszkiel KA, et al. Gray matter atrophy is related to long-term disability in multiple sclerosis. Ann Neurol. 2008;64(3):247–54.
52. Deloire-Grassin MS, Brochet B, Quesson B, Delalande C, Dousset V, Canioni P, et al. In vivo evaluation of remyelination in rat brain by magnetization transfer imaging. J Neurol Sci. 2000;178(1):10–6.
53. Rademacher J, Engelbrecht V, Burgel U, Freund H, Zilles K. Measuring in vivo myelination of human white matter fiber tracts with magnetization transfer MR. Neuroimage. 1999;9(4):393–406.
54. Schmierer K, Scaravilli F, Altmann DR, Barker GJ, Miller DH. Magnetization transfer ratio and myelin in postmortem multiple sclerosis brain. Ann Neurol. 2004;56(3):407–15.
55. Chen JT, Collins DL, Freedman MS, Atkins HL, Arnold DL. Local magnetization transfer ratio signal inhomogeneity is related to subsequent change in MTR in lesions and normal-appearing white-matter of multiple sclerosis patients. Neuroimage. 2005;25(4):1272–8.

56. Chen JT, Collins DL, Atkins HL, Freedman MS, Arnold DL. Magnetization transfer ratio evolution with demyelination and remyelination in multiple sclerosis lesions. Ann Neurol. 2008;63(2):254–62.

57. Chen JT, Kuhlmann T, Jansen GH, Collins DL, Atkins HL, Freedman MS, et al. Voxel-based analysis of the evolution of magnetization transfer ratio to quantify remyelination and demyelination with histopathological validation in a multiple sclerosis lesion. Neuroimage. 2007;36(4):1152–8.

58. Dwyer M, Bergsland N, Hussein S, Durfee J, Wack D, Zivadinov R. A sensitive, noise-resistant method for identifying focal demyelination and remyelination in patients with multiple sclerosis via voxel-wise changes in magnetization transfer ratio. J Neurol Sci. 2009;282(1–2):86–95.

59. Narayana PA. Magnetic resonance spectroscopy in the monitoring of multiple sclerosis. J Neuroimaging. 2005;15(4 Suppl):46S–57.

60. Inglese M, Grossman RI, Filippi M. Magnetic resonance imaging monitoring of multiple sclerosis lesion evolution. J Neuroimaging. 2005;15(4 Suppl):22S–9.

61. Rovaris M, Gass A, Bammer R, Hickman SJ, Ciccarelli O, Miller DH, et al. Diffusion MRI in multiple sclerosis. Neurology. 2005;65(10):1526–32.

62. Cercignani M, Inglese M, Pagani E, Comi G, Filippi M. Mean diffusivity and fractional anisotropy histograms of patients with multiple sclerosis. AJNR Am J Neuroradiol. 2001;22(5):952–8.

63. Goldberg-Zimring D, Mewes AU, Maddah M, Warfield SK. Diffusion tensor magnetic resonance imaging in multiple sclerosis. J Neuroimaging. 2005;15 (4 Suppl):68S–81.

64. Reddy H, Narayanan S, Arnoutelis R, Jenkinson M, Antel J, Matthews PM, et al. Evidence for adaptive functional changes in the cerebral cortex with axonal injury from multiple sclerosis. Brain. 2000;123(Pt 11):2314–20.

65. Parry AM, Scott RB, Palace J, Smith S, Matthews PM. Potentially adaptive functional changes in cognitive processing for patients with multiple sclerosis and their acute modulation by rivastigmine. Brain. 2003;126(Pt 12):2750–60.

66. Haacke EM, Mittal S, Wu Z, Neelavalli J, Cheng YC. Susceptibility-weighted imaging: technical aspects and clinical applications, part 1. AJNR Am J Neuroradiol. 2009;30:19–30.

67. Thomas B, Somasundaram S, Thamburaj K, Kesavadas C, Gupta AK, Bodhey NK, et al. Clinical applications of susceptibility weighted MR imaging of the brain – a pictorial review. Neuroradiology. 2008;50(2):105–16.

68. Ge Y, Zohrabian VM, Grossman RI. Seven-Tesla magnetic resonance imaging: new vision of microvascular abnormalities in multiple sclerosis. Arch Neurol. 2008;65(6):812–6.

69. Hammond KE, Lupo JM, Xu D, Metcalf M, Kelley DA, Pelletier D, et al. Development of a robust method for generating 7.0 T multichannel phase images of the brain with application to normal volunteers and patients with neurological diseases. Neuroimage. 2008;39(4):1682–92.

70. Haacke E, Makki M, Ge Y, et al. Characterizing iron deposition in multiple sclerosis lesions using susceptibility weighted imaging. J Magn Reson Imaging. 2009;29(3):537–44.

71. Mittal S, Wu Z, Neelavalli J, Haacke EM. Susceptibility-weighted imaging: technical aspects and clinical applications, part 2. AJNR Am J Neuroradiol. 2009;30(2):232–52.

72. Zivadinov R, Stosic M, Cox J, Ramasamy D, Dwyer M. The place of conventional MRI and newly emerging MRI techniques in monitoring different aspects of treatment outcome. J Neurol. 2008;255 Suppl 1:61–74.

Disease Modifying Agents in the Treatment of Multiple Sclerosis

Syed A. Rizvi

Keywords: Clinically isolated syndrome, Relapse, Neurodegeneration, Side effects, Stem cells, Plasmapheresis

Introduction

Numerous agents have been tested in multiple sclerosis and the vast majority of these have either failed to show a beneficial effect or produced undesirable side effects. In some cases, there was worsening of disease activity. Treatment strategies for multiple sclerosis over the last 16 years have undergone a profound change. Several treatment options are now available primarily targeting the inflammatory phase of the disease [clinically isolated syndrome (CIS), relapsing remitting multiple sclerosis (RRMS), and secondary progressive multiple sclerosis (SPMS) with relapses]. All currently approved disease-modifying agents (DMA) are moderately effective in reducing relapses and MRI activity. The treatment effect appears to be greater when these drugs are used soon after onset of symptoms. The effect on long-term disability seems to be modest if any. This chapter reviews both currently used agents (both FDA approved and off-label) and also discusses several promising agents in various phases of development.

Currently Approved Agents

Interferons

Interferons (IFN) act through cell receptors producing a variety of immunological and antiviral effects. Although the exact mechanism of action in multiple sclerosis is unknown, an anti-inflammatory effect may be the result of inhibition of interferon gamma, inhibition of T-cell activation, production of anti-inflammatory cytokines, reduced T-cell migration, decrease blood brain barrier permeability, or possibly other unknown mechanisms [1–3].

From: *Clinical Neuroimmunology: Multiple Sclerosis and Related Disorders*, Current Clinical Neurology,
Edited by: S.A. Rizvi and P.K. Coyle, DOI 10.1007/978-1-60327-860-7_7,
© Springer Science+Business Media, LLC 2011

IFN β-1b subcutaneous (S/Q) every other day (Betaseron/Betaferon) was the first disease modifying agent approved for the treatment of RRMS. In the pivotal trial of IFN β-1b involving 372 RRMS patients, two different doses were compared with placebo [4]. Both doses were found to be significantly better than placebo with about one-third greater reduction in relapse rate (8 MIU vs. placebo $p=0.0001$, 1.6 MIU vs. placebo $p=0.0101$, and 8 MIU vs. 1.6 MIU $p=0.0086$). IFN β-1b had a profound beneficial effect on MRI parameters [5, 6].

The pivotal trial for *IFN β-1a intramuscular (I/M)* once weekly (Avonex) involved 301 RRMS patients and also showed a relapse rate reduction of about one-third and a positive effect on MRI parameters [7–9]. Additionally, there was a significant beneficial effect on time to sustained disability, which was the primary endpoint. Further analysis of the study also revealed a beneficial effect on the rate of brain atrophy in the second year of treatment [10].

The definitive trial for *IFN β-1a subcutaneous (S/C)* three times weekly (Rebif) compared two different doses (6 MIU and 12 MIU) with placebo in 560 RRMS patients. In the 2-year controlled phase, both doses had a significant effect on relapse rate reduction (about one-third) (6 MIU = 1.82, 12 MIU = 1.73, and placebo = 2.56), disability measures, and MRI parameters [11, 12]. After 2 years, the placebo group was re-randomized to receive either the low-dose or the high-dose IFN β-1a. After 4 years, a dose response relationship was observed for some measures but not others [13]. The higher dose group continued to do better for up to 8 years when compared with the original placebo group [14].

Interferons are generally well tolerated and have a proven long-term safety record. Side effects are more frequent with the high-dose, high-frequency formulations and may include injection site reactions, flu-like symptoms, elevated liver enzymes, lymphopenia, and depression [15]. The efficacy of interferons can be compromised by the development of neutralizing antibodies, which are more common with the high-frequency formulations [16]. The exact relationship of development of neutralizing antibodies to the loss of efficacy is unclear.

Glatiramer Acetate

Glatiramer acetate (GA) is a synthetic molecule compound consisting of four amino acids (L-alanine, L-glutamic acid, L-tyrosine, and L-lysine). Although the precise mechanism of action of GA is unknown, there is some evidence that GA might compete with myelin basic protein for antigen binding that can result in phenotypic shift of Th1 cells to Th2 cells. These cells then cross the blood brain barrier and release anti-inflammatory cytokines and possibly neuroprotective factors [1, 17].

The pivotal trial of GA involving 251 RRMS patients showed a significant effect on relapse reduction (about one-third) compared with placebo [18, 19]. MRI parameters were not assessed in the pivotal study, but a follow-up imaging study demonstrated a significant reduction in MRI lesions when compared with placebo [20]. The MRI effects of GA are less pronounced compared with interferons and this may be secondary to its lack of direct effect on the blood brain barrier. GA appears to have an excellent long-term safety profile and continues to be effective in a subgroup of patients who have continued on GA for more than a decade [21].

Natalizumab

Natalizumab (Tysabri) is the first humanized monoclonal antibody to be approved for the treatment of worsening RRMS and is generally recommended for patients who are unable to tolerate or have had inadequate response to the first-line disease modifying agents [22]. Natalizumab has been shown to be effective both in the early relapsing remitting population and patients worsening on first-line therapy [23].

Natalizumab binds to alpha 4-antegrin thus inhibiting adhesion of leukocytes to vascular cell adhesion molecule (VCAM) receptor, preventing leukocyte migration into the CNS and subsequent inflammatory events [24]. Treatment with natalizumab results in a significant reduction of CD4/CD8 cells in the CNS and reversal of CD4/CD8 ratio similar to what is seen in AIDS patients. This can persist up to 6 months after discontinuation of natalizumab [25].

The efficacy of natalizumab has been evaluated in two large double-blinded placebo controlled randomized studies: the AFFIRM (Natalizumab Safety And Efficacy In Relapsing Remitting Multiple Sclerosis) and SENTINEL (Safety and Efficacy of Natalizumab in Combination with IFN β (beta)-1a in patients with Relapsing Remitting Multiple Sclerosis) [26, 27]. The primary end point in both these studies was the rate of relapse at 1 year and cumulative probability of disability progression sustained for 12 weeks at 2 years. In the AFFIRM trial, 942 patients (natalizumab = 627 and placebo = 315) were enrolled and natalizumab monotherapy reduced the risk of disability progression sustained for 12 and 24 weeks over 2 years by 42% and 54%, respectively, compared with placebo. Natalizumab reduced the analyzed relapse rate by 68% compared with placebo at 1 year and the reduction was maintained for greater than 2 years. In the SENTINEL study, natalizumab in combination with IFN β-1a reduced the risk of disability progression sustained for 12 weeks over 2 years by 24% compared with IFN β-1a alone. No significant difference was noted at 24 weeks. There was a 54% relative reduction in analyzed relapse rate at 1 year and 55% at 2 years when natalizumab was added to patients on IFN β-1a. In both studies, natalizumab had a profound effect on MRI measures but was unable to show a beneficial effect on rate of brain atrophy at 2 years, although a positive effect was noted in both trials in the second year of treatment [28]. Natalizumab was found to be even more effective in a subgroup of patients with highly active disease, both in the AFFIRM and in the SENTINAL trials [29]. In about 6% of patients persistent neutralizing antibodies developed resulting in loss of efficacy [30].

Natalizumab was found ineffective in the treatment of acute relapses [31]. When tested in combination with glatiramer acetate, it was found to be safe and well tolerated during 6 months of therapy and interestingly the incidence of persistent anti-natalizumab antibodies was higher (13%) [32]. In a small study in children, natalizumab was noted to be well tolerated and resulted in strong suppression of disease activity [33].

There has been a concern about rebound phenomenon after discontinuation of natalizumab. In a recent study of patients who discontinued natalizumab after being enrolled in the phase III trials, there was no evidence of clinical, radiographic or immunologic rebound phenomenon [25]. Several other studies have documented an increase in disease activity after discontinuation of natalizumab treatment, especially in patients who were resistant to other treatments prior to starting therapy with natalizumab [34–36].

Unfortunately, natalizumab was withdrawn from the market soon after its approval in November 2004 when two patients in the SENTINAL trial (both on combination treatment) developed progressive multifocal leukoencephalopathy (PML) [37, 38]. Another patient in a Crohn's disease trial was also found to have PML [39].

Natalizumab and PML

After an extensive analysis of the two pivotal study populations, no further cases of PML were discovered and the drug was subsequently reintroduced with a risk management plan Tysabri Outreach: Unified Commitment to Health (TOUCH) in June 2006 [40]. Currently >90,000 patients have been exposed to natalizumab and about 120 cases of PML have been documented with almost a 20% mortality rate. The risk of developing PML seems to be very low within the first 12 months of treatment (no cases of PML in MS patients with <12 months of treatment) and the risk seems to be higher with increasing duration of exposure. Patients exposed to prior immunosuppressive agents may be at increased risk as well.

Natalizumab may cause PML by reactivation of latent JC virus found in greater than 80% of individuals [41]. Although the exact mechanism is unknown, evidence points to impairment of immune surveillance. PML is usually seen in immunocompromised individuals such as patients infected with HIV and patients treated with aggressive immunosuppressive agents as well as other monoclonal antibodies including rituximab [42–44]. Although PML, in general, carries a grave prognosis, most of the data comes from the HIV literature. Early recognition, discontinuation of natalizumab and treatment with plasmapheresis, resulting in accelerated removal of natalizumab from the circulation may lead to a better outcome [45]. Other possible side effects include infusion and hypersensitivity reactions, liver failure, infections, and risk of secondary malignancy.

A newly developed assay to detect JC virus specific antibodies in MS patients is being tested in two separate studies to evaluate its potential utility for identifying patients at a higher risk for developing PML. In a preliminary trial, the overall seropositivity in the MS population was 53.6%, but more interestingly all 17 samples from patients who were eventually diagnosed with PML were positive for anti-JC virus antibodies [46]. If confirmed, the identification of patients with a significantly reduced risk of PML may result in a much more widespread use of natalizumab.

Fingolimod

Fingolimod (Gilenya) is the latest immunomodulating agent to be approved for the treatment of relapsing forms of MS. It is also the first oral disease modifying therapy for the treatment of MS. Fingolimod is a sphingosine-1-phosphate receptor modulator. It binds to four out of five S1P receptors on lymphocytes resulting in receptor internalization [47]. These receptors deliver a recognition signal for lymphocytes to egress the thymus and secondary lymphoid tissue. Lymphocytes including Th17 central memory T-cells are retained in the lymphoid tissue and prevented from reaching sites of inflammation [48]. Fingolimod can enter the CNS and may have a beneficial effect on glial cells [49]. A small study described strong expression of S1P receptor 1 and 3 in reactive astrocytes in active and chronic inactive MS lesions [50].

A 6-month phase II study showed that once daily oral treatment with fingolimod (1.25 or 5 mg) had a significant benefit on inflammatory measures of disease activity (MRI and relapse rate) and the effect seems to persist for at least 24 months [51]. In the TRANSFORMS study, patients treated with FTY720 had a 52% greater reduction of RR compared with IFNB-1a (I/M) [52]. Side effects of FTY720 include two deaths from disseminated herpes, several skin malignancies, macular edema, initial dose bradycardia, decrease in FEV, elevated liver enzymes, and a single case each of posterior reversible encephalopathy syndrome (PRES) and focal encephalitis [53]. In the recently reported FREEDOMS trial which involved >1,200 patients. FTY720 reduced the relapse rate by 54% in the 0.5 mg group and 60% in the 1.25 mg group compared with placebo ($p \leq 0.001$) [54]. There were positive effects on MRI, including reduction in rate of brain atrophy and a 30% reduction in disability progression. There were no unexpected adverse events and patients on the lower dose had very few side effects.

There remains a concern regarding potentially serious side effects including reactivation of latent infections, malignancies, macular edema, cardiopulmonary side effects, and delayed reconstitution of circulating lymphocyte counts after treatment with fingolimod [55]. The use of this drug may be limited at least initially, to patients with aggressive disease who fail to respond to other immunomodulating agents or are unable to tolerate injections. Other ongoing phase III trials in PPMS and RRMS may help clarify the risks and benefits associated with this novel disease modifying agents.

Mitoxantrone

Mitoxantrone binds to DNA and inhibits topoisomerase II. It has an effect on B- and T-cell function and decreases the secretion of TH1 cytokines [56, 57]. After several small trials with encouraging results, a phase III trial using two different doses (12 and 5 mg/m^2) was completed [58]. The higher dose had significantly more effect on a combined primary endpoint consisting of five clinical measures. The result led to the approval of mitoxantrone as a first chemotherapy drug for the treatment of worsening MS. Mitoxantrone has also been used as induction treatment and in combination with other immunomodulating agents [59, 60]. The results have been encouraging and in some cases long-lasting effects were seen. Unfortunately, the use of mitoxantrone is very limited because of dose-related cardiotoxicity and several reports of therapy-related leukemia [61–63]. Less cardiotoxic agents such as pixantrone and dexrazoxane (cardioprotective) are currently being studied [64, 65].

Treatment of Radiologically Isolated Syndrome

Several recent studies have raised awareness of patients with incidentally discovered MRI lesions suggestive of multiple sclerosis, the so-called radiologically isolated syndrome (RIS) [66]. These studies have documented a conversion rate to CIS of about 1/3 within a 5-year period. Many more patients (59%) continue to have radiological progression. Furthermore, the risk of an alternate diagnosis with characteristic MRI finding suggestive of MS seems to be extremely low. Patients with evidence of ongoing disease activity may be candidates for treatment.

Treatment of Clinically Isolated Syndrome

Several natural history and long-term longitudinal studies have provided useful information regarding progress in individual patients with multiple sclerosis. An increased rate of relapses in the first few years, poor recovery from relapses, high lesion burden on MRI, and an African-American race are all associated with a relatively poor long-term outcome. On the other hand, lack of bad prognostic indicators may not necessarily point toward a benign outcome. A recent large study noted that a significant proportion of patients who were noted to be benign at 10 years after diagnosis were no longer considered "benign" when followed for another 10 years [67]. Histopathological and advanced imaging studies have revealed that significant axonal loss occurs early in the course of MS and this loss of axons may be the principal determinate of fixed permanent disability [68–70]. Long-term MRI studies (10–20 years follow-up) have suggested that the lesion load on the initial MRI may be a prognostic indicator for long-term disability [71].

There is overwhelming evidence suggesting a better response to disease modifying treatments when used early in the disease course. Several studies have looked into the effect of these agents when initiated at the time of first clinical event (clinically isolated syndrome or CIS). These trials have demonstrated a beneficial effect on disease activity with a reduction in relapse rates and new MRI lesions in the critical first 2 years after the initial event. Other controlled trials have compared early versus late treatment and have demonstrated a beneficial effect of starting treatment early. It appears that in the early phases of multiple sclerosis there may be a window of opportunity to target the inflammatory component of the disease. However, it is unclear, if the benefit persists as the disease progresses.

In the BENEFIT study (Betaseron in Newly Emerging Multiple Sclerosis for Initial Treatment), 468 patients with a first clinical event were randomized to receive IFN β-1b vs. placebo [72, 73]. After 2 years, the treated group did much better with only 26% of treated patients converting to clinically definite multiple sclerosis (CDMS) versus 44% in the placebo group ($p<0.0001$). The patients in the placebo group who converted to CDMS were offered open-label IFN β-1b and were followed for an additional 3 years. After 5 years, early treatment with IFN β-1b reduced the risk of CDMS by 37%. Additional positive effects were noted on MRI, cognition, and disability (significant at 3 years only) [74]. In the CHAMPS study (Controlled High Risk Subjects Avonex Multiple Sclerosis Prevention Study trial), 383 patients with an initial mono-focal demyelinating event were randomized to receive IFN β-1a (I/M once weekly) or placebo [75]. The trial was stopped early after an interim analysis suggested a positive outcome. Thirty-five percent of the treated group converted to CDMS versus 50% in the placebo group ($p=0.002$). The benefit of early treatment was shown to persist for at least 5 years on relapses and MRI measures but not on disability [76]. In the ETOMS (Early Treatment of Multiple Sclerosis) trial, patients ($N=309$) treated with a low-dose IFN β-1a, 22 µg once weekly (S/C) were also less likely to have subsequent attacks compared with placebo (34% vs. 45%) [77]. The PRECISE study randomized mono-focal CIS patients to GA or placebo similar to the interferon CIS studies. Patients treated with GA had a reduced risk of developing CDMS (25% vs. 43%) [78]. A 5-year extension is currently evaluating early versus delayed treatment effect of GA.

Comparative Trials Involving GA and Interferons

Several trials have compared the efficacy of first-line disease modifying agents in a controlled setting sometimes with surprising results.

In the BEYOND (Betaseron Efficacy Yielding Outcomes of a New Dose) trial, two different doses of IFN β-1b were compared head-to-head with GA in 2,244 patients [79]. There was no difference between IFN β-1b and GA in relapse rate reduction (primary outcome). However, the higher-dose interferon had a slightly better effect on MRI (T2 lesions) compared with GA. Surprisingly, another study primarily looking at the MRI measures using triple GAD and 3-T MRI found no significant difference in the number of combined active lesion (primary outcome) between GA and IFN β-1b [80]. In the REGARD (Rebif vs. Glatiramer Acetate in Relapsing MS Disease) trial, there was no difference in the time of onset of clinical activity between IFN β-1a and GA, which was the primary outcome [81]. Patients on IFN β-1a had less MRI activity.

Interestingly, both REGARD and BEYOND patients had a significantly low prestudy and on study relapse rate suggesting a different study population when compared with the pivotal trials and a more robust effect of disease modifying agents on inflammatory measures when used early in the disease course [82].

Comparative studies involving different doses and frequency of interferons have suggested that the high-frequency formulations may be more effective in reducing relapses and MRI lesions when compared with once a week dosing, at least in the short term [83, 84]. A recently completed trial comparing two different doses of GA failed to show any beneficial effect of higher doses of GA.

Treatment of Worsening RRMS

It appears that greater than one-third of patients do not achieve an optimal response to an initial disease modifying agent and the percentage of patients failing may increase with time. There is currently no clear definition of a suboptimal response, but most specialists would consider an increase in relapse rate (compared with baseline) and the presence of new MRI activity as a sign of worsening disease. Possible options in managing these patients may include switching to alternate first-line or second-line agents, combination therapy or possibly enrollment in a clinical trial with an experimental agent (Table 7.1).

Recent data suggests that patients with mild worsening may be good candidates for switching to an alternate first-line agent with an excellent safety profile [85, 86]. An alternate option may be to use two agents with different mechanism of action. Combination treatment may broaden the spectrum of therapeutic target and, therefore, may produce better efficacy. Several small open label combination studies have suggested an added benefit when another agent is added to a platform therapy [87, 88] Since most of these trials were small and short lasting, no clear long-term conclusions can be drawn. Additionally, the combination of two different immunologically active agents may result in unexpected side effects, especially when used long term [89]. A large NIH funded trial is currently evaluating the effects of combining IFN β-1a (IM) and GA in RRMS patients (CombiRx study).

Table 7.1 Suggested treatment approach in MS patients.

Radiologically isolated syndrome (RIS)	Observation with periodic exams and MRI	Consider treatment in patients with persistent increase in lesion load on MRI
CIS and RRMS	IFN β-1b, IFN β-1a (i/m), IFN β-1a (s/c), or GA Fingolimod for patients unable to tolerate injections	Consider natalizumab, mitoxantrone, or cyclophosphamide for aggressive disease
Worsening RRMS or SPMS with relapses	Switch to alternate first-line agent Natalizumab or fingolimod	Consider combination of an IFN or GA and pulse steroids or azathioprine
	Short-term treatment with mitoxantrone or cyclophosphamide	Consider rituximab or alemtuzumab in patients unresponsive to approved therapy
SPMS without relapses or increase in lesion load	Pulse corticosteroids?	Consider enrollment in clinical trials
PPMS	Trial of pulse corticosteroids	Consider enrollment in clinical trials

Other options for patients failing on first-line agents include the use of natalizumab, fingolimod, cyclophosphamide, mitoxantrone, or investigational agents such as rituximab, alemtuzumab, and cladribine. Although they appear to be more effective, there is a risk of serious and unexpected side effects such as PML with natalizumab, idiopathic thrombocytopenic purpura (ITP) with alemtuzumab, cardiotoxicity, and leukemia with mitoxantrone and bladder cancer with cyclophosphamide.

Induction Treatment

The so-called second-line or more aggressive agents can be used as induction treatments in a subgroup of patients with very aggressive disease. These patients tend to have a fairly high frequency of relapses as well as MRI activity and tend to accumulate significant disability in a short period of time. Several studies have suggested that aggressive treatment early in the disease course can result in effective and prolonged suppression of disease activity [59, 90].

Treatment of SPMS

Almost 80% of patients eventually develop progressive disease after an initial inflammatory relapsing remitting MS phase. These patients may continue to experience relapses and develop new MRI lesions in the earlier phases of SPMS. Several trials have suggested a modest benefit of using disease modifying agents in this subgroup of patients with SPMS. Two large trials with IFN β-1b (European and North American Trials) produced mixed results [91, 92]. A retrospective analysis indicated that IFN β-1b is effective in the relapsing phase of SPMS, but the benefit in patients with purely degenerative SPMS and an EDSS > 6 was not convincing [93]. Similarly, both formulations of IFN β-1a failed to show a positive effect on SPMS patients without relapses [94, 95]. Unfortunately, there is no evidence that SPMS without relapses may benefit from any of the currently available disease-modifying agents.

Other Off-Label Agents Used in the Treatment of RRMS

Corticosteroids

Corticosteroids are considered as standard treatment for acute relapses [96, 97]. Corticosteroids decrease inflammation and stabilize the blood brain barrier, resulting in more rapid recovery from relapses [98]. The standard dose is 1 g of methylprednisolone (MP) daily for 3–5 days through I/V infusion, although other regimens also have been used. Some studies have suggested that oral forms are also equally effective [99, 100].

One randomized study noted decrease brain atrophy, decreased T1 lesion volume, and decreased progression in patients treated with pulse steroids for 5 years [101]. Pulse steroids may also have a beneficial effect on disease activity when used in combination with interferons [102]. Corticosteroids are also safe to use during pregnancy and may have a role in the postpartum period [103, 104]. Treatment with steroids may reduce the development of neutralizing antibodies to IFN [105].

Corticosteroids when used as short-term or long-term pulse therapy seem to be well tolerated. Unusual but serious side effects may include steroid-induced psychosis, mood disorders, reversible memory disturbance, and aseptic vascular necrosis.

Cyclophosphamide

Cyclophosphamide is an alkylating agent that binds to DNA and suppresses both B and T cells. It is commonly used as an antineoplastic agent and is also used to treat several immune-mediated disorders [106]. It was initially studied in multiple sclerosis patients greater than three decades ago with encouraging results, although the trials were small and unblinded. Two large trials in patients with progressive disease (The Northeast Cooperative Multiple Sclerosis Treatment Group and Canadian Cooperative Multiple Sclerosis Group) provided conflicting results. The Northeast Trial suggested some benefit in young patients with maintenance dosing, while the Canadian study failed to show any benefit of using cyclophosphamide [107, 108]. Several recent small studies have reported a beneficial effect on a subgroup of patients who are young and have aggressive disease [109–111]. It carries a significant risk of serious side effects such as hemorrhagic cystitis [112], bladder cancer [113], and azoospermia and should only be used in patients with fairly aggressive disease unresponsive to other agents.

Azathioprine

Azathioprine is an oral immunosuppressive agent used to treat several immune-based disorders, including myasthenia gravis and rheumatoid arthritis. Clinical trials testing azathioprine in MS have been relatively small and lacked standardized MRI measures [114] A meta-analysis involving 793 patients suggested a slight benefit at 2 years of treatment, but the authors concluded that this probably did not outweigh the potential risks for long-term serious side effects [115] Several recent, open-label studies suggest that azathioprine may be modestly beneficial in combination with other agents [116, 117].

Methotrexate

Methotrexate has been used in the treatment of several immune disorders as well as multiple sclerosis for many years. When tested in controlled studies in MS patients, the results have been unimpressive. One small trial suggested a benefit in progressive patients [118]. A four-arm trial comparing the effect of methotrexate alone and in combination with I/V MP when added to patients with worsening disease on IFN β-1a (I/M) was recently concluded and failed to show a beneficial effect of adding methotrexate to IFN β in patients with worsening disease [119].

Mycophenolate Mofetil

Mycophenolate mofetil (cellcept) is an immunosuppressive agent. It is increasingly being used in preventing organ transplant rejection [120] and has been found to be beneficial in Crohn's disease [121]. It also promotes recovery in experimental allergic encephalomyelitis (EAE) [122]. A phase II trial in a small number of patients resulted in disease stabilization when mycophenolate was used in combination with IFB β-1a [123]. Ongoing phase II/III trials are currently evaluating the safety and efficacy of mycophenolate both as monotherapy and in combination.

Plasmapheresis and IVIG

Although both intravenous immune globulin (IVIG) and plasmapheresis have been used successfully in a variety of central and peripheral inflammatory immune-based disorders, the results in MS trials have not been encouraging.

IVIG may work by neutralizing circulating antibodies against myelin antigens, downregulating antibody production or interfering with complement or macrophage-mediated damage [124] It has also been shown to produce remyelination in animal models [125]. A meta-analysis of four double-blinded studies reported a beneficial effect on annual relapse rate as well as change in EDSS scores [126]. Several other trials failed to show a beneficial effect [127, 128]. IVIG was also found to be useful in reducing relapses in the postpartum period and patients with acute relapses who are intolerant to steroids. One small study noted a benefit in patients with a first demyelinating event [129]. IVIG is also the only disease modifying agent that has shown to reduce the rate of brain volume loss in SPMS [130].

Plasmapheresis may work by removing circulating autoantibodies and may be useful in patients with severe relapses unresponsive to steroids [131–134].

Drugs Currently in Development

MS is a chronic and heterogeneous disease requiring elaborate studies to provide evidence-based data concerning safety, efficacy, and tolerability of new therapeutic approaches. Several new biologics are on the horizon providing an opportunity of a more personalized therapy with improved efficacy, reduced side effects, and better compliance. These agents target different pathways involved in the currently presumed pathophysiology of MS and potentially may profoundly improve our understanding of the disease process (Figure 7.1 and Table 7.2).

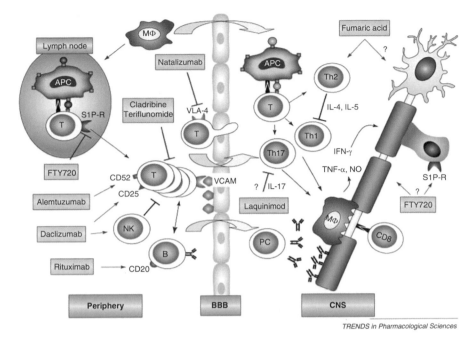

Figure 7.1 Schematic depiction of putative targets for the new MS treatment modalities. Interactions of immune cells are shown with *black arrows* and transmigration over the BBB is displayed with *yellow arrows*. *Red arrows* indicate therapeutic interactions with *pointed arrows* standing for targeting of specific cell types or molecules, T-shaped lines in *red* indicate blocking of pathways or receptors. Hypothetic mechanisms not proven in vivo are depicted with a *question mark*. Abbreviations: *APC* antigen-presenting cell, *B* B-cell, *BBB* blood–brain barrier, *CNS* central nervous system, *IL* interleukin, *INF-γ* interferon γ, *NK* natural killer cell, *NO* nitric oxide, *PC* plasma cell, *S1P-R* sphingosine-1-phosphate receptor, *Th* T-helper cell, *TNF-α* tumor necrosis factor α, *VCAM* vascular cell adhesion molecule-1 (with permission)
Source: Linker RA, Kieseier BC, Gold R. Identification and developement of new therapeutics for multiple sclerosis http: Trends Pharmacol Sci. 2008 Nov;29(11):558–65

Monoclonal Antibodies

Monoclonal antibodies (MCA) target specific antigens, which are responsible for selective biologic effects [135]. MCA have potent immunomodulating effects and have been used in neoplastic and inflammatory disorders for more than a decade. Apart from natalizumab, the first MCA to be approved in the treatment of multiple sclerosis, several others are in various stages of development.

Rituximab

Rituximab is a monoclonal antibody targeting CD20 positive B lymphocytes [136] resulting in rapid and sustained depletion of B-cells (6–9 months). Rituximab is currently approved in the treatment of NHL (non-Hodgkin's lymphoma) [137], refractory rheumatoid arthritis [138], and diffuse B cell lymphoma. Several case reports and smaller open label studies have found rituximab to be beneficial in the treatment of a range of neurological disorders including neuromyelitis optica [139], myasthenia gravis, demyelinating IgM neuropathy [140], multifocal motor neuropathy, paraneoplastic disorders as well as other systemic immune disorders. Treatment with rituximab results in selective depletion of CD20 positive B cells resulting in significant reduction of gadolinium-enhancing lesions (91%) and

Table 7.2 Emerging disease modifying agents in multiple sclerosis.

Agent	Mechanism of action	Route of administration	Clinical efficacy	Imaging	Safety concerns	Expected approval date
Cladribine	Immuno-suppressive	Oral, two or four 5-day cycles/year	Phase III CLARITY-58% reduction in ARR vs. placebo	>70% decrease in MRI measures compared with placebo	Bone marrow suppression, pregnancy category D, secondary malignancy	Unknown (recently rejected by FDA)
BG00012	Immunomodulator	Oral, once daily	Phase II 32% reduction in ARR, p=NS	69% reduction of new Gd-T1 lesions (weeks 12–24)	Flushing, pruritis, headache, GI side effects	2012–2013
Laquinimod	Immunomodulator	Oral, once daily	Phase II 33% reduction in ARR, p=NS Positive phase III (details pending)	40% reduction in Gd-T1 lesions	Elevation of LFT, chest pain	2012–2013
Teriflunomide	Immunosuppressant	Oral, once daily	Phase II 32% reduction in ARR, p=NS	61% reduction in Gd-T1 lesions	Elevation of LFT, neutropenia, alopecia	2012–2013
Alemtuzumab	Monoclonal antibody	Yearly infusions 5 consecutive days initially followed by 3 days at 12 months	Phase II 75% reduction in ARR compared with IFNB-1a SQ, improved mean disability score	Significant beneficial effect of lesion burden and brain volume when compared with IFNB-1a SQ	Graves disease, ITP, Goodpasture's syndrome, bone marrow suppression, infusion reaction	2013–2014
Ocrelizumab (rituximab)	Monoclonal antibody	IV infusion every 6–12 months	44% reduction in ARR	91% reduction in Gd-T1 lesions	PML, severe infusion reactions, infections	2014

clinical relapses (44%) as demonstrated in a phase II trial with 104 patients with relapsing multiple sclerosis treated with rituximab compared with placebo [141] Even though the existence of a humoral component in MS has been implicated for decades, the results of this trial provided solid evidence regarding the role of B cells in the immunopathology of multiple sclerosis [142, 143]. Rituximab may be useful in patients with aggressive RRMS who have failed to respond to other conventional therapies [144].

As with several other monoclonal antibodies, rituximab has been associated with fatal infusion reactions as well as other rare side effects including PML [145]. Rituximab was also studied in a large primary progressive multiple sclerosis population and was found to be ineffective in slowing down the disease progression when compared with placebo. Ocrelizumab, a humanized monoclonal antibody against CD20 is currently undergoing clinical trials in multiple sclerosis, B-cell malignancy [146] as well as other inflammatory disorders.

Alemtuzumab

Alemtuzumab is a humanized monoclonal antibody targeting CD52 cells resulting in prolonged depletion of lymphocytes [147]. The B-cells continue to return to normal in 3–6 months, while the T cells remain suppressed for a prolonged period [148]. Alemtuzumab is currently used for the treatment of B-cell lymphoma unresponsive to other standard treatments. Initial trials in MS suggested a beneficial effect in RRMS patients, while there was no significant beneficial effect in patients with secondary progressive MS [149, 150].

A recent phase II randomized trial (334 patients) compared two doses of alemtuzumab with IFN β-1a S/Q in patients with no prior treatment [151] Treatment with alemtuzumab resulted in a profound beneficial effect on relapse rate (0.10 vs. 0.36) when compared with IFN β-1a (75% reduction in relapse rate). Similarly, alemtuzumab was significantly better on disability measures as well as MRI measures. Adverse events were primarily related to autoimmunity, possibly because of an imbalance between the recovery of B cells and T cells. Six patients in the trial developed ITP and the first patient with ITP died of an intracranial hemorrhage. Other significant side effects include Goodpasture's syndrome (rare) and thyroid disease (23% of patients). Infections and malignancy including cervical dysplasia were more common in the alemtuzumab-treated group. The drug was generally well tolerated and is only infused once a year (over several days). Although the clinical efficacy of alemtuzumab looks to be very promising, given the low number of patients tested in controlled studies, there is a general concern regarding long-term autoimmune, infectious, and neoplastic complications. Two large phase III controlled trials (CARE-MS 1 and CARE-MS 2) are currently evaluating the effects of alemtuzumab in patients naive to treatment as well as patients worsening on first-line agents.

Daclizumab

Daclizumab is a humanized monoclonal antibody that binds to CD25 resulting in decreased IL-2-mediated stimulation of T cells [152]. Other possible mechanisms may include expansion of CD56 NK cells which may have an immunoregulatory function [153]. Daclizumab is currently used to prevent rejection of kidney transplants. After several smaller studies [154, 155] reported a beneficial effect on MS patients, a phase two trial involving 230 patients with active RRMS on IFN β-1a was conducted (CHOICE study).Patients were randomly assigned to two different S/Q doses of daclizumab in addition to the IFN and a third arm received IFN and placebo. Add-on daclizumab treatment reduced the number of Gad-enhancing lesions compared with IFN β alone. The drug was well tolerated with no serious or unexpected side effect. The long-term safety and efficacy is currently being evaluated in the phase IIB controlled study (SELECT study).

Oral Agents

Cladribine

Cladribine reduces lymphocyte counts selectively by getting incorporated into dividing cells leading to DNA damage and cell death. It has long-lasting effects and is currently approved for the treatment of hairy cell leukemia. When tested in the intravenous and subcutaneous forms, treatment of a mixed population of MS patients produced a clear beneficial effect on MRI parameters of inflammation, but its effects on clinical measures and MRI measures of degeneration were less pronounced [156–158].

The recently completed CLARITY study was a randomized, double-blinded, placebo-controlled trial involving 1,326 patients with relapsing-remitting MS. Patients were randomized in a 1:1:1 ratio to receive placebo or one of two dosing regimens of oral cladribine. The trial met its primary end point, with a 58% reduction in annualized relapse rates with the low dose and a 55% reduction with the high dose at 2 years [159] There was a statistically significant reduction in MRI activity as well as disability progression. A greater percentage of patients remained disease activity free over 96 weeks (placebo=16%, low dose=43%, and high dose=44.3%). The drug was well tolerated and only 2.6% of patients discontinued treatment because of blood and lymphatic system disorders. There were three isolated malignancies in the treatment arm and an additional case of choriocarcinoma detected in poststudy surveillance. There remains a concern about long-term immunosuppressive side effects. Cladribine was recently rejected by the FDA due to safety concerns. It is unclear if further studies are being planned to better understand the risks and benefits of this agent in the treatment of multiple sclerosis.

Teriflunomide

Teriflunomide is an inhibitor of mitochondrial dehydrogenase, an enzyme involved in pyrimidine synthesis. In a phase II study, teriflunomide (7 or 14 mg/day) reduced T1 enhancing and T2 lesions [160]. Teriflunomide is currently being tested in a large phase III trial (TEMSO study) as well as CIS and combination studies.

Laquinamod

Laquinamod has an unclear mode of action and is derived from roquinimex. When roquinimex was tested in the MS population, it produced serious side effects including myocardial infarction and death resulting in discontinuation of the trial [161]. Initial testing with Laquinamod in the RRMS population has produced positive results on MRI inflammatory measures and the effect seems to be sustained [162]. Laquinamod was found to be well tolerated with no serious side effects. Laquinamod is currently being evaluated in two large trials (ALLEGRO and BRAVO).

BG12 (Fumaric Acid)

Fumaric acid is an intermediary in the KREBS cycle. It is currently used as an immunomodulator in the treatment of psoriasis. An oral fumaric acid derivative BG00012 is currently being tested in RRMS. A phase II blinded placebo controlled trial revealed significant and dose-dependent reduction in MRI activity with a trend toward reduction in relapse rate [163] The drug seems to be safe and well tolerated. Two large phase III trials (DEFINE and CONFIRM) are currently evaluating the drug in the RRMS population.

Stem Cell Transplantation

Stem cell transplantation requires a collection of hematopoietic stem cells from the peripheral circulation followed by ablation of the immune system with chemotherapy agents followed by reinfusion of stem cells in the hope that the reconstituted immune system would be more tolerant to self-antigens. This idea is supported by several case reports of individual MS patients treated for malignancy and EAE animal models.

Several studies have looked at the effects of autologous hematopoietic stem cell transplantation and found encouraging results with prolonged periods of disease stabilization in patients with aggressive disease [164, 165]. However, stem cell transplantation is a difficult process and carries a significant mortality rate. There appears to be a direct neurotoxic effect and increased rate of brain atrophy [166–168]. Furthermore, the persistence of oligoclonal bands after the procedure may argue against a total reconstitution of the immune system.

Neuroprotection

It remains unclear, if degeneration in MS is a consequence of widespread inflammation or a primary and independent phenomenon. Treatment with standard immunomodulating agents have failed to show a meaningful effect on rate of brain atrophy. More aggressive treatment with potent anti-inflammatory agents and BMT seems to increase the rate of brain atrophy.

It is well known that remyelination occurs in MS and in some patients the remyelination is quite extensive [169, 170]. In the right environment, remyelination may be a quick process. Remyelination requires proliferation, migration, and differentiation of oligodendrocyte precursor cells (OPC) possibly mediated by a complex combination of signals including signals from the demyelinating neurons [171]. Persistent demyelination secondary to ongoing toxic insults can lead to permanent neuronal alteration within weeks [172]. The exact mechanism of neurotoxicity remains unknown although there seems to be some evidence suggesting mitochondrial dysfunction [173, 174]. It appears that the window of opportunity for therapeutic intervention is relatively short. A variety of agents thought to be neuroprotective have been tested in MS (Table 7.3).

The clinical trials involving presumed neuroprotective agents have either been inconclusive or failed to show any beneficial effect. The lack of a clear surrogate marker of demyelination and neuroprotection is a significant handicap in the development of neuroprotective agents.

Table 7.3 Possible neuroprotective agents in MS.

Drug	Reference
Minocycline	[175]
Riluzole	[176]
IVIG	[177]
Erythropoietin (EPO)	[178]
Growth Factor (IGF-1)	[179]
Antiepileptics	[180]

Treatment of PPMS

Primary progressive multiple sclerosis is characterized by late onset gradually progressive accumulation of disability. Several trials have failed to show a beneficial treatment effect in patients with PPMS [158, 181]. A recent trial with rituximab suggested a beneficial effect in a subgroup of patients with a significant inflammatory component. Further studies involving ocrelizumab (humanized MCA against CD20) are being planned. There is unfortunately no approved disease-modifying agent for the treatment of PPMS.

Conclusion

Over the last two decades, multiple disease-modifying agents have been approved for the treatment of relapsing forms of multiple sclerosis. The next generation of agents for the treatment of MS appear to be increasingly more effective therapeutic modalities targeting different proposed mechanisms of MS pathophysiology. These include monoclonal antibodies and several oral agents with novel mechanism of action. Unfortunately, increased efficacy may be associated with an increased risk of serious adverse events and only long-term data from controlled large-scale clinical trials will determine the extent of therapeutic efficacy and safety of these emerging therapies.

References

1. Yong VW. Differential mechanisms of action of interferon-beta and glatiramer acetate in MS. Neurology. 2002;59:802–8.
2. Yong VW, Chabot S, Stuve O, Williams G. Interferon beta in the treatment of multiple sclerosis: mechanisms of action. Neurology. 1998;51:682–9.
3. Kieseier BC, Seifert T, Giovannoni G, Hartung HP. Matrix metalloproteinases in inflammatory demyelination: targets for treatment. Neurology. 1999;53:20–5.
4. The IFNB Multiple Sclerosis Study Group. Interferon beta-1b is effective in relapsing-remitting multiple sclerosis. I. Clinical results of a multi-center, randomized, double-blind, placebo-controlled trial. Neurology. 1993;43:655–61.
5. Paty DW, Li DK, UBC MS/MRI Study Group and the IFNB Multiple Sclerosis Study Group. Interferon beta-1b is effective in relapsing-remitting multiple sclerosis. II. MRI analysis results of a multicenter, randomized, double-blind, placebo-controlled trial. Neurology. 1993;43:662–7.
6. The IFNB Multiple Sclerosis Study Group and the University of British Columbia MS/MRI Analysis Group. Interferon beta-1b in the treatment of multiple sclerosis: final outcome of the randomized controlled trial. Neurology. 1995;45:1277–85.

7. Jacobs LD, Cookfair DL, Rudick RA, Herndon RM, Richert JR, Slazar AM, et al. Intramuscular interferon beta-1a for disease progression in relapsing multiple sclerosis. Ann Neurol. 1996;39:285–94.

8. Rudick RA, Goodkin DE, Jacobs LD, Cookfair DL, Herndon RM, Richert JR, et al. Impact of interferon beta-1a on neurologic disability in relapsing multiple sclerosis. The Multiple Sclerosis Collaborative Research Group. Neurology. 1997;49(2):358–63.

9. Simon JH, Jacobs LD, Campion M, Wende K, Simonian N, Cookfair DL, et al. Magnetic resonance studies of intramuscular interferon beta-1a for relapsing multiple sclerosis. The Multiple Sclerosis Collaborative Research Group. Ann Neurol. 1998;43:79–87.

10. Rudick RA, Fisher E, Lee JC, et al. Use of the brain parenchymal fraction to measure whole brain atrophy in relapsing-remitting MS. Multiple Sclerosis Collaborative Research Group. Neurology. 1999;53:1698–704.

11. PRISMS Study Group. Randomized double-blind placebo-controlled study of interferon beta-1a in relapsing remitting multiple sclerosis. Lancet. 1998;352: 1498–504.

12. Li DK. Magnetic resonance imaging results of the PRISMS trial: a randomized, double-blind, placebo-controlled study of interferonbeta1a in relapsing-remitting multiple sclerosis. Prevention of relapses and disability by interferon-beta1a sub-cutaneously in multiple sclerosis. Ann Neurol. 1999;46:197–206.

13. PRISMS Study Group. PRISMS-4: Long-term efficacy of interferon-beta-1a in relapsing MS. Neurology. 2001;56:1628–36.

14. Kappos L, Traboulsee A, Constantinescu C, et al. Long-term subcutaneous interferon beta-1a therapy in patients with relapsing-remitting MS. Neurology. 2006;67:944–53.

15. Walther EU, Hohlfeld R. Multiple sclerosis: side effects of interferon therapy and their management. Neurology. 1999;53:1622–7.

16. Goodin DS, Frohman EM, Hurwitz B, et al. Neutralizing antibodies to interferon beta: assessment of their clinical and radiographic impact: an evidence report: report of the Therapeutics and Technology Assessment Subcommittee of the American Academy of Neurology. Neurology. 2007;68:977–84.

17. Farina C, Weber MS, Meinl E, Wekerle H, Hohlfeld R. Glatiramer acetate in multiple sclerosis: update on potential mechanisms of action. Lancet Neurol. 2005;4:567–75.

18. Johnson KP, Brooks BR, Cohen JA, Ford CC, Goldstein J, Lisak RP, et al. Copolymer 1 reduces relapse rate and improves disability in relapsing- remitting multiple sclerosis: results of a phase III multicenter, double-blind placebo-controlled trial. Neurology. 1995;45:1268–76.

19. Johnson KP, Brooks BR, Cohen JA, Ford CC, Goldstein J, Lisak RP, et al. Extended use of glatiramer acetate (Copaxone) is well tolerated and maintains its clinical effect on multiple sclerosis relapse rate and degree of disability. Copolymer 1 Multiple Sclerosis Study Group. Neurology. 1998;50:701–8.

20. Comi G, Filippi M, Wolinsky JS. European/Canadian multicenter, double- blind, randomized, placebo-controlled study of the effects of glatiramer acetate on magnetic resonance imaging-measured disease activity and burden in patients with relapsing multiple sclerosis. European/Canadian Glatiramer Acetate Study Group. Ann Neurol. 2001;49:290–7.

21. Ford C, Johnson KP, Lisak RP, et al. A prospective open,-label study of glatiramer acetate: over a decade of continuous use in multiple sclerosis patients. Mult Scler. 2006;12:309–20.

22. Goodin DS, Cohen BA, O'Connor P, Kappos L, Stevens JC. Assessment: the use of natalizumab (Tysabri) for the treatment of multiple sclerosis (an evidence-based review): report of the Therapeutics and Technology Assessment Subcommittee of the American Academy of Neurology. Neurology. 2008;71:766–73.

23. Putzki N, Kollia K, Woods S, Igwe E, Diener HC, Limmroth V. Natalizumab is effective as second line therapy in the treatment of relapsing remitting MS. Eur J Neurol. 2009;16:424–6.

24. Engelhardt B, Kappos L. Natalizumab: targeting alpha4-integrins in multiple sclerosis. Neurodegener Dis. 2008;5:16–22.

25. Stüve O, Cravens PD, Frohman EM, Phillips JT, Remington GM, von Geldern G, et al. Immunologic, clinical, and radiologic status 14 months after cessation of natalizumab therapy. Neurology. 2009;72:396–401.

26. Polman CH, O'Connor PW, Havrdova E, et al., AFFIRM Investigators. A randomized, placebo-controlled trial of natalizumab for relapsing multiple sclerosis. N Engl J Med. 2006;354:899–910.

27. Rudick RA, Stuart WH, Calabresi PA, et al., SENTINEL Investigators. Natalizumab plus interferon beta-1a for relapsing multiple sclerosis. N Engl J Med. 2006;354:911–23.

28. Miller DH, Soon D, Fernando KT, MacManus DG, Barker GJ, Yousry TA, et al. MRI outcomes in a placebo-controlled trial of natalizumab in relapsing MS. Neurology. 2007;68:1390–401.

29. Hutchinson M, Kappos L, Calabresi PA, Confavreux C, Giovannoni G, Galetta SL, et al. The efficacy of natalizumab in patients with relapsing multiple sclerosis: subgroup analyses of AFFIRM and SENTINEL. J Neurol. 2009;256(3):405–15.

30. Calabresi PA, Giovannoni G, Confavreux C, Galetta SL, Havrdova E, Hutchinson M, et al. The incidence and significance of anti-natalizumab antibodies: results from AFFIRM and SENTINEL. Neurology. 2007;69:1391–403.

31. O'Connor PW, Goodman A, Willmer-Hulme AJ, Libonati MA, Metz L, Murray RS, et al. Randomized multicenter trial of natalizumab in acute MS relapses: clinical and MRI effects. Neurology. 2004;62:2038–43.

32. Goodman AD, Rossman H, Bar-Or A, Miller A, Miller DH, Schmierer K, et al. Results of a phase 2, randomized, double-blind, placebo-controlled study. Neurology. 2009;72:806–12.

33. Ghezzi A, Pozzilli C, Grimaldi LM, Brescia Morra V, Bortolon F, Capra R, et al. Safety and efficacy of natalizumab in children with multiple sclerosis. Neurology. 2010;75(10):912–7.

34. Vellinga MM, Castelijns JA, Barkhof F, Uitdehaag BM, Polman CH. Postwithdrawal rebound increase in T2 lesional activity in natalizumab-treated MS patients. Neurology. 2008;70:1150–1.

35. Miravalle A, Jensen R, Kinkel RP. Immune reconstitution inflammatory syndrome in patients with multiple sclerosis following cessation of natalizumab therapy. Arch Neurol. 2011;68(2):186–91.

36. West TW, Cree BA. Natalizumab dosage suspension: are we helping or hurting? Ann Neurol. 2010;68(3):395–9.

37. Kleinschmidt-DeMasters BK, Tyler KL. Progressive multifocal leukoencephalopathy complicating treatment with natalizumab and interferon beta-1a for multiple sclerosis. N Engl J Med. 2005;353:369–74.

38. Langer-Gould A, Atlas SW, Green AJ, Bollen AW, Pelletier D. Progressive multifocal leukoencephalopathy in a patient treated with natalizumab. N Engl J Med. 2005;353:375–81.

39. Van Assche G, Van Ranst M, Sciot R, et al. Progressive multifocal leukoencephalopathy after natalizumab therapy for Crohn's disease. N Engl J Med. 2005;353:362–8.

40. Yousry TA, Major EO, Ryschkewitsch C, et al. Evaluation of patients treated with natalizumab for progressive multifocal leukoencephalopathy. N Engl J Med. 2006;354:924–33.

41. Khalili K, White MK, Lublin F, Ferrante P, Berger JR. Reactivation of JC virus and development of PML in patients with multiple sclerosis. Neurology. 2007;68:985–90.

42. Carson KR, Focosi D, Major EO, Petrini M, Richey EA, West DP, et al. Monoclonal antibody-associated progressive multifocal leucoencephalopathy in patients treated with rituximab, natalizumab, and efalizumab: a Review from the Research on Adverse Drug Events and Reports (RADAR) Project. Lancet Oncol. 2009;10(8):816–24.

43. Berger JR, Houff SA, Major EO. Monoclonal antibodies and progressive multifocal leukoencephalopathy. MAbs. 2009;1(6):583–9.

44. Berger JR. Progressive multifocal leukoencephalopathy and newer biological agents. Drug Saf. 2010;33(11):969–83.

45. Khatri BO, Man S, Giovannoni G, Koo AP, Lee J-C, Tucky B, et al. Effect of plasma exchange in accelerating natalizumab clearance and restoring leukocyte function. Neurology. 2009;72:402–9.

46. Gorelik L, Lerner M, Bixler S, Crossman M, Schlain B, Simon K, et al. Anti-JC virus antibodies: implications for PML risk stratification. Ann Neurol. 2010;68(3):295–303.

47. Brinkmann V, Davis MD, Heise CE, et al. The immune modulator FTY720 targets sphingosine 1-phosphate receptors. J Biol Chem. 2002;277:21453–7. 25:115–124.

48. Mehling M, Lindberg R, Raulf F, Kuhle J, Hess C, Kappos L, et al. Th17 central memory T cells are reduced by FTY720 in patients with multiple sclerosis. Neurology. 2010;75(5):403–10.

49. Sensken SC, Bode C, Gräler MH. Accumulation of fingolimod (FTY720) in lymphoid tissues contributes to prolonged efficacy. Pharmacol Exp Ther. 2009;328(3):963–9.

50. Van Doorn R, Van Horssen J, Verzijl D, Witte M, Ronken E, Van Het Hof B, et al. Sphingosine 1-phosphate receptor 1 and 3 are upregulated in multiple sclerosis lesions. Glia. 2010;58(12):1465–76.

51. O'Connor P, Comi G, Montalban X, Antel J, Radue EW, de Vera A, et al. Oral fingolimod (FTY720) in multiple sclerosis: two-year results of a phase II extension study. Neurology. 2009;72(1):73–9.

52. Cohen JA, Barkhof F, Comi G, Hartung HP, Khatri BO, Montalban X, et al. Oral fingolimod or intramuscular interferon for relapsing multiple sclerosis. N Engl J Med. 2010;362:402.

53. Leypoldt F, Münchau A, Moeller F, Bester M, Gerloff C, Heesen C. Hemorrhaging focal encephalitis under fingolimod (FTY720) treatment: a case report. Neurology. 2009;72(11):1022–4.

54. Kappos L, Radue EW, O'Connor P, Polman C, Hohlfeld R, Calabresi P, et al. A placebo-controlled trial of oral fingolimod in relapsing multiple sclerosis. N Engl J Med. 2010;362:387.

55. Johnson TA, Shames I, Keezer M, Lapierre Y, Haegert DG, Bar-Or A, et al. Reconstitution of circulating lymphocyte counts in FTY720-treated MS patients. Clin Immunol. 2010;137(1):15–20.

56. Neuhaus O, Wiendl H, Kieseier BC, Archelos JJ, Hemmer B, Stuve O, et al. Multiple sclerosis: mitoxantrone promotes differential effects on immunocompetent cells in vitro. J Neuroimmunol. 2005;168:128–37.

57. Kopadze T, Dehmel T, Hartung HP, Stuve O, Kieseier BC. Inhibition by mitoxantrone of in vitro migration of immunocompetent cells: a possible mechanism for therapeutic efficacy in the treatment of multiple sclerosis. Arch Neurol. 2006;63:1572–8.

58. Hartung HP, Gonsette R, Konig N, Kwiecinski H, Guseo A, Morrissey SP, et al. Mitoxantrone in progressive multiple sclerosis: a placebo-controlled, double blind, randomized multicentre trial. Lancet. 2002;360:2018–25.

59. Vollmer T, Panitch H, Bar-Or A, Dunn J, Freedman M, Gazda S, et al. Glatiramer acetate after induction therapy with mitoxantrone in relapsing multiple sclerosis. Mult Scler. 2008;14:663–70.

60. Edan G, Comi G, Lebrun D, Brassat C, Lubetzki C, Stankoff B, et al. The French-Italian Mitoxantrone-Interferon-beta trial: a 3-year randomized study. Mult Scler. 2007;13 Suppl 2:S22–3.
61. Goffette S, Van P V, Vanoverschelde JL, Morandini E, Sindic CJ. Severe delayed heart failure in three multiple sclerosis patients previously treated with mitoxantrone. J Neurol. 2005;252:1217–22.
62. Rizvi SA, Zwibel H, Fox EJ. Mitoxantrone for multiple sclerosis in clinical practice. Neurology. 2004;63:S25–7.
63. Ellis R, Boggild M. Therapy-related acute leukaemia with Mitoxantrone: what is the risk and can we minimise it? Mult Scler. 2009;15(4):505–8.
64. Gonsette RE, Dubois B. Pixantrone (BBR2778): a new immunosuppressant in multiple sclerosis with a low cardiotoxicity. J Neurol Sci. 2004;223:81–6.
65. Bernitsas E, Wei W, Mikol DD. Suppression of mitoxantrone cardiotoxicity in multiple sclerosis patients by dexrazoxane. Ann Neurol. 2006;59:206–9.
66. Okuda DT, Mowry EM, Beheshtian A, Waubant E, Baranzini SE, Goodin DS, et al. Incidental MRI anomalies suggestive of multiple sclerosis: the radiologically isolated syndrome. Neurology. 2009;72(9):800–5. Erratum in: Neurology. 2009;72(14):1284.
67. Sayao AL, Devonshire V, Tremlett H. Longitudinal follow-up of "benign" multiple sclerosis at 20 years. Neurology. 2007;68:496–500.
68. Trapp BD, Peterson J, Ransohoff RM, Rudick R, Mork S, Bo L. Axonal transection in the lesions of multiple sclerosis. N Engl J Med. 1998;338:278–85.
69. Trapp BD, Ransohoff R, Rudick R. Axonal pathology in multiple sclerosis: relationship to neurologic disability. Curr Opin Neurol. 1999;12:295–302.
70. De Stefano N, Narayanan S, Francis GS, et al. Evidence of axonal damage in the early stages of multiple sclerosis and its relevance to disability. Arch Neurol. 2001;58:65–70.
71. Fisniku LK, Brex PA, Altmann DR, Miszkiel KA, Benton CE, Lanyon R, et al. Disability and T2 MRI lesions: a 20-year follow-up of patients with relapse onset of multiple sclerosis. Brain. 2008;31:808–17.
72. Kappos L, Polman CH, Freedman MS, Edan G, Hartung HP, Miller DH, et al. Treatment with interferon beta-1b delays conversion to clinically definite and McDonald MS in patients with clinically isolated syndromes. Neurology. 2006;67:1242–9.
73. Kappos L, Freedman MS, Polman CH, Edan G, Hartung HP, Miller DH, et al. Effect of early versus delayed interferon beta-1b treatment on disability after a first clinical event suggestive of multiple sclerosis: a 3-year follow-up analysis of the BENEFIT study. Lancet. 2007;370:389–97.
74. Kappos L, Freedman MS, Polman CH, Edan G, Hartung HP, Miller DH, et al. Long-term effect of early treatment with interferon beta-1b after a first clinical event suggestive of multiple sclerosis: 5-year active treatment extension of the phase 3 BENEFIT trial. Lancet Neurol. 2009;8(11):987–97.
75. Jacobs LD, Beck RW, Simon JH, Kinkel RP, Brownscheidle CM, Murray TJ, et al. Intramuscular interferon beta-1a therapy initiated during a first demyelinating event in multiple sclerosis. CHAMPS Study Group. N Engl J Med. 2000;343:898–904.
76. Kinkel RP, Kollman C, O'Connor P, Murray TJ, Simon J, Arnold D, et al. IM interferon beta-1a delays definite multiple sclerosis 5 years after a first demyelinating event. Neurology. 2006;66:678–84.
77. Comi G, Filippi M, Barkhof F, Durelli L, Edan G, Fernandez O, et al. Effect of early interferon treatment on conversion to definite multiple sclerosis: a randomised study. Lancet. 2001;357:1576–82.
78. Comi G, Martinelli V, Rodegher M, Moiola L, Bajenaru O, Carra A, et al. Effect of glatiramer acetate on conversion to clinically definite multiple sclerosis in patients with clinically isolated syndrome (PreCISe study): a randomised, double-blind, placebo-controlled trial. Lancet. 2009;374:1503–11.

79. O'Connor P, Filippi M, Arnason B, Comi G, Cook S, Goodin D, et al. 250 mug or 500 mug interferon beta-1b versus 20 mg glatiramer acetate in relapsing-remitting multiple sclerosis: a prospective, randomised, multicentre study. Lancet Neurol. 2009;10:889–97.

80. Cadavid D, Wolansky LJ, Skurnick J, et al. Efficacy of treatment of MS with IFNβ-1b or glatiramer acetate by monthly brain MRI in the BECOME study. Neurology. 2009;72(23):1976–83.

81. Mikol DD, Barkhof F, Chang P, et al., on behalf of the REGARD Study Group. Comparison of subcutaneous interferon beta-1a with glatiramer acetate in patients with relapsing multiple sclerosis (the Rebif vs Glatiramer Acetate in Relapsing MS Disease [REGARD] study): a multicentre, randomised, parallel, open-label trial. Lancet Neurol 2008;7:903–914.

82. Klawiter EC, Cross AH, Naismith RT. The present efficacy of multiple sclerosis therapeutics: is the new 66% just the old 33%? Neurology. 2009;73:984–90.

83. Panitch H, Goodin DS, Francis G, et al. Randomized, comparative study of interferon beta-1a treatment regimens in MS: the EVIDENCE Trial. Neurology. 2002;59:1496–506.

84. Durelli L, Verdun E, Barbero P, et al. Every-other-day interferon beta-1b versus once-weekly interferon beta-1a for multiple sclerosis: results of a 2-year prospective randomised multicentre study (INCOMIN). Lancet. 2002;359:1453–60.

85. Caon C, Din M, Ching W, Tselis A, Lisak R, Khan O. Clinical course after change of immunomodulating therapy in relapsing-remitting multiple sclerosis. Eur J Neurol. 2006;13:471–4.

86. Hl Z. Glatiramer acetate in treatment-naive and prior interferon-beta-1b-treated multiple sclerosis patients. Acta Neurol Scand. 2006;113:378–86.

87. Fernandez O, Guerrero M, Mayorga C, et al. Combination therapy with interferon beta-1b and azathioprine in secondary progressive multiple sclerosis. A two-year pilot study. J Neurol. 2002;249:1058–62.

88. Lus G, Romano F, Scuotto A, Accardo C, Cotrufo R. Azathioprine and interferon beta(1a) in relapsing-remitting multiple sclerosis patients: increasing efficacy of combined treatment. Eur Neurol. 2004;51:15–20.

89. Birnbaum G, Cree B, Altafullah I, Zinser M, Reder AT. Combining beta interferon and atorvastatin may increase disease activity in multiple sclerosis. Neurology. 2008;71:1390–5.

90. Debouverie M, Taillandier L, Pittion-Vouyovitch S, Louis S, Vespignani H. Clinical follow-up of 304 patients with multiple sclerosis three years after mitoxantrone treatment. J Neurol. 2007;254(10):1370–5.

91. European Study Group on interferon beta-1b in secondary progressive MS Placebo-controlled multicentre randomised trial of interferon beta-1b in treatment of secondary progressive multiple sclerosis. Lancet. 1998;352:1491–7.

92. Panitch H, Miller A, Paty D, Weinshenker B. North American Study Group on Interferon beta-1b in secondary progressive MS interferon beta-1b in secondary progressive MS: results from a 3-year controlled study. Neurology. 2004;63:1788–95.

93. Kappos L, Weinshenker B, Pozzilli C, Thompson AJ, Dahlke F, Beckmann K, et al. European (EU-SPMS) Interferon beta-1b in Secondary Progressive Multiple Sclerosis Trial Steering Committee and Independent Advisory Board; North American (NA-SPMS) Interferon beta-1b in Secondary Progressive Multiple Sclerosis Trial Steering Committee and Independent Advisory Board Interferon beta-1b in secondary progressive MS: a combined analysis of the two trials. Neurology. 2004;63:1779–87.

94. SPECTRIMS Study Group. Randomized controlled trial of interferon-beta-1a in secondary progressive MS: clinical results. Neurology. 2001;56:1496–504.

95. Cohen JA, Cutter GR, Fischer JS, Goodman AD, Heidenreich FR, Kooijmans MF, et al. Benefit of interferon beta-1a on MSFC progression in secondary progressive MS. Neurology. 2002;59:679–87.

96. Frohman EM, Shah A, Eggenberger E, Metz L, Zivadinov R, Stuve O. Corticosteroids for multiple sclerosis: I. Application for treating exacerbations. Neurotherapeutics. 2007;4:618–26.

97. Thrower BW. Relapse management in multiple sclerosis. Neurologist. 2009;15(1):1–5. Review.

98. Gold R, Buttgereit F, Toyka KV. Mechanism of action of glucocorticosteroid hormones: possible implications for therapy of neuroimmunological disorders. J Neuroimmunol. 2001;117:1–8.

99. Alam SM, Kyriakides T, Lawden M, Newman PK. Methylprednisolone in multiple sclerosis: a comparison of oral with intravenous therapy at equivalent high dose. J Neurol Neurosurg Psychiatry. 1993;56:1219–20.

100. Barnes D, Hughes RA, Morris RW, Wade-Jones O, Brown P, Britton T, et al. Randomised trial of oral and intravenous methylprednisolone in acute relapses of multiple sclerosis. Lancet. 1997;349:902–6.

101. Zivadinov R, Rudick RA, De Masi R, Nasuelli D, Ukmar M, Pozzi-Mucelli RS, et al. Effects of IV methylprednisolone on brain atrophy in relapsing-remitting MS. Neurology. 2001;57:1239–47.

102. Sorensen PS, Mellgren SI, Svenningsson A, et al. NORdic trial of oral methylprednisolone as add-on therapy to interferon beta-1a for treatment of relapsing-remitting multiple sclerosis (NORMIMS study): a randomised, placebo-controlled trial. Lancet Neurol. 2009;8(6):519–29.

103. Ferrero S, Esposito F, Pretta S, et al. Fetal risks related to the treatment of multiple sclerosis during pregnancy and breastfeeding. Expert Rev Neurother. 2006;6(12):1823–31.

104. de Seze J, Chapelotte M, Delalande S, Ferriby D, Stojkovic T, Vermersch P. Intravenous corticosteroids in the postpartum period for reduction of acute exacerbations in multiple sclerosis. Mult Scler. 2004;10(5):596–7.

105. Pozzilli C, Antonini G, Bagnato F, Mainero C, Tomassini V, Onesti E, et al. Monthly corticosteroids decrease neutralizing antibodies to IFNbeta1 b: a randomized trial in multiple sclerosis. J Neurol. 2002;249(1):50–6.

106. Kovarsky J. Clinical pharmacology and toxicology of cyclophosphamide: emphasis on use in rheumatic diseases. Semin Arthritis Rheum. 1983;12:359–72.

107. Weiner HL, Mackin GA, Orav EJ, et al. Intermittent cyclophosphamide pulse therapy in progressive multiple sclerosis: final report of the Northeast Cooperative Multiple Sclerosis Treatment Group. Neurology. 1993;43:910–8.

108. The Canadian Cooperative Multiple Sclerosis Study Group. The Canadian cooperative trial of cyclophosphamide and plasma exchange in progressive multiple sclerosis. Lancet. 1991;337:441–6.

109. Weinstock-Guttman B. Treatment of fulminant multiple sclerosis with intervenous cyclophosphamide. Neurologist. 1997;3:178–85.

110. Khan OA, Zvartau-Hind M, Caon C, et al. Effect of monthly intravenous cyclophosphamide in rapidly deteriorating multiple sclerosis patients resistant to conventional therapy. Mult Scler. 2001;7:185–8.

111. Smith DR, Weinstock-Guttman B, Cohen JA, et al. A randomized blinded trial of combination therapy with cyclophosphamide in patients-with active multiple sclerosis on interferon beta. Mult Scler. 2005;11:573–82.

112. Stillwell TJ, Benson Jr RC. Cyclophosphamide-induced hemorrhagic cystitis. A review of 100 patients. Cancer. 1988;61:451–7.

113. De Ridder D, van Poppel H, Demonty L, et al. Bladder cancer in patients with multiple sclerosis treated with cyclophosphamide. J Urol. 1998;159:1881–4.

114. Yudkin PL, Ellison GW, Ghezzi A, Goodkin DE, Hughes RA, McPherson K, et al. Overview of azathioprine treatment in multiple sclerosis. Lancet. 1991;338(8774):1051–5.

115. Casetta I, Iuliano G, Filippini G. Azathioprine for multiple sclerosis. Cochrane Database Syst Rev. 2007;(4):CD003982. Review.

116. Pulicken M, Bash CN, Costello K, Said A, Cuffari C, Wilterdink JL, et al. Optimization of the safety and efficacy of interferon beta 1b and azathioprine combination therapy in multiple sclerosis. Mult Scler. 2005;11(2):169–74.

117. Markovic-Plese S, Bielekova B, Kadom N, Leist TP, Martin R, Frank JA, et al. Longitudinal MRI study: the effects of azathioprine in MS patients refractory to interferon beta-1b. Neurology. 2003;60(11):1849–51.

118. Goodkin DE, Rudick RA, VanderBrug Mendendorp S, et al. Low dose (7.5 mg) oral methotrexate reduces the rate of progression in chronic progressive multiple sclerosis. Ann Neurol. 1995;37:30–40.

119. Cohen JA, Imrey PB, Calabresi PA, et al. Results of the Avonex Combination Trial (ACT) in relapsing-remitting MS. Neurology. 2009;72:535–41.

120. Becker BN. Mycophenolate mofetil. Transplant Proc. 1999;31:2777–8.

121. Tan T, Lawrance IC. Use of mycophenolate mofetil in inflammatory bowel disease. World J Gastroenterol. 2009;15(13):1594–9.

122. Tran GT, Carter N, Hodgkinson SJ. Mycophenolate mofetil treatment accelerates recovery from experimental allergic encephalomyelitis. Int Immunopharmacol. 2001;1(9–10):1709–23.

123. Vermersch P, Waucquier N, Michelin E, Bourteel H, Stojkovic T, Ferriby D. G-SEP. Combination of IFN beta-1a (Avonex) and mycophenolate mofetil (Cellcept) in multiple sclerosis. Eur J Neurol. 2007;14(1):85–9.

124. Hartung HP. Advances in the understanding of the mechanism of action of IVIg. J Neurol. 2008;255 Suppl 3:3–6.

125. Trebst C, Stangel M. Promotion of remyelination by immunoglobulins: implications for the treatment of multiple sclerosis. Curr Pharm Des. 2006;12(2):241–9.

126. Sørensen P, Fazekas F, Lee M. Intravenous immunoglobulin G for the treatment of relapsing-remitting multiple sclerosis: a meta-analysis. Eur J Neurol. 2002;9(6):557–63.

127. Fazekas F, Lublin FD, Li D, et al. Intravenous immunoglobulin in relapsing-remitting multiple sclerosis: a dose-finding trial. Neurology. 2008;71:265–71.

128. Hommes O, Soerensen P, Fazekas F, et al. Intravenous immunoglobulin in secondary progressive multiple sclerosis: randomised, placebo-controlled trial. Lancet. 2004;364:1149–56.

129. Achiron A, Kishner I, Sarova-Pinhas I, et al. Intravenous immunoglobulin treatment following the first demyelinating event suggestive of multiple sclerosis: a randomized, double-blind, placebo-controlled trial. Arch Neurol. 2004;61:1515–20.

130. Lin X, Turner B, Constantinescu C. Cerebral volume change in secondary progressive multiple sclerosis: effects of intravenous immunoglobulins. J Neurol. 2002;249:I/169.

131. Lehmann HC, Hartung HP, Hetzel GR, Stuve O, Kieseier BC. Plasma exchange in neuroimmunological disorders: Part 1: Rationale and treatment of inflammatory central nervous system disorders. Arch Neurol. 2006;63:930–5.

132. Weinshenker BG. Therapeutic plasma exchange for acute inflammatory demyelinating syndromes of the central nervous system. J Clin Apher. 1999;14:144–8.

133. Llufriu S, Castillo J, Blanco Y, Ramió-Torrentà L, Río J, Vallès M, et al. Plasma exchange for acute attacks of CNS demyelination: predictors of improvement at 6 months. Neurology. 2009;73:949–53.

134. Schilling S, Linker RA, Konig FB, Koziolek M, Bahr M, Muller GA, et al. Plasma exchange therapy for steroid-unresponsive multiple sclerosis relapses: clinical experience with 16 patients. Nervenarzt. 2006;77:430–8.

135. Bielekova B, Becker BL. Monoclonal antibodies in MS: mechanisms of action. Neurology. 2010;74 Suppl 1:S31–40.

136. Liossis SN, Sfikakis PP. Rituximab-induced B cell depletion in autoimmune diseases: potential effects on T cells. Clin Immunol. 2008;127:280–5.

137. Fanale MA, Younes A. Monoclonal antibodies in the treatment of non-Hodgkin's lymphoma. Drugs. 2007;67:333–50.
138. Schuna AA. Rituximab for the treatment of rheumatoid arthritis. Pharmacotherapy. 2007;27:1702–10.
139. Cree BA et al. An open label study of the effects of rituximab in neuromyelitis optica. Neurology. 2005;64:1270–2.
140. Pestronk A et al. Treatment of IgM antibody associated polyneuropathies using rituximab. J Neurol Neurosurg Psychiatry. 2003;74:485–9.
141. Hauser SL et al. B-cell depletion with rituximab in relapsing-remitting multiple sclerosis. N Engl J Med. 2008;358:676–88.
142. Cepok S et al. Short-lived plasma blasts are the main B cell effector subset during the course of multiple sclerosis. Brain. 2005;128:1667–76.
143. Qin Y et al. Intrathecal B-cell clonal expansion, an early sign of humoral immunity, in the cerebrospinal fluid of patients with clinically isolated syndrome suggestive of multiple sclerosis. Lab Invest. 2003;83:1081–8.
144. Stuve O et al. Clinical stabilization and effective B-lymphocyte depletion in the cerebrospinal fluid and peripheral blood of a patient with fulminant relapsing-remitting multiple sclerosis. Arch Neurol. 2005;62:1620–3.
145. Carson KR, Evens AM, Richey EA, Habermann TM, Focosi D, Seymour JF, et al. Progressive multifocal leukoencephalopathy after rituximab therapy in HIV-negative patients: a report of 57 cases from the Research on Adverse Drug Events and Reports project. Blood. 2009;113(20):4834–40.
146. Hutas G. Ocrelizumab, a humanized monoclonal antibody against CD20 for inflammatory disorders and B-cell malignancies. Curr Opin Investig Drugs. 2008;9(11):1206–15.
147. Flynn JM, Byrd JC. Campath-1H monoclonal antibody therapy. Curr Opin Oncol. 2000;12:574–81.
148. Coles AJ, Cox A, Le Page E, et al. The window of therapeutic opportunity in multiple sclerosis: evidence from monoclonal antibody therapy. J Neurol. 2006;253:98–108.
149. Coles A, Deans J, Compston A. Campath-1H treatment of multiple sclerosis: lessons from the bedside for the bench. Clin Neurol Neurosurg. 2004;106:270–4.
150. Fox E et al. Two-years results with alemtuzumab in patients with active relapsing-remitting multiple sclerosis who have failed licensed beta interferon therapies. Mult Scler. 2007;13:A558.
151. Coles AJ, Compston DA, Selmaj KW, Lake SL, Moran S, Margolin DH, et al. Alemtuzumab vs. interferon beta-1a in early multiple sclerosis. N Engl J Med. 2008;359(17):1786–801.
152. Goebel J, Stevens E, Forrest K, Roszman TL. Daclizumab (Zenapax) inhibits early interleukin-2 receptor signal transduction events. Transpl Immunol. 2000;8:153–9.
153. Bielekova B, Catalfamo M, Reichert-Scrivner S, et al. Regulatory CD56 bright natural killer cells mediate immunomodulatory effects of IL 2R{alpha}-targeted therapy (daclizumab) in multiple sclerosis. Proc Natl Acad Sci USA. 2006;103:5941–594696.
154. Bielekova B, Richert N, Howard T, et al. Humanized anti-CD25 (daclizumab) inhibits disease activity in multiple sclerosis patients failing to respond to interferon {beta}. Proc Natl Acad Sci USA. 2004;101:8705–8.
155. Rose JW, Burns JB, Bjorklund J, Klein J, Watt HE, Carlson NG. Daclizumab phase II trial in relapsing and remitting multiple sclerosis: MRI and clinical results. Neurology. 2007;69:785–9.
156. Sipe JC et al. Cladribine improves relapsing-remitting MS: a double blind, placebo controlled study. Neurology. 1997;48 Suppl 2:A340.
157. Sipe JC et al. Development of cladribine treatment in multiple sclerosis. Mult Scler. 1996;1:343–7.

158. Rice GP, Filippi M, Comi G. Cladribine and progressive MS: clinical and MRI outcomes of a multicenter controlled trial. Cladribine MRI Study Group. Neurology. 2000;54:1145–55.

159. Giovannoni G, Comi G, Cook S, Rammohan K, Rieckmann P, Sorensen PS, et al. A placebo-controlled trial of oral cladribine for relapsing multiple sclerosis. N Engl J Med. 2010;362:416.

160. O'Connor PW et al. A phase II study of the safety and efficacy of teriflunomide in multiple sclerosis with relapses. Teriflunomide Multiple Sclerosis Trial Group; University of British Columbia MS/MRI Research Group. Neurology. 2006;66:894–900.

161. Noseworthy JH, Wolinsky JS, Lublin FD, Whitaker JN, Linde A, Gjorstrup P, et al. Linomide in relapsing and secondary progressive MS: part I: trial design and clinical results. North American Linomide Investigators. Neurology. 2000;54(9):1726–33.

162. Polman C et al. Treatment with laquinimod reduces development of active MRI lesions in relapsing MS. Neurology. 2005;64:987–91.

163. Kappos L et al. BG00012, a novel oral fumarate, is effective in patients with relapsing-remitting multiple sclerosis. Mult Scler. 2006;12:A325.

164. Mancardi G, Saccardi R. Auto logous haematopoietic stem-cell transplantation in multiple sclerosis. Lancet Neurol. 2008;7:626–36.

165. Roccatagliata L, Rocca MA, Valsasina P, Bonzano L, Sormani MP, Saccardi R, et al. The long-term effect of AHSCT on MRI measures of MS evolution: a five year follow-up study. Mult Scler. 2007;13:1068–70.

166. Inglese M et al. Brain tissue loss occurs after suppression of enhancement in patients with multiple sclerosis treated with autologous haematopoietic stem cell transplantation. J Neurol Neurosurg Psychiatry. 2004;75:643–4.

167. Chen JT et al. Brain atrophy after immunoablation and stem cell transplantation in multiple sclerosis. Neurology. 2006;66:1935–7.

168. Freedman MS, Atkins HL, Azzarelli B, Kolar OJ, Brück W. Autologous haematopoietic stem cell transplantation fails to stop demyelination and neurodegeneration in multiple sclerosis. Brain. 2007;130:1254–62.

169. Perier O, Gregoire A. Electron microscopic features of multiple sclerosis. Brain. 1965;88:937–52.

170. Patrikios P, Stadelmann C, Kutzelnigg A, Rauschka H, Schmidbauer M, Laursen H, et al. Remyelination is extensive in a subset of multiple sclerosis patients. Brain. 2006;129:3165–72.

171. Ishibashi T, Dakin KA, Stevens B, Lee PR, Kozlov LV, Stewart CL, et al. Astrocytes promote myelination in response to electrical impulses. Neuron. 2006;49:823–32.

172. Hoffmann K, Lindner M, Stangel M, Löscher W. Epileptic seizures and hippocampal damage after cupri-zone-induced demyelination in C56BL/6 mice. Exp Neurol. 2008;210:308–21.

173. Su KG, Banker G, Bourdette D, Forte M. Axonal degeneration in multiple sclerosis: the mitochondrial hypothesis. Curr Neurol Neurosci Rep. 2009;9(5): 411–7. Review.

174. Mahad D, Ziabreva I, Lassmann H, Turnbull D. Mitochondrial defects in acute multiple sclerosis lesions. Brain. 2008;131(Pt 7):1722–35.

175. Metz LM, Zhang Y, Yeung M, Patry DG, Bell RB, Stoian CA, et al. Minocycline reduces gadolinium-enhancing magnetic resonance imaging lesions in multiple sclerosis. Ann Neurol. 2004;55:756.

176. Kalkers NF, Barkhof F, Bergers E, van Schijndel R, Polman CH. The effect of the neuroprotective agent riluzole on MRI parameters in patients with progressive multiple sclerosis: a pilot study. Mult Scler. 2002;8:532–3.

177. Warrington AE, Asakura K, Bieber AJ, Ciric B, Van Keulen V, Kaveri SV, et al. Human monoclonal antibodies reactive to oligodendrocytes promote remyelination in a model of multiple sclerosis. Proc Natl Acad Sci USA. 2000;97:6820–5.

178. Ehrenreich H, Fischer B, Norra C, Schellenberger F, Stender N, Stiefel M, et al. Exploring human recombinant erythropoietin in chronic progressive multiple sclerosis. Brain. 2007;130:2577–88.
179. Frank JA, Richert N, Lewis B, Bash C, Howard T, Civil R, et al. A pilot study of recombinant insulin-like growth factor-1 in seven multiple sclerosis patients. Mult Scler. 2002;8:24–9.
180. Waxman SG. Mechanisms of disease: sodium channels and neuroprotection in multiple sclerosis-current status. Nat Clin Pract Neurol. 2008;4:159–69.
181. Leary SM, Miller DH, Stevenson VL, et al. Interferon beta-1a in primary progressive MS: an exploratory, randomized, controlled trial. Neurology. 2003;60: 44–51.

Pediatric Multiple Sclerosis

Lauren Krupp, Yashma Patel, and Vikram Bhise

Keywords: Optic neuritis, Initial demyclinating event, Cognition, Fatigue, Prognosis

Introduction

Pediatric multiple sclerosis (MS) has long been an under-recognized MS subgroup. Fortunately, the special diagnostic challenges, the clinical course, treatment, and special needs of this MS subgroup are receiving increased attention. Pediatric MS occurs in most of the world although the frequency varies. Differential diagnoses such as the distinction from acute disseminated encephalomyelitis (ADEM) differ from adults. The pathogenic mechanisms remain unclear with respect to pediatric MS. The strongest association of pediatric MS is with remote EBV infection, possibly reflecting heightened immune activation or reactivation of EBV. Certain clinical aspects of pediatric MS overlap with adults but there are often differences particularly in the younger children in clinical, radiologic, and laboratory manifestations. Unfortunately, there is a sizable proportion of children and adolescents who are very vulnerable to cognitive dysfunction in addition to other psychosocial stresses. The family unit is critically important in this age group and plays a different role than in adult MS. Management is complicated by the lack of clinical trials specific to children. Nonetheless, experience in evaluating and treating children has rapidly grown. The current review summarizes this experience.

Demographic Profile

Children before the age of 16 represent an estimated 2.7–5% of individuals with MS [1–4]. Among the youngest children (age 10 and younger), the frequency is much lower estimated to occur in 0.2–0.7% of cases [5–9]. In many studies which estimate prevalence, the data was collected retrospectively. Given the limitations of retrospective research, the reliability of the findings

From: *Clinical Neuroimmunology: Multiple Sclerosis and Related Disorders*, Current Clinical Neurology,
Edited by: S.A. Rizvi and P.K. Coyle, DOI 10.1007/978-1-60327-860-7_8,
© Springer Science+Business Media, LLC 2011

will need to be confirmed with more prospective studies. One prospective study of initial demyelinating events (IDE) of childhood found an incidence of 0.9% [10].

As in young adults with MS, pediatric MS displays an overall female preponderance. However, the gender ratio varies with the age of onset. In children with an onset of before 6 years, the female-to-male ratio is almost equal at 0.8:1. For an onset of between 6 and 10 years the ratio is 1.6:1, and for an onset over 10 years it is 2:1 [11]. The significant increase in the female preponderance in adolescence implies a hormonal influence on the risk of MS. A positive family history of MS among children with the disease ranges from 6 to 20% of individuals [1, 12].

The demographic findings in pediatric MS may differ from adults with MS. In an outpatient center in Boston, there was a higher proportion of African-Americans (AA) in the pediatric onset compared with the adult onset MS group (7.4% vs. 4.3%) [8]. AA pediatric MS cases may have a more severe presentation and course compared with Caucasians [13]. Demographic differences between pediatric and adult MS have been reported in other areas of North America as well. Among a sample seen at the Pediatric MS Center on Long Island in New York, a higher proportion of individuals of AA race, Hispanic ethnicity, and first generation Americans were present compared with adults with MS and other pediatric neurologic controls seen at the Center [14].

Risks for Developing MS

One of the most challenging aspects of pediatric MS is determining whether a child with an IDE will develop subsequent events consistent with MS or whether the IDE will remain a self-limited disorder such as an isolated optic neuritis (ON) or an isolated episode of ADEM.

Several studies from a variety of countries have addressed these issues. Table 8.1 summarizes IDE features suggestive of an ultimate diagnosis of MS [15–17]. A prospective study of 296 pediatric IDE patients found that after a mean observation period of 2.9 years, 57% experienced two or more episodes of demyelination [17]. Factors associated with an increased risk for a second

Table 8.1 Features of an initial demyelinating event of childhood which suggest subsequent attack consistent with MS.

ON
Monofocal onset
Family history of CNS demyelination
Intrathecal oligoclonal bands
Elevated IgG index
Absence of preceding infection
Absence of encephalopathy
Absence of seizures
Absence of meningismus or fever
MRI suggestive of MS

attack and an outcome of MS included age over 10 years, family history of CNS demyelination, optic neuritis, lack of change in mental status, and lack of isolated myelitis [18, 19]. Among a group of 52 children with an IDE followed for a mean of 5½ years, encephalopathy at presentation was absent from the 30% who developed MS further reinforcing the favorable prognosis when this finding is present. While, in general, a change in mental status goes along with a self-limited event, this is not a universal finding. As noted in the study from the Netherlands, there were patients with self-limited disease, i.e., ADEM who lacked encephalopathy [16].

As shown in Table 8.1, additional features suggestive of future MS following an IDE include a monofocal rather than polyfocal onset, absence of seizures, and lack of meningismus. In contrast, children who went on to develop MS are more likely to have in the cerebral spinal fluid (CSF) positive oligoclonal bands (OCB) and are more than twice as likely to have elevated IgG index 66% vs. 27% in the CSF [15–17, 20].

As with adults, pediatric ON when associated with an abnormal brain magnetic resonance imaging (MRI) is associated with an increased likelihood of MS [21]. In one prospective study of 36 patients with ON and abnormal brain MRI, a high proportion (36%) of children with ON were diagnosed with MS after a mean of 2.4 years [22]. The second attack confirming MS after childhood ON may occur many years after the initial attack and with time the risk of MS increases [16, 23]. Whether bilateral ON increases the risk of MS more than unilateral ON remains unclear [21, 24].

A number of MRI findings are closely associated with MS. The Barkhof criteria include the following features: ≥9 T2 lesions or ≥1 gadolinium enhancing lesion, ≥3 periventricular lesions, ≥1 juxtacortical lesion, ≥1 infratentorial or spinal cord lesion. The presence of at least three of these criteria is associated with an increased risk of MS in both adults and children [25]. Other criteria have also been established which increases the risk of a subsequent diagnosis of MS. The KIDMUS study from France found that the presence of one or more lesions perpendicular to the long axis of the corpus callosum and the sole presence of well-defined lesions were associated with increased MS risk [26]. A different set of criteria (Callen criteria) were established to distinguish MS from non-demyelinating disorders [27]. The Callen criteria require a minimum of two of the following: ≥5 T2 lesions, ≥2 periventricular lesions, or ≥1 brainstem lesion. Both Barkhof and KIDMUS MRI criteria share a high specificity and have a high positive predictive value for conversion to MS [27].

Clinical Features

Children can present with a variety of symptoms including ON, sensory deficits, weakness, gait disorders, and brainstem-related dysfunction. They are commonly polysymptomatic (50–70%), though a monosymptomatic (30–50%) presentation is not uncommon [7, 17, 28]. Of the children with a monosymptomatic presentation, 30% will have motor symptoms, 30% sensory symptoms, 25% brainstem symptoms, 10–22% present with ON, and 5–15% with ataxia [7, 28–30]. Isolated transverse myelitis is seen in less than 10% [1, 4, 17] and ADEM as an initial presentation of pediatric onset MS is seen in as high as 18–29% [11, 16, 17, 19, 20, 31]. Seizures are estimated to occur in 5% [30].

Visual evoked potentials were found to be abnormal retrospectively in 56% of 85 patients in whom only 40% had visual complaints in the past. Thus, ON may be underreported in pediatric MS especially in younger children who often have difficulties in verbalizing this symptom or who have not yet started to read [32].

Several clinical features differ from among the younger (usually 10 and under) relative to the postpubertal or adolescent MS patients. Younger patients have more seizures, more frequent ON, more brainstem or cerebellar involvement, and less spinal cord presentations. Younger patients also have more confluent disease on MRI and lesions that tend to vanish more quickly [11, 15, 33–35]. A study found that those under the age of 12 compared with those older than 12 years had a longer relapse-free interval and lower number of relapses in the first 2 years [6]. In children under the age of 10, the Barkhof criteria had a higher sensitivity than the KIDMUS criteria, but still lower than in older children [16, 26]. CSF in younger children is less often oligoclonal band positive and has a high proportion of neutrophils [36].

Fatigue is a consistent problem and has been reported in 40–70% of pediatric MS patients [37, 38]. A fatigue scale designed for children and adolescents showed that over half the children with pediatric MS reported fatigue and three quarters of their parents described fatigue in their children [39]. Using the fatigue severity scale (FSS), the frequency of fatigue was lower in children with MS [38]. Fatigue can be severe and can interfere with completing homework, performing well in school, and getting to classes in a timely fashion.

Mood disorders are another issue which requires special attention. In 12 patients who underwent psychiatric evaluation, almost half were diagnosed with depression or an anxiety disorder [40]. Using self-report measures, others have found low levels of depressive symptoms in children with MS [38]. Overall, health care providers should be attentive to changes in school performance and the possibility of depression or anxiety.

Children appear to be exceptionally vulnerable to cognitive disability. The most common impairments are found in complex attention, visuomotor integration, confrontation naming, receptive language, and executive function [40]. Verbal fluency tends to be relatively intact. One finding has been that duration of disease is associated with greater impairments [41]. In a more comprehensive study, 53% of the MS group failed at least two tests and 31% failed three tests of an extensive neuropsychological battery consisting of the following domains: intelligence quotient (IQ), verbal learning, visuospatial learning, attention and concentration, abstract reasoning, expressive language, and receptive language. These results showed significant cognitive dysfunction in pediatric MS relative to healthy controls though the only predictor was IQ [38]. Others have found that almost one-third of children with pediatric MS had deficits relative to normative samples [40]. Comprehensive longitudinal studies are required to determine the progression of cognitive deficits in children. Unfortunately, one small study of children on disease modifying therapy (DMT) found that declines over short periods such as 1–2 years are common [42] and this was further confirmed by a larger Italian study which suggested that as many as 70% of children decline in cognitive ability over 2 years [42, 43]. This is in contrast to adults where cognitive decline is more gradual.

Prognosis

Over time, children with MS develop repeated relapses and accumulate increasing disability. Annual relapse rates vary in different studies from 0.5 to 2.8 depending on differences in design (prospective vs. retrospective) and duration of follow-up [2, 8, 44, 45]. Overall, when compared with adults, children with MS have a higher rate of relapse within the first 2 years of disease but progress more gradually [7, 29, 33].

Overall, with increasing time disability accumulates and in one prospective study of 54 children, the mean EDSS was 3.8 after a period of 10 years. In several retrospective studies, the time to reach an EDSS of 6.0 from diagnosis varied from 19 to 29 years [6, 12]. The time to secondary progression in pediatric patients is twice as long as in adult patients. The mean duration associated with 50% risk of conversion to secondary progressive MS is 23 years in pediatric RR patients compared with 10 years in adult onset RR patients [6]. The risk of secondary progressive MS is associated with a higher frequency of relapses and shorter intervals between attacks in the first few years of disease [2, 7].

Certain characteristics are associated with a more severe prognosis. These include female sex, less than 1-year time interval to second attack, the absence of encephalopathy at disease onset, and secondary progressive disease. MRIs showing well-defined lesions or lesions perpendicular to the corpus callosum are also associated with a more severe prognosis [33]. In one prospective study which followed 197 children from the onset of their first MS attack, severe disease outcome was defined by the occurrence of a third MS attack or an EDSS of more than four which persisted for more than 12 months. Within the mean observation period of 5.5 years, severe disease outcome was recorded in 144/197 (73%) patients [33]. In other studies, the accumulation of disability within the first year of disease onset or a high frequency of relapses within the first 2 years of onset has been associated with higher EDSS scores [29].

Differential Diagnosis

Dissemination in time and space are essential features to the diagnosis of MS, as well as absence of non-neurological involvement or systemic disease. Numerous diseases may still mimic MS. Lesion pattern and distribution on MRI as well as clinical course and risk factors should be carefully taken into account to help exclude these diseases. Below is an overview of some of the more common disorders which need to be considered in the differential diagnosis of MS in children.

ADEM

The IDE of MS can be perhaps the most difficult diagnosis to differentiate from ADEM. As shown in Table 8.2, there are certain clinical, CSF, and radiological features more in favor of ADEM compared with MS. ADEM presents with multiple CNS lesions corresponding to neurological deficits, due to a post- or parainfectious demyelinating process [46]. Pathologically, ADEM represents a more localized pathological process with limited focal demyelination focused

Table 8.2 Features more common in ADEM versus MS.

Clinical	Younger age group (<10 years)
	Recent viral infection or vaccination
	Encephalopathy/meningismus
	Bulbar symptoms
	Seizures
	Single event which can fluctuate over 12 weeks
CSF	Pleocytosis
	Elevated protein
	No oligoclonal bands
MRI	Diffuse large bilateral lesions
	White and gray matter involvement
	Normal appearing white matter (NAWM) intact
	No T1 black holes
	Lesions typically resolve

in a perivenular location with macrophages and lymphocytes. In contrast, the multifocal demyelination in MS is more confluent and extensive with more macrophages [47]. Consistent with the pathology, on neuroimaging using magnetization transfer, the normal appearing white matter (NAWM) appears intact in ADEM where it is not in MS [48].

The International Pediatric MS Consensus definitions provide provisional diagnostic criteria for MS, ADEM, and other acquired demyelinating disorders of the central nervous system (CNS) [49]. The criteria for ADEM require multifocality and encephalopathy; however, this definition is likely to be too restrictive as some multifocal non-encephalopathic patients have a self-limited disease course as would occur in ADEM [16]. ADEM often includes prominent involvement of both white and gray matter on brain MRI. Rarely, a second inflammatory event may be seen in ADEM variants such as recurrent ADEM or multiphasic ADEM. However, unlike an MS attack, encephalopathy is present and the MRI shows characteristic features of ADEM as described below. The disease is subsequently self-limited without further events after the second episode [34, 49].

In a retrospective chart review study, comparing ADEM and MS, patients with ADEM were more likely to have nonspecific symptoms such as fever, headache, vomiting, meningismus, encephalopathy, and bulbar symptoms such as dysarthria and dysphagia [50]. A history of recent viral illness or vaccination usually is elicited in ADEM. Other important features include seizures, cranial neuropathies, and optic neuritis [15, 16, 51]. CSF studies tend to show a mild leukocytosis, elevated protein, and a lower frequency of OCB compared with MS.

Typically, the MRI in ADEM demonstrates multifocal lesions with indistinct margins distributed throughout the cerebral gray and white matters. Additional MRI features favoring ADEM are the presence of diffuse bilateral lesions, lack of two or more periventricular lesions, and lack of black holes. Efforts have been made to more formally distinguish MS and ADEM radiologically [52].

Differentiating ADEM from MS is a particular challenge in youngsters under 10 years. In this subgroup, even though the children are destined to have MS sometimes their initial MRI picture closely resembles ADEM. Often time and subsequent changes on MRI or clinical course reveal the correct diagnosis [53].

In the absence of a specific biomarker for either ADEM or MS, assessment of the paraclinical data and clinical course remain the most critical tools for the distinction.

Neuromyelitis Optica

Another inflammatory disorder of the CNS that can mimic MS is neuromyelitis optica (NMO), formerly referred to as Devic's disease. The criteria for the diagnosis require optic neuritis and transverse myelitis and either a longitudinally extensive lesion on spinal cord MRI or a positive NMO-IgG antibody titer [49]. The presence of brain involvement is not uncommon in children and does not exclude the diagnosis [54]. This disorder is discussed in detail in a separate chapter.

Infection and Other Disorders

Fever and CSF leukocytosis are the hallmarks of encephalitic or meningoencephalitic infectious processes in patients with acute presentations. CNS Lyme disease may manifest with multifocal white matter lesions and rarely a seemingly relapsing/remitting clinical course. Other infections to exclude would be HIV encephalomyelitis, HTLV-1, neurosyphilis, progressive multifocal leukoencephalopathy (PML), Whipple's disease, and subacute sclerosing panencephalitis.

Vascular and Inflammatory Disorders

CNS vasculitis and other autoimmune disorders can be difficult to distinguish from MS. The presence of systemic signs, abnormal serology, or beading on cerebral angiogram can suggest the diagnosis, as can elevated C-reactive protein or erythrocyte sedimentation rate (ESR). Unfortunately, in cases of isolated CNS vasculitis, the differential diagnosis is more difficult as there may be no laboratory or systemic abnormalities. In these cases, brain biopsy might establish the correct diagnosis. Autoimmune disorders such as systemic lupus erythematosus (SLE), Behçet disease, neurosarcoidosis, Sjogren's disease, and isolated CNS vasculitis can also present a varied, multifocal neurological clinical picture during or at the onset of disease. Vascular diseases mimicking MS in younger individuals are fortunately rare and would include moyamoya disease and cerebral autosomal dominant arteriopathy with subcortical infarcts and leukoencephalopathy (CADASIL). Other inflammatory disorders to distinguish from MS include macrophage activation syndrome (MAS) and Langerhans cell histiocytosis. MAS may resemble MS but most often affects very young children (usually 2 years old) and tends to have systemic involvement. This disorder may be related to hemophagocytic lymphohistiocytosis and consanguinity is not uncommon in these cases.

Neoplasms

Tumefactive presentation of MS on neuroimaging may mimic intracranial neoplasms, particularly CNS lymphoma [55, 56]. MRS studies performed along with routine MRI might help in the differential diagnosis in these instances.

Leukodystrophies

The leukodystrophies are another diagnostic group to consider when evaluating pediatric MS patients. They can be subdivided into myelination failure, delay, or breakdown, as well as those associated with malformations. Typical features are bilateral symmetric involvement of the white matter on MRI in a fairly homogenous manner. Adrenoleukodystrophy and adrenomyeloneuropathy tend to show preferential involvement of posterior head regions, namely the peritrigonal white matter, splenium of the corpus callosum, posterior limb of the internal capsule, the crus cerebri, and the cerebellar white matter [56].

Macrocrania with white matter dystrophy suggests either Alexander disease or Canavan disease. Early involvement of cortical U-fibers, as well as focal cystic changes on MRI is characteristic of Canavan disease, particularly in the Ashkenazi Jewish population. Alexander disease exhibits preference for frontal white matter, subependymal areas, and heads of the caudate nuclei, as well as widened lateral ventricles, sylvian fissures, and subarachnoid spaces. While the infantile onset of leukodystrophies is usually clearly differentiated from MS, those with a juvenile onset can overlap. For example, in juvenile cases of Alexander disease, the posterior fossa may be preferentially involved and the bilateral frontal white matter involvement less conspicuous. Persistent contrast enhancement can also occur [57]. A case of Pelizaeus Merzbacher has been described which overlapped considerably with MS both on clinical and radiologic manifestations. The patient's relapsing neurological problems were steroid responsive and the MRI showed features typical of MS. Further, the CSF was positive for OCB. The marked nystagmus led to testing of the proteolipid 1 protein abnormality and the correct diagnosis [58]. In general, progressive cognitive decline (as was present in the Pelizaeus Merzbacher case) is typical for the leukodystrophies but extremely rare in MS. The onset of a progressive course (such as Primary Progressive MS) represents only 1–3% of pediatric MS.

Degenerative and metabolic diseases can rarely mimic MS and include metachromatic leukodystrophy, Krabbe disease, Refsum disease, vanishing white matter disease, Wilson's disease, Fabry disease, vitamin B12 deficiency, folate deficiency, vitamin E deficiency, and celiac disease.

Mitochondrial Disorders

Mitochondrial disorders can also present with a relapsing pattern of events, but the course is typically progressive over time. Basal ganglia or brain stem involvement on MRI are good clues for the diagnosis of a mitochondrial disorder, such as Leigh syndrome. Further red flags, such as visual loss, bilateral hearing deficit, short stature, ophthalmoplegia (Kearns-Sayre), cardiac involvement (Kearns-Sayre), stroke-like events (MELAS), or myoclonic epilepsy (MERRF) can help hone in on the specific cytopathy.

Diagnostic Testing

A standard diagnostic evaluation beyond imaging and CSF should include: CBC, ESR, and ANA, while extended testing might include Lyme antibody titers, MR angiography, MR spectroscopy, evoked potentials, CSF lactate/

pyruvate, serum vitamin levels (B12, D, E, folate), anti-Ro, anti-La, serum angiotensin-converting enzyme, HIV, rapid plasma reagin, HTLV-1, serum EBV and mycoplasma titers, and NMO antibody. Many diagnosticians opt for an extended evaluation, particularly for diseases that are easily tested or amenable to treatment. Further laboratory testing for specific disorders in the differential diagnosis is more thoroughly reviewed elsewhere [56, 59].

Pathogenesis

Immunological, environmental, and genetic factors contribute to the development of MS in the pediatric age range as they do for adults. Certain epidemiologic associations suggest that molecular mimicry might lead to immune activation increasing MS risk. Exposure to remote EBV infection is more common among children who develop MS compared with a variety of controls including those with type 1 diabetes mellitus and other neurologic disorders [31]. Possible explanations include increased immune activation to the virus or reactivation of EBV infection. Other viruses have had variable associations or lack thereof with pediatric MS. For example, clinical infection with varicella is associated with a decreased relative risk of MS in one study but not in another [31, 60].

Vaccination has also been examined as a risk factor for the development of MS. The use of hepatitis vaccine is not associated with an increased risk of acute demyelinating events [61]. However, in a subgroup analysis, the most compliant patient group (with respect to vaccinations) had an increased MS risk if they had past vaccination with a particular brand of Hepatitis B vaccine (Engerix B). Another risk factor associated with pediatric MS is passive exposure to smoking [62]. The basis for this association is not known, but the authors speculate that toxins could lead to blood brain barrier breakdown, immune activation, or direct effect on the CNS.

In addition to the analysis of the role of viral infection or passive smoke exposure, the immune response to a variety of autoantigens has also been studied. There is no apparent difference in the response to myelin basic protein (MBP) among adult or pediatric cases [63]. In contrast, adults with MS more frequently have T-cell reactivity than children in their response to pancreatic antigens [64]. These differences in a more generalized non-organ-specific immune response may develop with increasing disease duration. Additional research will need not only to focus on the differences between pediatric and adult MS and the distinctions from other neurological or autoimmune controls, but also examine how immune activation fails to become a chronic disorder in ADEM as it does with pediatric MS.

Treatment

Communicating the Diagnosis

Being told of the diagnosis of MS can be traumatic for the patient and family. That the prognosis is uncertain and the condition rare contributes to the difficulty the family faces in adjustment. A number of considerations should go into the process of conveying the diagnosis. It is important to emphasize to the family that they are not alone and that online social network groups, support groups, and literature specific to the topic of pediatric MS are available. The National Multiple Sclerosis Society has programs for the families of children or teens with MS, and teen adventure summer programs or camps have been established in North America (see www.pediatricmscenter.org).

While conveying the diagnosis, the importance of treatment designed to modify the disease course can be emphasized. The rapid rate of progress in our understanding and in treatment options offers much hope.

Management of Relapses

The usual treatment for an acute relapse is with doses of parenteral methylprednisolone ranging from 10 to 30 mg/kg/day. In most instances, the maximum dose is 1,000 mg administered intravenously (IV) once daily in the morning for 3–5 days. An oral prednisone taper is optional. An alternative to IV corticosteroids is high-dose oral prednisone (same dose as IV therapy) which in adults may be as effective as IV treatment [65] and seems effective in managing acute relapses [66]. High-dose oral prednisone (up to 1,200 mg/day) has also been found to have good bioavailability compared with intravenous therapy [67]. However, high-dose prednisone has only been used in adults with MS and is untested in children or adolescents. Adverse effects of steroids such as insomnia, mood disturbance including psychosis, hyperglycemia, and hypertension need to be monitored. Prolonged steroid use can also possibly retard growth in youngsters. Despite its long-term risks, short courses of steroid therapy are reasonably safe and well tolerated by most children.

Plasmapheresis or intravenous immunoglobulins (IVIG) are options when IV steroids fail to improve a severe relapse. The use of either modality is based on its success in a limited number of cases of children or adults [68, 69]. Treatment with plasmapheresis is a consideration as it has been safely done on children with other immune-mediated disorders [69]. Alternatively, IVIG treatment can be used at a dose of 0.4 g/kg/day for 5 days and continued 1 day/month at 0.4 g/kg. This therapeutic approach has been studied in only small samples of ADEM and its variants [70, 71].

Treatment with Disease Modifying Therapy

Multiple studies have demonstrated the use of DMT in pediatric MS to be well tolerated. To the extent that efficacy can be established in the absence of placebo-controlled trials, the body of evidence supports treatment. In contrast, pediatric patients with an IDE and features highly suggestive of MS have not been studied with respect to treatment.

Overview of DMT

The bulk of studies demonstrating treatment efficacy is drawn from comparisons of pretreatment relapse frequency to that during treatment. However, a comparison of untreated to treated patients also favored treatment. In this study, 197 pediatric MS patients were followed after their MS defining event for a mean of 5.5 years. A total of 24 began interferon therapy a mean of 3.6 months after their relapse, whereas 73 remained untreated. Those treated had a relative reduction in relapses over the subsequent first 2 years on therapy with a hazard ratio of 0.40, $p < 0.01$. However, over the 4 years of follow-up, the benefit was less apparent [72].

IFN β-1a Intramuscular

IFN β-1a intramuscular (IM) injection at a dose of 30 μg once weekly is usually well tolerated in children with MS. In the largest study to date, a total of 53 children under the age of 16 were started on therapy and followed for a mean of 43±20 months [73]. Of this group, 19 discontinued treatment. Reasons for discontinuing were most often due to a switch to a possibly more effective therapy ($n=13$). The most common adverse events were similar to adults and included flu-like symptoms (33%), headache (29%), and myalgia (21%). Laboratory abnormalities were in most cases transient and most commonly included leukopenia, which was persistent in one patient and led to discontinuation. Overall, persistent adverse events developed in only 8%. For the total group, there was a drop in relapse rate from pretreatment to during therapy of 1.9–0.4 [73]. Similar positive treatment effects with IFN β-1a IM were noted in a small placebo-controlled study ($n=16$) which showed improvement in IFN β-1a IM relative to placebo over a 48-month period [74]. Others have also found good tolerability and improved relapse rate with treatment [75, 76].

The standard adult dose of 30 μg, IM once per week has been used effectively even in some children 10 years old and under. In our experience, a slow gradual titration of IFN β-1a IM is usually best tolerated. Depending on the age of the child, we have used the following schedule: ¼ dose×2–4 weeks, followed by ½ dose×2–4 weeks, followed by ¾ dose×2–4 weeks, and then the full dose. (The volume to be injected depends upon whether the prefilled or lyophilized form is being used.) The same injection sites used for adults can be used in children. In one case where the family of a 5-year-old girl misunderstood the instructions and on the first day of treatment injected a full dose, marked vomiting occurred for a day. Once the titration schedule was initiated, she tolerated the medication well but because of her small size did not go beyond a ½ dose.

Interferon β-1a Subcutaneous

Interferon β-1a subcutaneous (SC) injection has been administered to MS patients in the pediatric age range also with good effect. Among 51 children under the age of 16 begun on IFN β-1a SC therapy, treatment was well tolerated [44]. Six patients withdrew due to adverse events, two patients due to injection phobia, and one from suspected lack of efficacy. The mean annual relapse rate decreased from 1.9 prior to the initiation of therapy to 0.8. Adverse events were usually mild flu-like symptoms (65%) and laboratory changes similar to those reported in adults which included elevated transaminases (35%) and leukopenia (27%) [44]. Smaller studies of interferon β-1a SC have also noted good tolerability [73, 76, 77].

In a study of 24 children with a mean age of 9 who were treated for an average of 40 months, IFN β-1a SC was associated with two serious adverse events (arthritis and suicide attempt). More commonly side effects are minor. Among the 24 children studied these included flu-like symptoms (58%), myalgia (17%), and injection site reactions (75%) [77]. EDSS was decreased among children under 10 years old during therapy compared with pretreatment levels [77]. In the author's experience, the one serious adverse event that developed was with a teenager who continued to self-inject in an area of skin breakdown, developing a severe cellulitis which ultimately required skin grafts. Fortunately, the vast majority of children do extremely well with IFN β-1a SC. However, as is the case for all therapies, close monitoring of compliance and adverse events as well as laboratory testing is necessary.

The standard dose for IFN β-1a SC for children can be the same as adults: 44 μg three times a week with a minimum of 48 h between each dose. However, one study used 22 μg three times a week with good tolerability. The dosing schedule of IFN β-1a SC is somewhat simplified by the availability of different sized doses. For children depending on their age, we escalate at 8.8 μg three times a week × 2–4 weeks, 22 μg three times a week × 2–4 weeks, and 44 μg thereafter at three times a week.

Interferon β-1b

A multicenter collaborative effort to examine experience with IFN β-1b SC was completed among 43 individuals who all started on therapy prior to their 18th birthday [78]. There were no serious adverse events. Flu-like symptoms (35%), elevated LFTs (25%), and injection site reactions (21%) were the most frequent side effects. Most of the side effects were similar to those seen in adult MS patients. Only one patient discontinued treatment due to an adverse event: an injection site reaction. However, some patients switched to different therapies or failed to continue therapy due to poor adherence or continued disease progression [78].

This overall positive experience regarding ability to tolerate IFN β-1b SC is also supported by a case report [79]. One 7-year-old boy who experienced multiple relapses between ages 3 and 7 was started on IFN β-1b SC and tolerated the medication well. No subsequent relapses occurred during the 3-year follow-up period and there were no serious adverse events [79].

The standard dose of IFN β-1b SC is 1.0 cc (0.25 mg), self-administered every other day. It is important to titrate gradually and to monitor for adverse events and laboratory changes during this process. One approach is to begin a dose of ¼ cc × 2–4 weeks, followed by ½ cc × 2–4 weeks, followed by ¾ cc × 2–4 weeks, and then titrated to the full dose. The same injection sites used for adults can be used in children. There are no known drug interactions with the IFNs. The concurrent use of steroids and symptomatic therapies were not associated with adverse events in any of the adult clinical trials or pediatric studies.

Glatiramer Acetate

Glatiramer acetate (GA) represents another treatment option which has an advantage in that it does not require laboratory monitoring and is not associated with flu-like symptoms as possible adverse events. However, this advantage is somewhat counterbalanced by the need for daily SC administration, and as with the IFNs there exists a possibility of injection site reactions. In a web-based survey supported by Teva Neuroscience of MS patients, 96 subjects reported that they were 18 years or younger. Of these 96 individuals, 84 (88%) were prescribed a DMT. GA was the most frequently prescribed medication in 51% of respondents followed by IFN β-1a IM (28%). Only one patient on GA reported discontinuation due to side effects. A total of 86% of individuals were started on DMT within 6 months of diagnosis [80].

In a study of seven patients between ages 9 and 16 who were treated with GA, all tolerated the medication well at standard doses and without escalation. A total of 2/7 remained relapse free during a 2-year follow-up period while on treatment. The median pre-treatment relapse rate of 4 (range 2–6) dropped to 1 (range 0–4) the year following treatment and to 0 (range 0–4) in the subsequent year [81]. In another study examining children on different DMTs, there were seven patients treated with GA who were under the age of 16 [45]. In this group, the annual relapse rate decreased from 2.5 to 1.0 after mean treatment duration of 14.7 months [45]. The experience with GA is less well documented in pediatric MS compared with the other DMTs. However, the adult experience is informative. In controlled clinical trials of adults, the most commonly observed adverse experiences associated with the use of GA were: injection site reactions, vasodilation, chest pain, asthenia, infection, pain, nausea, arthralgia, anxiety, and hypertonia. These side effects have also been reported in children.

Dosing of GA for children is the same as in adults which is 1 cc SC (20 mg) daily and can be initiated at full dose from the onset of treatment. There are no known drug interactions with glatiramer acetate. The concurrent use of steroids and symptomatic therapies were not associated with adverse events in the pivotal clinical trials. GA is contraindicated in patients with known hypersensitivity to GA or mannitol.

Natalizumab in Pediatric MS

Several children treated with natalizumab have been reported [82, 83]. Patients were 12–13 years at the time of therapy and had failed first-line DMTs (interferons and glatiramer acetate). A dose of 5 mg/kg of body weight was administered with decrease in disease activity and in three patients in whom it was recorded, improved quality of life. All patients tolerated the treatment well, but none at the time of the report had been followed for more than 24 months. The potential development of PML remains a substantial concern in choosing this treatment option.

Breakthrough Disease

Unfortunately, many children treated with first-line DMTs experience break through disease and need to be switched to either another first-line treatment or second-line therapies. In a preliminary study of 164 treated children, 25% had breakthrough disease with initial DMT. Of these, eight children were switched to chemotherapy, two went on natalizumab, and two were treated with pulse IVIG [84].

Cyclophosphamide appears effective in children who are refractory to first-line treatments. In a recent study of 17 pediatric onset patients, annualized relapse rates decreased from 3.8 to 1.1 per year after 1 year of treatment. However, adverse events included bladder carcinoma in one patient and idiopathic thrombocytopenic purpura (ITP) in another [85].

Treatment Adherence

Compliance requires the family, patient, and physician to jointly acknowledge the disease and treatment. Poor adherence can result from poor family dynamics, limited education about the disease, and incomplete understanding of the purpose of therapy. Among older children, responsibility shifts from the parents toward the adolescent. However, teens for which there is parental involvement have better compliance [76]. Reasons for poor adherence among teens include: anger, loss of control, or failure to recognize that the therapy is designed to alter the disease course rather than provide symptomatic relief. Interventions to increase adherence to DMT include open discussions with the patient and parents, review of the treatment options including side effect profiles, and balancing the teen's need for autonomy with parental preference.

Symptom Management

There are no specific studies of symptomatic management in pediatric MS. Therefore, most of the following suggestions are based on adult studies and anecdotal reports. Most of the common MS symptoms associated with adult MS also occur in children [86]. These include problems with fatigue, cognitive impairment, mood disturbance, paroxysmal spasms, bladder/bowel dysfunction, and motor impairments.

Fatigue

While there are no studies addressing treatment of fatigue in pediatric MS, there are a few clinical trials examining the efficacy of fatigue therapies in adults with MS [87–92]. The most numerous address the role of amantadine, but a recent Cochrane database review concluded that there is inadequate data to address the efficacy of this agent for fatigue [93]. Studies concerning modafinil have yielded conflicting results [94, 95]. However, given the frequency of sleep problems in MS, it is not surprising that this agent might be effective for some patients with MS-related fatigue. Non-pharmacologic approaches include exercise, conservation of energy, improved sleep hygiene, and rescheduling the more demanding academic activities in the early morning when fatigue is often less severe. On the other hand, keeping children and teens socially engaged and involved in sports activities to the extent possible are important to self-image. Often, parents need reassurance that sports are appropriate for MS.

Cognition

There are a few studies demonstrating consistent benefits with either pharmacologic or non-pharmacologic interventions for cognitive deficits in adults. However, no studies have been done in children. Among adults, a randomized control clinical trial demonstrated that donepezil 10 mg/day was associated with improved memory [96]. Whether or not such treatment should be considered in cognitively impaired children is unknown. Cognitive rehabilitation has shown some benefits on overall cognitive functioning in adults with MS [97] but has not been studied in children.

Depression

The use of antidepressant therapy has not been examined in children with pediatric MS but has been studied in children with major depression [98]. The one agent with the most consistent benefit is fluoxetine. The usual dose ranges from 10 to 40 mg [98]. The other selective serotonin reuptake inhibitors (SSRIs) have shown less consistent results [98]. While there is a risk of suicide in teenagers treated for depression, the risk of untreated depression is also severe. Some untreated as well as treated children are severely depressed to the point of expressing suicidal ideation and have required psychiatric hospitalization.

Urinary/Bowel Dysfunction

Urinary dysfunction is a critical issue for individuals with MS affecting both adults and children of both genders. Among children participating in open discussions regarding their MS, many admitted they were reluctant to disclose this problem to their health care providers. Special awareness and specific questioning are important in assessing the problem. As reviewed elsewhere, between 32 and 97% of adults with MS experience symptoms of urinary dysfunction which are most often detrusor and sphincter disorders [99]. These symptoms most often appear on average 6 years after the onset of the disease (ranges from 5 to 9.5 years) [99]. Medications commonly used in adults are oxybutynin, tolterodine, and solifenacin succinate.

Bowel problems in MS are infrequently studied especially in the pediatric population. A few studies of adult MS have shown bowel dysfunction prevalence of 45–68% and this was more common with longer duration of disease [100, 101]. The most common bowel problem is constipation. Other problems include diarrhea and fecal incontinence. Several medications used to treat other symptoms of MS can precipitate or exacerbate constipation and they should be adjusted accordingly. Increasing water intake, high fiber-balanced diet, bulk formers, and exercise are a few non-medical interventions useful in the treatment of constipation. If this fails, stool softeners, oral laxatives, suppositories, and enemas have been successful in relief of constipation in adults with MS [102].

Spasticity

Spasticity is a problem that can be addressed with multidisciplinary treatment. Physical therapy and exercise are helpful in adults and should be considered for children as well. In children, oral baclofen (0.36–1.5 mg/kg) can be used in MS as well as in those with other neurological disorders. However, very young patients have a risk of seizures with baclofen [103]. The experience of intrathecal baclofen in patients with cerebral palsy (25–50 μg/day) is in general positive and in severely spastic MS children might be a consideration for those failing oral baclofen [104]. Another oral therapy effective for spasticity is tizanidine (2–24 mg/day).

Paroxysmal Spasms

Paroxysmal spasms are most typically characterized by trigeminal neuralgia and can occur in children with MS as they can in adults. For trigeminal neuralgia the most consistently effective medication in adults with the disease is carbamazepine [105].

Motor Impairments

Motor problems are common in pediatric MS. Physical therapy and exercises are the main therapeutic interventions. In adults, the medication Fampridine-SR has been associated with improved walking speed and strength [106]. This medication has not been studied in children.

Supporting the Family

MS affects the entire family including parents, siblings, and grandparents. Support, education, and reassurance are needed. We believe that the diagnosis should be shared with both the parents and the patient regardless of the age. There are a variety of different support systems available to assist in breaking the diagnosis to the family. Educational materials available through the National Multiple Sclerosis Society (NMSS) include "Children get MS too: A Guide for Parents," "Children and Teens with MS: A Network for Families," and "Mighty Special Kids – An Activity Book for Children with MS." More information, additional services, and online networking for parents and teens are available at the website of the NMSS which is www.NationalMSsociety. org/pediatricms or by phone 1 866 – KIDS WMS (866 543 7967). Additional information can also be found at www.pediatricmscenter.org.

Conclusion

Pediatric MS is a chronic disorder whose risk following an initial clinical attack varies with the specific features. Clearly some patients whose presentation resembles ADEM will subsequently be reclassified as MS. The differential diagnosis and clinical features differ slightly from adults with the disease and is most distinctive in the youngest patients. The management includes educating and reassuring the family, using medications to modify the disease course, and addressing the daily symptoms and psychosocial consequences of the disease. Most children appear to do reasonably well and do not develop a progressive course until decades later [6]. However, ongoing support and assistance in transitioning to adulthood as the children become older are all critical aspects to the care of this MS subgroup.

References

1. Duquette P, Murray TJ, Pleines J, et al. Multiple sclerosis in childhood: clinical profile in 125 patients. J Pediatr. 1987;111:359–63.
2. Boiko A, Vorobeychik G, Paty D, Devonshire V, Sadovnick D. Early onset multiple sclerosis: a longitudinal study. Neurology. 2002;59:1006–10.
3. Ghezzi A, Deplano V, Faroni J, et al. Multiple sclerosis in childhood: clinical features of 149 cases. Mult Scler. 1997;3:43–6.
4. Sindern E, Haas J, Stark E, Wurster U. Early onset MS under the age of 16: clinical and paraclinical features. Acta Neurol Scand. 1992;86:280–4.
5. Ruggieri M, Polizzi A, Pavone L, Grimaldi LM. Multiple sclerosis in children under 6 years of age. Neurology. 1999;53:478–84.
6. Renoux C, Vukusic S, Mikaeloff Y, et al. Natural history of multiple sclerosis with childhood onset. N Engl J Med. 2007;356:2603–13.

7. Simone IL, Carrara D, Tortorella C, et al. Course and prognosis in early-onset MS: comparison with adult-onset forms. Neurology. 2002;59:1922–8.
8. Chitnis T, Glanz B, Jaffin S, Healy B. Demographics of pediatric-onset multiple sclerosis in an MS center population from the Northeastern United States. Mult Scler. 2009;15:627–31.
9. Compston A. McAlpine's multiple sclerosis. 3rd ed. London: Churchill Livingston; 1998.
10. Banwell B, Kennedy J, Sadovnick D, et al. Incidence of acquired demyelination of the CNS in Canadian children. Neurology. 2009;72:232–9.
11. Banwell B, Ghezzi A, Bar-Or A, Mikaeloff Y, Tardieu M. Multiple sclerosis in children: clinical diagnosis, therapeutic strategies, and future directions. Lancet Neurol. 2007;6:887–902.
12. Deryck O, Ketelaer P, Dubois B. Clinical characteristics and long term prognosis in early onset multiple sclerosis. J Neurol. 2006;252:720–3.
13. Boster AL, Endress CF, Hreha SA, Caon C, Perumal JS, Khan OA. Pediatric-onset multiple sclerosis in African-American black and European-origin white patients. Pediatr Neurol. 2009;40:31–3.
14. Krupp L. Racial and ethnic findings in pediatric MS: an update. Neurology. 2008;S70:A135.
15. Dale RC, de Sousa C, Chong WK, Cox TC, Harding B, Neville BG. Acute disseminated encephalomyelitis, multiphasic disseminated encephalomyelitis and multiple sclerosis in children. Brain. 2000;123(Pt 12):2407–22.
16. Neuteboom RF, Boon M, Catsman Berrevoets CE, et al. Prognostic factors after a first attack of inflammatory CNS demyelination in children. Neurology. 2008;71:967–73.
17. Mikaeloff Y, Suissa S, Vallee L, et al. First episode of acute CNS inflammatory demyelination in childhood: prognostic factors for multiple sclerosis and disability. J Pediatr. 2004;144:246–52.
18. Dale RC, Brilot F, Banwell B. Pediatric central nervous system inflammatory demyelination: acute disseminated encephalomyelitis, clinically isolated syndromes, neuromyelitis optica, and multiple sclerosis. Curr Opin Neurol. 2009;22:233–40.
19. Mikaeloff Y, Caridade G, Husson B, Suissa S, Tardieu M. Acute disseminated encephalomyelitis cohort study: prognostic factors for relapse. Eur J Paediatr Neurol. 2007;11:90–5.
20. Dale RC, Pillai SC. Early relapse risk after a first CNS inflammatory demyelination episode: examining international consensus definitions. Dev Med Child Neurol. 2007;49:887–93.
21. Bonhomme GR, Waldman AT, Balcer LJ, et al. Pediatric optic neuritis: brain MRI abnormalities and risk of multiple sclerosis. Neurology. 2009;72:881–5.
22. Wilejto M, Shroff M, Buncic JR, Kennedy J, Goia C, Banwell B. The clinical features, MRI findings, and outcome of optic neuritis in children. Neurology. 2006;67:258–62.
23. Lucchinetti CF, Kiers L, O'Duffy A, et al. Risk factors for developing multiple sclerosis after childhood optic neuritis. Neurology. 1997;49:1413–8.
24. Alper G, Wang L. Demyelinating optic neuritis in children. J Child Neurol. 2009;24:45–8.
25. McDonald WI, Compston A, Edan G, et al. Recommended diagnostic criteria for multiple sclerosis: guidelines from the International Panel on the diagnosis of multiple sclerosis. Ann Neurol. 2001;50:121–7.
26. Mikaeloff Y, Adamsbaum C, Husson B, et al. MRI prognostic factors for relapse after acute CNS inflammatory demyelination in childhood. Brain. 2004;127:1942–7.
27. Callen DJ, Shroff MM, Branson HM, et al. MRI in the diagnosis of pediatric multiple sclerosis. Neurology. 2009;72:961–7.

28. Ozakbas S, Idiman E, Baklan B, Yulug B. Childhood and juvenile onset multiple sclerosis: clinical and paraclinical features. Brain Dev. 2003;25:233–6.
29. Ghezzi A, Pozzilli C, Liguori M, et al. Prospective study of multiple sclerosis with early onset. Mult Scler. 2002;8:115–8.
30. Gusev E, Boiko A, Bikova O, et al. The natural history of early onset multiple sclerosis: comparison of data from Moscow and Vancouver. Clin Neurol Neurosurg. 2002;104:203–7.
31. Banwell B, Krupp L, Kennedy J, et al. Clinical features and viral serologies in children with multiple sclerosis: a multinational observational study. Lancet Neurol. 2007;6:773–81.
32. Pohl D, Rostasy K, Treiber-Held S, Brockmann K, Gartner J, Hanefeld F. Pediatric multiple sclerosis: detection of clinically silent lesions by multimodal evoked potentials. J Pediatr. 2006;149:125–7.
33. Mikaeloff Y, Caridade G, Assi S, Suissa S, Tardieu M. Prognostic factors for early severity in a childhood multiple sclerosis cohort. Pediatrics. 2006;118:1133–9.
34. Tenembaum S, Chamoles N, Fejerman N. Acute disseminated encephalomyelitis: a long-term follow-up study of 84 pediatric patients. Neurology. 2002;59:1224–31.
35. Chabas D, Castillo-Trivino T, Mowry EM, Strober JB, Glenn OA, Waubant E. Vanishing MS T2-bright lesions before puberty: a distinct MRI phenotype? Neurology. 2008;71:1090–3.
36. Chabas D, Ness J, Belman A, et al. Younger children with pediatric MS have a distinct CSF inflammatory profile at disease onset. Neurology. 2010;74(5):399–405.
37. MacAllister WS, Krupp LB. Multiple sclerosis-related fatigue. Phys Med Rehabil Clin N Am. 2005;16:483–502.
38. Amato MP, Goretti B, Ghezzi A, et al. Cognitive and psychosocial features of childhood and juvenile MS. Neurology. 2008;70:1891–7.
39. MacAllister W, Milazzo M, Troxell RM, et al. Fatigue and quality of life in pediatric multiple sclerosis. Ann Neurol. 2006;60:S39.
40. MacAllister WS, Belman AL, Milazzo M, et al. Cognitive functioning in children and adolescents with multiple sclerosis. Neurology. 2005;64:1422–5.
41. Banwell BL, Anderson PE. The cognitive burden of multiple sclerosis in children. Neurology. 2005;64:891–4.
42. MacAllister WS, Christodoulou C, Milazzo M, Krupp LB. Longitudinal neuropsychological assessment in pediatric multiple sclerosis. Dev Neuropsychol. 2007;32:625–44.
43. Amato M. Cognitive and psychosocial features of childhood and juvenile multiple sclerosis: a reappraisal after 2 years. Neurology. 2009;3:A97.
44. Pohl D, Rostasy K, Gartner J, Hanefeld F. Treatment of early onset multiple sclerosis with subcutaneous interferon beta-1a. Neurology. 2005;64:888–90.
45. Ghezzi A, Amato MP, Capobianco M, et al. Disease-modifying drugs in childhood-juvenile multiple sclerosis: results of an Italian co-operative study. Mult Scler. 2005;11:420–4.
46. Tenembaum S, Chitnis T, Ness J, Hahn JS. Acute disseminated encephalomyelitis. Neurology. 2007;68:S23–36.
47. Wingerchuk DM, Lucchinetti CF. Comparative immunopathogenesis of acute disseminated encephalomyelitis, neuromyelitis optica, and multiple sclerosis. Curr Opin Neurol. 2007;20:343–50.
48. Filippi M, Rocca MA. MRI evidence for multiple sclerosis as a diffuse disease of the central nervous system. J Neurol. 2005;252 Suppl 5:v16–24.
49. Krupp LB, Banwell B, Tenembaum S. Consensus definitions proposed for pediatric multiple sclerosis and related disorders. Neurology. 2007;68:S7–12.
50. Brass SD, Caramanos Z, Santos C, Dilenge ME, Lapierre Y, Rosenblatt B. Multiple sclerosis vs acute disseminated encephalomyelitis in childhood. Pediatr Neurol. 2003;29:227–31.

51. Tenembaum S, Chitnis T, Ness J, Hahn JS, Group IPMS. Acute disseminated encephalomyelitis. Neurology. 2007;68:S23–36.
52. Callen DJ, Shroff MM, Branson HM, et al. Role of MRI in the differentiation of ADEM from MS in children. Neurology. 2009;72:968–73.
53. Hynson JL, Kornberg AJ, Coleman LT, Shield L, Harvey AS, Kean MJ. Clinical and neuroradiologic features of acute disseminated encephalomyelitis in children. Neurology. 2001;56:1308–12.
54. Banwell B, Tenembaum S, Lennon VA, et al. Neuromyelitis optica-IgG in childhood inflammatory demyelinating CNS disorders. Neurology. 2008;70: 344–52.
55. Hahn CD, Shroff MM, Blaser SI, Banwell BL. MRI criteria for multiple sclerosis: evaluation in a pediatric cohort. Neurology. 2004;62:806–8.
56. Hahn JS, Pohl D, Rensel M, Rao S. Differential diagnosis and evaluation in pediatric multiple sclerosis. Neurology. 2007;68:S13–22.
57. Van der Knaap MS. Magnetic resonance of myelination and myelin disorders. 3rd ed. New York: Springer; 2005.
58. Gorman MP, Golomb MR, Walsh LE, et al. Steroid-responsive neurologic relapses in a child with a proteolipid protein-1 mutation. Neurology. 2007;68:1305–7.
59. Chitnis T. Pediatric multiple sclerosis. Neurologist. 2006;12:299–310.
60. Mikaeloff Y, Caridade G, Suissa S, Tardieu M. Clinically observed chickenpox and the risk of childhood-onset multiple sclerosis. Am J Epidemiol. 2009; 169:1260–6.
61. Mikaeloff Y, Caridade G, Suissa S, Tardieu M. Hepatitis B vaccine and the risk of CNS inflammatory demyelination in childhood. Neurology. 2009;72:873–80.
62. Mikaeloff Y, Caridade G, Tardieu M, Suissa S. Parental smoking at home and the risk of childhood-onset multiple sclerosis in children. Brain. 2007;130:2589–95.
63. Correale J, Tenembaum SN. Myelin basic protein and myelin oligodendrocyte glycoprotein T-cell repertoire in childhood and juvenile multiple sclerosis. Mult Scler. 2006;12:412–20.
64. Banwell B, Bar-Or A, Cheung R, et al. Abnormal T-cell reactivities in childhood inflammatory demyelinating disease and type 1 diabetes. Ann Neurol. 2008;63:98–111.
65. Barnes D, Hughes RA, Morris RW, et al. Randomised trial of oral and intravenous methylprednisolone in acute relapses of multiple sclerosis. Lancet. 1997;349:902–6.
66. Martinelli V, Pulizzi A, Annovazzi P, Rocca M, Rodegher M, et al. A short-term MRI study comparing high-dose oral versus intravenous methylpredisolone in MS relapse. Neurology. 2008;70:A83–4.
67. Morrow SA, Stoian CA, Dmitrovic J, Chan SC, Metz LM. The bioavailability of IV methylprednisolone and oral prednisone in multiple sclerosis. Neurology. 2004;63:1079–80.
68. Weinshenker BG, O'Brien PC, Petterson TM, Noseworthy JH. A randomized trial of plasma exchange in acute central nervous system inflammatory demyelinating disease. Ann Neurol. 1999;46:878–86.
69. Duzova A, Bakkaloglu A. Central nervous system involvement in pediatric rheumatic diseases: current concepts in treatment. Curr Pharm Des. 2008;14: 1295–301.
70. Hahn JS, Siegler DJ, Enzmann D. Intravenous gammaglobulin therapy in recurrent acute disseminated encephalomyelitis. Neurology. 1996;46:1173–4.
71. Nishikawa M, Ichiyama T, Hayashi T, Ouchi K, Furukawa S. Intravenous immunoglobulin therapy in acute disseminated encephalomyelitis. Pediatr Neurol. 1999;21:583–6.
72. Mikaeloff Y, Caridade G, Tardieu M, Suissa S. Effectiveness of early beta interferon on the first attack after confirmed multiple sclerosis: a comparative cohort study. Eur J Paediatr Neurol. 2008;12:205–9.

73. Ghezzi A, Amato MP, Capobianco M, et al. Treatment of early-onset multiple sclerosis with intramuscular interferonbeta-1a: long-term results. Neurol Sci. 2007;28:127–32.

74. Pakdaman H, Fallah A, Sahraian MA, Pakdaman R, Meysamie A. Treatment of early onset multiple sclerosis with suboptimal dose of interferon beta-1a. Neuropediatrics. 2006;37:257–60.

75. Waubant E, Hietpas J, Stewart T, et al. Interferon beta-1a in children with multiple sclerosis is well tolerated. Neuropediatrics. 2001;32:211–3.

76. Mikaeloff Y, Moreau T, Debouverie M, et al. Interferon-beta treatment in patients with childhood-onset multiple sclerosis. J Pediatr. 2001;139:443–6.

77. Tenembaum SN, Segura MJ. Interferon beta-1a treatment in childhood and juvenile-onset multiple sclerosis. Neurology. 2006;67:511–3.

78. Banwell B, Reder AT, Krupp L, et al. Safety and tolerability of interferon beta-1b in pediatric multiple sclerosis. Neurology. 2006;66:472–6.

79. Adams AB, Tyor WR, Holden KR. Interferon beta-1b and childhood multiple sclerosis. Pediatr Neurol. 1999;21:481–3.

80. Krupp L, Pardo L, Vitt D. Clinical features and disease-modifying therapy experience in paediatric multiple sclerosis. Mult Scler. 2004;10:S178.

81. Kornek B, Bernert G, Balassy C, Geldner J, Prayer D, Feucht M. Glatiramer acetate treatment in patients with childhood and juvenile onset multiple sclerosis. Neuropediatrics. 2003;34:120–6.

82. Borriello G, Prosperini L, Luchetti A, Pozzilli C. Natalizumab treatment in pediatric multiple sclerosis: a case report. Eur J Paediatr Neurol. 2009;13(1):67–71.

83. Huppke P, Stark W, Zurcher C, Huppke B, Bruck W, Gartner J. Natalizumab use in pediatric multiple sclerosis. Arch Neurol. 2008;65:1655–8.

84. Yeh EA, Waubant E, Krupp L, Ness J, Chitnis T, Kuntz N, Ramanathan M, Belman A, Chabas D, Gorman M, Rodriguez M, Rinker J, Weinstock-Guttman B. MS Therapies in Pediatric MS Patients With Refractory Disease. Archives of Neurology 2011;68(4):437–444.

85. Makhani N, Gorman MP, Branson HM, Stazzone L, Banwell BL, Chitnis T. Cyclophosphamide therapy in pediatric multiple sclerosis. Neurology. 2009;72:2076–82.

86. Krupp LB, Rizvi SA. Symptomatic therapy for underrecognized manifestations of multiple sclerosis. Neurology. 2002;58:S32–9.

87. Murray TJ. Amantadine therapy for fatigue in multiple sclerosis. Can J Neurol Sci. 1985;12:251–4.

88. Krupp LB, Coyle PK, Doscher C, et al. Fatigue therapy in multiple sclerosis: results of a double-blind, randomized, parallel trial of amantadine, pemoline, and placebo. Neurology. 1995;45:1956–61.

89. A randomized controlled trial of amantadine in fatigue associated with multiple sclerosis. The Canadian MS Research Group. Can J Neurol Sci. 1987;14:273–8.

90. Rammohan KW, Lynn DJ. Modafinil for fatigue in MS: a randomized placebo-controlled double-blind study. Neurology. 2005;65:1995–7. author reply 1995–7.

91. Zifko UA, Rupp M, Schwarz S, Zipko HT, Maida EM. Modafinil in treatment of fatigue in multiple sclerosis. Results of an open-label study. J Neurol. 2002;249:983–7.

92. Weinshenker BG, Penman M, Bass B, Ebers GC, Rice GP. A double-blind, randomized, crossover trial of pemoline in fatigue associated with multiple sclerosis. Neurology. 1992;42:1468–71.

93. Pucci E, Branas P, D'Amico R, Giuliani G, Solari A, Taus C. Amantadine for fatigue in multiple sclerosis. Cochrane Database Syst Rev. 2007;(1):CD002818.

94. Rammohan KW, Rosenberg JH, Lynn DJ, Blumenfeld AM, Pollak CP, Nagaraja HN. Efficacy and safety of modafinil (Provigil) for the treatment of fatigue in multiple sclerosis: a two centre phase 2 study. J Neurol Neurosurg Psychiatry. 2002;72:179–83.

95. Stankoff B, Waubant E, Confavreux C, et al. Modafinil for fatigue in MS: a randomized placebo-controlled double-blind study. Neurology. 2005;64:1139–43.

96. Krupp LB, Christodoulou C, Melville P, Scherl WF, MacAllister WS, Elkins LE. Donepezil improved memory in multiple sclerosis in a randomized clinical trial. Neurology. 2004;63:1579–85.

97. O'Brien AR, Chiaravalloti N, Goverover Y, Deluca J. Evidenced-based cognitive rehabilitation for persons with multiple sclerosis: a review of the literature. Arch Phys Med Rehabil. 2008;89:761–9.

98. Cheung AH, Emslie GJ, Mayes TL. The use of antidepressants to treat depression in children and adolescents. CMAJ. 2006;174:193–200.

99. de Seze M, Ruffion A, Denys P, Joseph PA, Perrouin-Verbe B. The neurogenic bladder in multiple sclerosis: review of the literature and proposal of management guidelines. Mult Scler. 2007;13:915–28.

100. Chia YW, Fowler CJ, Kamm MA, Henry MM, Lemieux MC, Swash M. Prevalence of bowel dysfunction in patients with multiple sclerosis and bladder dysfunction. J Neurol. 1995;242:105–8.

101. Nortvedt MW, Riise T, Frugard J, et al. Prevalence of bladder, bowel and sexual problems among multiple sclerosis patients two to five years after diagnosis. Mult Scler. 2007;13:106–12.

102. DasGupta R, Fowler CJ. Bladder, bowel and sexual dysfunction in multiple sclerosis: management strategies. Drugs. 2003;63:153–66.

103. Hansel DE, Hansel CR, Shindle MK, et al. Oral baclofen in cerebral palsy: possible seizure potentiation? Pediatr Neurol. 2003;29:203–6.

104. Sgouros S, Seri S. The effect of intrathecal baclofen on muscle co-contraction in children with spasticity of cerebral origin. Pediatr Neurosurg. 2002;37:225–30.

105. Gronseth G, Cruccu G, Alksne J, et al. Practice parameter: the diagnostic evaluation and treatment of trigeminal neuralgia (an evidence-based review). Report of the Quality Standards Subcommittee of the American Academy of Neurology and the European Federation of Neurological Societies. Neurology. 2008;71(15):1183–90.

106. Goodman AD, Cohen JA, Cross A, et al. Fampridine-SR in multiple sclerosis: a randomized, double-blind, placebo-controlled, dose-ranging study. Mult Scler. 2007;13:357–68.

Is Multiple Sclerosis a Vascular Disease?

Mahesh V. Jayaraman and Syed A. Rizvi

Keywords: Cerebrospinal venous insufficiency, Angioplasty, Venous congestion, Disability, Clinical trials

Introduction

Multiple sclerosis (MS) is widely recognized as a progressive, inflammatory neurogenerative disease, for which the causative agent(s) or triggers are not well known. A recent hypothesis is that MS is caused, at least to some extent, by chronic venous insufficiency of the extracranial venous drainage. In this chapter, we explore the historical and modern perspectives on possible vascular etiologies to multiple sclerosis, parallels from other cerebrovascular diseases, and identify future areas of exploration.

Historical Perspectives

In 1863, Dr. Eduard Rindflcisch described inflammatory lesions surrounding small vessels [1], leading him to suggest that "...this leads us to search for the primary cause of the disease in an alteration of individual vessels and their ramifications." Years later, Dr. James Dawson also noted demyelination around inflamed vessels [2]. Later in the century, interest turn toward identifying a possible viral or environmental trigger to the autoimmune process, as a unifying mechanism for the vascular theory was never confirmed. Vascular thrombosis has also been implicated as a causative factor [3] for multiple sclerosis.

Normal Venous Drainage of the Brain and Spinal Cord

Before considering the possible vascular, and more precisely venous, etiologies proposed for MS, we must first briefly understand the normal venous drainage pathways of the brain and spinal cord.

From: *Clinical Neuroimmunology: Multiple Sclerosis and Related Disorders*, Current Clinical Neurology, Edited by: S.A. Rizvi and P.K. Coyle, DOI 10.1007/978-1-60327-860-7_9, © Springer Science+Business Media, LLC 2011

The intracranial venous drainage is divided into two main systems: the superficial system and the deep system. The superficial venous system primarily comprises of venous drainage of the cortex, with venules coalescing to form cortical veins along the surface of the brain, eventually draining into the superior sagittal sinus (SSS) and the transverse sinuses. The deep venous drainage system consists of the territory, which eventually drains into the Vein of Galen and subsequently the straight sinus. Anatomically, this primarily includes the deep gray nuclei and thalamus, corpus callosum, periventricular white matter, mesial temporal lobe, diencephalon, and rostral brainstem [4, 5]. The deep and superficial systems unite at the torcular herophili, and both systems eventually drain through the jugular veins. Important collaterals exist at the jugular bulb between the proximal internal jugular veins (IJV) and the condylar venous confluence, with connections to anterior, posterior, and lateral condylar veins which connect to the vertebral venous plexus [6].

Important differences in venous drainage exist between supine and upright positions [7–9]. In the supine position, the primary venous drainage of the brain is the jugular venous system. In contrast, the vertebral venous system occupies that role in the upright position. Various theories for this difference have been postulated [10], but suffice it to say that understanding this difference has major implications with respect to any vascular theories of MS. It also has been shown that in control patients, the jugular veins will collapse as patients are gradually moved from supine to upright positions [7].

The venous drainage of the spinal cord is more complex. Small collecting veins eventually coalesce to form multiple anterior and posterior spinal veins lying on the surface of the cord within the arachnoid mater. These eventually communicate with the vertebral venous plexus, a large valveless venous system with potentially multidirectional flow, which is continuous from the skull base to the sacrum [11, 12]. Multiple routes of venous efflux from the vertebral venous plexus exist, but among the primary drainage of the external vertebral venous system are the azygous and hemiazygous veins, which typically drain into the superior vena cava.

Vascular and Perfusion Abnormalities in MS Patients

The availability of noninvasive brain perfusion imaging using MR perfusion sparked interest in evaluating patients with MS. One of the early studies evaluated whole brain MR perfusion imaging in 17 patients with relapsing–remitting MS (RRMS) and 17 control patients [13]. This study showed that normal appearing white matter (NAWM) in MS patients had prolonged mean transit time (MTT) and decreased cerebral blood flow (CBF) when compared with age-matched controls. The conclusion from their research was that "We interpret our findings of diminished perfusion in NAWM as evidence that MS has a primary vascular pathogenesis." Further research from the same group has shown elevated CBF and cerebral blood volume (CBV) in enhancing lesions, while non-enhancing lesions showed variable appearances. Another group performed longitudinal evaluation with monthly perfusion MRI in RRMS patients and showed that regional increases in CBF and CBV preceded the development of new contrast enhancement in a lesion by up to 3 weeks [14].

The same group that published the initial MR perfusion papers further studied this relationship using 3 Tesla (3T) MRI, in 11 controls and 22 MS patients [15]. They found greater CBF decrease in primary progressive MS (PPMS) when compared with RRMS, and also found strong correlation between estimated disease severity score (EDSS) and periventricular CBF ($r = -0.48$ and $p = 0.0016$). Studies have also shown correlation between degree of CBF decrease and decline in neuropsychological testing [16] and fatigue [17]. Perhaps, most important in supporting a potential vascular etiology for MS was a study evaluating 12 patients with clinically isolated syndrome (CIS), 12 patients with RRMS, and 12 healthy controls. That study showed decreased CBF in NAWM in both CIS and RRMS patients compared with controls and decreased CBF in deep gray nuclei in RRMS patients compared with controls [18]. This could imply that the vascular disturbances are present at disease onset and are progressive rather than static.

Confirming the early pathologic descriptions, Tan showed that high-resolution MR venography can demonstrate central veins in almost all MS plaques [19]. They evaluated 15 MS patients who had a total of 95 lesions, 43 periventricular, and 52 focal deep white matter. In all but one of the lesions, a central vein was identified, and the veins ran along the long axis of ovoid lesions. They felt that this technique allowed for in vivo confirmation of the previously described veno-centric nature of MS plaques. Global differences in venous visibility have also been shown in MS patients compared with controls [20]. However, that study showed diminished visibility of cerebral veins in MS patients compared with controls when using susceptibility-weighted imaging (SWI) MR technique. This may be somewhat counterintuitive to what one would expect if indeed a venous occlusive process was present, where perhaps more rather than less veins would be visualized.

The CCSVI Hypothesis

A vascular etiology for multiple sclerosis has been recently reevaluated in detail by Paolo Zamboni and colleagues. They performed a specialized ultrasound protocol combining extracranial and transcranial Doppler (TCD) techniques, coining the term chronic cerebrospinal venous insufficiency (CCSVI) [21]. A total of 65 MS patients and 235 control patients were scanned. Four specific parameters were found to be abnormal in patients with MS and absent in control patients:

1. Reflux of flow in the IJV and/or vertebral veins (VV) in sitting and supine posture (71% of MS, 0% of controls, $p < 0.0001$).
2. Reflux in the deep cerebral veins, as assessed by TCD (61% of MS, 0% of controls, $p < 0.0001$).
3. High-resolution B-mode evidence of IJV stenosis (37% of MS, 0% of controls, $p < 0.0001$).
4. Flow not detectable by Doppler in the IJVs and/or VVs (52% of MS, 3% of controls, $p < 0.0001$).
5. Reverted postural control of the main cerebral venous outflow pathways (55% of MS, 11% of controls, $p < 0.0001$).

Patients were considered to have an abnormal ultrasound, if any two of the five above criteria were present, with 100% of MS patients and 0% of controls meeting those criteria. Venography confirmed stenosis of either jugular vein

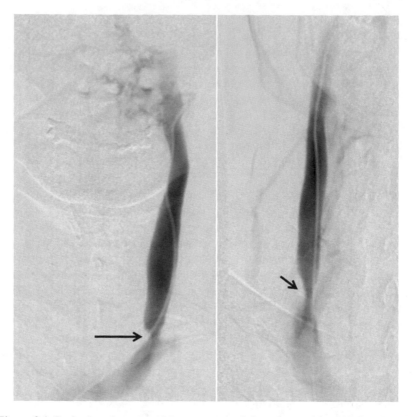

Figure 9.1 Examples of extracranial venous stenosis in patients with multiple sclerosis. Two anterior–posterior projection images from selective jugular venography in two different patients with RRMS show focal, high-grade stenosis (*arrows*) of the inferior aspect of the internal jugular vein, just above its junction with the subclavian vein

in 91% of patients and the azygous vein in 86% of MS patients. Venography was also performed in 48 control patients, and none showed any stenosis. They further divided the venographic patterns of occlusion and collateral flow into four types and found some correlation between type of MS and flow pattern, most notably for PPMS. Examples of venous stenoses in patients with multiple sclerosis are shown in Figures 9.1–9.3.

While provocative, Zamboni's results have not been consistently duplicated by other centers. Among the many criticisms of their ultrasound technique are the fact that one sonographer scanned every patient in this study, calling into question the reproducibility of this technique. Doepp et al. studied 56 MS and 20 control patients using Zamboni's protocol and were unable to duplicate Zamboni's results [22]. However, at least one other small series has confirmed Zamboni's findings [23]. At this present time, there does not appear to be sufficient conclusive evidence that there are reproducible differences on ultrasound between MS and control patients. Whether this is a function of the ultrasound technique or a true lack of difference is yet to be determined.

Even if one were to presume that there was a venous outlet component to multiple sclerosis, it would be necessary to integrate that theory with the known autoimmune and inflammatory background of MS. Zamboni proposes that

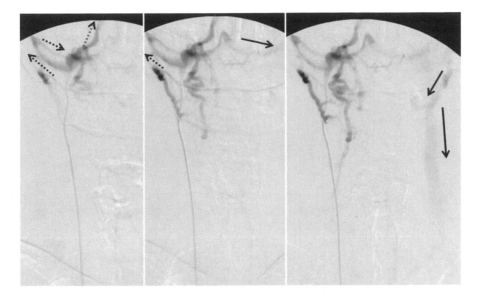

Figure 9.2 High-grade stenosis of the jugular vein with retrograde intracranial flow in a patient with SPMS. These sequential images from a selective right internal jugular venogram demonstrate retrograde flow in the right sigmoid and transverse sinuses (*dashed arrows*, first image) and the inferior petrosal sinus (*double dashed arrows*, first image). The second image shows flow across the left transverse sinus (*solid arrow*), and the third image shows eventual flow down the left jugular vein (*arrows*)

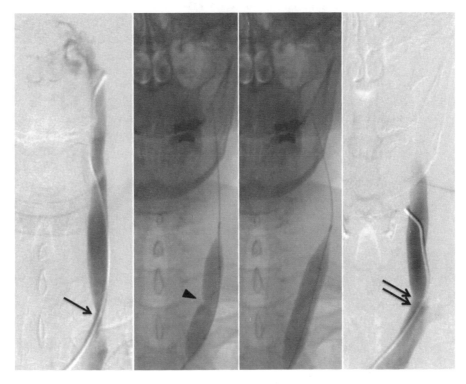

Figure 9.3 Angioplasty for focal jugular stenosis of the inferior left internal jugular vein in a patient with RRMS. First image shows a focal narrowing of the lower jugular vein (*arrow*). When the angioplasty balloon is initially inflated, a "waist" is seen in the balloon at the area of narrowing (*arrowhead*, second image). This waist is treated with further dilatation of the balloon, and final image shows no residual stenosis (*double arrows*, fourth image)

there is local, perivenular erythrocyte extravasation secondary to CCSVI, which results in iron overload and activation of the immune response [24], drawing parallels from chronic venous disease in the lower extremities [25]. In essence, Zamboni suggests that venous occlusive disease with local extravasation of erythrocytes may be the elusive trigger that starts the autoimmune cascade.

Zamboni then took the next step and treated 65 patients with percutaneous transluminal angioplasty (PTA) of the jugular and azygous stenosis [26]. This study included 35 RRPS, 20 SPMS, and 10 PPMS patients, who all underwent selective venography based on abnormal ultrasound criteria as described previously. All patients were treated with angioplasty alone (no stents were placed). Statistically significant reduction in venous pressures was documented post-angioplasty. Clinical outcome measures included relapse rates, percentage of patients relapse free, and quality of life measures (MSQOL). Among the 35 RRMS patients, there was no statistically significant reduction in annualized relapse rate (0.9 pre vs. 0.7 post), but there was a reduction in percentage of patients who were relapse free during the mean 18 months of follow-up (27% pre vs. 50% post PTA, $p < 0.0014$). Significant differences in MSQOL measures and MSFC were also seen for RRMS patients. Among SP and PPMS patients, the only quality of life measure which met statistical significance was the mental health component of the MSQOL (60 pre vs. 78 post PTA, $p < 0.01$). Restenosis was a substantial problem, with 47% of treated IJVs having restenosis documented on ultrasound, typically 8–9 months postprocedure. Azygous vein patency was high, with only 4% of patients restenosing at this location on follow-up venography performed at 18 months. Zamboni also went to further describe that no relapses occurred in patients who were normal by ultrasound at 18 months.

There are many criticisms of this study. First of all, there was no control group of MS patients, and evaluation (both clinical and imaging) was not blinded. In addition, the pretreatment and posttreatment medications were not controlled. The annualized relapse rate in treated RRMS patients (0.7 relapses/year) is higher than that has been shown in recent trials of medical therapy [27, 28]. Zamboni's results have prompted many patients to seek out and undergo venography and angioplasty with or without stent placement, but at the time of this writing, no other peer reviewed series of endovascular therapy for MS exists in the literature.

Angioplasty of central venous stenosis has been performed by Interventional Radiologists for many years with an extremely favorable safety profile, which is one of the features that makes this potential breakthrough treatment attractive. Serious adverse events in patients undergoing venous angioplasty are extremely rare [29–35], with most of the literature focusing on patients with surgically created hemodialysis fistulae. However, as was the case with Zamboni's series, restenosis was a common problem, and it is uncertain whether stent placement will improve upon long-term patency rates.

Parallels from Other Cerebrovascular Diseases

Parallels of venous hypertension causing pathology can be drawn from other cerebrovascular disease. We will evaluate what is known about venous hypertension in dural arteriovenous fistulae (dAVF), pial arteriovenous malformations (AVM), and in idiopathic intracranial hypertension (IIH).

Dural arteriovenous fistulae are acquired connections between dural arterial branches (such as the middle meningeal artery) and a venous structure. The recipient venous structure can either be a major venous sinus or be a cortical vein. Several classification systems exist [36–38], but the common thread is that the venous drainage of the lesion rather than the arterial supply is the defining factor in determining the natural history of the lesion. In general, lesions that drain directly into the major sinuses with no retrograde cortical venous flow have more benign natural histories, while those with retrograde cortical venous drainage have a more aggressive course, especially when presenting with hemorrhage. A broad range of clinical presentations exist, and nonhemorrhagic lesions can present with focal neurologic deficits related to venous hypertension in the area of the fistula [39–42], including myelopathy [39, 43–46], dementia [40, 47–49], even parkinsonism [50]. Many of these are reversible following treatment of the lesion with resolution of venous hypertension. In addition, white matter lesions in the territories affected with venous hypertension can be seen and are also reversible following treatment [47–49, 51, 52]. In patients with spinal dural fistulae, the presenting symptoms of myelopathy follow a characteristic pattern of ascending leg weakness, rather than in a haphazard fashion, and urinary symptoms are also frequently present [53, 54]. A similar pattern of ascending leg weakness with urinary symptoms is also seen in progressive MS patients.

Perfusion imaging has also been performed in dural fistulas, demonstrating locally elevated MTT in areas of venous hypertension which resolves following treatment [55]. More regional areas of abnormal perfusion have been shown even in the absence of retrograde cortical venous drainage [51].

In contrast to dAVF, pial AVMs are acquired lesions which represent abnormal tangle of vessels with dilated arterial supply directly into small veins without a normal intervening capillary bed. The natural history of these lesions is also influenced by the venous drainage, with higher rates of hemorrhage in patients with venous outlet stenoses or exclusively deep venous drainage [56, 57]. Perhaps, the deep venous system is less tolerant of venous hypertension, and many of the periventricular white matter lesions in MS are seen in the drainage territory of the deep venous system.

The final entity in which we will explore the association of venous hypertension is IIH, a condition in which symptoms of elevated intracranial pressure are present, without a space occupying lesion to account for such elevation. The feared long-term consequences of IIH are primarily visual, where prolonged papilledema can lead to optic atrophy [58, 59]. Recently, patients with IIH have been found to have stenoses of the major dural sinuses, typically in the distal transverse sinus region. Catheter venography has confirmed these narrowings and pressure measurements across the stenosis clearly demonstrate elevated pressure proximal to the lesion. Placement of stents in these lesions appears to resolve the stenosis and lower the venous pressure in the sinus [58–61]. The mechanism by which this causes IIH is unknown, but small studies have shown that CSF opening pressure normalized following stent placement, leading many to consider stenting a primary treatment modality for IIH refractory to medical therapy with acetazolamide [61]. One of the proposed mechanisms of action is that lowering the venous pressure reduces the gradient across which CSF resorption occurs in the arachnoid villi, facilitating greater CSF resorption.

This does raise several questions regarding venous outflow obstruction and MS. If indeed venous obstruction can cause IIH, why do those patients not have white matter lesions? Furthermore, why don't MS patients have elevated intracranial pressure? One possible answer is that occlusions within the cranial vault (such as in IIH) are subject to the Monroe–Kellie doctrine and that bilateral transverse sinus stenosis with elevated venous pressures in the IIH patient result in poor CSF resorption. In contrast, extracranial occlusions may not result in the same degree of CSF hydrodynamic disturbance. In addition, stenosis above the level of the jugular bulb results in constant intracranial venous hypertension, but because of the previously described postural changes in venous drainage, occlusion or stenosis of the extracranial jugular system may result in intermittent venous hypertension, seen only when supine. Regardless, questions such as these remain to be answered.

Unanswered Questions About CCSVI

If indeed the CCSVI hypothesis is involved in the pathogenesis of MS, many unanswered questions remain. MS has known geographic, racial, and gender predeliction. How does this model of venous disease integrate with those known epidemiologic factors? Is there a "double hit" model where the combination of CCSVI and one other factor are necessary to develop MS? Or is it possible that CCSVI is the result of MS rather than the cause of it? Zamboni's model of differing areas of obstruction in RRMS vs. PPMS is intriguing, but will need further validation. Is CCSVI a static or progressive process, and if so, when is the optimal therapeutic window? If indeed angioplasty is effective for CCSVI, what about restenosis – should they be treated and when?

Conclusion

From the earliest days of MS, researchers have searched for the elusive trigger(s) for this progressively debilitating disease. The earliest pathologic descriptions have documented a venocentric pattern, which has now been replicated in vivo using high-resolution MR techniques. Several studies have demonstrated whole brain and regional perfusion abnormalities in MS patients compared with controls. Parallels of venous hypertensive disease causing focal and diffuse neurologic symptoms, and white matter lesions, have been seen in intracranial and spinal dural arteriovenous fistulae, and treatment of the venous hypertension in these patients results in improvement or resolution of both the focal symptoms and imaging lesions. The CCSVI hypothesis integrates several of these threads into a common theory, where chronic venous insufficiency of the CNS triggers the inflammatory cascade.

Further study exploring this hypothesis appears to be warranted and should focus on several areas: Are there abnormalities in CNS venous drainage in MS patients when compared with controls? Which imaging modalities are able to accurately quantify these abnormalities? Does the location or pattern of these lesions correlate topographically with the location of demyelinating plaques? If indeed preliminary studies confirm venous outflow abnormalities, will treating these lesions with angioplasty and/or stent placement result in symptomatic change or alter progression of the disease? All of these questions remain unanswered but should be one of our main areas of MS research.

References

1. Rindfleisch E. Histologisches Detail zur grauen Degeneration von Gehirn und Ruckermark. Arch Pathol Anatl Physiol Klin Med (Virchow). 1863;26:474–83.
2. Dawson J. The histology of disseminated sclerosis. Trans R Soc Edinb. 1916;50: 517–740.
3. Putnam T. The pathogenesis of multiple sclerosis: a possible vascular factor. N Engl J Med. 1933;209:786–90.
4. Andeweg J. Consequences of the anatomy of deep venous outflow from the brain. Neuroradiology. 1999;41:233–41.
5. Andeweg J. The anatomy of collateral venous flow from the brain and its value in aetiological interpretation of intracranial pathology. Neuroradiology. 1996;38:621–8.
6. San Millan Ruiz D, Gailloud P, Rufenacht DA, et al. The craniocervical venous system in relation to cerebral venous drainage. AJNR Am J Neuroradiol. 2002;23:1500–8.
7. Doepp F, Schreiber SJ, von Munster T, et al. How does the blood leave the brain? A systematic ultrasound analysis of cerebral venous drainage patterns. Neuroradiology. 2004;46:565–70.
8. Schreiber SJ, Lurtzing F, Gotze R, et al. Extrajugular pathways of human cerebral venous blood drainage assessed by duplex ultrasound. J Appl Physiol. 2003;94:1802–5.
9. Valdueza JM, von Munster T, Hoffman O, et al. Postural dependency of the cerebral venous outflow. Lancet. 2000;355:200–1.
10. Dawson EA, Secher NH, Dalsgaard MK, et al. Standing up to the challenge of standing: a siphon does not support cerebral blood flow in humans. Am J Physiol Regul Integr Comp Physiol. 2004;287:R911–4.
11. Zamboni P, Consorti G, Galeotti R, et al. Venous collateral circulation of the extracranial cerebrospinal outflow routes. Curr Neurovasc Res. 2009;6:204–12.
12. Tobinick E, Vega CP. The cerebrospinal venous system: anatomy, physiology, and clinical implications. MedGenMed. 2006;8:53.
13. Law M, Saindane AM, Ge Y, et al. Microvascular abnormality in relapsing-remitting multiple sclerosis: perfusion MR imaging findings in normal-appearing white matter. Radiology. 2004;231:645–52.
14. Wuerfel J, Bellmann-Strobl J, Brunecker P, et al. Changes in cerebral perfusion precede plaque formation in multiple sclerosis: a longitudinal perfusion MRI study. Brain. 2004;127:111–9.
15. Adhya S, Johnson G, Herbert J, et al. Pattern of hemodynamic impairment in multiple sclerosis: dynamic susceptibility contrast perfusion MR imaging at 3.0 T. Neuroimage. 2006;33:1029–35.
16. Inglese M, Adhya S, Johnson G, et al. Perfusion magnetic resonance imaging correlates of neuropsychological impairment in multiple sclerosis. J Cereb Blood Flow Metab. 2008;28:164–71.
17. Inglese M, Park SJ, Johnson G, et al. Deep gray matter perfusion in multiple sclerosis: dynamic susceptibility contrast perfusion magnetic resonance imaging at 3 T. Arch Neurol. 2007;64:196–202.
18. Varga AW, Johnson G, Babb JS, et al. White matter hemodynamic abnormalities precede sub-cortical gray matter changes in multiple sclerosis. J Neurol Sci. 2009;282:28–33.
19. Tan IL, van Schijndel RA, Pouwels PJ, et al. MR venography of multiple sclerosis. AJNR Am J Neuroradiol. 2000;21:1039–42.
20. Ge Y, Zohrabian VM, Osa EO, et al. Diminished visibility of cerebral venous vasculature in multiple sclerosis by susceptibility-weighted imaging at 3.0 Tesla. J Magn Reson Imaging. 2009;29:1190–4.
21. Zamboni P, Galeotti R, Menegatti E, et al. Chronic cerebrospinal venous insufficiency in patients with multiple sclerosis. J Neurol Neurosurg Psychiatry. 2009; 80:392–9.

22. Doepp F, Paul F, Valdueza JM, et al. No cerebrocervical venous congestion in patients with multiple sclerosis. Ann Neurol. 2010;68:173–83.
23. Al-Omari MH, Rousan LA. Internal jugular vein morphology and hemodynamics in patients with multiple sclerosis. Int Angiol. 2010;29:115–20.
24. Singh AV, Zamboni P. Anomalous venous blood flow and iron deposition in multiple sclerosis. J Cereb Blood Flow Metab. 2009;29:1867–78.
25. Zamboni P. The big idea: iron-dependent inflammation in venous disease and proposed parallels in multiple sclerosis. J R Soc Med. 2006;99:589–93.
26. Zamboni P, Galeotti R, Menegatti E, et al. A prospective open-label study of endovascular treatment of chronic cerebrospinal venous insufficiency. J Vasc Surg. 2009;50:1348–58.e1–3.
27. O'Connor P, Filippi M, Arnason B, et al. 250 microg or 500 microg interferon beta-1b versus 20 mg glatiramer acetate in relapsing-remitting multiple sclerosis: a prospective, randomised, multicentre study. Lancet Neurol. 2009;8:889–97.
28. Polman CH, O'Connor PW, Havrdova E, et al. A randomized, placebo-controlled trial of natalizumab for relapsing multiple sclerosis. N Engl J Med. 2006;354: 899–910.
29. Ozyer U, Harman A, Yildirim E, et al. Long-term results of angioplasty and stent placement for treatment of central venous obstruction in 126 hemodialysis patients: a 10-year single-center experience. AJR Am J Roentgenol. 2009;193:1672–9.
30. Kim YC, Won JY, Choi SY, et al. Percutaneous treatment of central venous stenosis in hemodialysis patients: long-term outcomes. Cardiovasc Intervent Radiol. 2009;32:271–8.
31. Nael K, Kee ST, Solomon H, et al. Endovascular management of central thoracic veno-occlusive diseases in hemodialysis patients: a single institutional experience in 69 consecutive patients. J Vasc Interv Radiol. 2009;20:46–51.
32. Bakken AM, Protack CD, Saad WE, et al. Long-term outcomes of primary angioplasty and primary stenting of central venous stenosis in hemodialysis patients. J Vasc Surg. 2007;45:776–83.
33. Maya ID, Saddekni S, Allon M. Treatment of refractory central vein stenosis in hemodialysis patients with stents. Semin Dial. 2007;20:78–82.
34. Trerotola SO, Stavropoulos SW, Shlansky-Goldberg R, et al. Hemodialysis-related venous stenosis: treatment with ultrahigh-pressure angioplasty balloons. Radiology. 2004;231:259–62.
35. Quinn SF, Schuman ES, Demlow TA, et al. Percutaneous transluminal angioplasty versus endovascular stent placement in the treatment of venous stenoses in patients undergoing hemodialysis: intermediate results. J Vasc Interv Radiol. 1995;6:851–5.
36. Zipfel GJ, Shah MN, Refai D, et al. Cranial dural arteriovenous fistulas: modification of angiographic classification scales based on new natural history data. Neurosurg Focus. 2009;26:E14.
37. Cognard C, Gobin YP, Pierot L, et al. Cerebral dural arteriovenous fistulas: clinical and angiographic correlation with a revised classification of venous drainage. Radiology. 1995;194:671–80.
38. Borden JA, Wu JK, Shucart WA. A proposed classification for spinal and cranial dural arteriovenous fistulous malformations and implications for treatment. J Neurosurg. 1995;82:166–79.
39. Hahnel S, Jansen O, Geletneky K. MR appearance of an intracranial dural arteriovenous fistula leading to cervical myelopathy. Neurology. 1998;51:1131–5.
40. Hurst RW, Bagley LJ, Galetta S, et al. Dementia resulting from dural arteriovenous fistulas: the pathologic findings of venous hypertensive encephalopathy. AJNR Am J Neuroradiol. 1998;19:1267–73.
41. Brunereau L, Gobin YP, Meder JF, et al. Intracranial dural arteriovenous fistulas with spinal venous drainage: relation between clinical presentation and angiographic findings. AJNR Am J Neuroradiol. 1996;17:1549–54.

42. Davies MA, TerBrugge K, Willinsky R, et al. The validity of classification for the clinical presentation of intracranial dural arteriovenous fistulas. J Neurosurg. 1996;85:830–7.
43. Kim NH, Cho KT, Seo HS. Myelopathy due to intracranial dural arteriovenous fistula: a potential diagnostic pitfall. Case report. J Neurosurg. 2011;114(3):830–3.
44. Stevens EA, Powers AK, Morris PP, et al. Occult dural arteriovenous fistula causing rapidly progressive conus medullaris syndrome and paraplegia after lumbar microdiscectomy. Spine J. 2009;9:e8–12.
45. Akkoc Y, Atamaz F, Oran I, et al. Intracranial dural arteriovenous fistula draining into spinal perimedullary veins: a rare cause of myelopathy. J Korean Med Sci. 2006;21:958–62.
46. Renner C, Helm J, Roth H, et al. Intracranial dural arteriovenous fistula associated with progressive cervical myelopathy and normal venous drainage of the thoracolumbar cord: case report and review of the literature. Surg Neurol. 2006;65:506–10.
47. Waragai M, Takeuchi H, Fukushima T, et al. MRI and SPECT studies of dural arteriovenous fistulas presenting as pure progressive dementia with leukoencephalopathy: a cause of treatable dementia. Eur J Neurol. 2006;13:754–9.
48. Yamakami I, Kobayashi E, Yamaura A. Diffuse white matter changes caused by dural arteriovenous fistula. J Clin Neurosci. 2001;8:471–5.
49. Zeidman SM, Monsein LH, Arosarena O, et al. Reversibility of white matter changes and dementia after treatment of dural fistulas. AJNR Am J Neuroradiol. 1995;16:1080–3.
50. Lee PH, Lee JS, Shin DH, et al. Parkinsonism as an initial manifestation of dural arteriovenous fistula. Eur J Neurol. 2005;12:403–6.
51. Fujita A, Nakamura M, Tamaki N, et al. Haemodynamic assessment in patients with dural arteriovenous fistulae: dynamic susceptibility contrast-enhanced MRI. Neuroradiology. 2002;44:806–11.
52. Willinsky R, Goyal M, terBrugge K, et al. Tortuous, engorged pial veins in intracranial dural arteriovenous fistulas: correlations with presentation, location, and MR findings in 122 patients. AJNR Am J Neuroradiol. 1999;20:1031–6.
53. Saladino A, Atkinson JL, Rabinstein AA, et al. Surgical treatment of spinal dural arteriovenous fistulae: a consecutive series of 154 patients. Neurosurgery. 2010;67(5):1350–7. discussion 1357-8.
54. Prieto R, Pascual JM, Gutierrez R, et al. Recovery from paraplegia after the treatment of spinal dural arteriovenous fistula: case report and review of the literature. Acta Neurochir (Wien). 2009;151:1385–97.
55. Lagares A, Millan JM, Ramos A, et al. Perfusion computed tomography in a dural arteriovenous fistula presenting with focal signs: vascular congestion as a cause of reversible neurologic dysfunction. Neurosurgery. 2010;66:E226–7. discussion E227.
56. Stefani MA, Porter PJ, terBrugge KG, et al. Large and deep brain arteriovenous malformations are associated with risk of future hemorrhage. Stroke. 2002;33:1220–4.
57. Stefani MA, Porter PJ, terBrugge KG, et al. Angioarchitectural factors present in brain arteriovenous malformations associated with hemorrhagic presentation. Stroke. 2002;33:920–4.
58. Donnet A, Metellus P, Levrier O, et al. Endovascular treatment of idiopathic intracranial hypertension: clinical and radiologic outcome of 10 consecutive patients. Neurology. 2008;70:641–7.
59. Higgins JN, Cousins C, Owler BK, et al. Idiopathic intracranial hypertension: 12 cases treated by venous sinus stenting. J Neurol Neurosurg Psychiatry. 2003;74:1662–6.
60. Bussiere M, Falero R, Nicolle D, et al. Unilateral transverse sinus stenting of patients with idiopathic intracranial hypertension. AJNR Am J Neuroradiol. 2010;31:645–50.
61. Arac A, Lee M, Steinberg GK, et al. Efficacy of endovascular stenting in dural venous sinus stenosis for the treatment of idiopathic intracranial hypertension. Neurosurg Focus. 2009;27:E14.

10

Multiple Sclerosis: The Next 20 Years

Howard L. Weiner

Keywords: Heterogeneity, Biomarkers, Lesions, Innate immune system, Cytotoxic, Immunotherapy, Cure

Introduction

Although one cannot predict where science will be in two decades from now, based on our current understanding and the work being done, it is possible to speculate on where the field of multiple sclerosis will be in 2030. I discuss below, four important areas which I believe will change our understanding and treatment of the disease in the next 20 years.

Understanding the Heterogeneity of MS

Although MS is classified as a single disease, it is clear that there are different subtypes and most likely different pathological processes. Thus, MS is more a syndrome than a single disease entity and the MS syndrome has both clinical and pathologic heterogeneity [1, 2]. The clinical heterogeneity is reflected in the different types and stages of the disease. One of the clear examples is the recent identification of antibodies as being linked to neuromyelitis optica (NMO). Although NMO has not been classically considered MS, it is classified as a demyelinating disease and many of the treatment approaches to MS are applied to NMO. NMO appears to be an MS variant associated with antibodies to the aquaporin receptor [3, 4]. An important question is the degree to which there are different pathologic subtypes to MS whose etiology, although still in the immune realm, is driven by different mechanism, for example, is there a type of MS that is more mediated by CD8 cells and linked to a specific viral infection? There may be a type of MS linked to immune repertoire that is driven by defects in regulatory cells and there may be different immune mechanisms such as Th1 type MS vs. Th17 type MS. There are rare malignant forms including Marburg's variant, tumefactive MS, and Balo's concentric

From: *Clinical Neuroimmunology: Multiple Sclerosis and Related Disorders*, Current Clinical Neurology, Edited by: S.A. Rizvi and P.K. Coyle, DOI 10.1007/978-1-60327-860-7_10, © Springer Science+Business Media, LLC 2011 sclerosis. An unanswered question relates to why benign forms of MS exist [5, 6]. Although some cases of MS are defined as benign, and progress with prolonged follow-up [7], there are clearly benign forms of the disease. By definition, patients with benign MS do not enter the progressive phase. The ability to identify benign or malignant MS early in the course of the illness is very important for treatment strategies. We compared brain parenchymal fraction over a 2-year period in benign vs. early relapsing remitting MS matched for age and EDSS and found that patients with benign MS had less loss of BPF [8]. The key to understanding MS subtypes will depend on linking specific mechanisms to specific disease categories, clinical course, and response to therapy. Genetic factors appear linked to disease susceptibility and a better understanding of these factors may also distinguish different subgroups. For example, an HLA-DR2 dose effect may be associated with a more severe form of the disease [9]. Thus, a major change in the future will be understanding the heterogeneity of the disease.

Development of Biomarkers

One of the major advances that can be expected in the future is the development of reliable biomarkers. Despite the availability of approved drugs for MS and many more in the pipeline, biomarkers are needed to address the heterogeneity of MS and devise appropriate treatment strategies. The two major areas related to biomarkers are magnetic resonance imaging and immune biomarkers.

Magnetic Resonance Imaging

MRI has served as the primary biomarker for MS [10] and although conventional imaging does not always link strongly to clinical outcomes, every FDA-approved MS drug showed positive results on MRI. Because of MRI, the first drug for MS (betaseron) was approved when it was shown that treatment markedly reduced new and enhancing lesions on MRI, clearly demonstrating a biologic effect. Since then MRI has served as a cornerstone, a biomarker, for the development of drugs for MS. In general, the classic pathway for drug development is a Phase II study showing that the drug being tested effects gadolinium enhancing lesions on the MRI. Despite the success and importance of MRI as a biomarker for testing drugs in Phase II for relapsing forms of MS, much is needed to advance MRI as a biomarker accepted by the FDA as a surrogate.

MRI and pathologic studies have shown gray matter atrophy in MS, which is linked to cognitive impairment [11]. In addition, cortical foci of demyelination, microglial activation, leptomeningeal inflammation, iron deposition, and neuronal loss occur in the gray matter. The degree to which current therapy attenuate gray matter destruction is not known. It is likely that the processes affecting the gray matter are highly clinically relevant and will ultimately provide new therapeutic targets. MRI has also shown diffuse involvement of the normal appearing white matter including demyelination, inflammation, and axonal injury not seen by conventional imaging [12] but which can be visualized by magnetization transfer, diffusion-weighted, and spectroscopic imaging. These changes can precede overt gadolinium-enhancing lesions by months and result from early migration of lymphocytes into the brain.

Although there are studies demonstrating atrophy, gray matter changes, and iron deposition, these have not yet been successfully applied to MS as a workable biomarker. Spinal cord dysfunction is primarily responsible for gait impairment in MS, the major disabling feature of the illness and better spinal cord imaging should improve clinical MRI correlation [13]. Spinal cord atrophy may occur early and the clinical heterogeneity of MS and benign forms of MS may relate to atrophy and spinal cord involvement. MRI studies using double inversion-recovery imaging to detect cortical lesions suggests the importance of gray matter sparing in predicting a benign clinical course [11]. In the future, more sophisticated imaging should give a better picture of the disease at different stages and become a validated biomarker.

One of the most important areas is cellular imaging, currently there are ways to image a microglia, but these are comparatively primitive. With new techniques and new ligands identified for PET imaging, it should be possible to understand different inflammatory components of the disease and different stages. These studies combined with a better understanding of neurodegeneration should allow for the monitoring and development of drugs related to disease progression by MRI.

Immune Biomarkers

A crucial area that could revolutionize treatment and drug development in MS is the development of a blood test (blood biomarker) linked to disease stage and activity. Although there are many changes in the blood that have been identified, there is no validated blood test that can serve as an immune profile of disease stage. With more sophisticated immune measures, we anticipate biomarkers in the blood to provide an immune profile of the MS patient. Similar approaches may be developed for the spinal fluid, although it is not easy to perform multiple spinal taps on MS patients. With many drugs currently on the market and more to be developed, it is becoming increasing difficult to perform placebo-controlled trials and in the future the use of the blood biomarkers to serve as surrogates for the development of new drugs will be crucial.

We and others have shown immune measures that are associated with disease activity and MRI activity [14–16] and RNA profiling is beginning to identify gene expression patterns associated to different forms of MS and disease progression [17, 18]. In a new approach, we performed antigen microarray analysis to characterize patterns of low-affinity antibody reactivity in MS serum against a panel of CNS protein and lipid autoantigens and heat shock proteins. Using informatic analysis for validation, we found unique autoantibody signatures that distinguished RR, SPMS, PPMS MS from healthy controls and other neurologic or autoimmune diseases [19]. RRMS was characterized by autoantibodies to heat shock proteins that were not observed in PPMS or SPMS. In addition, RRMS, SPMS, and PPMS were characterized by unique patterns of reactivity to CNS antigens (Figure 10.1). We also examined sera from patients with different immunopathologic patterns of MS as determined by brain biopsy [1] and we identified unique antibody patterns to lipids and CNS-derived peptides that were linked to type I and type II patterns. The demonstration of unique serum immune signatures linked to different stages and pathologic processes in MS provides a new avenue to understand disease heterogeneity, to monitor MS and to characterize immunopathogenic

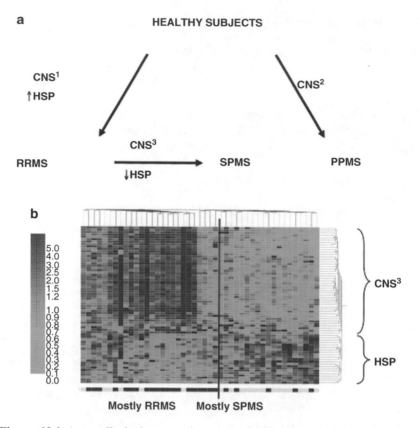

Figure 10.1 Autoantibody immune signatures of MS in the peripheral blood as revealed by antigen arrays. (**a**) Schematic depiction of immune signatures associated with RRMS, SPMS, and PPMS. (**b**) Heatmap depicting antibody reactivities against myelin antigens and heat shock proteins in SPMS vs. RRMS

mechanisms and therapeutic targets in the disease. Furthermore, based on the antigen arrays, we have found increased levels of oxysterols in the blood of MS patients with unique patterns for relapsing remitting and progressive MS [20]. Oxysterols may serve as a serum biomarker for progressive forms of MS.

Understanding the Relationship Between Relapsing Remitting and Progressive MS

In most instances, MS begins as a relapsing remitting disease that in many patients becomes secondary progressive. Approximately 10% of patients begin with a primary progressive form of the disease. Although primary progressive MS differs clinically and in response to treatment from relapsing MS [21], it is somehow related as there are families in which one member has relapsing MS and another the primary progressive form. Not all patients enter the secondary progressive stage and those that do not generally have a more benign form of the disease. Early stages of MS are associated with relapses and gadolinium enhancement on MRI which decrease with time even without treatment. It is not clear why this happens though it may relate to changes that occur in the adaptive and innate immune system over the course of the illness (Figure 10.2). The progressive forms of the disease are the most disabling and are likely similar in terms of pathogenic mechanisms. Epidemiologic studies have raised the question whether relapses are related to or are independent from the development of progressive MS [22]. Some argue that MS is primarily a degenerative process with secondary inflammation. This raises the central question: will strong anti-inflammatory therapy given early prevent the onset of progression? A major advance that we can expect over the next 20 years is an understanding of the progressive forms of MS, development of treatments that affect progression and ways to monitor it. Understanding progression will probably involve a better understanding of the innate immune system in MS and mechanisms of neurodegeneration.

The Innate Immune System

The innate immune system consists of monocytes, dendritic cells, and microglia. It is becoming increasingly recognized that the innate immune system plays an important role in the immunopathogenesis of MS. Although the secondary progressive phase of MS is related to neuorodegenerative changes in the CNS, it is now clear that the peripheral innate immune system changes when patients transition from the relapsing remitting to the progressive stage. We have observed this in our studies of IL-12, IL-18, and dendritic cells [23–26]. Furthermore, chronic microglial activation occurs in MS [27]. This leads to a different view of the immunopathogenesis of MS that integrates both limbs of the immune system and links them to different disease stages and processes. Thus, the adaptive immune system drives acute inflammatory events (attacks, gadolinium enhancement on MRI), whereas innate immunity drives progressive aspects of MS (Figure 10.2). This raises important questions regarding the pathogenesis and treatment of different stages of MS. Of note, there do not appear to be abnormalities of CD4+CD25+ regulatory T cells in secondary progressive MS [28]. It is not known the degree to which the adaptive and innate immune systems affect each other in MS. As discussed below, a major question is whether aggressive and early anti-inflammatory treatment will prevent the secondary progressive form of the disease. There is some evidence that this is occurring; studies are beginning to show that treatment with interferons delays the onset of progressive stage [29]. Of note, there is a form of EAE driven by the innate, rather than the adaptive immune system [30]. There are no specific therapies designed to affect the innate immune system in MS and scientists are only beginning to investigate the innate immune system in MS and characterize it as relates to disease stage and response to therapy. Furthermore, as the adaptive immune system, there are different classes of innate immune responses, e.g., protective and tolerogenic vs. pathogenic and pro-inflammatory. We have found increased osteopontin expression in dendritic cells in relapsing MS [31].

Neurodegeneration in MS

Axonal and myelin loss are prominent pathologic features of MS [32] and can be directly caused by immune cells, e.g., cytotoxic CD8 cells damaging neurons or macrophages stripping myelin from the axon [33]; or can result from release of toxic intermediates, e.g., glutamate and nitric oxide.

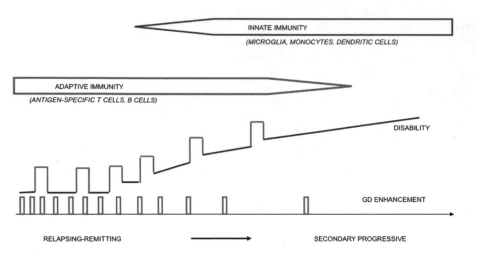

IMMUNE STATUS AND DISEASE COURSE IN MS

INNATE IMMUNITY
(MICROGLIA, MONOCYTES, DENDRITIC CELLS)

ADAPTIVE IMMUNITY
(ANTIGEN-SPECIFIC T CELLS, B CELLS)

DISABILITY

GD ENHANCEMENT

RELAPSING-REMITTING   SECONDARY PROGRESSIVE

Figure 10.2 Immune status and disease course in multiple sclerosis. MS involves a relapsing–remitting followed by a secondary progressive phase. The relapsing–remitting phase is characterized by clinical attacks, gadolinium enhancement on MRI, minimal disability and is driven by the adaptive immune response. The secondary progressive phase is characterized by progressive accumulation of disability in the absence of clinical attacks and is driven by the innate immune system

These intermediates can trigger immune cascades that further enhance inflammatory-mediated CNS damage. Thus, glutamate and nitric oxide can lead to enhanced expression of CCL2 on astrocytes which, in turn, leads to infiltration of CD11b cells and additional tissue damage [34]. AMPA antagonists have been shown to have an ameliorating affect in acute EAE models [35, 36] and we have found that a carbon-based fullerene linked to an NMDA receptor with anti-excitotoxic properties slows progression and prevents axonal damage in the spinal cord in a model of chronic progressive EAE [34]. Although the compound is not an immune compound, it reduces infiltration of CD11b cells into the CNS. Another important component of neurodegeneration relates to changes in Na channels and these are targets of therapy [37]. Thus development of compounds to affect these processes and biomarkers that link to them is crucial to our understanding of the progressive forms of the disease.

Curing MS

Great strides have been made in our understanding and treatment of MS and given this progress, we must now ask what would it mean to cure MS and what is needed to achieve this goal [38]. When one examines the question, it becomes clear that there are three definitions of "cure" as it relates to MS: (1) halt progression of the disease, (2) reverse neurologic deficits, and (3) develop a strategy to prevent MS. We are making progress in halting or slowing progression of MS have approaches that may help reverse neurologic deficits and for the first time are beginning to develop strategies to prevent MS.

Immunotherapy to Halting Disease Activity and Progression

One could argue that a cure is a treatment that eradicates MS. This may be true for an infection or tumor but not for MS, in which there is an inherent defect of the immune system and chronic inflammation of the brain. If, however, one treated MS at the clinical onset and prevented disease progression for the remainder of the patient's life, it would be considered a cure. There may be patients that are being "cured" with current therapy though they may have less severe forms of the disease. Interferons and glatiramer acetate are only partially effective in MS, with stronger effects observed with natalizumab and alemtuzumab [39, 40]. This raises a central question: will aggressive and early immunotherapy prevent the secondary progressive form of the disease? With the strong anti-inflammatory effects of a drug such as alemtuzumab, this question could be addressed in the future, though widespread testing may be prohibited by side effects. Other approaches of aggressive immunotherapy at disease onset to test this hypothesis includes bone marrow transplantation, non-ablative chemotherapy utilizing cyclophosphamide [41], or induction with a drug such as cyclophosphamide or mitoxantrone followed by maintenance immune modulation [42].

Because the immune damage to myelin and axons initiates secondary pathways of CNS damage, non-immune-based therapy may be required to control disease progression. The presence of gluatamate and nitric oxide leads to axon injury and demyelination which in itself can set up an inflammatory response on astrocytes that express CCL2 and lead to the infiltration of CD11B cells.

Thus, a complex disease such as MS will require treatment(s) that have an effect on multiple pathways including the suppression of Th1/Th17 responses, induction of T regs, altering traffic of cells into the CNS and protecting axons and myelin from degeneration initiated by inflammation, and affecting the innate immune system. If multiple drugs are required to achieve this effect, one must be certain that one treatment does not interfere with the other. It may also be that one must first suppress Th1 and Th17 responses before inducing T regs. Because of disease heterogeneity, there will be responders and nonresponders to each "effective" therapy. Finally, the earlier treatment is initiated the more likely it is to be effective.

Inherent in the concept of curing MS by halting progression, is the ability to demonstrate that progression has been halted in a group of patients and to identify those factors associated with preventing the onset of progressive disease. We have initiated the CLIMB natural history study in which 1,000 patients with new onset MS will be followed over a 20-year period with clinical evaluation, MRI imaging, and immune and genetic markers, to identify which factors are associated with disease progression [43].

Repairing a Damaged Nervous System

There is evidence of repair in the CNS of those with MS, though the mechanisms involved are not well understood. Furthermore, it has been shown in animal models that reducing inflammation promotes repair even with non-specific immunosuppressants such as cyclophosphamide [44]. Blocking molecules that inhibit axonal (Nogo) or myelin (Lingo-1) growth may promote repair and treatment of animal models with anti-Lingo-1, anti-Nogo, or antibodies reacting with oligodendrocytes have shown positive effects [45–47]. Furthermore, treatments that affect sodium channels may not only affect nerve conduction but also have effects in microglia activation [48]. Nonetheless, it must be emphasized that when severe neuronal and oligodendrocyte loss occurs, it is unlikely that one would be able to significantly reverse neurologic deficits. Of note, stem cell therapy may be inhibited by CNS inflammation [49].

Preventing MS

If MS is triggered in the environment in susceptible individuals, it may be possible to prevent MS, though one must first be able to identify those at risk. Autoantibody signatures in the serum have the potential to identify those at risk [19]. Some believe vaccination against EBV virus or treating children at high risk to develop MS with vitamin D may be initial approaches.

Conclusion

If one views MS in 20-year increments, clear patterns emerge and each 20-year period can be viewed as a specific era. 1970–1990 was the era of establishing the role of the immune system in MS and showing that MS was not caused by a specific MS virus. 1990–2010 was the era of FDA-approved anti-inflammatory drugs for the treatment of relapsing forms of MS. I believe that 2010–2030 will be the era in which we understand and develop therapy to treat and/or prevent the progressive forms of MS. Furthermore, it will be an era in which we develop biomarkers for individual patient profiling and as tools to test new drugs. Looking forward, the era of 2030–2050 will be one of trials to prevent MS and consolidating our ability at nervous system repair.

References

1. Lassmann H, Bruck W, Lucchinetti CF. The immunopathology of multiple sclerosis: an overview. Brain Pathol. 2007;17:210–8.
2. Breij EC, Brink BP, Veerhuis R, et al. Homogeneity of active demyelinating lesions in established multiple sclerosis. Ann Neurol. 2008;63:16–25.
3. Hinson SR, Roemer SF, Lucchinetti CF, et al. Aquaporin-4-binding autoantibodies in patients with neuromyelitis optica impair glutamate transport by down-regulating EAAT2. J Exp Med. 2008;205:2473–81.
4. Misu T, Fujihara K, Kakita A, et al. Loss of aquaporin 4 in lesions of neuromyelitis optica: distinction from multiple sclerosis. Brain. 2007;130:1224–34.
5. Ramsaransing GS, De Keyser J. Benign course in multiple sclerosis: a review. Acta Neurol Scand. 2006;113:359–69.
6. Pittock SJ, McClelland RL, Mayr WT, et al. Clinical implications of benign multiple sclerosis: a 20-year population-based follow-up study. Ann Neurol. 2004;56:303–6.
7. Hawkins SA, McDonnell GV. Benign multiple sclerosis? Clinical course, long term follow up, and assessment of prognostic factors. J Neurol Neurosurg Psychiatry. 1999;67:148–52.
8. Gauthier S, Berger AM, Liptak Z, et al. Benign MS is characterized by a lower rate of brain atrophy as compared to early MS. Arch Neurol. 2009;66(2):234–7.
9. Barcellos LF, Oksenberg JR, Begovich AB, et al. HLA-DR2 dose effect on susceptibility to multiple sclerosis and influence on disease course. Am J Hum Genet. 2003;72:710–6.
10. Bakshi R, Neema M, Healy B, et al. Predicting clinical progression in multiple sclerosis with the magnetic resonance disease severity scale. Arch Neurol. 2008;65(11):1449–53.

11. Pirko I, Lucchinetti CF, Sriram S, et al. Gray matter involvement in multiple sclerosis. Neurology. 2007;68:634–42.
12. Miller DH, Thompson AJ, Filippi M. Magnetic resonance studies of abnormalities in the normal appearing white matter and grey matter in multiple sclerosis. J Neurol. 2003;250:1407–19.
13. Agosta F, Filippi M. MRI of spinal cord in multiple sclerosis. J Neuroimaging. 2007;17 Suppl 1:46S–9.
14. Comabella M, Balashov K, et al. Elevated interleukin-12 in progressive multiple sclerosis correlates with disease activity and is normalized by pulse cyclophosphamide therapy. J Clin Invest. 1998;102:671–8.
15. Khoury SJ, Guttmann CR, Orav EJ, et al. Longitudinal MRI in multiple sclerosis: correlation between disability and lesion burden. Neurology. 1994;44:2120–4.
16. Khoury SJ, Guttmann CR, Orav EJ, et al. Changes in activated T cells in the blood correlate with disease activity in multiple sclerosis. Arch Neurol. 2000;57: 1183–9.
17. Achiron A, Gurevich M, Friedman N, et al. Blood transcriptional signatures of multiple sclerosis: unique gene expression of disease activity. Ann Neurol. 2004;55:410–7.
18. Corvol JC, Pelletier D, Henry RG, et al. Abrogation of T cell quiescence characterizes patients at high risk for multiple sclerosis after the initial neurological event. Proc Natl Acad Sci USA. 2008;105:11839–44.
19. Quintana F, Farez M, Viglietta V, et al. Antigen microarrays identify unique serum autoantibody signatures associated with different clinical forms and pathologic subtypes of multiple sclerosis. Proc Natl Acad Sci USA. 2008;105(48):18889–94.
20. Farez MF, Quintana FJ, Gandhi R, Izquierdo G, Lucas M, Weiner HL. Toll-like receptor 2 and poly(ADP-ribose) polymerase 1 promote central nervous system neuroinflammation in progressive EAE. Nat Immunol. 2009;10:958–64.
21. Miller DH, Leary SM. Primary-progressive multiple sclerosis. Lancet Neurol. 2007;6:903–12.
22. Confavreux C, Vukusic S, Moreau T, et al. Relapses and progression of disability in multiple sclerosis. N Engl J Med. 2000;343:1430–8.
23. Balashov KE, Smith DR, Khoury SJ, et al. Increased interleukin 12 production in progressive multiple sclerosis: induction by activated CD4+ T cells via CD40 ligand. Proc Natl Acad Sci USA. 1997;94:599–603.
24. Karni A, Koldzic DN, Bharanidharan P, et al. IL-18 is linked to raised IFN-gamma in multiple sclerosis and is induced by activated CD4(+) T cells via CD40-CD40 ligand interactions. J Neuroimmunol. 2002;125:134–40.
25. Karni A, Abraham M, Monsonego A, et al. Innate immunity in multiple sclerosis: myeloid dendritic cells in secondary progressive multiple sclerosis are activated and drive a proinflammatory immune response. J Immunol. 2006;177:4196–202.
26. Vaknin-Dembinsky A, Balashov K, Weiner HL. IL-23 is increased in dendritic cells in multiple sclerosis and down-regulation of IL-23 by antisense oligos increases dendritic cell IL-10 production. J Immunol. 2006;176:7768–74.
27. Kutzelnigg A, Lucchinetti CF, Stadelmann C, et al. Cortical demyelination and diffuse white matter injury in multiple sclerosis. Brain. 2005;128:2705–12.
28. Venken K, Hellings N, Hensen K, et al. Secondary progressive in contrast to relapsing-remitting multiple sclerosis patients show a normal CD4+CD25+ regulatory T-cell function and FOXP3 expression. J Neurosci Res. 2006;83:1432–46.
29. Trojano M, Pellegrini F, Fuiani A, et al. New natural history of interferon-beta-treated relapsing multiple sclerosis. Ann Neurol. 2007;61:300–6.
30. Furtado GC, Pina B, Tacke F, et al. A novel model of demyelinating encephalomyelitis induced by monocytes and dendritic cells. J Immunol. 2006;177:6871–9.
31. Gopal M, Mittal A, Weiner H. Increased osteopontin expression in dendritic cells amplifies IL-17 production by CD4+ T cells in experimental autoimmune encephalomyelitis and in multiple sclerosis. J Immunol. 2008;181(11):7480–8.

32. Bjartmar C, Wujek JR, Trapp BD. Axonal loss in the pathology of MS: consequences for understanding the progressive phase of the disease. J Neurol Sci. 2003;206:165–71.
33. Trapp BD, Wujek JR, Criste GA, et al. Evidence for synaptic stripping by cortical microglia. Glia. 2007;55:360–8.
34. Basso AS, Frenkel D, Quintana FJ, et al. Reversal of axonal loss and disability in a mouse model of progressive multiple sclerosis. J Clin Invest. 2008;118:1532–43.
35. Pitt D, Werner P, Raine CS. Glutamate excitotoxicity in a model of multiple sclerosis. Nat Med. 2000;6:67–70.
36. Smith T, Groom A, Zhu B, et al. Autoimmune encephalomyelitis ameliorated by AMPA antagonists. Nat Med. 2000;6:62–6.
37. Waxman SG. Mechanisms of disease: sodium channels and neuroprotection in multiple sclerosis-current status. Nat Clin Pract Neurol. 2008;4:159–69.
38. Weiner H. Curing MS how science is solving the mysteries of multiple sclerosis. New York: Crown; 2004. p. 309.
39. Rudick RA, Stuart WH, Calabresi PA, et al. Natalizumab plus interferon beta-1a for relapsing multiple sclerosis. N Engl J Med. 2006;354:911–23.
40. Coles AJ, Compston DA, Selmaj KW, et al. Alemtuzumab vs. interferon beta-1a in early multiple sclerosis. N Engl J Med. 2008;359:1786–801.
41. Krishnan C, Kaplin AI, Brodsky RA, et al. Reduction of disease activity and disability with high-dose cyclophosphamide in patients with aggressive multiple sclerosis. Arch Neurol. 2008;65:1044–51.
42. Le Page E, Leray E, Taurin G, et al. Mitoxantrone as induction treatment in aggressive relapsing remitting multiple sclerosis: treatment response factors in a 5 year follow-up observational study of 100 consecutive patients. J Neurol Neurosurg Psychiatry. 2008;79:52–6.
43. Gauthier SA, Glanz BI, Mandel M, et al. A model for the comprehensive investigation of a chronic autoimmune disease: the multiple sclerosis CLIMB study. Autoimmun Rev. 2006;5:532–6.
44. Rodriguez M, Lindsley MD. Immunosuppression promotes CNS remyelination in chronic virus-induced demyelinating disease. Neurology. 1992;42:348–57.
45. Mi S, Hu B, Hahm K, et al. LINGO-1 antagonist promotes spinal cord remyelination and axonal integrity in MOG-induced experimental autoimmune encephalomyelitis. Nat Med. 2007;13:1228–33.
46. Karnezis T, Mandemakers W, McQualter JL, et al. The neurite outgrowth inhibitor Nogo A is involved in autoimmune-mediated demyelination. Nat Neurosci. 2004;7:736–44.
47. Warrington AE, Asakura K, Bieber AJ, et al. Human monoclonal antibodies reactive to oligodendrocytes promote remyelination in a model of multiple sclerosis. Proc Natl Acad Sci USA. 2000;97:6820–5.
48. Craner MJ, Damarjian TG, Liu S, et al. Sodium channels contribute to microglia/macrophage activation and function in EAE and MS. Glia. 2005;49:220–9.
49. Pluchino S, Muzio L, Imitola J, et al. Persistent inflammation alters the function of the endogenous brain stem cell compartment. Brain. 2008;131:2564–78.

Part II

Other CNS Inflammatory Disorders

11

Acute Disseminated Encephalomyelitis

Patricia K. Coyle

Keywords: Acute disseminated encephalomyelitis, Leukoencephalitis, Perivenous, Intravenous immunoglobulins, Steroids

Introduction

Acute disseminated encephalomyelitis (ADEM), also called postinfectious encephalitis/encephalomyelitis, is an immune-mediated inflammatory and demyelinating multifocal disorder of the central nervous system (CNS). It is typically monophasic [1]. In most patients, ADEM follows within a few days to weeks of a triggering infection or more rarely vaccination (Table 11.1). A minority of patients have no identifiable prior event. ADEM does not represent an ongoing CNS infection.

ADEM is predominantly a pediatric disorder. The average age at onset is 6–8 years [2, 3]. ADEM is much less common in adults, where it can occur at any age but particularly affects young adults. It is rare in the very young (ages 2–3 years) and in the elderly. The incidence in children is reported to range from 0.07 to 0.64 cases per 100,000 population per year [4–7]. Most series show a slight male predominance. ADEM is said to account for at least 8%, and perhaps as high as 20%, of acute encephalitis cases [8].

Pathology

The pathologic hallmark of ADEM is widespread white and gray matter perivenous inflammation with demyelination [9]. The inflammatory infiltrate is made up of predominantly lymphocytes and monocytes/macrophages. Inflammation results in subsequent "sleeve-like" demyelination, with axons relatively spared [10]. In a recent pathology study, perivenous demyelination was associated with a distinct pattern of cortical microglial activation without myelin loss [9]. Perivenous lesions can coalesce to form larger demyelinated lesions. This neuropathology is quite distinct from multiple sclerosis (MS)

From: *Clinical Neuroimmunology: Multiple Sclerosis and Related Disorders*, Current Clinical Neurology,
Edited by: S.A. Rizvi and P.K. Coyle, DOI 10.1007/978-1-60327-860-7_11,
© Springer Science+Business Media, LLC 2011

Table 11.1 Triggering events for postinfectious encephalitis/encephalomyelitis.

- Exanthematous viral infections (more historical)
  - Measles (0.1%), varicella zoster virus, rubella, smallpox
- Other viruses (HIV, HTLV-1, hepatitis, other herpesviruses)
- Viral respiratory tract infection
- Viral gastroenteritis
- Nonspecific febrile illness
- Bacterial infection
  - Group a beta-hemolytic streptococci
  - *Borrelia burgdorferi*
  - Campylobacter, leptospira, chlamydia, legionella
  - Mycoplasma pneumoniae
- Rickettsial infection
  - *Rickettsia rickettsii*
- Aseptic meningitis
- Vaccination ($\leq$1–5 cases per million)
  - Rabies, pertussis, diphtheria
  - Tetanus-polio, measles-mumps-rubella, influenza, smallpox, hepatitis B, Japanese B encephalitis, hog vaccine, yellow fever
- Animal/insect bites
- Viper bite with anti-venom therapy
- Neoplastic process
  - Leukemia, non-Hodgkin's lymphoma
- Organ transplant

or acute viral encephalitis. MS involves confluent demyelination [9]. Gross pathology can involve brain congestion and swelling, with engorged blood vessels within the white matter. Microscopically, this is associated with hyperemia, endothelial swelling, vessel wall infiltration by inflammatory cells, and perivascular edema [11].

Acute hemorrhagic leukoencephalitis (AHLE), a hyperacute variant of ADEM discussed below, shows a somewhat different pathology, with prominent neutrophil infiltration, punctate petechial and ring-like hemorrhages, and necrotizing vasculitis [12].

Clinical Features

At least 70% of patients report an antecedent prodromal event, with symptoms beginning 2–30 days later [8]. Most often this is infection, with less than 5% following vaccination [13]. Viral infection is the commonest trigger, but nonviral pathogens and rare noninfectious exposures are also reported [14, 15]. The classic clinical picture of ADEM involves multifocal neurologic deficits superimposed on diffuse encephalopathy (Table 11.2) [16]. A key feature is impaired level of consciousness. Drowsiness, lethargy, stupor, or coma is much more suggestive for an ADEM diagnosis than is simple irritability or

Table 11.2 Clinical features of postinfectious encephalitis/encephalomyelitis.

- Encephalopathy (drowsiness/lethargy, stupor/coma)
- Fever
- Headache
- Motor deficits
- Ataxia
- Sensory abnormalities
- Seizures (focal or generalized)
- Optic neuritis (unilateral or bilateral)
  - Bilateral may need to rule out neuromyelitis optica-Devic spectrum disorder
- Transverse myelitis
- Bladder, bowel disturbances
- Language abnormalities
- Cranial neuropathy/brainstem deficits
- Visual field defects
- Radicular, neuropathic features
- Meningismus

mood disturbance. Cognitive deficits are seen [17]. Multifocal deficits can involve motor, sensory, visual, coordination, and gait disturbances. Ataxia and language disturbance may be more common in children than adults [16, 18]. Lower urinary tract dysfunction can be seen in 33% and may persist [19]. It is also common to have neurologic abnormalities outside the brain itself. Spinal cord is involved in up to 67% of cases and is more often seen in adults [8, 10]. Peripheral nervous system involvement (polyradiculoneuropathy) occurs in 5–44% [8, 20], perhaps reflecting that ADEM is part of a much broader immune-mediated neurologic spectrum that includes Guillain–Barre syndrome. Unusual clinical manifestations include acute psychosis, cerebellar mutism, various movement disorders, and Kluver–Bucy syndrome [21–25]. ADEM can certainly present with a picture that suggests mass lesion with increased intracranial pressure. It has also developed following aseptic meningitis [26]. Sustained high fever and hyponatremia were noted in these meningitis patients.

Based on recently proposed diagnostic criteria (see below), clinical features may fluctuate, and new features may appear over a 3-month period and are still considered one episode. Perhaps 5% up to 25% of ADEM patients have more than one attack, with as many as four episodes over a 32-month period [27].

Diagnosis

Diagnosis depends on a consistent clinical and laboratory picture, with other possibilities ruled out. Core laboratory tests involve blood work, neuroimaging, and cerebrospinal fluid (CSF) evaluation. The International Pediatric MS Study Group proposed formal consensus definition criteria for pediatric ADEM (Table 11.3) [28]. They also recognized and defined recurrent (80%)

Table 11.3 Proposed pediatric postinfectious encephalitis/encephalomyelitis ADEM diagnostic criteria [28].

- Monophasic ADEM
  - Acute or subacute onset; involves multifocal CNS areas; clinical onset polysymptomatic with encephalopathy (behavioral changes; altered consciousness)
  - Acute event covers 3 months (include new/fluctuating clinical, MRI features)
  - Brain MRI predominantly supra or infratentorial focal/multifocal lesions; ≥1–2 cm; GM (basal ganglia, thalamus) frequently involved; MRI rarely can show single large (1–2 cm) WM lesion
  - Spinal cord MRI may show confluent intramedullary lesion(s) with variable enhancement
  - No prior episodes; no better explanation
- Recurrent ADEM
  - New ADEM episode involving same clinical/MRI areas, ≥3 months after first episode (if treated, ≥1 month after steroid therapy)
  - No new MRI lesions (may get larger)
  - No better explanation
- Multiphasic ADEM
  - New ADEM episode involving new clinical/MRI areas, ≥3 months after ADEM onset (if treated ≥1 month after completing steroids)
  - Brain MRI shows new lesions, with partial/complete resolution of old lesions)

WM white matter; *GM* gray matter.

and multiphasic (20%) variants [27]. The ADEM criteria require polysymptomatic onset with encephalopathy. These diagnostic criteria have not been uniformly accepted and are likely to be revised. In a recent pathologic verification study, they showed 80% sensitivity and 91% specificity [9]. Many studies have not used any formal standards and have entered patients with CNS inflammatory syndromes of unknown etiology, with or without encephalopathy. In such series, up to 58% of ADEM may not have encephalopathy [29].

The diagnosis in adults is more problematic, since it is fairly easy to include multifocal clinically isolated syndrome (CIS) (representing the first attack of relapsing MS) in ADEM series, unless encephalopathy is required. Encephalopathy is virtually never seen in MS relapses. In one series of 60 patients over age 15, who presented with an acute demyelinating syndrome, ADEM was differentiated from MS by meeting at least two of three critical criteria: atypical clinical symptoms for MS, absent CSF oligoclonal bands, or gray matter involvement [30].

ADEM should be considered in anyone who presents with a suggestive neurologic syndrome. Recent illness or vaccination increases likelihood of this diagnosis, but is not required. The rare postvaccinal cases typically follow a primary rather than revaccination [10].

Neuroimaging is central for the diagnosis of ADEM. Although brain CT may show patchy areas of low attenuation in white matter, with focal or diffuse cortical enhancement, it is normal in about 70% of patients and is much less sensitive than magnetic resonance imaging (MRI) [31]. Brain MRI with and without contrast should be carried out in all patients, unless contraindicated. Normal brain MRI probably excludes a diagnosis of classic ADEM, although imaged lesions may be delayed for several weeks [32]. MRI typically shows multiple T2/FLAIR hyperintense lesions involving white matter and also gray matter. ADEM lesions may (but do not have to) lack sharp borders. The classical imaging features for ADEM are symmetric bilateral lesions, relative periventricular sparing, and deep gray matter involvement. Deep gray matter (basal ganglia and thalamus) involvement is reported in 15–60% of adult cases [33]. Bilateral thalamic involvement is reported in 12% of pediatric cases [34]. In a recent study, MRI criteria were evaluated to differentiate ADEM from MS; the so-called Callen MS-ADEM criteria had the best sensitivity (75%) and specificity (91%) [35]. They involved meeting at least two of the following three criteria: absence of a diffuse bilateral lesion pattern, presence of black holes, and two or more periventricular lesions. Lesions affect subcortical white matter predominantly, although middle cerebellar peduncle and periventricular involvement can be seen [36]. Diffuse extensive supratentorial white matter involvement has also been seen [33]. Sometimes there can be a single tumefactive lesion, which can even be confined to the brainstem [7].

Contrast enhancement is not that helpful. Although very suggestive when it involves all lesions, there may be enhancement of only a subset of lesions or none may enhance. There can be rare presentations with multiple ring enhancing lesions [37].

Follow-up brain MRI 6 months after presentation should show partial or complete resolution of lesions, with no new lesions [10]. Spinal cord MRI may be abnormal as well. Cord lesions in ADEM are more likely to involve the thoracic region and may be diffuse and longitudinally extensive [38, 39].

There are limited reports using nonconventional MRI techniques. It would be helpful if a unique diagnostic imaging signature could be developed. Using diffusion MRI, apparent diffusion coefficient (ADC) was reported as decreased in early ADEM lesions and increased in later stages [36]. In another small series, diffusion tensor imaging signal was reported as abnormal in ADEM vs. MS basal ganglia [40]. Using MR spectroscopy, acute and chronic phases of ADEM showed distinct patterns. Reduced N-acetyl aspartate to creatine ratios were noted in supratentorial normal appearing white matter, while choline to creatine ratios were increased acutely, but decreased back towards normal later. Myoinositol to creatine ratios were decreased acutely, but increased in the chronic phase consistent with gliosis. Elevated lipids and lactate were noted in the acute phase for all subjects, but later normalized [41]. Elevated glutamine/glutamate was present in 67% acutely, then dropped. The authors suggested that the decrease in myoinositol during the acute phase might distinguish ADEM from MS [41].

CSF is routinely examined as part of the diagnostic workup. It helps exclude direct infection. CSF can be normal in up to 33% of cases [8]. Most often there is a low-grade mononuclear pleocytosis, with mildly elevated protein and normal glucose. Rarely neutrophils may predominate. All cultures and stains, and any PCR or antigen tests, should be negative. CSF pressure may be elevated. Positive oligoclonal bands or elevated intrathecal IgG production are reported in a minority of cases. ADEM can be associated with oligoclonal bands in both CSF and serum [8]. If positive, they are transient and not persistently abnormal. Myelin basic protein (MBP) is often elevated in CSF, as a nonspecific acute injury marker.

With regard to other laboratory testing, about 50% of patients show peripheral leukocytosis or elevated acute phase reactants [18]. Electroencephalogram (EEG) generally shows diffuse background slowing [16]. Brain biopsy is rarely necessary, but may be indicated in confusing cases (particularly with continued deterioration).

Differential Diagnosis

The differential diagnosis of ADEM involves principally other causes of encephalitis or encephalomyelitis, stupor, or brain MRI white matter lesions (Table 11.4) [1, 42–47]. The differential is influenced somewhat by age, since conditions such as mitochondrial disorders are more likely in the young while toxic abuse is more likely in adults.

Table 11.4 Differential diagnosis of postinfectious encephalitis/encephalomyelitis.

- Acute infectious encephalitis/encephalomyelitis
  - Viruses (herpes viruses, West Nile virus)
  - Bacteria (legionnaires, listeria, tuberculosis)
  - Parasites (amebae)
- Brain abscess
- Systemic disorders
  - Autoimmune connective tissue disease
  - Neurosarcoidosis
- Vasculitis
- Neoplastic and paraneoplastic disorders
  - Lymphoma, angioendotheliomatosis, gliomatosis cerebri
- Multiple sclerosis
  - Tumefactive
  - Marburg variant
- Toxic leukoencephalopathy
  - Inhaled heroin ("chasing the dragon")
  - Carbon monoxide
- Mitochondrial disorders
- Metabolic disorders
  - Central and extrapontine myelinolysis
  - Marchiafava–Bignami disease
  - Wernicke–Korsakoff encephalopathy
- Posterior reversible encephalopathy syndrome

Management

Symptomatic management involves general supportive measures, such as assuring airway and venous access, controlling fever, and treating electrolyte imbalance. Seriously ill patients or those who decompensate should be managed in an ICU setting, since increased intracranial pressure is a major concern in severe cases. Appropriate measures are taken to prevent venous thrombosis, and any seizures are treated.

There are no randomized controlled trials for the treatment of ADEM. Glucocorticoids are standard therapy based on Class III evidence [48]. The most typical dose is one gram intravenous (IV) methylprednisolone for 3–7 days. Occasionally, higher doses (up to 2 g) are used. Plasma exchange (typically seven exchanges) can be considered in steroid unresponsive patients. The expected response rate is at least 44% [49]. Males, those with preserved reflexes, and those who receive early (within 21 days) plasma exchange appear to do better. In one study early treatment, and improvement at discharge, predicted good response 6 months postexchange [50]. Treatment with intravenous immune globulin (IVIG) can also be considered in steroid resistant patients, typically 1–2 g/kg over 2–5 days [31, 51]. IVIG is preferred to plasma exchange for postvaccinal ADEM [10, 52]. Peripheral nervous system involvement, milder onset disability, and lower CSF albumin have predicted IVIG treatment response [8]. IV cyclophosphamide has also been used for patients who continue to deteriorate. Rarely aggressive surgical decompression or hypothermia may be needed to control brain swelling [53–55].

Prognosis

With the exception of the AHLE hyperacute variant, ADEM overall has a good prognosis. Mortality rate is less than 5% in pediatric series, but has been reported as high as 8–25% in adults requiring ICU admission [33, 56]. Most patients make a good recovery from ADEM, though there may be permanent deficits in 10–30% including cognitive deficits [24, 25, 29, 57]. In a pediatric series, initially severe course was associated with cognitive and visual spatial deficits years later [58]. Adults are reported to have a worse disease course and outcome than children [18]. In one small series of eight patients, brainstem involvement was associated with poorer outcome [59]. Peripheral nervous system involvement may also be associated with poorer recovery and higher risk of relapse [27]. Seizures and coma are also suggested to indicate worse prognosis [16, 24]. Other features associated with poorer outcome were older age onset, female gender, increased CSF protein, and spinal cord involvement [20]. In another very small series (two patients), decreased ADC in the internal capsule, consistent with cytotoxic edema, predicted poor motor outcome [60]. Patients with relapsing attacks are reported to have a good outcome in long-term (9–13 years) follow-up [61].

ADEM Spectrum Overlap Disorders

ADEM can be considered part of a spectrum of CNS disorders (Table 11.5). As discussed previously, ADEM is typically monophasic but can involve repeat episodes in 5–25% of cases. A repeat episode must occur beyond 3 months.

Table 11.5 Postinfectious encephalitis/encephalomyelitis CNS spectrum overlap disorders.

- Multiphasic ADEM
- Recurrent ADEM
- Acute hemorrhagic leukoencephalitis
- Acute necrotizing encephalopathy
- Bickerstaff brainstem encephalitis
- Pediatric MS

Table 11.6 Management of acute hemorrhagic leukoencephalitis.

- Admit to ICU
- Ensure airway, breathing, oxygenation, IV access
- Control fever, seizures
- Monitor and control intracranial pressure (intracranial transducers, sedation,
  hypothermia, other measures)
- Glucocorticoids; consider concomitant plasma exchange or IVIG
- Surgical decompression to control swelling
- Consider IV cyclophosphamide for ongoing process

By convention, when the episode involves new areas it is called multiphasic ADEM; when the same areas are involved, it is recurrent ADEM.

AHLE (Hurst syndrome) is a very rare disorder. It is the hyperacute and most severe form of ADEM [62, 63]. AHLE typically follows nonspecific respiratory tract infection. Clinical onset involves fever, confusion proceeding to stupor and coma, seizures, and focal neurologic deficits that mimic a rapidly expanding mass lesion within the brain. Mortality approaches 70% and occurs within days, with severe morbidity in survivors. MRI shows large hemispheric white matter lesions, with relative sparing of gray matter (although basal ganglia and thalamus may be involved, as can brainstem/cerebellum and spinal cord) [12]. There may be limited MRI enhancement despite evidence of edema and hemorrhage. On diffusion MRI, both acute and subacute lesions showed increased ADC values [12]. CSF shows pleocytosis with RBCs. Neuropathology involves polymorphonuclear cell infiltration with fibrinoid necrosis of small blood vessels, perivascular exudates, microhemorrhages, and cerebral edema. Myelin loss occurs in the setting of relative preservation of axons. There are no formal guidelines on treatment, but one can formulate a reasonable approach based on small case series (Table 11.6). Therapy requires aggressive treatment of increased intracranial pressure and other complications [31]. Corticosteroids with plasma exchange, IVIG, and/or immunosuppressants (cyclophosphamide) may be tried, and surgical intervention and hypothermia may be needed for severe cases [53–55, 64, 65]. Clinical improvement has been noted within 2 days of starting plasma exchange.

Acute necrotizing encephalopathy, formally characterized in 1995, is a rare disease which follows influenza, parainfluenza, human herpesvirus-6, measles, or mycoplasma infections [66, 67]. Young children under the age of 5, particularly from an Asian background (Japan and Taiwan), seem to be preferentially vulnerable [68]. The clinical syndrome is fulminant, with fever and altered mental status within 1–4 days of the viral febrile illness, progressing to within 24–72 h. Seizures, (often refractory to treatment) are common and mortality is 30–70%, typically due to cardiorespiratory issues [69]. Brain MRI shows multiple symmetric lesions involving the thalami, brainstem tegmentum, cerebellum, periventricular white matter, and putamen [68]. The differential diagnosis includes Reye syndrome, Leigh's disease (subacute necrotizing encephalomyelopathy), Wernicke encephalopathy, Sandhoff disease, cerebrovascular event, or tumor [70]. CSF shows increased protein without pleocytosis and has been PCR positive for virus in only a minority of cases. Serum aminotransferases but not blood ammonia may be elevated. Postmortem studies show tissue necrosis, vascular changes with petechial hemorrhages, local vessel congestion, microthrombi, and vasogenic edema [69]. Some patients show high circulating levels of interleukin 6 and tumor necrosis factor [66]. Corticosteroids administered within 24 h of onset may be associated with better outcome, at least when brainstem is not involved [70]. An autosomal dominant disorder, involving recurrent bouts of acute necrotizing encephalopathy, has been associated with missense mutations in the Ran-binding protein 2 (RANBp2) gene on chromosome 2. This gene codes for a nuclear pore component [68, 71]. Acute necrotizing encephalopathy shows many similarities to AHLE. It is interesting to speculate whether it is an expression of AHLE in the very young.

Bickerstaff brainstem encephalitis is characterized by ophthalmoparesis, ataxia, and other CNS features including impaired consciousness. It appears to be part of a very broad neuroimmune spectrum which includes Guillain–Barre Syndrome, especially the Miller Fisher variant [72, 73]. Reflexes in these brainstem encephalitis patients may be increased, normal, or even absent. Patients can show central motor and sensory abnormalities. A proportion (up to 66%) has anti-GQ1b antibodies [74]. CSF shows cytoalbuminologic dissociation most often, but 32% do have a pleocytosis. Brain MRI is abnormal in up to 30%, with T2 hyperintense lesions most often within brainstem [75]. Bickerstaff brainstem encephalitis is treated with either IVIG or plasma exchange [76]. Outcome is generally good with spontaneous recovery, but several deaths have occurred [77].

MS is the major acquired CNS inflammatory demyelinating disease. It is certainly in the differential diagnosis for ADEM, but can also be considered part of this immune-mediated spectrum. This is especially true for pediatric MS and also for adult-onset MS. Pediatric MS is discussed in a separate chapter. When compared with ADEM, pediatric MS is not monophasic. It has onset typically over age 10, shows female predominance, and no triggering event. It is more likely to have a monosymptomatic vs. polysymptomatic onset, and is much less likely to involve any encephalopathic features, bilateral optic neuritis, fever, headache, meningismus, or seizures [29, 78]. Family history of MS also favors MS over ADEM [29]. However, up to 20% of pediatric MS patients experience ADEM as their initial event, then go on to clearcut MS [79, 80]. These children tend to be under 10 years. Laboratory distinctions are helpful. In MS, the CSF is more likely to show oligoclonal bands which persist, without increased protein or pleocytosis. Brain MRI is much more likely to show periventricular perpendicular and corpus callosum ovoid lesions with well-defined margins, without gray matter or brainstem/cerebellar macroscopic lesions [29, 78].

MS MRI lesions increase over time and do not resolve the way ADEM lesions do. MS spinal cord MRI lesions are never longitudinally extensive (extending three or more vertebral segments) except in rare pediatric cases. MRI diffusion weighted imaging shows MS vs. ADEM differences. ADC values within the corpus callosum were consistently elevated in MS compared with ADEM or neurosarcoidosis patients, consistent with nonrestricted water diffusion due to demyelination.

For adult onset MS, multifocal CIS can be confused with ADEM, but a key feature is the lack of encephalopathy as a component of the CIS presentation.

Etiology

ADEM is considered an immune-mediated CNS syndrome. It is believed that myelin components are generally the autoimmune targets. Several hypotheses have been proposed. The first is based on molecular mimicry. In this scenario, an environmental pathogen or external vaccination, it contains antigenic epitopes that cross react with myelin components and results in a misdirected systemic immune attack against the CNS. This would be akin to the major animal model for MS, experimental allergic/autoimmune encephalomyelitis, because it involves a systemic immune pathogenesis. This hypothesis is partially supported by early reports that rabies vaccines developed in CNS tissues had an excessive high rate of postinfectious sequelae.

A second hypothesis involves a transient infection of the CNS, which results in blood brain barrier damage, with the release of sequestered myelin antigens to the systemic immune system. This is temporally linked to a secondary organ-specific immune attack against the CNS. A third hypothesis requires a critically timed two-hit infection, with the second infection reactivating previously primed autoreactive lympocytes. In a limited number of cases, there is one final interesting observation: a mutation in the SCNIA sodium channel has been associated with postvaccination ADEM [10, 81, 82].

T cells sensitized to MBP have been reported in ADEM. In an immunologic study of ADEM, most patients showed lymphocyte proliferation to MBP [83]. Some patients show antibodies to glycolipids such as galactocerebroside as well as myelin proteins. IgG antibodies to native myelin oligodendrocyte glycoprotein (MOG) (but not to proteolipid protein or aquaporin 4) are present in a subset of ADEM patients and were also noted in CIS patients [84]. IgM antibodies to MOG were only found in 3 of 19 ADEM cases. In another series involving 19 children with ADEM vs. 25 with CIS, 28 other neurologic disease patients, and 30 healthy controls, IgM to EBV early antigen was present in 16% of ADEM cases only. Serum IgG to EBV was no different between ADEM and controls, but titers were higher in CIS patients. High-IgG titers to native MOG were found only in the ADEM and CIS cohorts and were unrelated to the EBV antibody response [85]. There has been a particular interest in anti-MOG antibodies because they demyelinate in vitro. In another recent study, antibodies to MOG were more frequent in ADEM and pediatric MS vs. encephalitis and control children, while anti-MBP antibodies did not differentiate these groups [86]. This anti-MOG antibody exclusivity to demyelinating disorders is not mirrored in adults, however. Only 30% were positive for anti-MOG antibodies. One recent study suggested that Pediatric MS patients who had a first episode of ADEM were more likely to show anti-MBP antibodies [87].

Cytokines are implicated as well [88], and lesion formation is said to involve cytokines such as interleukin 2 (IL-2), interferon-γ, and tumor necrosis factor [89]. In a study of chemokines and cytokines in ADEM, MS, and healthy control subjects, ADEM showed elevated CSF levels of chemokines involved in neutrophil and T helper 2-cell attraction [90]. There was no difference in serum cytokine/chomokine levels.

Human leucocyte antigen alleles have been studied a little bit in ADEM, and in various populations have been similar (but not identical) to those associated with MS [91]. A recent child with biopsy-documented ADEM showed two heterozygous mutations of the polymerase gamma gene, consistent with mitochondrial disease [92]. The significance of this association in a single case is unclear.

Conclusion

ADEM is an important neuroimmune syndrome that is part of a spectrum of CNS inflammatory demyelinating diseases. It is distinct from MS, and carries overall a good prognosis with the exception of the hyperacute AHLE variant. The immunopathogenesis is not well understood, which limits the development of preventive strategies and definitive therapies.

Diagnostic paradigms continue to be refined. Management involves appropriate supportive care, and early institution of immunomodulatory therapies such as corticosteroids, plasma exchange, and IVIG. Aggressive management is always justified to control increased intracranial pressure, since such patients can ultimately do very well once this monophasic syndrome has ended.

References

1. Young NP, Weinshenker BG, Lucchinetti CF. Acute disseminated encephalomyelitis: current understanding and controversies. Semin Neurol. 2008;28:84–94.
2. Mikaeloff Y, Suissa S, Vallee L, et al. First episode of acute CNS inflammatory demyelination in childhood: prognostic factors for multiple sclerosis and disability. J Pediatr. 2004;144:246–52.
3. Torisu H, Kira R, Ishizaki Y, et al. Clinical study of childhood acute disseminated encephalomyelitis, multiple sclerosis, and acute transverse myelitis in Fukuoka Prefecture, Japan. Brain Dev. 2010;32:454–62.
4. Leake JA, Albani S, Kao AS, et al. Acute disseminated encephalomyelitis in childhood: epidemiologic, clinical and laboratory features. Pediatr Infect Dis J. 2004;23:756–64.
5. Pohl D, Hennemuth I, von Kries R, et al. Paediatric multiple sclerosis and acute disseminated encephalomyelitis in Germany: results of a nationwide survey. Eur J Pediatr. 2007;166:405–12.
6. Banwell B, Kennedy J, Sadovnick D, et al. Incidence of acquired demyelination of the CNS in Canadian children. Neurology. 2009;20:232–9.
7. VanLandingham M, Hanigan W, Vedanarayanan V, et al. An uncommon illness with a rare presentation: neurosurgical management of ADEM with tumefactive demyelination in children. Childs Nerv Syst. 2010;26:655–61.
8. Sonneville R, Klein IF, Wolff M. Update on investigation and management of postinfectious encephalitis. Curr Opin Neurol. 2010;23:300–4.
9. Young NP, Weinshenker BG, Parisi JE, et al. Perivenous demyelination: association with clinically defined acute disseminated encephalomyelitis and comparison with pathologically confirmed multiple sclerosis. Brain. 2010;133:333–48.

10. Huynh W, Cordato DJ, Kehdi E, et al. Post-vaccination encephalomyelitis: literature review and illustrative case. J Clin Neurosci. 2008;15:1315–22.
11. Garg RK. Acute disseminated encephalomyelitis. Review. Postgrad Med J. 2003;79:11–7.
12. Lee HY, Chang KH, Kim JH, et al. Serial MR imaging findings of acute hemorrhagic leukoencephalitis: a case report. AJNR Am J Neuroradiol. 2005;26:1996–9.
13. Bennetto L, Scolding N. Inflammatory/post-infectious encephalomyelitis. J Neurol Neurosurg Psychiatry. 2004;75:i22–8.
14. De Lau LM, Siepman DA, Remmers MJ, et al. Acute disseminated encephalomyelitis following legionnaires disease. Arch Neurol. 2010;67:623–6.
15. Tripathy S, Routray PK, Mohapatra AK, et al. Acute demyelinating encephalomyelitis after anti-venous therapy in Russell's viper bite. J Med Toxicol. 2010;6:318–21.
16. Panicker JN, Nagaraja D, Kovoor JM, et al. Descriptive study of acute disseminated encephalomyelitis and evaluation of functional outcome predictors. J Postgrad Med. 2010;56:12–6.
17. Deery B, Anderson V, Jacobs R, et al. Childhood MS and ADEM: investigation and comparison of neurocognitive features in children. Dev Neuropsychol. 2010;35:508–21.
18. Ketelslegers IA, Visser IER, Neuteboom RF, et al. Disease course and outcome of acute disseminated encephalomyelitis is more severe in adults than in children. Mult Scler. 2011;17(4):441.
19. Panicker JN, Nagaraja D, Kovoor JME, et al. Lower urinary tract dysfunction in acute disseminated encephalomyelitis. Mult Scler. 2009;15:1118–22.
20. Marchioni E, Ravaglia S, Piccolo G, et al. Postinfectious inflammatory disorders: subgroups based onprospective follow-up. Neurology. 2005;65:1057–65.
21. Nasr JT, Andriola MR, Coyle PK. ADEM: literature review and case report of acute psychosis presentation. Pediatr Neurol. 2000;22:8–18.
22. Krishnakumar P, Jayakrishnan MP, Beegum MN, et al. Acute disseminated encephalomyelitis presenting as acute psychotic disorder. Indian Pediatr. 2008;45:999–1001.
23. Har-Gil M, Evrani M, Watemberg N. Torticollis as the only manifestation of acute disseminated encephalomyelitis. J Child Neurol. 2010;25:1415–8.
24. Jha S, Ansari MK. Partial Kluver-Bucy syndrome in a patient with acute disseminated encephalomyelitis. J Clin Neurosci. 2010;17:1436–8.
25. Parrish JB, Weinstock-Guttman B, Yeh EA. Cerebellar mutism in pediatric acute disseminated encephalomyelitis. Pediatr Neurol. 2010;42:259–66.
26. Fujiki F, Tsuboi Y, Hori T, et al. Aseptic meningitis as initial presentation of acute disseminated encephalomyelitis. J Neurol Sci. 2008;272:129–31.
27. Marchioni E, Tavazzi E, Minoli L, et al. Acute disseminated encephalomyelitis. Curr Infect Dis Rep. 2008;10:307–14.
28. Krupp LB, Banwell B, Tenembaum S, et al. Consensus definitions proposed for pediatric multiple sclerosis and related disorders. Neurology. 2007;68:S7–12.
29. Alper G, Heyman R, Wang L. Multiple sclerosis and acute disseminated encephalomyelitis diagnosed in children after long-term follow up: comparison of presenting features. Dev Med Child Neurol. 2009;51:480–6.
30. De Seze J, Debouverie M, Zephir H, et al. Acute fulminant demyelinating disease. A descriptive study of 60 patients. Arch Neurol. 2007;64:1426–32.
31. Sonneville R, Klein I, de Broucker T, et al. Post-infectious encephalitis in adults: diagnosis and management. J Infect. 2009;58:321–8.
32. Honkaniemi J, Dastidar P, Kahara U, et al. Delayed MR imaging changes in acute disseminated encephalomyelitis. AJNR Am J Neuroradiol. 2001;22:1117–24.
33. Sonneville R, Demeret S, Klein I, et al. Acute disseminated encephalomyelitis in the intensive care unit: clinical features and outcome of 20 adults. Intensive Care Med. 2008;34:528–32.

34. Dardiotis E, Kountra P, Kapsalaki E, et al. Acute disseminated encephalomyelitis with bilateral thalamic necrosis. J Child Neurol. 2009;24:1001–4.
35. Ketelslegers IA, Neuteboom RF, Boon M, et al. A comparison of MRI criteria for diagnosing pediatric ADEM and MS. Neurology. 2010;74:1412–5.
36. Balasubramanya KS, Kovoor JME, Jayakumar PN, et al. Diffusion-weighted imaging and proton MR spectroscopy in the characterization of acute disseminated encephalomyelitis. Neuroradiology. 2007;49:177–83.
37. Kamel MH, Kelleher M, O'Riordan C, et al. CT and MRI ring sign may be due to demyelination: diagnostic pitfall. Br J Neurosurg. 2007;21:309–11.
38. Farber RS, DeVilliers L, Miller A, et al. Differentiating multiple sclerosis from other causes of demyelination using diffusion weighted imaging of the corpus callosum. J Magn Reson Imaging. 2009;30:732–6.
39. Yiu EM, Komberg AJ, Ryan MM, et al. Acute transverse myelitis and aucte disseminated encephalomyelitis in childhood: spectrum or separate entities. J Child Neurol. 2009;24:287–96.
40. Holtmannspotter M, Inglese M, Rovaris M, et al. A diffusion tensor MRI study of basal ganglia from patients with ADEM. J Neurol Sci. 2003;206:27–30.
41. Ben Sira L, Miller E, Artzi M, et al. H-MRS for the diagnosis of acute disseminated encephalomyelitis: insight into the acute-disease stage. Pediatr Radiol. 2010;40:106–13.
42. Borhani Haghighi A, Ashjazadeh N. Acute disseminated encephalomyelitis-like manifestations in a patient with neuro-Behcet disease. Neurologist. 2009;15:282–4.
43. Centers for Disease Control and Prevention. Balamuthia mandrillaris transmitted through organ transplantation. MMWR Morb Mortal Wkly Rep. 2010;59:1165–70.
44. Goraya J, Marks H, Khurana D, et al. Subacute sclerosing panencephalitis (SSPE) presenting as acute disseminated encephalomyelitis in a child. J Child Neurol. 2009;24:899–903.
45. Richard HT, Harrison JF, Abel TW, et al. Pediatric gliomatosis cerebri mimicking acute disseminated encephalomyelitis. Pediatrics. 2010;126:79–82.
46. Summerfield R, Al-Saleh A, Robbins SE. Small cell lung carcinoma presenting with acute disseminated encephalomyelitis. Br J Radiol. 2010;83:e54–7.
47. Zadro I, Brinar VV, Barun B, et al. Primary diffuse meningeal melanomatosis. Neurologist. 2010;16:117–9.
48. Tunkel AR, Glaser CA, Bloch KC, et al. The management of encephalitis: clinical practice guidelines by the Infectious Diseases Society of America. Clin Infect Dis. 2008;47:303–27.
49. Weinshenker BG, O'Brien PC, Petterson TM, et al. A randomized trial of plasma exchange in acute central nervous system inflammatory demyelinating disease. Ann Neurol. 1999;46:878–86.
50. Llufriu S, Castillo J, Blanco Y, et al. Plasma exchange for acute attacks of CNS demyelination: predictor of improvement at 6 months. Neurology. 2009;73:949–53.
51. Ravaglia S, Piccolo G, Ceroni M, et al. Severe steroid-resistant post-infectious encephalomyelitis general features and effects of IVIG. J Neurol. 2007;254:1518–23.
52. Van Dam CN, Syed S, Eron JJ, et al. Severe postvaccinia encephalitis with acute disseminated encephalomyelitis: recovery with early intravenous immunoglobulin, high-dose steroids, and vaccinia immunoglobulin. Clin Infect Dis. 2009;48:47–9.
53. Takata T, Hirakawa M, Sakurai M, et al. Fulminant forms of acute disseminated encephalomyelitis: successful treatment with hypothermia. J Neurol Sci. 1999;165:94–7.
54. Payne ET, Rutka JT, Ho TK, et al. Treatment leading to dramatic recovery in acute hemorrhagic leukoencephalitis. J Child Neurol. 2007;22:109–13.
55. Ahmed AI, Eynon CA, Kinton L, et al. Decompressive craniectomy for acute disseminated encephalomyelitis. Neurocrit Care. 2010;13:393–5.

56. Absoud M, Parslow RC, Wassmer E, et al. Severe acute disseminated encephalomyelitis: a pediatric intensive care population-based study. Mult Scler. 2010;27:1–4.
57. Schwarz S, Mohr A, Knauth M, et al. Acute disseminated encephalomyelitis: a follow-up study of 40 adult patients. Neurology. 2001;56:1313–8.
58. Rostasy K, Nagl A, Lutjen S, et al. Clinical outcome of children presenting with a severe manifestation of acute disseminated encephalomyelitis. Neuropediatrics. 2009;40:211–7.
59. Donmez FY, Asian H, Coskun M. Evaluation of possible prognostic factors of fulminant acute disseminated encephalomyelitis (ADEM) on magnetic resonance imaging with fluid-attenuated inversion recovery (FLAIR) and diffusion-weighted imaging. Acta Radiol. 2009;50:334–9.
60. Kawashima S, Matsukawa N, Ueki Y, et al. Predicting the motor outcome of acute disseminated encephalomyelitis by apparent diffusion coefficient imaging: two case reports. J Neurol Sci. 2009;280:123–6.
61. Mar S, Lenox J, Benzinger T, et al. Long-term prognosis of pediatric patients with relapsing acute disseminated encephalomyelitis. J Child Neurol. 2010;25:681–8.
62. Hurst EW. Acute hemorrhagic leukoencephalitis: a previously undefined entity. Med J Aust. 1941;2:1–6.
63. Lann MA, Lovell MA, Kleinschmidt-DeMasters BK. Acute hemorrhagic leukoencephalitis: a critical entity for forensic pathologists to recognize. Am J Forensic Med Pathol. 2010;31:7–11.
64. Leake JA, Billman GF, Nespeca MP, et al. Pediatric acute hemorrhagic leukoencephalitis: report of a surviving patient and review. Clin Infect Dis. 2002;34:699–703.
65. Ryan LJ, Bowman R, Zantek ND, et al. Use of therapeutic plasma exchange in the management of acute hemorrhagic leukoencephalitis: a case report and review of the literature. Transfusion. 2007;47:981–6.
66. Martin A, Reade EP. Acute necrotizing encephalopathy progressing to brain death in a pediatric patient with novel influenza A (H1N1) infection. Clin Infect Dis. 2010;50:e50–2.
67. Wang GF, Li W, Li K. Acute encephalopathy and encephalitis caused by influenza virus infection. Curr Opin Neurol. 2010;23:305–11.
68. Gika AD, Rich P, Gupta S, et al. Recurrent acute necrotizing encephalopathy following influenza A in a genetically predisposed family. Dev Med Child Neurol. 2010;52:99–102.
69. Manara R, Franzoi M, Cogo P, et al. Acute necrotizing encephalopathy: combined therapy and favorable outcome in a new case. Childs Nerv Syst. 2006;22:1231–6.
70. Yadav S, Das CJ, Kumar V, et al. Acute necrotizing encephalopathy. Indian J Pediatr. 2010;77:307–9.
71. Neilson DE, Adams MD, Orr CMD, et al. Infection-triggered familial or recurrent cases of acute necrotizing encephalopathy caused by mutations in a component of the nuclear pore, RANBP2. Am J Hum Genet. 2009;84:44–51.
72. Kimoto K, Koga M, Odaka M, et al. Relationship of bacterial strains to clinical syndromes of campylobacter-associated neuropathies. Neurology. 2006;28:1837–43.
73. Roos RP, Soliven B, Goldenberg F, et al. An elderly patient with Bickerstaff brainstem encephalitis and transient episodes of brainstem dysfunction. Arch Neurol. 2008;65:821–4.
74. Steer AC, Starr M, Kornberg AJ. Bickerstaff brainstem encephalitis associated with mycoplasma pneumoniae infection. J Child Neurol. 2006;21:533–4.
75. Odaka M, Yuki N, Yamada M, et al. Bickerstaff's brainstem encephalitis: clinical features of 62 cases and a subgroup associated with Guillain-Barre syndrome. Brain. 2003;126:2279–90.
76. Mori M, Kuwabara S. Fisher syndrome. Curr Treat Options Neurol. 2011;13:71–8.
77. Yuki N. Fisher syndrome and Bickerstaff brainstem encephalitis (Fisher-Bickerstaff syndrome). J Neuroimmunol. 2009;21:1–9.

78. Atzori M, Battistella PA, Perini P, et al. Clinical and diagnostic aspects of multiple sclerosis and acute monophasic encephalomyelitis in pediatric patients: a single centre prospective study. Mult Scler. 2009;15:363–70.
79. Banwell B, Krupp L, Kennedy L, et al. Clinical features and viral serologies in children with multiple sclerosis: a multinational observational study. Lancet Neurol. 2007;6:773–81.
80. Visudtibhan A, Tuntiyathorn L, Vaewpanich J, et al. Acute disseminated encephalomyelitis: a 10-year cohort study in Thai children. Eur J Pediatr Neurol. 2010;14:513–8.
81. Berkovic SF, Harkin L, McMahon JM, et al. De-novo mutations of the sodium channel gene SCN1a an alleged vaccine encephalopathy retrospective study. Lancet Neurol. 2006;5:488–92.
82. Sell E, Minassian BA. Demystifying vaccination-associated encephalopathy. Lancet Neurol. 2006;5:465–6.
83. Johnson RT, Griffin DE, Hirsch RL, et al. Measles encephalomyelitis – clinical and immunologic studies. N Engl Med. 1984;310:137–41.
84. Brilot F, Dale RC, Selter RC, et al. Antibodies to native myelin oligodendrocyte glycoprotein in children with inflammatory demyelinating central nervous system disease. Ann Neurol. 2009;66:833–42.
85. Selter RC, Brilot F, Grummel V, et al. Antibody responses to EBV and native MOG in pediatric inflammatory demyelinating CNS diseases. Neurology. 2010;74:1711–5.
86. Lalive PH, Hausler MG, Maurey H, et al. Highly reactive anti-myelin oligodendrocyte glycoprotein antibodies differentiate demyelinating diseases from viral encephalitis in children. Mult Scler J. 2010. doi:10:1-6.
87. O'Connor KC, Lopez-Amaya C, Gagne D, et al. Anti-myelin antibodies modulate clinical expression of childhood multiple sclerosis. J Neuroimmunol. 2010;223:92–9.
88. Kadhim H, De Prez C, Gazagnes MD, et al. In situ cytokine immune responses in acute disseminated encephalomyelitis: insights into pathophysiologic mechanisms. Hum Pathol. 2003;3:293–7.
89. Sabayan B, Zolghadrasli A. Vasculitis and rheumatologic diseases may play a role in the pathogenesis of acute disseminated encephalomyelitis (ADEM). Med Hypotheses. 2007;69:322–4.
90. Franciotta D, Zardini E, Ravaglia S, et al. Cytokines and chemokines in cerebrospinal fluid and serum of adult patients with acute disseminated encephalomyelitis. J Neurol Sci. 2006;247:202–7.
91. Alves-Leon SV, Veluttini-Pimentel ML, Gouveia ME, et al. Acute disseminated encephalomyelitis. Arq Neuropsiquiatr. 2009;67:643–51.
92. Harris MO, Walsh LE, Hattab EM, et al. Is it ADEM, POLG, or both? Arch Neurol. 2010;67:493–6.

Neuromyelitis Optica Spectrum Disorders

Dean M. Wingerchuk

Keywords: Neuromyelitis optica, Aquaporin, Area postrema, Myelitis, Optic neuritis

Introduction

The nosology of neuromyelitis optica has evolved dramatically over the past decade but only after more than a century of slowly accumulating knowledge about the disorder. It has historically been defined as a severe, monophasic disease consisting of optic neuritis and myelitis occurring in close temporal proximity and without brain involvement [1, 2].

Albutt first recognized an association between optic neuropathy and spinal cord disease in the late nineteenth century [3]. Devic and his student Gault solidified the concept with their case descriptions and the entity became known as Devic's syndrome or Devic's disease [4, 5]. During the next hundred years or so, neuromyelitis optica merited only a paragraph (or a footnote) in chapters detailing the clinical and pathological features of central nervous system demyelinating diseases. It was something of a curiosity or item for academic debate: Is it a distinct disease or simply an unusual phenotype of multiple sclerosis recognizable by its propensity to attack the optic nerves and spinal cord in a particularly severe manner, while sparing the brain? [1, 2] Some experts argued that it was a multiple sclerosis variant because of the lack of pathological changes that suggest otherwise (indeed, inflammation, and demyelination are present) and because optic neuritis and myelitis are common features of typical multiple sclerosis. Others noted features such as a monophasic course (in some cases) and the particularly severe inflammatory changes in the spinal cord and optic nerve, often with necrosis, and postulated that neuromyelitis optica was either distinct or a topographically restricted form of acute disseminated encephalomyelitis [6]. Interesting observations in the later part of the twentieth century included the tendency for neuromyelitis optica to coexist

From: *Clinical Neuroimmunology: Multiple Sclerosis and Related Disorders*, Current Clinical Neurology,
Edited by: S.A. Rizvi and P.K. Coyle, DOI 10.1007/978-1-60327-860-7_12,
© Springer Science+Business Media, LLC 2011

with other systemic autoimmune disorders, the low prevalence of oligoclonal bands in cerebrospinal fluid, and unusual pathological characteristics such as the presence of thickened, hyalinized blood vessels in the vicinity of cord lesions. None of these characteristics were sufficiently specific or reproducible to settle the issue, even in the latter years of the twentieth century, but there was increasing speculation that the disorder is mediated predominantly by humoral autoimmunity [7–10].

The explosive increase in interest in neuromyelitis optica can be traced to the discovery, reported in 2004 by Lennon and colleagues, of the serum autoantibody known as NMO-IgG [11]. This marker, which is highly specific for neuromyelitis optica and rarely detected in prototypic multiple sclerosis, is also implicated in its pathogenesis. Numerous investigative groups throughout the world, studying patient groups of diverse ethnic and racial backgrounds, have confirmed its high specificity. Furthermore, NMO-IgG has informed us about the "neuromyelitis optica spectrum" of disorders, which includes patients with isolated recurrent optic neuritis, isolated "longitudinally extensive" transverse myelitis (defined below), and Asian optic-spinal multiple sclerosis [12]. Increasing evidence suggests that NMO-IgG titers are associated with disease activity, raising the possibility that it may be useful as a biomarker of treatment response. The target of NMO-IgG is aquaporin-4, an astrocyte water channel not found on oligodendrocytes or in association with myelin [13]. Investigations into the role of NMO-IgG and this unexpected antigenic target in the pathobiology of neuromyelitis optica are intensifying as we attempt to better understand the mechanisms underlying initiation and propagation of the disease.

Epidemiology and Clinical Features of Neuromyelitis Optica

Neuromyelitis optica predominantly affects women, but has a later median age of onset (late fourth decade) than multiple sclerosis (late third decade) [8]. The disease also differs from multiple sclerosis in its propensity to affect people of nonwhite racial background. It makes up a sizeable proportion of all cases of CNS demyelinating disease in peoples of Asian, African-American, or Hispanic background [8, 14–17]. Furthermore, there are groups such as native North Americans or aboriginal peoples in which the existing and scarce reported cases of CNS demyelinating disease have clinical and pathological features of NMO [18]. Therefore, the occurrence of optic or severe myelitis in a patient of non-Caucasian ancestry should increase diagnostic suspicion for neuromyelitis optica. The prevalence of neuromyelitis optica is unclear, but estimates range from approximately one to three cases per 100,000 population in studies from Martinique, Japan, and Mexico [16, 17, 19].

Neuromyelitis optica remains a clinical diagnosis. The diagnosis should be entertained for patients who present with first-ever optic neuritis attacks or who have experienced recurrent isolated optic neuritis, especially if their brain MRI does not reveal typical lesions of multiple sclerosis. The occurrence of bilateral simultaneous or sequential optic neuritis in rapid succession is also suggestive [20]. Other clinical features of neuromyelitis optica-related optic neuritis attacks, such as pain, pattern of visual loss, and examination findings, do not differ from MS-related attacks [8].

Myelitis events are usually severe. Clinically, they may be "complete" with bilateral loss of sensorimotor and sphincter function, but they can be

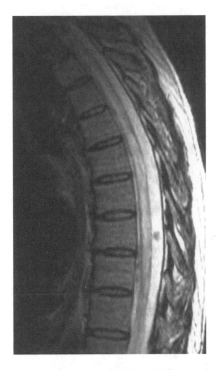

Figure 12.1 Sagittal T2-weighted cervical spine MRI scan demonstrates a longitudinally extensive transverse myelitis (LETM) lesion typical of a neuromyelitis optica spectrum disorder

incomplete, asymmetric, and even mild. The typical severe myelitis attack is usually associated with a "longitudinally extensive" spinal cord MRI lesion, leading to use of the term "longitudinally extensive transverse myelitis" or LETM and the abnormality occupies the central portion of the spinal cord (Figure 12.1). In contrast, cord lesions in MS are smaller, usually unilateral, and more likely to result in milder, asymmetric clinical syndromes [21, 22]. MS lesions have a propensity to affect the dorsal spinal cord, causing recognizable sensory patterns such as a partial Brown-Séquard syndrome or a "useless hand" phenomenon in which proprioceptive sensation loss renders an upper extremity useless despite normal motor function. L'hermitte's sign (paresthesias in the spine or limbs elicited by neck flexion) often accompanies myelitis attacks in both neuromyelitis optica and MS. Paroxysmal tonic spasms, however, seem more common in neuromyelitis optica [8].

Additional clinical myelitis-related events that should raise suspicion for NMO are the occurrence of hiccoughs or respiratory failure. Misu and colleagues reported that NMO-related longitudinally extensive myelitis may extend into the medulla, resulting in persistent hiccough [23]. This symptom occurred in 17% of 47 NMO patients but in no MS controls. The occurrence of hiccoughs was associated with MRI evidence of a lesion involving the pericanal region of the medulla, likely affecting the area postrema and medial and lateral portions of the nucleus tractus solitarius. Such extensive myelitic lesions may also interrupt medullary centers involved in neuromuscular control of respiration, a rare event in typical multiple sclerosis [8, 24].

Key Investigations in Neuromyelitis Optica

Brain MRI scans are typically normal at disease onset or demonstrate only nonspecific white matter abnormalities that do not meet MS criteria [25–27]. A normal brain MRI in the setting of a new, severe myelitis, or optic neuritis event raises the possibility of neuromyelitis optica. A minority of patients have signature lesions that suggest neuromyelitis optica; these include focal abnormalities in areas such as the thalamus, hypothalamus, and adjacent to the third and fourth ventricles [28–32].

Spinal cord MRI is very helpful in neuromyelitis optica diagnosis. The presence of a longitudinally extensive, centrally based lesion that extends contiguously over three or more vertebral segments strongly suggests a neuromyelitis optica spectrum disorder in the absence of another specific explanation (such as neoplasm, sarcoidosis, etc.) In contrast, myelitis attacks in typical MS are usually small, focal, asymmetric, often dorsal cord lesions that measure 0.5–2 vertebral segments in craniocaudal length [21, 22].

A longitudinally extensive lesion may appear to break up into several shorter fragments or shrink to a length of less than three vertebral segments, therefore, awareness of the temporal relationship of a given scan to a clinical attack is important.

Cerebrospinal fluid abnormalities in neuromyelitis optica are variable but may be dramatic during an acute attack, with $50–1,000 \times 10^6$ WBC/L and a neutrophilic predominance. These findings are useful (specificity >95%) but unfortunately are not very sensitive (less than 30%) for diagnosis [8]. In contrast, MS is usually associated with a modest pleocytosis ($5–25 \times 10^6$ WBC/L) that dominated by lymphocytes. Furthermore, whereas about 85% of people with MS have unique oligoclonal bands in their CSF, only about 20–30% of those with neuromyelitis optica have detectable bands [8].

Definition of Neuromyelitis Optica

The aforementioned clinical and laboratory data have led to incremental refinement of diagnostic criteria for neuromyelitis optica. Revised diagnostic criteria proposed by Mayo Clinic investigators in 2006 incorporate clinical, laboratory, and neuroimaging features that, in combination, accurately distinguish neuromyelitis optica from MS (Table 12.1) [33]. To achieve a conclusive diagnosis, a patient must have experienced both optic neuritis and acute myelitis. In addition, at least two of three supportive features must be present. One of the supportive criteria is the detection of a longitudinally extensive (>3 segment) spinal cord lesion in association with an acute myelitis event. This is a very strong indicator of neuromyelitis optica in adults but may be somewhat less predictive in children [34]. A normal brain MRI at disease onset, or one revealing lesions that do not meet criteria for multiple sclerosis, is another supportive criterion. Finally, NMO-IgG seropositivity is strongly supportive of the diagnosis. Note that the diagnosis of neuromyelitis optica may be confirmed without NMO-IgG testing or if NMO-IgG is negative (if the other two supportive criteria are fulfilled). However, the very high specificity of the autoantibody marker makes testing highly desirable and seropositivity results in a more confident diagnosis. The criteria are 99% sensitive and 90% specific for neuromyelitis optica in patients presenting with clinical optic neuritis and

Table 12.1 Current diagnostic criteria for neuromyelitis optica.

Criteria	Mayo Clinic [33]	National MS Society [36]
Required	Optic neuritis	Optic neuritis
	Myelitis	Myelitis, associated with:
		Spinal cord MRI T2 lesion >3 vertebral segments, and includes T1 hypointensity, during acute attack
		No evidence for sarcoidosis, vasculitis, and clinically manifest lupus, Sjogren's syndrome, or other explanation for the syndrome
Supportive	Require 2 of 3:	Require 1 of 2:
	Initial brain MRI normal or not compatible with typical MS	Initial brain MRI normal or not compatible with typical MS
	Cord MRI T2 lesion >3 vertebral segments during acute attack	See required section
	Positive serology for NMO-IgG (aquaporin-4 antibodies)	Positive test for NMO-IgG/aquaporin-4 antibodies in serum or CSF

myelitis syndromes as the expression of CNS demyelinating disease [33]. These results have been replicated by others [35].

In 2008, a National Multiple Sclerosis Society task force proposed alternative criteria for NMO that are generally aligned with the Mayo Clinic criteria [36]. The task force criteria require the presence of a longitudinally extensive spinal cord lesion, whereas the Mayo Clinic criteria utilize this as a supportive feature. By requiring the cord lesion, the task force criteria may fail to capture some patients (including NMO-IgG seropositive patients) who experienced a prior LETM event but have an atypical MRI, and MRI that was performed late in the course of the myelitis (at which point the lesion may have evolved and become smaller), or whose imaging results are not available for review. The task force criteria also exclude patients with clinical evidence of an active systemic autoimmune disease, even though NMO-IgG seropositive neuromyelitis optica may coexist with systemic autoimmune disease. The two sets of diagnostic criteria would likely have a high level of agreement though they have not been formally evaluated against one another. From a practical perspective, clinicians will likely be able to use either set of criteria to correctly identify (or have high suspicion of) neuromyelitis optica and move forward with appropriate therapy.

Neuromyelitis Optica Spectrum Disorders

The discovery of NMO-IgG contributed to recognizing that several other clinical scenarios fall within the spectrum of neuromyelitis optica, even though they fail to meet the full criteria noted above (Table 12.2) [12]. This section outlines the evidence supporting the notion of "Neuromyelitis Optica Spectrum Disorders."

Table 12.2 NMO spectrum disorders [12].

- Neuromyelitis optica (Mayo Clinic criteria, 2006) [33]
- Limited forms of NMO
  - "Idiopathic" single or recurrent events of longitudinally extensive myelitis
    (≥3 vertebral segment spinal cord MRI lesion)
  - Bilateral simultaneous or recurrent optic neuritis
- Asian optic-spinal MS
- Optic neuritis or longitudinally extensive myelitis associated with systemic
  autoimmune disease
- Optic neuritis or myelitis associated with characteristic NMO brain lesion pattern (hypothalamic, periventricular, brainstem involvement)
- Other distinct clinical features in a patient seropositive for NMO-IgG
  - Intractable vomiting or hiccoughs
  - Posterior reversible encephalopathy syndrome

First, the long-held belief that neuromyelitis optica completely spared the brain has been dismissed. Brain lesions are especially common in children and may be the presenting syndrome of the disease [37]. Although most patients have a normal brain MRI at disease onset, more than 60% accrue brain white matter lesions over time. In some patients, brain lesions are detected in sites of relatively high expression of aquaporin-4, including the hypothalamus and regions adjacent to the third and fourth ventricles [28, 29]. Second, the NMO-IgG seropositivity rate is about 50% in patients with recurrent LETM and approximately 25% in patients with simultaneous bilateral or sequential events of optic neuritis [11]. Such seropositive patients are at high risk for relapse and subsequent conversion to confirmed neuromyelitis optica. NMO-IgG seropositive patients who experience their first-ever event of LETM have a 56% risk of LETM recurrence or optic neuritis (confirmed neuromyelitis optica) over the subsequent 12 months [38]. Seropositive patients with recurrent optic neuritis tend to have worse visual outcome and a high risk of developing LETM, approaching 50% at 10 years [39]. These data suggest that single or recurrent events of LETM, bilateral simultaneous optic neuritis, and recurrent optic neuritis are, at least in some cases, limited or incompletely developed forms of neuromyelitis optica.

Third, NMO-IgG appears to be a highly specific marker for Asian optic-spinal MS. In a Japanese cohort, 58% of patients with optic-spinal MS were NMO-IgG seropositive compared with none of the "conventional" or "Western" MS phenotype [11]. Other groups have confirmed the high prevalence and specificity of NMO-IgG for an optic-spinal disease phenotype among Asians [40, 41]. Although debate continues because of differences in case definition and ascertainment, these data suggest that clinically diagnosed neuromyelitis optica and Asian optic-spinal multiple sclerosis are the same disease in many or most instances.

Fourth, NMO-IgG has clarified to some degree the relationship between neuromyelitis optica and other systemic autoimmune disorders such as systemic lupus erythematosus (SLE) and Sjögren's syndrome. Although the diagnostic criteria put forth by the National Multiple Sclerosis Society specifically exclude patients with these and other systemic autoimmune diseases, recent evidence supports the notion that SLE and Sjogren's syndrome (and their associated autoantibodies) coexist with, rather than cause, the neuromyelitis optica clinical syndrome [36, 42]. For example, patients with clinically defined SLE or Sjogren's syndrome who do not have symptoms or signs of optic nerve and spinal cord disease are uniformly NMO-IgG seronegative. In addition, NMO-IgG is detected more commonly in patients with NMO symptoms who have clinical or serological evidence for SLE or SS than in those who do not. These findings suggest that individuals with neuromyelitis optica may harbor an overall tendency toward developing autoimmune diseases.

The expanded spectrum of neuromyelitis optica disorders means that clinicians should consider the evaluation of NMO-IgG in any child or adult patient with LETM, recurrent isolated myelitis with normal brain MRI, isolated bilateral or sequential optic neuritis, unusual brain lesions, or a compatible clinical syndrome described above.

Clinical Course of Neuromyelitis Optica

Most patients, probably about 90%, experience a relapsing course with repeated episodes of optic neuritis, myelitis, or other clinical features [12]. Morbidity remains high in neuromyelitis optica from the standpoint of neurological impairment as well as potential medical complications of immobility, such as pneumonia and deep vein thrombosis. However, it is likely that the current prognosis for neuromyelitis optica is substantially better than the outcomes we reported on patients observed at Mayo Clinic dating back to the 1950s. In that cohort, we noted a 33% mortality rate owing to severe myelitis events that resulted in respiratory failure and other medical complications [8].

An important recent observation is that neuromyelitis optica patients uncommonly develop secondary progressive disease of the type noted so frequently with multiple sclerosis [43]. The natural history of the neuromyelitis optica is usually that of stepwise deterioration in motor, sensory, visual, and bowel/bladder function as a result of cumulative attack-related neurological injury [8, 20, 43]. The corollary of this observation would seem to be that effective attack prevention will likely stabilize the disease over the long term.

Pathology of Neuromyelitis Optica

Affected optic nerves and spinal cord specimens reveal extensive or multifocal softening and swelling [44]. Lesions are associated with inflammatory demyelination with patchy areas of gray and white matter necrosis, whereas perivascular inflammation is variable. Chronic lesions are characterized by gliosis, cystic degeneration, cavitation, and atrophy. Hyalinized medium-caliber spinal cord arteries may be associated with cord necrosis and a macrophage-predominant inflammatory infiltrate [44–46].

Immunopathological evaluation of active neuromyelitis optica lesions reveals a vasculocentric pattern of complement activation together with infiltration of eosinophils and neutrophils. Lucchinetti and colleagues postulated that CNS blood vessels may be a primary disease target because of the colocalization of immunoglobulin, C9neo antigen (a marker of the terminal lytic complement complex), and activated macrophages in the perivascular region [44]. These findings also suggested a major role for complement activation in the pathogenesis of the disease.

The discovery of NMO-IgG was followed quickly by identification of its target antigen, aquaporin-4. There are more than a dozen members of the aquaporin family of water channels and they are important for fluid balance and cell water homeostasis [47]. Aquaporin-4 is the most common type found in the CNS, where it is anchored within astrocyte foot process membranes by the dystroglycan complex and faces the abluminal surface of blood vessels (within the "glia limitans"), somewhat similar to the distribution of immune complexes noted above.

Studies of aquaporin-4 in MS and neuromyelitis optica have demonstrated differences that are likely relevant to the primary pathogenesis of each disorder [48]. Loss of aquaporin-4 expression is stage-dependent in MS but occurs in all neuromyelitis optica lesions regardless of stage of demyelination, region of involvement or degree of necrosis. Typical neuromyelitis optica lesions are associated with vasculocentric immune complex deposition and aquaporin-4 loss, active demyelination, and vascular hyperplasia with hyalinization [44, 48]. An interesting additional finding in neuromyelitis optica is the detection of a unique lesion type with inflammation, vasculocentric loss of aquaporin-4 along with immunoglobulin deposition, and complement activation but no evidence of demyelination. Such lesions were found in the spinal cord and especially in the area postrema, a region which lacks a blood–brain barrier and which might be implicated in attacks of intractable nausea, vomiting, and hiccough. Although aquaporin-4 is expressed throughout the CNS, it is not clear why neuromyelitis optica lesions favor regions such as the optic nerve, brain stem, and spinal cord. It is possible that regional differences in expression, access by autoantibody, or orientation of the water channel could influence where lesions develop. The pathology of brain lesions in neuromyelitis optica cases reveals similar findings, suggesting that they are owing to the same mechanisms and one disease rather than representing overlap between neuromyelitis optica and MS.

Is NMO-IgG/Anti-aquaporin-4 Pathogenic?

Several lines of evidence suggest a primary role for aquaporin-4-specific autoantibody as the initiator of the NMO lesion. In addition to the observations that brain lesions coincide with regions of high aquaporin-4 expression and the pathological data summarized above, in vitro evidence shows that NMO-IgG binds selectively to the surface of living cell membranes expressing aquaporin-4. This binding initiates two potentially competing events: (1) rapid downregulation of aquaporin-4 via endocytosis/degradation and (2) activation of the lytic complement cascade [49]. The relative predominance of one or the other event may dictate the clinical expression and therapeutic response.

It is not yet clear whether and how these events result in demyelination. Possible mechanisms of demyelination include oligodendrocyte injury at the paranode (where they are in direct contact with aquaporin-4-containing astrocytic foot processes) or a result of axonal injury due to changes in the ionic microenvironment at the internode [49]. Glutamate toxicity is another potential mechanism; binding of NMO-IgG to astrocytic aquaporin-4 also downregulates the excitatory neurotransmitter transporter EAAT2 [50]. This could alter glutamate homeostasis, injuring oligodendrocytes.

Therapy

Treatment recommendations for neuromyelitis optica, both for acute attacks and attack prevention, rest upon multicenter experience and published case series [51]. There are no randomized controlled trials focusing specifically on neuromyelitis optica.

Treatment of Attacks

Intravenous corticosteroids are the standard of care, first-line treatment for optic neuritis and myelitis attacks. A typical regimen calls for 1,000 mg methylprednisolone infusions administered daily for 5 consecutive days [51]. A brief postinfusion oral prednisone taper is optional. However, if the attack prevention treatment plan will include an immunosuppressive regimen with a delayed onset of action, a higher dose of oral prednisone (40–60 mg daily) may be initiated after completion of the infusion.

Steroid-refractory attacks sometimes occur in neuromyelitis optica. Rescue therapy with plasmapheresis is indicated in this scenario. Evidence from a small, randomized, controlled trial of evidence supports intervention with plasmapheresis (seven exchanges of approximately 55 mL/kg each, administered every other day for 14 days) [52]. In that crossover trial of true versus sham plasmapheresis, patients with severe clinical deficits (paraplegia, quadriplegia, and coma) due to idiopathic CNS demyelinating disease, meaningful clinical improvement occurred in significantly more plasmapheresis patients (42%) than sham exchange patients (6%). Assessment of responders revealed that the subgroup of NMO patients were among the most likely to respond. This finding was further supported by a retrospective review in which six of ten NMO patients experienced moderate or marked clinical improvement of myelitis-related symptoms and signs within days after starting plasmapheresis [53]. Some patients with severe visual loss may improve after plasmapheresis [54]. Therefore, plasmapheresis therapy should be considered if a severe attack of myelitis or optic neuritis does not respond promptly to corticosteroids. Progressive, ascending cervical myelitis, which can threaten respiratory function, is a situation in which plasmapheresis should be initiated as soon as it is evident that corticosteroid treatment is not having a significant clinical impact [8].

Therapy for Attack Prevention

Patients with neuromyelitis optica develop virtually all of their permanent neurological disability from the effects of optic neuritis and myelitis attacks [43]. In most instances, brain-related symptoms are mild and transient and a secondary progressive course, unlike in typical MS, is uncommon. Therefore, treatments directed toward attack prevention are the primary means to protect neurological function for patients with neuromyelitis optica spectrum disorders and should be instituted as early in the disease course as possible. At present, this means starting treatment when a relapsing course has declared itself (i.e., two or more attacks). As noted above, the detection of NMO-IgG seropositivity in new-onset patients with longitudinally extensive myelitis appears to portend a high risk of relapse within 1 year and it is advisable to start attack prevention therapy in that patient group after the sentinel myelitis attack [38].

Multicenter experience suggests that standard immunomodulatory therapies approved for MS, such as beta-interferons and glatiramer acetate, are ineffective or may even aggravate neuromyelitis optica, despite a single case report of apparent glatiramer acetate benefit [55, 56]. A recent report indicated that interferon beta-1b benefited Japanese MS, but the trial was not powered to specifically evaluate the optic-spinal subgroup, therefore, there remain no convincing data for beta-interferon efficacy in NMO patients [57].

Clinical experience, coupled with the current understanding of the immunopathological features of neuromyelitis optica, has led to widespread concurrence that long-term attack suppression is best achieved with chronic immunosuppression. There are numerous options, including general immunosuppressant medications given by oral (azathioprine, mycophenolate, and methotrexate) or parenteral (mitoxantrone, methotrexate, cyclophosphamide, and others) routes. More targeted therapies, such as the anti-CD20 B cell-depleting drug rituximab, are also now used extensively.

For several years, a standard preventative approach included azathioprine (2–3 mg/kg daily) in combination with oral prednisone (beginning at 1 mg/kg/day), similar to the approach described in an observational case series of seven patients, but using higher doses [58]. The therapeutic goal is to achieve azathioprine monotherapy by via slow prednisone taper once azathioprine effects are evident (reduced peripheral WBC count and elevation in mean corpuscular volume), usually within 4–6 months. A similar approach can be used for the oral immunosuppressant mycophenolate mofetil, using a target dose of 1,000 mg twice daily. The advantage of mycophenolate may be better tolerability, but the duration of the delayed onset of action is probably similar to that of azathioprine [59]. Unfortunately, some patients treated with oral therapies seem to exhibit corticosteroid dependency because they experience breakthrough relapses when the prednisone dosage is reduced below 5–15 mg/day [51]. Because many relapsing NMO patients are young and otherwise healthy, steroid dependence for clinical remission represents a reason to consider alternative immunosuppressive therapies.

The recognition that neuromyelitis optica pathogenesis is likely driven primarily by antibody-mediated mechanisms led to evaluation of the chimeric murine/human anti-CD20 monoclonal protein rituximab as a potential treatment. Rituximab depletes peripheral B cells [60]. Eight patients with active, relapsing neuromyelitis optica that failed to respond to other therapies (including interferons, glatiramer acetate, azathioprine, intravenous immune globulin, mitoxantrone, and plasmapheresis) appeared to respond to rituximab treatment [61]. Each was given four weekly 375 mg/m^2 intravenous rituximab infusions. Six of eight patients maintained relapse-free status over the next 12 months (range of follow-up 6–18 months) and median attack rate declined from 2.6 attacks/patient/year to 0 attacks/patient/year ($p=0.0078$). Seven of the patients experienced significant recovery; the median Expanded Disability Status Scale scores were 7.5 before treatment and 5.5 at follow-up ($p=0.013$). Rituximab was well tolerated in this case series (there were no adverse events) but, in addition to its long-term immunosuppressive effect, is associated with risk of infusion-related reactions (fever, chills/rigors, urticaria, angioedema, bronchospasm, and hypotension), cardiac arrhythmias, and rash. In a larger series of 25 patients from several centers, results were generally favorable, but several patients had breakthrough attacks after receiving rituximab and adverse events included severe infection and death [62]. There are no additional data concerning the safety or efficacy of long-term rituximab therapy for neuromyelitis optica.

There are fewer data concerning the benefit of other immunosuppressive approaches for relapse prevention. Mitoxantrone, a synthetic anthracenedione chemotherapeutic agent approved for use in rapidly worsening secondary progressive or relapsing-remitting MS [63, 64], appears beneficial, as does methotrexate, but the number of treated patients reported to date is very small [65, 66]. Some clinicians utilize cyclophosphamide for severe MS despite unconvincing evidence for efficacy; its effects on B cells make it worthy of exploration for NMO, but there are no reported data. Repeated infusions of intravenous immune globulin have been reported to stabilize otherwise refractory cases [67]. Maintenance plasmapheresis is also worth exploring. Future investigations will likely focus on therapies that modulate or suppress the important steps in antibody and complement-mediated pathobiology of the disease, probably utilizing combinations of available therapies that utilize different mechanisms (e.g., intravenous immune globulin in combination with a general immunosuppressant).

Conclusion

The collective evidence from such diverse sources as systematic immunopathological studies and fundamental clinical observations demonstrate that neuromyelitis optica is a distinct disease. The concept of spectrum of neuromyelitis optica disorders is now generally accepted, solidified by the numerous studies worldwide that have replicated the very high specificity of NMO-IgG and its clinical associations. The discovery that NMO-IgG targets aquaporin-4 will accelerate achievement of necessary next steps such as development of an animal model of neuromyelitis optica and determining whether NMO-IgG is indeed the primary effector of the disease. Completion of these goals will fuel greater understanding of underlying pathogenic mechanisms, more accurate and earlier clinical diagnosis, and development of more effective therapies for this enigmatic and disabling disease.

References

1. Cree BA, Goodin DS, Hauser SL. Neuromyelitis optica. Semin Neurol. 2002;22(2):105–22.
2. de Seze J. Neuromyelitis optica. Arch Neurol. 2003;60(9):1336–8.
3. Allbutt T. On the ophthalmoscopic signs of spinal disease. Lancet. 1870;1:76–8.
4. Gault F. De la neuromyelite optique aigue [thesis]. Lyon; 1894.
5. Devic E. Myelite subaigue compliquee de nevrite optique. Bull Med. 1894;35:18–30.
6. Modi G, Mochan A, Modi M, Saffer D. Demyelinating disorder of the central nervous system occurring in black South Africans. J Neurol Neurosurg Psychiatry. 2001;70(4):500–5.
7. O'Riordan JI, Gallagher HL, Thompson AJ, Howard RS, Kingsley DP, Thompson EJ, et al. Clinical, CSF, and MRI findings in Devic's neuromyelitis optica. J Neurol Neurosurg Psychiatry. 1996;60(4):382–7.

8. Wingerchuk DM, Hogancamp WF, O'Brien PC, Weinshenker BG. The clinical course of neuromyelitis optica (Devic's syndrome). Neurology. 1999;53(5):1107–14.

9. Weinshenker BG. Neuromyelitis optica: what it is and what it might be. Lancet. 2003;361(9361):889–90.

10. de Seze J, Lebrun C, Stojkovic T, Ferriby D, Chatel M, Vermersch P. Is Devic's neuromyelitis optica a separate disease? A comparative study with multiple sclerosis. Mult Scler. 2003;9(5):521–5.

11. Lennon VA, Wingerchuk DM, Kryzer TJ, Pittock SJ, Lucchinetti CF, Fujihara K, et al. A serum autoantibody marker of neuromyelitis optica: distinction from multiple sclerosis. Lancet. 2004;364(9451):2106–12.

12. Wingerchuk DM, Lennon VA, Lucchinetti CF, Pittock SJ, Weinshenker BG. The spectrum of neuromyelitis optica. Lancet Neurol. 2007;6:810–5.

13. Lennon VA, Kryzer TJ, Pittock SJ, Verkman AS, Hinson SR. IgG marker of optic-spinal multiple sclerosis binds to the aquaporin-4 water channel. J Exp Med. 2005;202(4):473–7.

14. Kira J. Multiple sclerosis in the Japanese population. Lancet Neurol. 2003;2: 117–27.

15. Papais-Alvarenga RM, Miranda-Santos CM, Puccioni-Sohler M, de Almeida AM, Oliveira S, Basilio De Oliveira CA, et al. Optic neuromyelitis syndrome in Brazilian patients. J Neurol Neurosurg Psychiatry. 2002;73(4):429–35.

16. Cabre P, Heinzlef O, Merle H, et al. MS and neuromyelitis optica in Martinique (French West Indies). Neurology. 2001;56(4):507–14.

17. Rivera JF, Kurtzke JF, Alatriste Booth VJ, Corona T. Characteristics of Devic's disease (neuromyelitis optica) in Mexico. J Neurol. 2008;255:710–5.

18. Mirsattari SM, Johnston JB, McKenna R, Del Bigio MR, Orr P, Ross RT, et al. Aboriginals with multiple sclerosis: HLA types and predominance of neuromyelitis optica. Neurology. 2001;56(3):317–23.

19. Kuroiwa Y, Igata A, Itahara K, Koshijima S, Tsubaki T, Toyokura Y. Nationwide survey of multiple sclerosis in Japan. Clinical analysis of 1,084 cases. Neurology. 1975;25:845–51.

20. Wingerchuk DM, Weinshenker BG. Neuromyelitis optica: clinical predictors of a relapsing course and survival. Neurology. 2003;60(5):848–53.

21. Thielen KR, Miller GM. Multiple sclerosis of the spinal cord: magnetic resonance appearance. J Comput Assist Tomogr. 1996;20:434–8.

22. Bot JC, Barkhof F, Polman CH, Lycklama a Nijeholt GJ, deGroot V, Bergers E, et al. Spinal cord abnormalities in recently diagnosed MS patients: added value of spinal MRI examination. Neurology. 2004;62(2):226–33.

23. Misu T, Fujihara K, Nakashima I, Sato S, Itoyama Y. Intractable hiccup and nausea with periaqueductal lesions in neuromyelitis optica. Neurology. 2005; 65(9): 1479–82.

24. Pittock SJ, Weinshenker BG, Wijdicks EF. Mechanical ventilation and tracheostomy in multiple sclerosis. J Neurol Neurosurg Psychiatry. 2004;75(9):1331–3.

25. McDonald WI, Compston A, Edan G, Goodkin D, Hartung HP, Lublin FD, et al. Recommended diagnostic criteria for multiple sclerosis: guidelines from the International Panel on the diagnosis of multiple sclerosis. Ann Neurol. 2001;50(1):121–7.

26. Barkhof F, Filippi M, Miller DH, Scheltens P, Campi A, Polman CH, et al. Comparison of MRI criteria at first presentation to predict conversion to clinically definite multiple sclerosis. Brain. 1997;120(Pt 11):2059–69.

27. Tintore M, Rovira A, Martinez MJ, Rio J, Diaz-Villoslada P, Brieva L, et al. Isolated demyelinating syndromes: comparison of different MR imaging criteria to predict conversion to clinically definite multiple sclerosis. AJNR Am J Neuroradiol. 2000;21(4):702–6.

28. Pittock SJ, Lennon VA, Krecke K, Wingerchuk DM, Lucchinetti CF, Weinshenker BG. Brain abnormalities in neuromyelitis optica. Arch Neurol. 2006;63(3):390–6.

29. Pittock SJ, BG W, Lucchinetti CF, Wingerchuk DM, Corboy JR, Lennon VA. Neuromyelitis optica brain lesions localized to sites of high aquaporin 4 expression. Arch Neurol. 2006;63:964–8.
30. Vernant JC, Cabre P, Smadja D, Merle H, Caubarrere I, Mikol J, et al. Recurrent optic neuromyelitis with endocrinopathies: a new syndrome. Neurology. 1997;48(1):58–64.
31. Fardet L, Genereau T, Mikaeloff Y, Fontaine B, Seilhean D, Cabane J. Devic's neuromyelitis optica: study of nine cases. Acta Neurol Scand. 2003;108(3):193–200.
32. Poppe AY, Lapierre Y, Melancon D, Lowden D, Wardell L, Fullerton LM, et al. Neuromyelitis optica with hypothalamic involvement. Mult Scler. 2005;11(5):617–21.
33. Wingerchuk DM, Lennon VA, Pittock SJ, Lucchinetti CF, Weinshenker BG. Revised diagnostic criteria for neuromyelitis optica. Neurology. 2006;66:1485–9.
34. Banwell B, Tenembaum S, Lennon VA, et al. Neuromyelitis optica-IgG in childhood inflammatory demyelinating CNS disorders. Neurology. 2008;70:344–52.
35. Saiz A, Zuliani L, Blanco Y, et al. Revised diagnostic criteria for neuromyelitis optica (NMO). Application in a series of suspected patients. J Neurol. 2007;254:1233–7.
36. Miller DH, Weinshenker BG, Filippi MF, et al. Differential diagnosis of suspected multiple sclerosis: a consensus approach. Mult Scler. 2008;14:1157–74.
37. McKeon A, Lennon VA, Lotze T, et al. CNS aquaporin-4 autoimmunity in children. Neurology. 2008;71:93–100.
38. Weinshenker BG, Wingerchuk DM, Vukusic S, et al. Neuromyelitis optica IgG predicts relapse after longitudinally extensive transverse myelitis. Ann Neurol. 2006;59:566–9.
39. Matiello M, Jacob A, Pittock SJ, Lennon VA, Lucchinetti CF, Wingerchuk DM, et al. NMO-IgG predicts the outcome of recurrent optic neuritis. Neurology. 2008;70:2197–200.
40. Nakashima I, Fujihara K, Miyazawa I, et al. Clinical and MRI features of Japanese patients with multiple sclerosis positive for NMO-IgG. J Neurol Neurosurg Psychiatry. 2006;77:1073–5.
41. Takahashi T, Fujihara K, Nakashima I, et al. Anti-aquaporin-4 antibody is involved in the pathogenesis of NMO: a study on antibody titre. Brain. 2007;130 (Pt 5):1235–43.
42. Pittock SJ, Lennon VA, de Seze J, et al. Neuromyelitis optica and non-organ-specific autoimmunity. Arch Neurol. 2008;65:78–83.
43. Wingerchuk DM, Lennon VA, Pittock SJ, Lucchinetti CF, Weinshenker BG. A secondary progressive clinical course is uncommon in neuromyelitis optica. Neurology. 2007;68:603–5.
44. Lucchinetti CF, Mandler RN, McGavern D, Bruck W, Gleich G, Ransohoff RM, et al. A role for humoral mechanisms in the pathogenesis of Devic's neuromyelitis optica. Brain. 2002;125(Pt 7):1450–61.
45. Ortiz de Zarate JC, Tamaroff L, Sica RE, Rodriguez JA. Neuromyelitis optica versus subacute necrotic myelitis. II. Anatomical study of two cases. J Neurol Neurosurg Psychiatry. 1968;31(6):641–5.
46. Lefkowitz D, Angelo JN. Neuromyelitis optica with unusual vascular changes. Arch Neurol. 1984;41(10):1103–5.
47. Agre P, Kozono D. Aquaporin water channels: molecular mechanisms for human diseases. FEBS Lett. 2003;555(1):72–8.
48. Roemer SF, Parisi JE, Lennon VA, et al. Pattern specific loss of aquaporin 4 immunoreactivity distinguishes neuromyelitis optica from multiple sclerosis. Brain. 2007;130:1194–205.
49. Hinson SR, Pittock SJ, Lucchinett iCF, et al. Pathologic potential of IgG binding to water channel extracellular domain in neuromyelitis optica. Neurology. 2007;69:1–11.
50. Hinson SR, Roemer SF, Lucchinetti CF, et al. Aquaporin-4 binding autoantibodies in patients with neuromyelitis optica impair glutamate transport by downregulating EAAT2. J Exp Med. 2008;205:2473–81.

51. Wingerchuk DM, Weinshenker BG. Neuromyelitis optica. Curr Treat Options Neurol. 2008;10:55–66.
52. Weinshenker BG, O'Brien PC, Petterson TM, Noseworthy JH, Lucchinetti CF, Dodick DW, et al. A randomized trial of plasma exchange in acute central nervous system inflammatory demyelinating disease. Ann Neurol. 1999;46(6):878–86.
53. Keegan M, Pineda AA, McClelland RL, Darby CH, Rodriguez M, Weinshenker BG. Plasma exchange for severe attacks of CNS demyelination: predictors of response. Neurology. 2002;58(1):143–6.
54. Ruprecht K, Klinker E, Dintelmann T, Rieckmann P, Gold R. Plasma exchange for severe optic neuritis: treatment of 10 patients. Neurology. 2004;63(6):1081–3.
55. Papeix C, Deseze J, Pierrot-Deseilligny C, et al. French therapeutic experience of Devic's disease: a retrospective study of 33 cases. Neurology. 2005;64:A328.
56. Bergamaschi R, Uggetti C, Tonietti S, Egitto MG, Cosi V. A case of relapsing neuromyelitis optica treated with glatiramer acetate. J Neurol. 2003;250(3):359–61.
57. Saida T, Tashiro K, Itoyama Y, Sato T, Ohashi Y, Zhao Z. Interferon beta-1b is effective in Japanese RRMS patients: a randomized, multicenter study. Neurology. 2005;64(4):621–30.
58. Mandler RN, Ahmed W, Dencoff JE. Devic's neuromyelitis optica: a prospective study of seven patients treated with prednisone and azathioprine. Neurology. 1998;51(4):1219–20.
59. Jacob A, Weinshenker B, Matiello M, et al. Mycophenolate treatment of neuromyelitis optica: retrospective analysis of 25 cases. Mult Scler. 2007;13 Suppl 2:S244.
60. Silverman GJ, Weisman S. Rituximab therapy and autoimmune disorders: prospects for anti-B cell therapy. Arthritis Rheum. 2003;48(6):1484–92.
61. Cree BA, Lamb S, Morgan K, Chen A, Waubant E, Genain C. An open label study of the effects of rituximab in neuromyelitis optica. Neurology. 2005;64(7):1270–2.
62. Jacob A, Weinshenker BG, Violich I, et al. Treatment of neuromyelitis optica with rituximab: retrospective analysis of 25 patients. Arch Neurol. 2008;65:1443–8.
63. Hartung HP, Gonsette R, Konig N, Kwiecinski H, Guseo A, Morrissey SP, et al. Mitoxantrone in progressive multiple sclerosis: a placebo-controlled, double-blind, randomised, multicentre trial. Lancet. 2002;360(9350):2018–25.
64. Goodin DS, Arnason BG, Coyle PK, Frohman EM, Paty DW. The use of mitoxantrone (Novantrone) for the treatment of multiple sclerosis: report of the Therapeutics and Technology Assessment Subcommittee of the American Academy of Neurology. Neurology. 2003;61(10):1332–8.
65. Weinstock-Guttman B, Ramanathan M, Lincoff N, et al. Study of mitoxantrone for the treatment of recurrent neuromyelitis optica (Devic disease). Arch Neurol. 2006;63:957–63.
66. Minagar A, Sheremata WA. Treatment of Devic's disease with methotrexate and prednisone. Int J MS Care (Serial Online). 2000;2(4):39–43.
67. Bakker J, Metz L. Devic's neuromyelitis optica treated with intravenous gamma globulin (IVIG). Can J Neurol Sci. 2004;31(2):265–7.

The Neuroimmunology of Cancer

Enrico C. Lallana, William F. Hickey, and Camilo E. Fadul

Keywords: Gliomas, Immunology, Nervous system, Paraneoplastic syndromes

Introduction

Decreased immune surveillance is thought to be one of the mechanisms by which neoplastic cells are able to thrive. When cancer is located in the nervous system, an immune privileged site, its ability to evade detection, and targeting by immune cells may contribute to its aggressive behavior. Furthermore, high-grade gliomas, the most frequent and lethal primary brain tumors, induce both a local and systemic state of immune suppression that hampers efforts to manipulate the immune system as an effective therapeutic modality. On the other hand, there are rare instances when the immune response elucidated against systemic cancer causes nervous system injury without direct spread of the tumor. Although the neural injury is thought to be mediated by an autoimmune process, in most cases it is uncertain if it is caused by a humoral response, a cellular response, or a combination of both. This chapter reviews concepts related to the unique relationship between the nervous and immune systems, when cancer is present, as well as immune therapeutic modalities employed when the neural structures are affected directly by a primary tumor or indirectly in the case of paraneoplastic neurologic syndromes. The distinct immunologic characteristics of the central nervous system (CNS) become more unique and complex in the setting of neoplastic disease. In 2008, approximately 1,437,180 new cancer cases, including 21,810 arising from the nervous system, were diagnosed in the USA [1]. Gliomas, the most frequent type of brain tumors, are characterized by the infiltration of normal cerebral tissue, but this rarely results in systemic metastases. The tumor microenvironment shows a meager inflammatory response often accompanied by systemic immune suppression. These alterations might be considered epiphenomena unrelated to tumor pathogenesis, but experimental and clinical observations suggest that the immune system plays an important role in glioma biology. Our current concept of glioma immunobiology lends strong support to the idea

From: *Clinical Neuroimmunology: Multiple Sclerosis and Related Disorders*, Current Clinical Neurology,
Edited by: S.A. Rizvi and P.K. Coyle, DOI 10.1007/978-1-60327-860-7_13,
© Springer Science+Business Media, LLC 2011

of manipulating the immune system as a therapeutic approach for primary brain tumors. Glioma immunotherapy has evolved over the years, unfortunately as yet, without a major success. Nevertheless, extraneural or systemic neoplasms can trigger an immune response that in rare instances have repercussions in the nervous system. These interactions indirectly cause clinical syndromes that are aptly termed paraneoplastic neurologic syndromes. In some cases, antibodies have been identified as the element responsible for the phenomenon, but as primary tumors of the brain and spinal cord, the role that the immune system plays in the pathogenesis of these syndromes has not been clearly elucidated.

In spite of these ample gaps in knowledge, there have been great strides in the past decade that enhance our understanding of the immune system, the nervous system, and their intricate interaction. This chapter reviews current glioma and immunology concepts as a basis to appreciate why these CNS tumors represent such a challenge to the immune system. The insight gained allows the development of antineoplastic treatments that exploit one or several of the interactions between such neoplasms and the immune system. The rationale, design, and outcome of the most important immunotherapeutic approaches to gliomas will be described, followed by a discussion on future initiatives to optimize their use in combination with other therapeutic modalities. Finally, possible pathogenic mechanisms, immunologic/clinical findings, and outcomes of paraneoplastic neurologic syndromes will be presented.

Glioma Immunobiology

Classification

According to the World Health Organization (WHO) classification of tumors [2], gliomas fall under the category of neuroepithelial tumors which comprise 39.2% of all primary nervous system tumors [3]. Gliomas are classified and named according to their precursor cells into astrocytic, oligodendroglial, and ependymal cell and mixed (usually a combination of astrocytic and oligodendroglial components). Astrocytic tumors or astrocytomas are the most common and for clinical purposes, classified according to their degree of differentiation or grade (Table 13.1). Pilocytic astrocytoma is a well-differentiated usually focal glial tumor (WHO grade I) and often cured with complete resection. WHO grade II includes diffuse infiltrating oligodendrogliomas, astrocytomas, and gliomas of mixed histology. The term high-grade glioma comprises the

Table 13.1   Grading of the most common gliomas.

WHO grade	Histology
Grade I	Pilocytic astrocytoma
Grade II	Diffuse astrocytoma
	Oligodendroglioma
	Mixed glioma (oligoastrocytoma)
Grade III	Anaplastic astrocytoma
	Anaplastic oligodendroglioma
	Anaplastic mixed glioma (oligoastrocytoma)
Grade IV	Glioblastoma multiforme

anaplastic oligodendroglioma and anaplastic astrocytoma (WHO grade III), as well as the more aggressive and common glioma called glioblastoma (WHO grade IV).

Molecular Immunobiology

The blood–brain barrier (BBB) poses a special obstacle to immune responses and standard therapies in the CNS, but is not impermeable. The endothelial cells of the BBB are connected by tight rather than gap junctions that restrict movement of most cells and substances, but activated T-lymphocytes are known to traffic in and out of the CNS parenchyma and under some circumstances may do so even prior to antigenic stimulation [4, 5]. This lymphocyte migration is highly restricted through cell adhesion molecules, chemokines, cytokines, and matrix metalloproteinases [6]. The migration through endothelial cells is mediated by the interactions of leukocyte functional antigen-1 (LFA 1) and intercellular adhesion molecule-1 (ICAM-1), and between very late activation antigen-4 (VLA-4) and vascular cell adhesion molecule-1 (VCAM-1) [7]. Following these interactions, there is an upregulation of protein expression of matrix metalloproteinases for breakdown of extracellular matrix components allowing the entry of the T-cell into the CNS [8].

Transforming growth factor-beta (TGF-β) is an important cytokine in the maintenance of the BBB. It is found in leptomeningeal cells [9] and has the ability to suppress proliferation of T-lymphocytes migrating into the CNS [10]. In vitro migration of leukocytes across endothelial cell and astrocytes layers is suppressed by TGF-β, suggesting that it is a critical factor in limiting CNS immune surveillance. Other cytokines that inhibit immune activity are interleukin-10 (IL-10), prostaglandin (PG) E2, and gangliosides [11–13]. These cytokines' effects are counter to that of IL-1, IFN-γ, and TNF-α which are proinflammatory cytokines that have the ability to activate leukocytes behind the BBB [14].

The BBB, inhibitory cytokines, and the absence of traditional lymphatic drainage all constitute the inherent factors of the normal CNS that inhibit immune responses. Despite this apparent decreased activity, immune surveillance and immune responses do occur in the CNS. This knowledge has paved the way for researchers to better understand the molecular mechanisms involved in the interaction between gliomas and the nervous system. Genomics and proteomics have identified glioma-associated antigens that have been the subject of scrutiny due to their potential for recognition by the immune system. Epidermal growth factor receptor (EGFR) is one such antigen and it is known to be amplified and/or rearranged in malignant gliomas. The most common mutant form, EGFR type III variant (EGFRvIII) [15], is active and enhances tumorigenic activity in glioma models [16]. Antibodies created to target EGFRvIII can inhibit DNA synthesis, reduce cellular proliferation, and induce autonomous, complement-mediated, and antibody-dependent cell-mediated cytotoxicity [17]. Other glioma antigens that are involved in growth factor cell signaling include platelet-derived growth factor (PDGF), phosphatase and tensin homologue (PTEN), and vascular endothelial growth factor (VEGF). Several melanoma antigens such as gp100, melanoma antigen encoding gene 1 (MAGE-1), MAGE-E1, and MAGE-3 are expressed in gliomas and are potential targets for immunotherapy. Tenascin, Her2/neu, and gp240 are just a few of the many additional cell surface antigens that have been identified and are being studied as possible targets [18].

Immune Defects Associated with Gliomas (Table 13.2)

The expression of MHC-I in the nervous system is restricted to endothelial and parenchymal cells and is downregulated in different types of tumor cells [19] including gliomas [20]. While MHC-I downregulation has been a demonstrated process wherein tumors evade immune detection [19], it remains a controversial topic in gliomas. There are studies that have shown normal or elevated MHC-I expression by tumors [21–23] suggesting a wide variability of MHC-I expression and/or adaptive changes in the expression of the molecule.

The presentation of antigens to lymphocytes by APCs occurs via MHC-II molecules. Perivascular cells and to a lesser extent microglia express macrophage cell surface markers including MHC antigens and appear to be the APCs in the nervous system [24]. Microglial cells have been demonstrated in elevated numbers in rat [25] and human gliomas [26, 27]. While MHC-II expression is limited to APCs, neoplastic astrocytes have been shown to upregulate MHC-II expression in the presence of cytokines [28, 29]. Not surprisingly, in the CNS environment, APCs are ineffective in producing a sufficient immune response against the tumors due to secretion of soluble inhibitory factors resulting in a blunted immune response and low numbers of T-cells to recognized antigen [30].

Activation of lymphocytes requires a co-stimulatory signal in addition to the MHC-antigen interaction. This signal is also provided by the APC through binding of T-cell surface proteins such as CD40, CD28, and B7 family of molecules. After successful activation, the lymphocytes undergo clonal expansion stimulated by the presence of cytokines such as IFN-γ and interleukin 2 (IL-2). This adaptive immune response then proceeds to effect humoral and cell-mediated immunity. Of course, these processes do not progress normally in malignant glioma patients due to their impaired cellular immune responses [31, 32].

Malignant gliomas have the potential to impair lymphocyte proliferation and T-cell cytotoxicity by producing soluble inhibitory factors [33] such as TGF-β [34] and IL-10 [35]. TGF-β has a complex role in the development of gliomas and is thought to both stimulate and inhibit tumor cell growth. It may initially stunt tumor growth by the inhibition of proliferation [36] and DNA synthesis, but gliomas eventually lose their response to this action [37]. On the other hand, TGF-β supports tumors by positively influencing cell-to-extracellular matrix interactions and by increasing expression of integrin molecules that are vital to adhesion and invasion of glioma cells [38]. Additionally, TGF-β has been implicated in the increased expression of VEGFs, which stimulate angiogenesis in the growing tumor cells [39]. As TGF-β, IL-10 has been implicated in enhancing glioma cell proliferation and migration [40].

Table 13.2 Immune defects associated with glioma.

Microenvironment	Systemic
Decreased expression of MHC I	Increased population of T-regs
Decreased T-cell population	Downregulation of IL-2 expression
Elevated levels of TGF-β, IL-10	Inhibition of IFN-γ
Secretion of IL-6 and IL-8	

Gliomas are known to secrete the cytokine IL-6 [41] which has been demonstrated in an animal glioma model to serve as an oncofetal protein responsible for the rapid proliferation of fetal and tumor cells [42]. Likewise, IL-8 cytokine secretion in glioblastoma has also been demonstrated in vivo [43]. IL-8 is thought to be responsible for altering leukocyte chemotactic activity. Most recently, it has been shown to have significant tumorigenic properties [44] that enhance endothelial cell proliferation and survival and to induce the expression of cytokines that positively influence angiogenesis [45].

The immunological defects in patients with malignant gliomas are not limited to the CNS as systemic immune suppression has been well documented. Abnormalities in the number and function of T-cells have been thought to be responsible for much of the underlying immune deficiency. Regulatory T-cells (T-regs), or CD4$^+$ CD25$^+$ FOXP3$^+$ T-cells, modulate the immune response by the inhibition of effector T-cells; thus they are particularly helpful in the prevention of autoimmunity. Depletion of this population has been shown to be associated with autoimmune disease [46] and increased numbers linked with neoplastic disease [47–49]. T-regs infiltrate gliomas [50] and are disproportionately elevated in the blood of patients with these tumors [51]. They inhibit T-cell activation and proliferation through downregulation of IL-2 expression, inhibition of IFN-γ, and diversion of the clonal expansion of CD4$^+$ cells to more CD4$^+$CD25$^+$ cells [52]. Removal of this population reverses the inhibition on CD4$^+$ cells and has been shown to potentiate an antitumor response [51].

Immune Therapy for Gliomas

The complex interaction of the immune system and malignant gliomas not only highlights the deficiencies of the immune response but also provides insight into possible strategies in developing passive and active therapeutic modalities to combat these tumors (Table 13.3). Passive therapy aims for immediate response from administration or transfer of immune effectors such as antibodies and activated T-cells. Active immune therapy endeavors to improve or increase the patient's own immune response by the introduction of cytokines or tumor-associated antigens. These strategies have the potential for not only eradicating the tumor anywhere in the body (in both passive and active immunotherapy), but also giving the patient lifelong immunity to recurrence (in active immunotherapy).

Table 13.3 Types of immune therapy.

Passive immunotherapy	
Antibody-mediated immunotherapy	Use of antibodies to target tumor-associated antigens
Adoptive transfer	Administration of lymphocytes to provoke an immune response
Active immunotherapy	
Active nonspecific immunotherapy	Administration of cytokines to stimulate immune response
Active-specific immunotherapy	Vaccination with antigens to generate an immune response

Passive Immunotherapy

Antibody-Mediated Immunotherapy

The emergence of monoclonal antibodies resulted in a new class of therapeutic agents in the fight against cancer. These antibodies target tumor-associated antigens and facilitate tumor death through (1) complement dependent lysis, (2) opsonization, whereby antigen binding by antibodies leads to phagocytosis, and (3) antibody-dependent cellular cytotoxicity.

Antibodies to EGFR were used in several trials in an attempt to induce an antitumor effect. A phase I study by Faillot et al. [53] demonstrated good tolerance to the therapy and Stragliotto et al. [54] followed this with a phase I/II trial and found minimal toxicities. Unfortunately, no measurable tumor regression was seen in any of the 13 patients evaluated. Intratumoral injection of the antibody was attempted by Wersall et al. [55], to achieve high tumor cell antigen saturation by antibody, which was thought to be lacking when given intravenously. This resulted in significant tumor necrosis in several patients, but it also caused intolerable inflammatory reaction prompting discontinuation of the trial. In another iteration of anti-EGFR therapy, Quang and Brady [56] used radioactive iodine-125-labeled monoclonal antibody 425 (^{125}I-MAb 425), which binds to a protein on the external domain of the human EGFR [57]. A total of 180 patients with malignant gliomas were treated and followed for 5 years. They were able to demonstrate increased survival in patients under 40 years old and with good performance status.

Another anti-EGFR agent, cetuximab (Erbitux; ImClone Systems), has demonstrated preclinical antitumor activity when combined with radiation in the treatment of glioblastoma patients with known EGFR amplification [58] and is currently being investigated in phase II trials. PDGF, VEGF, and other receptors are being researched as targets for monoclonal antibodies, but they are beyond the scope of this review.

Adoptive Transfer

The adoptive transfer strategy relies on the premise that lymphocytes can be harvested and expanded ex vivo and later on be administered to the patient to provoke a specific immune response. Young and colleagues' initial trial utilizing non-activated immune cells was unsuccessful in prolonging survival in their subjects [59]. Subsequently, lymphocytes were harvested and stimulated with IL-2, resulting in what is called lymphokine-activated killer (LAK) cell. The LAK cells appeared to be effective in prolonging survival in animals harboring glioma cell lines [60, 61], but clinical trials showed mixed results but with no clear benefit [62–64]. The next iteration of this strategy resulted in a more antigen-specific immune response by harvesting tumor-infiltrating lymphocytes and stimulating then in vitro with IL-2. Although this strategy resulted in negative results in animal models [63], in a small phase I clinical trial tumor infiltrating lymphocytes expanded ex vivo with IL-2 were injected directly in the tumoral cavity via a reservoir. Six patients with recurrent high-grade glioma were treated with one complete response and two partial responses that persisted on follow-up of more than 3 years [65]. Following this, researchers switched to using extracranial subcutaneous implantation of irradiated tumor cells along with an adjuvant to enhance the immune response. The lymphocytes were then harvested from the draining lymph nodes, stimulated and administered intravenously to the patient. A phase I trial by Plautz et al. [66] revealed promising results, but poor tumor-specific trafficking and disappearance of transferred T-cells limited further studies using this approach.

Active Immunotherapy

Active Nonspecific Immunotherapy

Administration of cytokines has been used to influence the immune response to one that tips the balance toward tumor lysis. Systemic and intratumoral administration of IL-2 was attempted in several trials but was limited by the appearance of cerebral edema and other toxicities [67]. TNF-α infusion was tested in small case series and showed some activity [68, 69], but no convincing evidence of its efficacy has ever been published. IFN-α combined with surgery versus combination with surgery and radiation was given to patients with malignant brain tumors and showed initial promising results [70]. Unfortunately, a follow-up trial revealed unacceptable neurotoxicity [71]. Studies using IFN-β [72, 73] and IFN-γ [74, 75], likewise, revealed no significant improvement in clinical measures of efficacy. In summary, cytokine infusion has so far resulted in immune response limited by unacceptable toxicity, resulting in disappointment of this approach's potential to positively influence antitumor immune responses.

Active-specific Immunotherapy

This type of therapy typically relies on vaccination, wherein the patients' immune system is challenged with an antigen to generate an effective T-cell immune response against tumor. Ideally, these antigens should have one or more epitopes that can bind with MHC and be presented to CD8$^+$ cell. Recent advances have resulted in the discovery of glioma-associated antigens that can elicit a T-cell response which are currently being studied [18, 76, 77].

Early vaccination strategies relied on the use of autologous tumor cell vaccines and were largely ineffective. Likely limiting factors included poor antigen presenting capabilities of tumor cells, downregulation or failure of upregulation of expression of MHC, and absence of co-stimulatory signals from the APC.

A newer approach that allows for direct manipulation of the APC has been the modality most frequently reported in vaccination therapy. While perivascular and microglial cells are the main APCs in the CNS, they are technically difficult to harvest and attention has been directed to DCs. These cells are harvested and isolated from the peripheral circulation and activated with tumor-derived material such as eluted peptides or tumor lysate. The use of DCs and tumor-derived material appear to circumvent the limitations seen in autologous tumor cell vaccination outlined above. Initial in vitro studies have shown good evidence of antitumor immune responses [78–80]. Phase I studies in malignant gliomas have demonstrated its safety and tolerability [81–84] paving the way for additional trials. Liau et al. [85] published the results of their phase I trial using eluted tumor peptides to activate DCs in 12 patients. The patients were given intradermal vaccinations and followed for 5 years. The therapy resulted in one objective clinical response and six measurable systemic antitumor cytotoxic responses. They demonstrated some correlation between increased T-cell infiltrate of tumor samples obtained after vaccination, decreased TGF-β

expression, and increased survival. Yamanaka et al. [86] used tumor lysate to load their DC and they have reported in their phase I/II trial: one patient with partial response, three patients with minor response, ten patients with stable disease, with the other ten patients progressing despite therapy. They were also able to show increased survival when compared with a control population, especially in patients who received both intradermal and intratumoral administration of DC.

A novel approach to vaccination currently under investigation administers the specific mutant antigen EGFRvIII (chemically conjugated peptide called PEPvIII) [87] to produce an immune response. The studies have not been published formally, but Sampson reported this technique in a review article [88] and his preliminary results in abstracts. In the initial clinical trial, 16 patients with malignant astrocytomas were treated with the intradermal injection of autologous DCs pulsed with PEPvIII conjugated with keyhole limpet hemocyanin (PEPvIII–KLH) after surgical resection and radiation. A robust immune response specific for KLH, PEPvIII, and EGFRvIII was seen. The median time to tumor progression (TTP) in the glioblastoma subset was 47 weeks and median overall survival (OS) was 111 weeks. In response to the inevitable need for a large-scale trial, they simplified their technique by direct PEPvIII–KLH vaccination combined with granulocyte macrophage-colony stimulating factor (GM-CSF) stimulation. The subsequent phase I study enrolled only glioblastoma multiforme patients who received standard treatment with radiation and temozolomide. Median TTP was reported to be 12 months and median OS exceeded 18 months [89]. The subsequent phase II study was split into two arms, and patients were divided to receive either standard dose temozolomide (200 mg/m^2 for 5 of 28 days) or continuous dose temozolomide (100 mg/m^2 for 21 of 28 days) after standard radiation and concurrent temozolomide chemotherapy. There were no significant differences found in either regimen in terms of their PFS (16.6 months) or OS (not reached) [90]. These promising results led to a phase III trial that is underway.

Future Initiatives

Although most therapeutic approaches based on cell and peptide manipulation can induce an antitumor response against gliomas, their impact in overall survival and clinical response remains to be demonstrated. One of the issues is how to optimize the use of immunotherapy within the multimodality therapy strategy for patients with high-grade tumors. Maximum feasible surgical resection seems to offer a clear advantage not only since less tumor volume provides optimal conditions for other treatment modalities to be more effective, but also by the fact that the immune suppressive environment appears to correlate directly with tumor burden [85]. The addition of chemotherapy to immune therapy would appear to be counter intuitive, but several studies have shown that patients who received this combination seem to have a better outcome [85, 91]. A mechanism for an additive effect of immune therapy and chemotherapy is unknown but thought to be related to a decrease of T-regs, allowing the therapy to have a better chance to overcome the immune suppressive state [85]. Another explanation is that vaccination sensitizes tumor cells to chemotherapy [92, 93]. More aggressive or selective immune depleting strategies to enhance the effect of immune therapy have not been used for brain tumors. High-grade gliomas are extremely vascularized tumors as the result of angiogenesis factors, such as VEGF, that are known to interfere with the antitumor immune response. As a result, antiangiogenesis drugs in combination with immunotherapy approaches are being explored. In the future, it is possible that the optimal multimodality therapy for high-grade gliomas includes maximum feasible surgical resection followed by a combination of chemotherapy, immunotherapy, and antiangiogenesis agents.

As previously discussed the adoptive transfer of lymphocytes targeting specific antigens expressed by glioma cells has not been very successful. Despite the poor responses seen in gliomas, there have been promising reports in the use of adoptive transfer therapy for other tumors such as melanoma [94] when using non-myeloablative lymphocyte-depleting chemotherapy before adoptive transfer of tumor-specific T-cells. They were able to demonstrate tumor regression with this strategy, highlighting that the ablation of regulatory T-cells may be a factor in successful clonal expansion and persistence of transferred lymphocytes. Since melanoma and gliomas share antigens, it is possible that, in the future, expanded lymphocytes that are targeted to specific tumor-associated antigens would be an effective therapy for gliomas.

Paraneoplastic Syndromes and the CNS

Systemic cancer has far reaching effects in the body and can affect the nervous system by direct invasion through metastasis or by indirect or non-metastatic complications. Indirect effects of cancer include hypercoagulability, immune suppression, metabolic derangement, and nutritional deficiencies. These typically cause cerebrovascular disease, nervous system infection, encephalopathy, and seizures. A unique remote effect of systemic cancer on the nervous system is classified under the category of paraneoplastic syndromes. This concept was probably introduced as early as 1888, by Hermann Oppenheim, when he observed unexplained neurological symptoms in two cancer patients without the evidence of nervous system involvement of their tumor at necropsy [95]. He proposed that these neurologic disorders were caused by an infection or secretion of toxic substances from their respective tumors. Today, we use the term "paraneoplastic syndrome" for a group of disorders caused by a remote cancer that is not a direct result of the tumor mass or its metastasis [96]. Paraneoplastic syndromes often antedate the diagnosis of cancer by months or even years [97] and with few exceptions, cause irreversible damage to the nervous system without effective treatment.

The exact pathogenesis of paraneoplastic syndromes is unknown, although most authors believe that it is immune mediated. The demonstration of antineuronal or onconeural antibodies in the serum and cerebrospinal fluid of patients with paraneoplastic syndromes offers the best support for this theory. These antibodies are believed to be a product of an immune response to antigens expressed by the tumor early in its development. These onconeural antigens are analogous to normally expressed antigens in the nervous system and are recognized in the peripheral circulation as foreign by the immune system [98, 99]. The resultant immune response then causes significant injury not only to the tumor but also to nervous system elements.

Table 13.4 Common paraneoplastic syndromes.

Paraneoplastic syndrome	Associated neoplasm	Antibodies
Paraneoplastic cerebellar degeneration	Breast, gynecological	Anti-Yo (cdr2 or PCA1), anti-Ri (ANNA-2)
	SCLC	Anti-Hu (ANNA-1)
	Hodgkin's lymphoma	Anti-Tr
Paraneoplastic encephalomyelitis	SCLC	Anti-Hu, anti-CV2,
	Thymoma	Anti-CV2
	Testicular	Anti-Ma2
Opsoclonus/myoclonus	Breast, gynecological, lung	Anti-Ri
Lamber–Eaton myasthenic syndrome	SCLC	Anti-VGCC, anti-AGNA

The detection of antineuronal antibodies is the basis of commercially available tests that have been validated for the diagnosis of paraneoplastic disorders (Table 13.4). Many researchers believe that these antibodies have a direct pathogenic role in the development of paraneoplastic syndromes, but there is also strong evidence for T-cell-mediated immune response in its pathogenesis.

Humoral-Mediated Paraneoplastic Syndromes

Lambert–Eaton myasthenic syndrome (LEMS) and myasthenia gravis (MG) are the two disorders that are clearly humorally mediated [96]. P/Q type voltage-gated calcium channel (P/Q VGCC) antibodies are invariably demonstrated in patients with paraneoplastic LEMS and acetylcholine receptor antibodies are seen in majority of patients with MG. Both antibodies target cell surface receptors and their interaction directly results in the generation of neurologic symptoms. It is important to note that these antibodies and syndromes frequently occur without cancer. In fact, a patient diagnosed with LEMS has an approximately 62% chance of having small-cell lung cancer (SCLC) which declines significantly after 2 years [100]. In MG patients, the incidence of thymic tumors is estimated to be about 10%.

Antibodies to voltage-gated potassium channels (VGKC) are present in paraneoplastic neuromyotonia [101] and are directly linked to the reduction of potassium currents causing hyperexcitability [102]. Reversible limbic encephalitis has been associated with the presence of anti-VGKC antibodies which can be seen with or without the presence of cancer [103, 104]. A more severe form of encephalitis has recently been linked with the presence of N-methyl-D-aspartate (NMDA) antibodies and associated with ovarian teratoma [105, 106]. Interestingly, these tumors can contain immature or mature CNS tissue.

Additional disorders and associated antibodies include cerebellar ataxia (associated with mGluR1 antibody [107]) in Hodgkin's lymphoma, cancer-associated retinopathy (antibodies to recoverin [108]), stiff-person syndrome (amphiphysin antibody [109]), and autonomic neuropathy (glutamic acid decarboxylase antibody [110]).

T-Cell-Mediated Paraneoplastic Syndromes

In contrast to the theory citing a direct pathogenic role for antibodies, certain paraneoplastic syndrome antibodies react only with intracellular antigens. This suggests that a more complex immune reaction, involving a T-cell-mediated response is necessary for the pathogenesis of neural cell injury. A T-cell-mediated response would also explain the lack of efficacy of plasmapheresis and infusion of intravenous immunoglobulin in many of the well-characterized paraneoplastic syndromes. In addition, T-cell infiltrates have been demonstrated in the brain [111, 112] of paraneoplastic syndrome patients, suggesting that they may play an active role in the pathogenesis. However, the most compelling evidence of T-cell response is seen in paraneoplastic cerebellar degeneration (PCD) associated with anti-Yo (also known as anti-cdr2). Albert and associates were able to show increased population of cdr2-specific cytotoxic T-cells in the blood of three patients with PCD. They were also able to model in vitro cross-presentation of apoptotic cells by DC leading to an active cytotoxic T-cell response [113]. In a follow-up study by the same group, activated cdr2-specific T-cells were found in PCD patients' cerebrospinal fluid, giving additional support for a T-cell-mediated immune response [114]. Although these findings suggest that T-cells may be pathogenic in many of these syndromes, by no means are they conclusive. In a prior attempt to prove T-cell mediation, Tanaka et al. published two papers [115, 116] attempting to create an animal model of PCD. In the first experiment, they actively immunized animals with recombinant anti-cdr2 protein with different MHC proteins. The second study involved passive transfer of PCD patients' lymphocytes to immunodeficient mice. Neither of these studies was able to produce cerebellar degeneration in the animals.

Paraneoplastic Neurologic Syndromes

Paraneoplastic Cerebellar Degeneration

PCD is classically associated with ovarian and breast cancer [117], SCLC [118], Hodgkin's lymphoma [119], but it can be seen in association with any malignancy. The neurologic symptoms often precede the diagnosis of cancer by several months to a year. Given the narrow differential diagnosis of a pan-cerebellar syndrome, a diligent search for the underlying malignancy must be undertaken, if no underlying cause can be found. This disease is characterized by an insidious onset and subacute progression to a pan-cerebellar syndrome. Initial symptoms include a nonspecific dizziness associated with nausea, vomiting, and visual disturbance. Within several weeks, incoordination, ataxia with dysarthria, and dysphagia appear. The disorder is unrelentingly progressive until the patient is severely disabled by the cerebellar dysfunction, after which some stability of symptoms may occur. Physical findings include nystagmus with oscillopsia, appendicular and gait ataxia, cerebellar dysarthria, extensor plantar responses as well as occasional transient myoclonus and opsoclonus. Some subjects are found to have cognitive impairment and emotional lability [117].

Routine laboratory and imaging findings are typically unrevealing. Early cerebrospinal fluid analysis may show a mild pleocytosis, increased protein, and IgG, but in most cases it is normal [96]. Magnetic resonance imaging (MRI) scans are normal at the onset and over time may reveal cerebellar atrophy. There is one case report of cerebellar edema seen on MRI during the course of the disease and another describing focal fluid-attenuated inversion recovery (FLAIR) and T1 post-contrast hyperintensities in the temporal lobe and cerebellum [120].

The characteristic pathologic feature of PCD is Purkinje cell loss in the cerebellum associated with leukocytic infiltration [121]. The classic syndrome is associated with the Anti-Yo (anti-cdr2) antibodies that are seen in breast and gynecologic malignancies. This antibody interacts with the cdr2 antigen that is expressed in the cytoplasm of the cerebellar Purkinje cells and in breast and ovarian tumors associated with PCD [98, 122]. In SCLC, the cerebellar syndrome is usually part of an encephalomyelitis syndrome and is associated with anti-VGCC, anti-Hu, and other antibodies [123]. In Hodgkin's disease-associated PCD, the antineuronal anti-Tr antibody is present in the CSF [124, 125]. In contrast to most paraneoplastic syndromes, Hodgkin's disease-associated PCD often manifests clinically after the tumor diagnosis.

Paraneoplastic Encephalomyelitis

Most paraneoplastic encephalomyelitis cases occur in association with SCLC, affecting as the name denotes, multiple structures of the nervous system with clinical signs and symptoms suggesting a more diffuse disorder. Limbic encephalitis is a form of this disease that presents with personality changes, irritability, depression, memory loss, or even dementia progressing in a matter of days to weeks. Seizures are also a prominent feature of this syndrome, which are often complex partial or generalized in nature [126]. A variant of encephalomyelitis presents with somnolence, cataplexy, unexplained weight gain, and various hormonal abnormalities signifying hypothalamic involvement. Certain cases have a prominent brainstem involvement with or without limbic or diencephalic signs and symptoms. These patients present with Parkinsonism, dystonia, bradykinesia, vertical gaze paralysis, sleep-related symptoms, and cranial neuropathies [127]. Occasionally, patients present with a subacute myelitis [128], but often the spinal cord involvement occurs as part of a more diffuse syndrome. In some cases, the symptoms are localized to a certain location and presenting with very focal symptoms. A curious case of orgasmic epilepsy without any other symptoms in a woman with SCLC has been reported [129].

The CSF often shows pleocytosis and elevation of protein. MRI reveals T2 hyperintensities in either or both temporal lobes and other areas. Electroencephalogram regularly shows cerebral dysfunction such as focal or generalized slowing, epileptic discharges, and even periodic lateralized epileptiform discharges (PLEDS) [127, 130].

The antineuronal nuclear antibody type 1(ANNA1 or anti-Hu) antibodies are present in both serum and CSF, in about 50% of SCLC patients with limbic encephalitis and sensory neuronopathy. Less frequently, anti-CV2 (anti-CRMP5) antibody that recognizes a neuronal cytoplasmic antigen called collapsin response-mediator brain protein (CRMP) is seen and found to be associated with SCLC and thymoma [131]. Anti-Ma2 is another antineuronal antibody that is usually seen in patients with diencephalic and brainstem encephalitis and testicular cancer [132].

Opsoclonus/Myoclonus

Opsoclonus/myoclonus is best known as a presenting symptom of approximately 2% of children with neuroblastoma [133]. In adults, it arises in relation to fallopian or breast cancer. The prominent findings are the presence of involuntary irregular, large amplitude conjugate saccades in random directions (opsoclonus) and focal or diffuse random, small amplitude and rapid contraction, and relaxation of muscles also occurring at random (myoclonus) accompanied by cerebellar and brainstem dysfunction. Brain MRI is usually unremarkable and CSF analysis can show pleocytosis infrequently.

Children with neuroblastoma often have antineuronal antibodies, but none of these have been consistently associated with the same antigen [134, 135]. Researchers have demonstrated activity against cerebellar granular neurons in animal models [136] and membrane antigens of child neuroblastoma [137]. In adults, the syndrome is frequently associated with an anti-RNA binding protein called anti-Ri antibody.

Lambert–Eaton Myasthenic Syndrome

The LEMS most frequently involves axial and lower extremity muscle weakness and fatigability. The patients' symptoms reflect the distribution of weakness and often involve difficulty arising from a chair, climbing stairs, or walking. In some patients, repetitive movements can increase the strength of the muscle group temporarily. Unlike myasthenia gravis, ptosis, diplopia, dysphagia, and dysarthria are not very common. Other symptoms include dryness of the mouth, constipation, and impotence. The onset of symptoms is insidious and is often accompanied by fatigue. The weakness progresses over weeks to months and the diagnosis typically precedes the diagnosis of cancer. Examination of the patient reveals proximal muscle weakness in the shoulder and pelvic girdle muscles with decreased deep-tendon reflexes.

Electromyography will show the classic incremental response on repetitive stimulation. The typical finding is diminished compound muscle action potential (CMAP), which increases more than 100% on repetitive stimulation of about 50 Hz. This is in contrast to myasthenia gravis which usually shows normal CMAPs and a decremental response on repetitive nerve stimulation at 10 Hz.

LEMS occurs in patients with SCLC and has an incidence of about 2% [138] and SCLC is found in patients with LEMS in about 40–62% [100, 139]. It has also been described with other neuroendocrine carcinomas such as carcinoid, large cell neuroendocrine carcinoma, and lymphoproliferative disorders including lymphoma [140, 141]. The antibody associated with paraneoplastic LEMS is anti-P/Q VGCC which can be seen in patients with SCLC. The antibody can also be found in low titers in SCLC patients without evidence of LEMS. It is associated with prolonged survival in SCLC when present along with LEMS but not in patients who do not manifest the myasthenic syndrome [142]. Anti-glial nuclear antibody (AGNA) is also found in SCLC patient with LEMS [143]. LEMS is discussed in more detail in a separate chapter (neuromuscular disorders).

Treatment

The treatment of paraneoplastic syndromes relies mostly in the treatment of the underlying cancer and when suspected an exhaustive search for an occult tumor cannot be overemphasized. Treatment of the tumor is essential for long-term survival as well as for prevention of progression of the neurologic syndrome [144]. In some syndromes, cancer treatment can improve the neurological condition associated with its paraneoplastic response. Remissions of paraneoplastic opsoclonus/myoclonus, LEMS, and paraneoplastic encephalomyelitis have been reported after successful treatment of the tumor [145–147].

Immunosuppressive therapy should be considered depending on the type of paraneoplastic syndrome. The treatment is typically effective with syndromes that have a physiologic rather than anatomic pathogenesis. The functional abnormality in LEMS is the reduction of acetylcholine release due to the inhibition of VGCC receptors in the pre-synaptic nerve terminal [148]. LEMS patient has been effectively treated with prednisone, plasmapheresis, and intravenous immunoglobulin G (IVIgG). In other syndromes, there is little benefit to immunosuppressants. However, stabilization of neurologic symptoms can be achieved and in some situations, improvement. Neuroblastoma-associated opsoclonus/myoclonus has been shown to be responsive to tumor treatment combined with ACTH. Other therapies to modify elements of the immune response that have been reported to have positive outcomes are dexamethasone [149], IVIgG [150], plasmapheresis [151], prednisone [150], and rituximab [152]. In syndromes that affect the CNS, the efficacy of immunotherapy is unclear [144]. In PCD, immune treatments are generally ineffective owing to the widespread loss of Purkinje cells early in the course of the disease. There have been, however, reports of improvement in PCD [153–156] with immune therapy, but these are usually associated with antibodies other than anti-Yo or anti-Hu. Paraneoplastic encephalomyelitis, such as most cases of PCD, is poorly responsive to immunotherapy.

Conclusion

The clinician must have a high index of suspicion for paraneoplastic neurologic symptoms whenever the patient's neurologic symptoms resemble any of the syndromes we have outlined here. Making the correct diagnosis early after the onset of symptoms will allow for a possible early diagnosis of cancer and enable the patient to receive treatment for both the cancer and the paraneoplastic syndrome.

References

1. Jemal A, Siegel R, Ward E, et al. Cancer statistics, 2008. CA Cancer J Clin. 2008;58(2):71–96.
2. Louis DN, Ohgaki H, Wiestler OD, et al. The 2007 WHO classification of tumours of the central nervous system. Acta Neuropathol. 2007;114(2):97–109.
3. CBTRUS (2008) Statistical report: primary brain tumors in the United States, 2000–2004. Central Brain Tumor Registry of the United States, Hindsdale, IL.
4. Owens T, Tran E, Hassan-Zahraee M, Krakowski M. Immune cell entry to the CNS – a focus for immunoregulation of EAE. Res Immunol. 1998;149(9):781–9. discussion 844–6, 855–60.
5. Hickey WF. Leukocyte traffic in the central nervous system: the participants and their roles. Semin Immunol. 1999;11(2):125–37.

6. Pachter JS, de Vries HE, Fabry Z. The blood-brain barrier and its role in immune privilege in the central nervous system. J Neuropathol Exp Neurol. 2003;62(6): 593–604.

7. Greenwood J, Wang Y, Calder VL. Lymphocyte adhesion and transendothelial migration in the central nervous system: the role of LFA-1, ICAM-1, VLA-4 and VCAM-1. off. Immunology. 1995;86(3):408–15.

8. Romanic AM, Graesser D, Baron JL, Visintin I, Janeway Jr CA, Madri JA. T cell adhesion to endothelial cells and extracellular matrix is modulated upon transendothelial cell migration. Lab Invest. 1997;76(1):11–23.

9. Johnson MD, Gold LI, Moses HL. Evidence for transforming growth factor-beta expression in human leptomeningeal cells and transforming growth factor-beta-like activity in human cerebrospinal fluid. Lab Invest. 1992;67(3):360–8.

10. Taylor AW, Streilein JW. Inhibition of antigen-stimulated effector T cells by human cerebrospinal fluid. Neuroimmunomodulation. 1996;3(2–3):112–8.

11. Aloisi F, De Simone R, Columba-Cabezas S, Levi G. Opposite effects of interferon-gamma and prostaglandin E2 on tumor necrosis factor and interleukin-10 production in microglia: a regulatory loop controlling microglia pro- and anti-inflammatory activities. J Neurosci Res. 1999;56(6):571–80.

12. Irani DN, Lin KI, Griffin DE. Brain-derived gangliosides regulate the cytokine production and proliferation of activated T cells. J Immunol. 1996;157(10):4333–40.

13. Maca RD. The effects of prostaglandins on the proliferation of cultured human T lymphocytes. Immunopharmacology. 1983;6(4):267–77.

14. Hickey WF, Vass K, Lassmann H. Bone marrow-derived elements in the central nervous system: an immunohistochemical and ultrastructural survey of rat chimeras. J Neuropathol Exp Neurol. 1992;51(3):246–56.

15. Ekstrand AJ, Sugawa N, James CD, Collins VP. Amplified and rearranged epidermal growth factor receptor genes in human glioblastomas reveal deletions of sequences encoding portions of the N- and/or C-terminal tails. Proc Natl Acad Sci USA. 1992;89(10):4309–13.

16. Ding H, Shannon P, Lau N, et al. Oligodendrogliomas result from the expression of an activated mutant epidermal growth factor receptor in a RAS transgenic mouse astrocytoma model. Cancer Res. 2003;63(5):1106–13.

17. Sampson JH, Crotty LE, Lee S, et al. Unarmed, tumor-specific monoclonal antibody effectively treats brain tumors. Proc Natl Acad Sci USA. 2000;97(13):7503–8.

18. Zhang JG, Eguchi J, Kruse CA, et al. Antigenic profiling of glioma cells to generate allogeneic vaccines or dendritic cell-based therapeutics. Clin Cancer Res. 2007;13(2 Pt 1):566–75.

19. Restifo NP, Esquivel F, Kawakami Y, et al. Identification of human cancers deficient in antigen processing. J Exp Med. 1993;177(2):265–72.

20. Ito A, Shinkai M, Honda H, Wakabayashi T, Yoshida J, Kobayashi T. Augmentation of MHC class I antigen presentation via heat shock protein expression by hyperthermia. Cancer Immunol Immunother. 2001;50(10):515–22.

21. Saito T, Tanaka R, Yoshida S, Washiyama K, Kumanishi T. Immunohistochemical analysis of tumor-infiltrating lymphocytes and major histocompatibility antigens in human gliomas and metastatic brain tumors. Surg Neurol. 1988;29(6):435–42.

22. Miyagi K, Ingram M, Techy GB, Jacques DB, Freshwater DB, Sheldon H. Immunohistochemical detection and correlation between MHC antigen and cell-mediated immune system in recurrent glioma by APAAP method. Neurol Med Chir (Tokyo). 1990;30(9):649–55.

23. Friese MA, Platten M, Lutz SZ, et al. MICA/NKG2D-mediated immunogene therapy of experimental gliomas. Cancer Res. 2003;63(24):8996–9006.

24. Gehrmann J, Matsumoto Y, Kreutzberg GW. Microglia: intrinsic immuneffector cell of the brain. Brain Res Brain Res Rev. 1995;20(3):269–87.

25. Hickey WF. Basic principles of immunological surveillance of the normal central nervous system. Glia. 2001;36(2):118–24.

26. Roggendorf W, Strupp S, Paulus W. Distribution and characterization of microglia/macrophages in human brain tumors. Acta Neuropathol. 1996;92(3): 288–93.
27. Rossi ML, Hughes JT, Esiri MM, Coakham HB, Brownell DB. Immunohistological study of mononuclear cell infiltrate in malignant gliomas. Acta Neuropathol. 1987;74(3):269–77.
28. Hong LL, Johannsen L, Krueger JM. Modulation of human leukocyte antigen DR expression in glioblastoma cells by interferon gamma and other cytokines. J Neuroimmunol. 1991;35(1–3):139–52.
29. Reder AT, Lascola CD, Flanders SA, et al. Astrocyte cytolysis by MHC class II-specific mouse T cell clones. Transplantation. 1993;56(2):393–9.
30. Gabrilovich DI, Chen HL, Girgis KR, et al. Production of vascular endothelial growth factor by human tumors inhibits the functional maturation of dendritic cells. Nat Med. 1996;2(10):1096–103.
31. Brooks WH, Netsky MG, Normansell DE, Horwitz DA. Depressed cell-mediated immunity in patients with primary intracranial tumors. Characterization of a humoral immunosuppressive factor. J Exp Med. 1972;136(6):1631–47.
32. Mahaley Jr MS, Brooks WH, Roszman TL, Bigner DD, Dudka L, Richardson S. Immunobiology of primary intracranial tumors. Part 1: studies of the cellular and humoral general immune competence of brain-tumor patients. J Neurosurg. 1977;46(4):467–76.
33. McVicar DW, Davis DF, Merchant RE. In vitro analysis of the proliferative potential of T cells from patients with brain tumor: glioma-associated immunosuppression unrelated to intrinsic cellular defect. J Neurosurg. 1992;76(2):251–60.
34. Kuppner MC, Hamou MF, Sawamura Y, Bodmer S, de Tribolet N. Inhibition of lymphocyte function by glioblastoma-derived transforming growth factor beta 2. J Neurosurg. 1989;71(2):211–7.
35. Wagner S, Czub S, Greif M, et al. Microglial/macrophage expression of interleukin 10 in human glioblastomas. Int J Cancer. 1999;82(1):12–6.
36. Hunter KE, Sporn MB, Davies AM. Transforming growth factor-betas inhibit mitogen-stimulated proliferation of astrocytes. Glia. 1993;7(3):203–11.
37. Rich JN, Zhang M, Datto MB, Bigner DD, Wang XF. Transforming growth factor-beta-mediated p15(INK4B) induction and growth inhibition in astrocytes is SMAD3-dependent and a pathway prominently altered in human glioma cell lines. J Biol Chem. 1999;274(49):35053–8.
38. Paulus W, Baur I, Huettner C, et al. Effects of transforming growth factor-beta 1 on collagen synthesis, integrin expression, adhesion and invasion of glioma cells. J Neuropathol Exp Neurol. 1995;54(2):236–44.
39. Koochekpour S, Merzak A, Pilkington GJ. Vascular endothelial growth factor production is stimulated by gangliosides and TGF-beta isoforms in human glioma cells in vitro. Cancer Lett. 1996;102(1–2):209–15.
40. Huettner C, Czub S, Kerkau S, Roggendorf W, Tonn JC. Interleukin 10 is expressed in human gliomas in vivo and increases glioma cell proliferation and motility in vitro. Anticancer Res. 1997;17(5A):3217–24.
41. Van Meir E, Sawamura Y, Diserens AC, Hamou MF, de Tribolet N. Human glioblastoma cells release interleukin 6 in vivo and in vitro. Cancer Res. 1990;50(20):6683–8.
42. Goswami S, Gupta A, Sharma SK. Interleukin-6-mediated autocrine growth promotion in human glioblastoma multiforme cell line U87MG. J Neurochem. 1998;71(5):1837–45.
43. Van Meir E, Ceska M, Effenberger F, et al. Interleukin-8 is produced in neoplastic and infectious diseases of the human central nervous system. Cancer Res. 1992;52(16):4297–305.
44. Brat DJ, Bellail AC, Van Meir EG. The role of interleukin-8 and its receptors in gliomagenesis and tumoral angiogenesis. Neuro-oncol. 2005;7(2):122–33.

45. Li A, Dubey S, Varney ML, Dave BJ, Singh RK. IL-8 directly enhanced endothelial cell survival, proliferation, and matrix metalloproteinases production and regulated angiogenesis. J Immunol. 2003;170(6):3369–76.

46. Sakaguchi S, Sakaguchi N, Asano M, Itoh M, Toda M. Immunologic self-tolerance maintained by activated T cells expressing IL-2 receptor alpha-chains (CD25). Breakdown of a single mechanism of self-tolerance causes various autoimmune diseases. J Immunol. 1995;155(3):1151–64.

47. Ichihara F, Kono K, Takahashi A, Kawaida H, Sugai H, Fujii H. Increased populations of regulatory T cells in peripheral blood and tumor-infiltrating lymphocytes in patients with gastric and esophageal cancers. Clin Cancer Res. 2003;9(12):4404–8.

48. Ling KL, Pratap SE, Bates GJ, et al. Increased frequency of regulatory T cells in peripheral blood and tumour infiltrating lymphocytes in colorectal cancer patients. Cancer Immun. 2007;7:7.

49. Liyanage UK, Moore TT, Joo HG, et al. Prevalence of regulatory T cells is increased in peripheral blood and tumor microenvironment of patients with pancreas or breast adenocarcinoma. J Immunol. 2002;169(5):2756–61.

50. El Andaloussi A, Lesniak MS. An increase in CD4+CD25+FOXP3+ regulatory T cells in tumor-infiltrating lymphocytes of human glioblastoma multiform. Neuro-oncol. 2006;8(3):234–43.

51. Fecci PE, Mitchell DA, Whitesides JF, et al. Increased regulatory T-cell fraction amidst a diminished CD4 compartment explains cellular immune defects in patients with malignant glioma. Cancer Res. 2006;66(6):3294–302.

52. Zheng SG, Wang JH, Gray JD, Soucier H, Horwitz DA. Natural and induced CD4+CD25+ cells educate CD4+CD25- cells to develop suppressive activity: the role of IL-2, TGF-beta, and IL-10. J Immunol. 2004;172(9):5213–21.

53. Faillot T, Magdelenat H, Mady E, et al. A phase I study of an anti-epidermal growth factor receptor monoclonal antibody for the treatment of malignant gliomas. Neurosurgery. 1996;39(3):478–83.

54. Stragliotto G, Vega F, Stasiecki P, Gropp P, Poisson M, Delattre JY. Multiple infusions of anti-epidermal growth factor receptor (EGFR) monoclonal antibody (EMD 55,900) in patients with recurrent malignant gliomas. Eur J Cancer. 1996;32A(4):636–40.

55. Wersall P, Ohlsson I, Biberfeld P, et al. Intratumoral infusion of the monoclonal antibody, mAb 425, against the epidermal-growth-factor receptor in patients with advanced malignant glioma. Cancer Immunol Immunother. 1997;44(3):157–64.

56. Quang TS, Brady LW. Radioimmunotherapy as a novel treatment regimen: 125I-labeled monoclonal antibody 425 in the treatment of high-grade brain gliomas. Int J Radiat Oncol Biol Phys. 2004;58(3):972–5.

57. Sunada H, Magun BE, Mendelsohn J, MacLeod CL. Monoclonal antibody against epidermal growth factor receptor is internalized without stimulating receptor phosphorylation. Proc Natl Acad Sci USA. 1986;83(11):3825–9.

58. Eller JL, Longo SL, Kyle MM, Bassano D, Hicklin DJ, Canute GW. Anti-epidermal growth factor receptor monoclonal antibody cetuximab augments radiation effects in glioblastoma multiforme in vitro and in vivo. Neurosurgery. 2005;56:155–62. discussion 162.

59. Young H, Kaplan A, Regelson W. Immunotherapy with autologous white cell infusions ("lymphocytes") in the treatment of recurrrent glioblastoma multiforme: a preliminary report. Cancer. 1977;40(3):1037–44.

60. Kruse CA, Lillehei KO, Mitchell DH, Kleinschmidt-DeMasters B, Bellgrau D. Analysis of interleukin 2 and various effector cell populations in adoptive immunotherapy of 9L rat gliosarcoma: allogeneic cytotoxic T lymphocytes prevent tumor take. Proc Natl Acad Sci USA. 1990;87(24):9577–81.

61. Tzeng JJ, Barth RF, Clendenon NR, Gordon WA. Adoptive immunotherapy of a rat glioma using lymphokine-activated killer cells and interleukin 2. Cancer Res. 1990;50(14):4338–43.

62. Merchant RE, Grant AJ, Merchant LH, Young HF. Adoptive immunotherapy for recurrent glioblastoma multiforme using lymphokine activated killer cells and recombinant interleukin-2. Cancer. 1988;62(4):665–71.

63. Barba D, Saris SC, Holder C, Rosenberg SA, Oldfield EH. Intratumoral LAK cell and interleukin-2 therapy of human gliomas. J Neurosurg. 1989;70(2):175–82.

64. Kruse CA, Mitchell DH, Lillehei KO, et al. Interleukin-2-activated lymphocytes from brain tumor patients. A comparison of two preparations generated in vitro. Cancer. 1989;64(8):1629–37.

65. Quattrocchi KB, Miller CH, Cush S, et al. Pilot study of local autologous tumor infiltrating lymphocytes for the treatment of recurrent malignant gliomas. J Neurooncol. 1999;45(2):141–57.

66. Plautz GE, Touhalisky JE, Shu S. Treatment of murine gliomas by adoptive transfer of ex vivo activated tumor-draining lymph node cells. Cell Immunol. 1997;178(2):101–7.

67. Merchant RE, Ellison MD, Young HF. Immunotherapy for malignant glioma using human recombinant interleukin-2 and activated autologous lymphocytes. A review of pre-clinical and clinical investigations. J Neurooncol. 1990;8(2):173–88.

68. Fukushima T, Yamamoto M, Ikeda K, et al. Treatment of malignant astrocytomas with recombinant mutant human tumor necrosis factor-alpha (TNF-SAM2). Anticancer Res. 1998;18(5D):3965–70.

69. Yoshida J, Wakabayashi T, Mizuno M, et al. Clinical effect of intra-arterial tumor necrosis factor-alpha for malignant glioma. J Neurosurg. 1992;77(1):78–83.

70. Jereb B, Petric J, Lamovec J, Skrbec M, Soss E. Intratumor application of human leukocyte interferon-alpha in patients with malignant brain tumors. Am J Clin Oncol. 1989;12(1):1–7.

71. Jereb B, Petric-Grabnar G, Klun B, Lamovec J, Skrbec M, Soos E. Addition of IFN-alpha to treatment of malignant brain tumors. Acta Oncol. 1994;33(6): 651–4.

72. von Wild KR, Knocke TH. The effects of local and systemic interferon beta (Fiblaferon) on supratentorial malignant cerebral glioma – a phase II study. Neurosurg Rev. 1991;14(3):203–13.

73. Yung WK, Prados M, Levin VA, et al. Intravenous recombinant interferon beta in patients with recurrent malignant gliomas: a phase I/II study. J Clin Oncol. 1991;9(11):1945–9.

74. Priestman TJ, Bleehen NM, Rampling R, Stenning S, Nethersell AJ, Scott J. A phase II evaluation of human lymphoblastoid interferon (Wellferon) in relapsed high grade malignant glioma. Medical Research Council Brain Tumour Working Party. Clin Oncol (R Coll Radiol). 1993;5(3):165–8.

75. Farkkila M, Jaaskelainen J, Kallio M, et al. Randomised, controlled study of intratumoral recombinant gamma-interferon treatment in newly diagnosed glioblastoma. Br J Cancer. 1994;70(1):138–41.

76. Hatano M, Eguchi J, Tatsumi T, et al. EphA2 as a glioma-associated antigen: a novel target for glioma vaccines. Neoplasia. 2005;7(8):717–22.

77. Schmitz M, Wehner R, Stevanovic S, et al. Identification of a naturally processed T cell epitope derived from the glioma-associated protein SOX11. Cancer Lett. 2007;245(1–2):331–6.

78. Celluzzi CM, Mayordomo JI, Storkus WJ, Lotze MT, Falo Jr LD. Peptide-pulsed dendritic cells induce antigen-specific CTL-mediated protective tumor immunity. J Exp Med. 1996;183(1):283–7.

79. Zitvogel L, Mayordomo JI, Tjandrawan T, et al. Therapy of murine tumors with tumor peptide-pulsed dendritic cells: dependence on T cells, B7 costimulation, and T helper cell 1-associated cytokines. J Exp Med. 1996;183(1):87–97.

80. Ribas A, Butterfield LH, Hu B, et al. Generation of T-cell immunity to a murine melanoma using MART-1-engineered dendritic cells. J Immunother. 2000; 23(1):59–66.

81. Kikuchi T, Akasaki Y, Irie M, Homma S, Abe T, Ohno T. Results of a phase I clinical trial of vaccination of glioma patients with fusions of dendritic and glioma cells. Cancer Immunol Immunother. 2001;50(7):337–44.
82. Yu JS, Wheeler CJ, Zeltzer PM, et al. Vaccination of malignant glioma patients with peptide-pulsed dendritic cells elicits systemic cytotoxicity and intracranial T-cell infiltration. Cancer Res. 2001;61(3):842–7.
83. Yamanaka R, Abe T, Yajima N, et al. Vaccination of recurrent glioma patients with tumour lysate-pulsed dendritic cells elicits immune responses: results of a clinical phase I/II trial. Br J Cancer. 2003;89(7):1172–9.
84. Rutkowski S, De Vleeschouwer S, Kaempgen E, et al. Surgery and adjuvant dendritic cell-based tumour vaccination for patients with relapsed malignant glioma, a feasibility study. Br J Cancer. 2004;91(9):1656–62.
85. Liau LM, Prins RM, Kiertscher SM, et al. Dendritic cell vaccination in glioblastoma patients induces systemic and intracranial T-cell responses modulated by the local central nervous system tumor microenvironment. Clin Cancer Res. 2005;11(15):5515–25.
86. Yamanaka R, Homma J, Yajima N, et al. Clinical evaluation of dendritic cell vaccination for patients with recurrent glioma: results of a clinical phase I/II trial. Clin Cancer Res. 2005;11(11):4160–7.
87. Wikstrand CJ, Hale LP, Batra SK, et al. Monoclonal antibodies against EGFRvIII are tumor specific and react with breast and lung carcinomas and malignant gliomas. Cancer Res. 1995;55(14):3140–8.
88. Sampson JH, Archer GE, Mitchell DA, Heimberger AB, Bigner DD. Tumor-specific immunotherapy targeting the EGFRvIII mutation in patients with malignant glioma. Semin Immunol. 2008;20(5):267–75.
89. Heimberger AB, Hussain SF, Aldape K, et al. Tumor-specific peptide vaccination in newly diagnosed patients with GBM. J Clin Oncol. 2006;24(18S):2529 (Abstracts).
90. Sampson JH, Archer GE, Bigner DD, et al. Effect of EGFRvIII-targeted vaccine (CDX-110) on immune response and TTP when given with simultaneous standard and continuous temozolomide in patients with GBM. J Clin Oncol. 2008;26(Suppl):2001. doi:2001 (Meeting Abstracts).
91. Wheeler CJ, Das A, Liu G, Yu JS, Black KL. Clinical responsiveness of glioblastoma multiforme to chemotherapy after vaccination. Clin Cancer Res. 2004;10(16):5316–26.
92. Liu G, Akasaki Y, Khong HT, et al. Cytotoxic T cell targeting of TRP-2 sensitizes human malignant glioma to chemotherapy. Oncogene. 2005;24(33):5226–34.
93. Wheeler CJ, Black KL, Liu G, et al. Vaccination elicits correlated immune and clinical responses in glioblastoma multiforme patients. Cancer Res. 2008;68(14):5955–64.
94. Dudley ME, Wunderlich JR, Yang JC, et al. Adoptive cell transfer therapy following non-myeloablative but lymphodepleting chemotherapy for the treatment of patients with refractory metastatic melanoma. J Clin Oncol. 2005;23(10):2346–57.
95. Oppenheim H. Ueber Hirnsymptome bei Carcinomatose ohne nachweisbare Veranderungen im Gehirn. Charite Annalen. 1888;13:335–44.
96. Posner JB, DeAngelis LM. Neurologic complications of cancer. 2nd ed. New York: Oxford University Press; 2009.
97. Darnell RB, Posner JB. Paraneoplastic syndromes involving the nervous system. N Engl J Med. 2003;349(16):1543–54.
98. Furneaux HM, Rosenblum MK, Dalmau J, et al. Selective expression of Purkinje-cell antigens in tumor tissue from patients with paraneoplastic cerebellar degeneration. N Engl J Med. 1990;322(26):1844–51.
99. Dalmau J, Furneaux HM, Cordon-Cardo C, Posner JB. The expression of the Hu (paraneoplastic encephalomyelitis/sensory neuronopathy) antigen in human normal and tumor tissues. Am J Pathol. 1992;141(4):881–6.

100. O'Neill JH, Murray NM, Newsom-Davis J. The Lambert-Eaton myasthenic syndrome. A review of 50 cases. Brain. 1988;111(Pt 3):577–96.

101. Shillito P, Molenaar PC, Vincent A, et al. Acquired neuromyotonia: evidence for autoantibodies directed against K+ channels of peripheral nerves. Ann Neurol. 1995;38(5):714–22.

102. Tomimitsu H, Arimura K, Nagado T, et al. Mechanism of action of voltage-gated K+ channel antibodies in acquired neuromyotonia. Ann Neurol. 2004;56(3): 440–4.

103. Buckley C, Oger J, Clover L, et al. Potassium channel antibodies in two patients with reversible limbic encephalitis. Ann Neurol. 2001;50(1):73–8.

104. Vincent A, Buckley C, Schott JM, et al. Potassium channel antibody-associated encephalopathy: a potentially immunotherapy-responsive form of limbic encephalitis. Brain. 2004;127(Pt 3):701–12.

105. Dalmau J, Tuzun E, Wu HY, et al. Paraneoplastic anti-N-methyl-D-aspartate receptor encephalitis associated with ovarian teratoma. Ann Neurol. 2007;61(1):25–36.

106. Iizuka T, Sakai F, Ide T, et al. Anti-NMDA receptor encephalitis in Japan: long-term outcome without tumor removal. Neurology. 2008;70(7):504–11.

107. Coesmans M, Smitt PA, Linden DJ, et al. Mechanisms underlying cerebellar motor deficits due to mGluR1-autoantibodies. Ann Neurol. 2003;53(3):325–36.

108. Maeda A, Maeda T, Ohguro H, Palczewski K, Sato N. Vaccination with recoverin, a cancer-associated retinopathy antigen, induces autoimmune retinal dysfunction and tumor cell regression in mice. Eur J Immunol. 2002;32(8):2300–7.

109. Sommer C, Weishaupt A, Brinkhoff J, et al. Paraneoplastic stiff-person syndrome: passive transfer to rats by means of IgG antibodies to amphiphysin. Lancet. 2005;365(9468):1406–11.

110. Vernino S, Low PA, Fealey RD, Stewart JD, Farrugia G, Lennon VA. Autoantibodies to ganglionic acetylcholine receptors in autoimmune autonomic neuropathies. N Engl J Med. 2000;343(12):847–55.

111. Bernal F, Graus F, Pifarre A, Saiz A, Benyahia B, Ribalta T. Immunohistochemical analysis of anti-Hu-associated paraneoplastic encephalomyelitis. Acta Neuropathol. 2002;103(5):509–15.

112. Blumenthal DT, Salzman KL, Digre KB, Jensen RL, Dunson WA, Dalmau J. Early pathologic findings and long-term improvement in anti-Ma2-associated encephalitis. Neurology. 2006;67(1):146–9.

113. Albert ML, Darnell JC, Bender A, Francisco LM, Bhardwaj N, Darnell RB. Tumor-specific killer cells in paraneoplastic cerebellar degeneration. Nat Med. 1998;4(11):1321–4.

114. Albert ML, Austin LM, Darnell RB. Detection and treatment of activated T cells in the cerebrospinal fluid of patients with paraneoplastic cerebellar degeneration. Ann Neurol. 2000;47(1):9–17.

115. Tanaka K, Tanaka M, Igarashi S, Onodera O, Miyatake T, Tsuji S. Trial to establish an animal model of paraneoplastic cerebellar degeneration with anti-Yo antibody. 2. Passive transfer of murine mononuclear cells activated with recombinant Yo protein to paraneoplastic cerebellar degeneration lymphocytes in severe combined immunodeficiency mice. Clin Neurol Neurosurg. 1995;97(1):101–5.

116. Tanaka M, Tanaka K, Onodera O, Tsuji S. Trial to establish an animal model of paraneoplastic cerebellar degeneration with anti-Yo antibody. 1. Mouse strains bearing different MHC molecules produce antibodies on immunization with recombinant Yo protein, but do not cause Purkinje cell loss. Clin Neurol Neurosurg. 1995;97(1):95–100.

117. Peterson K, Rosenblum MK, Kotanides H, Posner JB. Paraneoplastic cerebellar degeneration. I. A clinical analysis of 55 anti-Yo antibody-positive patients. Neurology. 1992;42(10):1931–7.

118. Hammack JE, Kimmel DW, O'Neill BP, Lennon VA. Paraneoplastic cerebellar degeneration: a clinical comparison of patients with and without Purkinje cell cytoplasmic antibodies. Mayo Clin Proc. 1990;65(11):1423–31.

119. Hammack J, Kotanides H, Rosenblum MK, Posner JB. Paraneoplastic cerebellar degeneration. II. Clinical and immunologic findings in 21 patients with Hodgkin's disease. Neurology. 1992;42(10):1938–43.

120. McHugh JC, Tubridy N, Collins CD, Hutchinson M. Unusual MRI abnormalities in anti-Yo positive "pure" paraneoplastic cerebellar degeneration. J Neurol. 2008;255(1):138–9.

121. Verschuuren J, Chuang L, Rosenblum MK, et al. Inflammatory infiltrates and complete absence of Purkinje cells in anti-Yo-associated paraneoplastic cerebellar degeneration. Acta Neuropathol. 1996;91(5):519–25.

122. Chen YT, Rettig WJ, Yenamandra AK, et al. Cerebellar degeneration-related antigen: a highly conserved neuroectodermal marker mapped to chromosomes X in human and mouse. Proc Natl Acad Sci USA. 1990;87(8):3077–81.

123. Shams'ili S, Grefkens J, de Leeuw B, et al. Paraneoplastic cerebellar degeneration associated with antineuronal antibodies: analysis of 50 patients. Brain. 2003;126(Pt 6):1409–18.

124. Bernal F, Shams'ili S, Rojas I, et al. Anti-Tr antibodies as markers of paraneoplastic cerebellar degeneration and Hodgkin's disease. Neurology. 2003;60(2):230–4.

125. Graus F, Dalmau J, Valldeoriola F, et al. Immunological characterization of a neuronal antibody (anti-Tr) associated with paraneoplastic cerebellar degeneration and Hodgkin's disease. J Neuroimmunol. 1997;74(1–2):55–61.

126. Gultekin SH, Rosenfeld MR, Voltz R, Eichen J, Posner JB, Dalmau J. Paraneoplastic limbic encephalitis: neurological symptoms, immunological findings and tumour association in 50 patients. Brain. 2000;123(Pt 7):1481–94.

127. Dalmau J, Graus F, Villarejo A, et al. Clinical analysis of anti-Ma2-associated encephalitis. Brain. 2004;127(Pt 8):1831–44.

128. Pittock SJ, Lucchinetti CF. Inflammatory transverse myelitis: evolving concepts. Curr Opin Neurol. 2006;19(4):362–8.

129. Fadul CE, Stommel EW, Dragnev KH, Eskey CJ, Dalmau JO. Focal paraneoplastic limbic encephalitis presenting as orgasmic epilepsy. J Neurooncol. 2005;72(2):195–8.

130. Lawn ND, Westmoreland BF, Kiely MJ, Lennon VA, Vernino S. Clinical, magnetic resonance imaging, and electroencephalographic findings in paraneoplastic limbic encephalitis. Mayo Clin Proc. 2003;78(11):1363–8.

131. Yu Z, Kryzer TJ, Griesmann GE, Kim K, Benarroch EE, Lennon VA. CRMP-5 neuronal autoantibody: marker of lung cancer and thymoma-related autoimmunity. Ann Neurol. 2001;49(2):146–54.

132. Rosenfeld MR, Eichen JG, Wade DF, Posner JB, Dalmau J. Molecular and clinical diversity in paraneoplastic immunity to Ma proteins. Ann Neurol. 2001;50(3):339–48.

133. Rudnick E, Khakoo Y, Antunes NL, et al. Opsoclonus-myoclonus-ataxia syndrome in neuroblastoma: clinical outcome and antineuronal antibodies-a report from the Children's Cancer Group Study. Med Pediatr Oncol. 2001;36(6): 612–22.

134. Antunes NL, Khakoo Y, Matthay KK, et al. Antineuronal antibodies in patients with neuroblastoma and paraneoplastic opsoclonus-myoclonus. J Pediatr Hematol Oncol. 2000;22(4):315–20.

135. Connolly AM, Pestronk A, Mehta S, Pranzatelli 3rd MR, Noetzel MJ. Serum autoantibodies in childhood opsoclonus-myoclonus syndrome: an analysis of antigenic targets in neural tissues. J Pediatr. 1997;130(6):878–84.

136. Blaes F, Fuhlhuber V, Korfei M, et al. Surface-binding autoantibodies to cerebellar neurons in opsoclonus syndrome. Ann Neurol. 2005;58(2):313–7.

137. Korfei M, Fuhlhuber V, Schmidt-Woll T, Kaps M, Preissner KT, Blaes F. Functional characterisation of autoantibodies from patients with pediatric opsoclonus-myoclonus-syndrome. J Neuroimmunol. 2005;170(1–2):150–7.

138. Seute T, Leffers P, ten Velde GP, Twijnstra A. Neurologic disorders in 432 consecutive patients with small cell lung carcinoma. Cancer. 2004;100(4):801–6.

139. Tim RM, Massey JM, Sanders DB. Lambert-Eaton Myasthenic Syndrome (LEMS): clinical and electrodiagnostic features and response to therapy in 59 patients. Ann N Y Acad Sci. 1998;84:823–6.

140. Argov Z, Shapira Y, Averbuch-Heller L, Wirguin I. Lambert-Eaton myasthenic syndrome (LEMS) in association with lymphoproliferative disorders. Muscle Nerve. 1995;18(7):715–9.

141. Burns TM, Juel VC, Sanders DB, Phillips II LH. Neuroendocrine lung tumors and disorders of the neuromuscular junction. Neurology. 1999;52(7):1490–1.

142. Wirtz PW, Lang B, Graus F, et al. P/Q-type calcium channel antibodies, Lambert-Eaton myasthenic syndrome and survival in small cell lung cancer. J Neuroimmunol. 2005;164(1–2):161–5.

143. Graus F, Vincent A, Pozo-Rosich P, et al. Anti-glial nuclear antibody: marker of lung cancer-related paraneoplastic neurological syndromes. J Neuroimmunol. 2005;165(1–2):166–71.

144. Keime-Guibert F, Graus F, Broet P, et al. Clinical outcome of patients with anti-Hu-associated encephalomyelitis after treatment of the tumor. Neurology. 1999;53(8):1719–23.

145. Douglas CA, Ellershaw J. Anti-Hu antibodies may indicate a positive response to chemotherapy in paraneoplastic syndrome secondary to small cell lung cancer. Palliat Med. 2003;17(7):638–9.

146. Bataller L, Graus F, Saiz A, Vilchez JJ. Clinical outcome in adult onset idiopathic or paraneoplastic opsoclonus-myoclonus. Brain. 2001;124(Pt 2):437–43.

147. Chalk CH, Murray NM, Newsom-Davis J, O'Neill JH, Spiro SG. Response of the Lambert-Eaton myasthenic syndrome to treatment of associated small-cell lung carcinoma. Neurology. 1990;40(10):1552–6.

148. Lang B, Newsom-Davis J, Prior C, Wray D. Antibodies to motor nerve terminals: an electrophysiological study of a human myasthenic syndrome transferred to mouse. J Physiol. 1983;344(1):335–45.

149. Ertle F, Behnisch W, Al Mulla NA, et al. Treatment of neuroblastoma-related opsoclonus-myoclonus-ataxia syndrome with high-dose dexamethasone pulses. Pediatr Blood Cancer. 2008;50(3):683–7.

150. Russo C, Cohen SL, Petruzzi MJ, de Alarcon PA. Long-term neurologic outcome in children with opsoclonus-myoclonus associated with neuroblastoma: a report from the Pediatric Oncology Group. Med Pediatr Oncol. 1997;28(4):284–8.

151. Yiu VWY, Kovithavongs T, McGonigle LF, Ferreira P. Plasmapheresis as an effective treatment for opsoclonus-myoclonus syndrome. Pediatr Neurol. 2001;24(1):72–4.

152. Pranzatelli MR, Tate ED, Travelstead AL, Longee D. Immunologic and clinical responses to rituximab in a child with opsoclonus-myoclonus syndrome. Pediatrics. 2005;115(1):e115–9.

153. Stark E, Wurster U, Patzold U, Sailer M, Haas J. Immunological and clinical response to immunosuppressive treatment in paraneoplastic cerebellar degeneration. Arch Neurol. 1995;52(8):814–8.

154. David YB, Warner E, Levitan M, Sutton DM, Malkin MG, Dalmau JO. Autoimmune paraneoplastic cerebellar degeneration in ovarian carcinoma patients treated with plasmapheresis and immunoglobulin. A case report. Cancer. 1996;78(10):2153–6.

155. Cocconi G, Ceci G, Juvarra G, et al. Successful treatment of subacute cerebellar degeneration in ovarian carcinoma with plasmapheresis. A case report. Cancer. 1985;56(9):2318–20.

156. Counsell CE, McLeod M, Grant R. Reversal of subacute paraneoplastic cerebellar syndrome with intravenous immunoglobulin. Neurology. 1994;44(6):1184–5.

Infections of the Central Nervous System

Najam Zaidi, Melissa Gaitanis, John N. Gaitanis, Karl Meisel, and Syed A. Rizvi

Keywords: Encephalitis, Meningitis, Brain abscess, Seizures, Progressive multifocal leukoencephalopathy, Neurocysticercosis

Introduction

Infections of the central nervous system (CNS) may be acute (days) or chronic (months to years). The CNS is sequestered from the rest of the body. The blood brain barrier (BBB) excludes most microorganisms and also vital immune cells including phagocytes, antibodies, and complement. Once this barrier is breached, pathogens in the subarachnoid space may grow logarithmically. In this chapter, we discuss the immune response and clinical manifestations of common bacterial, viral, fungal, and parasitic infections of the CNS.

Bacterial Infections

Meningitis

Meningitis is inflammation of the leptomeninges, the tissues surrounding the brain and spinal cord. Bacterial meningitis occurs when bacteria invade the arachnoid mater and the cerebral spinal fluid (CSF) in the subarachnoid space and the cerebral ventricles. Neurological injury results from both the invading organism and the inflammatory response that ensues. Prompt recognition and treatment is required if death and significant morbidity are to be avoided. Approximately 1.2 million cases of bacterial meningitis occur annually worldwide [1]. Bacterial meningitis can be community-acquired or nosocomial. In developed countries, the major causes of community-acquired bacterial meningitis are *Streptococcus pneumoniae* and *Neisseria meningitidis*. Hospital-acquired bacterial meningitis is more likely to be caused by staphylococci and aerobic gram-negative bacilli. Other uncommon causes include Listeria monocytogenes and *Streptococcus agalactiae*.

From: *Clinical Neuroimmunology: Multiple Sclerosis and Related Disorders*, Current Clinical Neurology,
Edited by: S.A. Rizvi and P.K. Coyle, DOI 10.1007/978-1-60327-860-7_14,
© Springer Science+Business Media, LLC 2011

Preventive administration of several different types of vaccines has dramatically reduced the incidence of bacterial meningitis.

Clinical Features

Patients with bacterial meningitis become ill very early in the disease course. The median duration from symptom onset to illness severe enough to warrant inpatient admission and care is only 24 hours [2]. The classic triad of symptoms includes fever, nuchal rigidity, and change in mental status. All patients have at least one of these three symptoms. Headache is common and is described as severe and generalized. Seizures and focal neurologic deficits may also be seen at presentation. Complications include the formation of brain abscesses, hydrocephalus, adrenal insufficiency, and vasculitis.

Treatment

The treatment of acute bacterial meningitis always begins with supportive care. Adequate ventilation and cardiac perfusion must first be assured. Intravenous access needs to be established and the administration of fluids may be required for hypotension. Hypoglycemia and acidosis must be corrected if present. If seizures develop, an anticonvulsant should be initiated. As supportive care is taking place, an empiric treatment regime should be initiated. The initial choice of antibiotics can be modified once cultures and sensitivities have returned. Empiric therapy is based on historical information about the patient. There are three requirements for empiric antibiotic therapy in bacterial meningitis: the choice of medication must be effective against the infecting organism, it must enter the CSF, and the dose should be timed to optimize efficacy based on the pharmacodynamic properties of the antimicrobial [3].

In adults and children with pneumococcal meningitis and children with *H. influenzae*, dexamethasone may be considered as an adjuvant therapy to prevent hearing loss and other neurological sequelae [4].

Mechanisms of Brain Injury

Bacterial meningitis is a life-threatening condition requiring immediate diagnosis and treatment, if brain injury is to be avoided. Even patients with good outcomes suffer significant long-term neuropsychological impairment [5]. Neurological injury results not only from direct invasion by the pathogen but also from the resulting immunologic response.

Invasion into the Central Nervous System: Invasion of the CNS occurs in one of two ways: bacteria colonizing the nasopharynx invade the bloodstream and thus disseminate and seed the CNS or by direct extension through bone. The latter occurs from skull defects caused by trauma or infection, whereas the former happens when bacteria evade the immune system and colonize mucosal spaces. Pneumococci use their polysaccharide capsule to impede phagocytosis and prevent activation of the complement system [6]. Bacteria also evade attack by cleavage of IgA antibodies with proteases [6]. Meningococci colonize the nasopharynx by binding to mucosal CD46 and CD66 proteins [7] and *Streptococcus pneumoniae* binds to polymeric immunoglobulin receptors of epithelial cells [6].

Before entering the CNS, bacteria must first enter the bloodstream from the mucosal spaces. A high level of bacteremia is needed for CNS invasion to occur. Entry into the CNS requires transit across the blood brain barrier (BBB), which is composed of tight junction proteins along capillary endothelial cells that limit the movement of solutes. To cross the BBB, bacteria must either move through the interior of endothelial cells (transcytosis) or between them (paracellular). Transcytosis is a common way for *H. influenzae* and pneumococci to cross the endothelium, whereas meningococci are presumed to enter the CNS in a paracellular fashion [8].

Bacterial Components Contributing to Injury: When bacteria die following antibiotic treatment, the resulting breakdown products act to stimulate cytokines and promote leukocyte migration into the CNS [6]. Higher densities of bacterial compounds result in greater concentrations of inflammatory mediators, and an increased chance of neurological sequelae. Of all the compounds found in bacteria, lipopolysaccharides are perhaps the strongest inducer of inflammation [6]. Bacterial DNA also stimulates genes needed for the immune response and may, therefore, contribute to inflammation [9]. Pneumolysin, a cholesterol-dependent cytolysin found in the cell wall of *Streptococcus pneumoniae* also induces bacterial injury, inflammation, and apoptosis in mammalian cells [10]. It is toxic to endothelial cells and contributes to cell death by causing an influx of extracellular calcium and mitochondrial injury [11, 12].

Role of the Immune System in Neurological Injury: Host defense against bacterial invasion requires recognition of the microbe and activation of the immune system. Such recognition occurs via molecules that are not present in humans and are unique to bacteria, fungi, and viruses. These compounds stimulate the immune system through the activation of toll-like receptors (TLRs) [13]. TLRs are central regulators of the innate immune response. Each subclass of TLRs responds to specific types of compounds. For example, TLR9 is stimulated by short segments of bacterial DNA, which differs from human DNA in that the content of unmethylated cytosine–guanosine (CpG) dinucleotides is 20 times higher in bacteria [14]. TLR4, on the other hand, is activated lipopolysaccharides found in the outer membrane of Gram-negative bacteria (i.e., endotoxin). Pneumolysin also activates TLR4. TLR2 is important in mediating host responses to the cell wall components of Gram-positive bacteria. Mice deficient in TLR2 are more susceptible to infection from *S. pneumoniae* and have reduced bacterial clearance.

Once these unique bacterial compounds bind to TLRs, they activate the myeloid differentiation primary response protein, MyD88 [15]. MyD88 induces inflammatory responses via NF-kappa-B and cytokine activation and is necessary for generating an immune response to bacterial meningitis. Patients with MyD88 deficiency develop recurrent pyogenic bacterial infections [16].

Once activated, microglia and leukocytes release reactive oxygen species and nitrogen intermediates (i.e., nitric oxide). These free radicals are important in host defense and also contribute to neuronal injury. Oxygen- and nitrogen-free radicals promote the formation of peroxynitrite [6], which causes membrane peroxidation, breakdown of protein structure, DNA damage, and ultimately cell death [1, 6]. Reactive oxygen species also promote vasospasm and vasculitis [6].

Strategies to Reduce Inflammation and Improve Neurological Outcome: Since an overly vigorous inflammatory response contributes to neurological injury, strategies for treating meningitis include the use of anti-inflammtory agents. One strategy is to use nonbacteriolytic agents. By reducing bacterial breakdown products, these treatments reduce the proinflammatory response and may, therefore, reduce neuronal damage. Pretreatment with the nonbacteriolytics rifampicin and daptomycin reduce CSF inflammation and resulting brain injury in experimental models [17, 18]. A different approach is to use the anti-inflammatory proteins IL-10 and transforming growth factor (TGF)-1b [19]. These proteins inhibit the production of proinflammatory cytokines and downregulate inflammatory activity within the CNS. Future treatments that selectively interfere with the TLR cascade in a way that reduces inflammation without limiting the ability of the host to kill invading organisms might also be an option in the future [6]. Further studies will be needed to determine the clinical utility of such approaches. One strategy that is better studied is the use of corticosteroids. A recent meta-analysis on the subject reviewed 24 trials that included 4,041 participants [20]. The overall mortality rate was similar in the corticosteroid and placebo groups. Short-term neurological sequelae were reduced in those patients receiving corticosteroids, and a significant reduction was seen in the rate of hearing loss with the use of corticosteroids.

Neuroborreliosis

Lyme disease, caused by the spirochete *Borrelia bugdorfori*, is transmitted by the bite of the *Ixodes scapularis* tick. Endemic to North America, higher rates of disease are usually encountered in the northeast, mid-Atlantic, and northcentral states throughout the year during the non-winter months. Early epidemiologic studies reported 10–15% of patients with untreated Lyme disease developing neurologic manifestations [21, 22].

Early in the disease, a primary erythema migrans (EM) rash (or >1 lesion if dissemination has occurred) may be present. Lesion(s) become apparent an average of 7–14 days after tick exposure. Neurologic symptoms may occur early in the disease, while the EM rash is still present but more typically 1–2 months after the initial infection. Acute Lyme disease can result in inflammation in the peripheral nerves, the meningeal lining, or parenchyma of the brain itself. It can cause acute lymphocytic meningitis, cranial neuritis, radiculitis, encephalomyelitis, pseudotumor cerebri, and cerebellitis.

Late neurologic Lyme disease may present as encephalomyelitis, peripheral neuropathy, or encephalopathy. Encephalomyelitis can be monophasic and slowly progressive, principally involving white matter. Lyme encephalomyelitis may be confused clinically with multiple sclerosis. Late neurologic Lyme disease-associated peripheral neuropathy typically presents as a mild, diffuse, "stocking glove" process. Patients typically complain of intermittent limb paresthesias and pain. The most frequent abnormality found on neurologic examination is reduced vibratory sensation of the distal lower extremities. Electrophysiologic studies may show findings consistent with a mild confluent mononeuritis multiplex [23]. Nerve biopsy reveals small perivascular collections of lymphocytes, without spirochetes.

Mechanism of Injury

Borrelia burgdorferi spirochetes express lipoproteins on the outer membrane of the borrelial cell wall that are proinflammatory. *B. burgdorferi*-specific T cells cross-react with self-antigens, suggesting that molecular mimicry is responsible for autoimmune mechanisms leading to chronic disease manifestation. The spirochete attaches to the endothelial lining of blood vessel walls where it releases inflammatory mediators which recruit leukocytes to the perivascular tissue. Vascular or perivascular inflammation results and impairment of the blood–brain barrier may ensue, allowing penetration of *B. burgdorferi* into the CNS [24].

Neurologic evaluation that may include lumbar puncture should be performed for patients in whom there is a clinical suspicion of neurologic involvement. In early neurologic disease with meningitis or radiculopathy, intravenous antibiotics (ceftriaxone 2 g daily for 4 weeks) are recommended. In early disease with isolated cranial nerve disease (without meningitis), oral antibiotics are recommended (po doxycycline 100 mg BID in adults for 2–4 weeks). Adults or children with late neurologic disease affecting the central or peripheral nervous system should be treated with intravenous therapy [25]. A minority of treated patients may experience fatigue and other vague symptoms for a prolonged period (post-Lyme syndrome).

Syphilis

Syphilis is caused by the bacterium *Treponema pallidum*, a spirochetal organism.

Clinically, syphilis is classified as primary (chancre lesion), secondary (skin rash and mucous membrane lesions), or tertiary (late and latent stages). Despite these classifications, CNS involvement may occur at any of these stages.

Early neurosyphilis affects the CSF, cerebral blood vessels, and meninges. It occurs within weeks to a few years after primary infection, can coexist with primary and secondary syphilis, and may be asymptomatic. Ten to twenty percent of patients with primary syphilis have signs of early involvement of the CNS, with cellular and protein abnormalities in the CSF [26]. Symptomatic forms of early neurosyphilis include meningitis, with or without cranial nerve or eye involvement, and meningovascular disease or stroke [27]. Syphilitic uveitis or other ocular manifestations are associated with neurosyphilis and should be managed and treated according to the recommendations for the treatment of neurosyphilis.

Tertiary lesions are caused by obliterative small vessel endarteritis, which usually involves the vasa vasorum. For purposes of classification most cases of tertiary syphilis are "late" as opposed to "latent." Meningovascular syphilis is a common manifestation of symptomatic neurosyphilis, accounting for 42–61% of cases [28]. Heubner's arteritis in meningovascular syphilis is an inflammatory infiltration of the adventitia of medium to large arteries that causes progressive stenosis. Most often, meningovascular syphilis involves the middle cerebral artery. The vasculopathy may be purely intracranial, or it may be both extracranial and intracranial.

Latent neurosyphilis is a disease beyond the immune tertiary stage and evolves into an organism-laden stage of fulminant anergic necrotizing encephalitis, affecting meninges and brain or spinal cord parenchyma. Latent neurosyphilis is now much less common due to treatment at earlier stages. Clinical presentations may be general paresis (chronic progressive dementia), rapidly progressive dementia with psychotic features, and tabes dorsalis (spinal cord disorder with sensory ataxia and bowel or bladder dysfunction). Its diagnosis is rare in the antibiotic era but may present in those with coexistent human immunodeficiency virus (HIV) infection. In the immunocompetent host, it often occurs years to decades after primary infection. HIV patients tend to be diagnosed with neurosyphilis early in the course of disease, prompting concern for increased risk of neurologic complications in this group of patients [29]. CSF examination should be performed on all HIV patients with a diagnosis of syphilis of unknown duration, late latent syphilis, neurologic signs or symptoms, or suspected treatment failure.

Patients with neurosyphilis are treated with Penicillin G for 10–14 days. Alternate treatments include Procaine penicillin or ceftriaxone [30].

Viral Infections

Encephalitis

The worldwide incidence of viral encephalitis is 3.5–7.4 cases per 100,000 patient years with about 100 possible pathogens. It is suspected that up to 85% of encephalitic cases are from unknown viral pathogens [31]. Therefore, the search for the etiology in a patient presenting with encephalitis is a challenge. It is important to recognize the immunological state of the patient, possible exposures, common viruses, geographical variations, and outbreaks with seasonal patterns. In addition, conditions such as postinfectious encephalitis (acute disseminated encephalomyelitis [ADEM]), vasculitis, collagen vascular disorders, other infectious agents (bacteria, fungal, and parasitic), and paraneoplastic syndromes can present similar to viral encephalitis and need to be considered.

Clinical Features
It is important to distinguish encephalitis from meningitis because it may narrow the differential of possible viral organisms. Encephalitis is a distinct pathologic diagnosis from meningitis. The clinical difference is the constellation of symptoms indicating brain parenchyma inflammation including neurological deficits of motor, speech or sensory function, personality changes, altered mental status, or seizures. Often it may be difficult to distinguish between meningitis and encephalitis, if the patient presents only with confusion. Therefore, some authors suggest reserving meningitis for only those patients who have fever, headache, photophobia, and nuchal rigidity [32]. If a patient exhibits more than meningeal symptoms, it is appropriate to use the term meningoencephalitis as viral infections often involve both the meninges and brain parenchyma.

Diagnosis
The diagnostic evaluation should be guided by the clinical context. An investigation for viral etiologies of encephalitis involves a complete blood count, renal and hepatic function, coagulation studies, chest X-ray, neuroimaging, serum IgM titers, and CSF studies. An MRI of the brain is recommended; however, if unavailable then a CT is necessary. Routine CSF studies of opening pressure, glucose, protein, cell count with differential, and Gram stain is standard practice. A typical viral CSF result would be a mild mononuclear pleocytosis with perhaps an early polymorphonuclear cell component, elevated protein, normal glucose, and possibly RBCs, if there was hemorrhagic development. Additional PCR studies are needed for herpes simplex virus (HSV)-1 and -2, varicella

zoster virus (VZV), Epstein–Barr virus (EBV), West Nile virus (WNV), and enteroviruses. If the patient is immunocompromised, then CSF PCR can be ordered for cytomegalovirus, JC virus, and human herpesvirus 6. CSF may be sent for specific IgM levels for West Nile virus, St. Louis encephalitis virus, and VZV. Serologic testing is performed for HIV, EBV, St. Louis encephalitis virus, Eastern equine encephalitis virus, La Crosse virus, and VZV. Other diagnostic tests to consider would be culture or direct fluorescent antibody (DFA) of skin lesions for HSV and VZV [33].

Immune Response to Viral Infection

The immune response to a virus is initially protective, but if continued may lead to neurological dysfunction. Any resident CNS cell can detect a viral invasion because of pattern recognition receptors (PRR). A TLR is a type of PRR that once activated will induce IFN-α/β, IL-1β, and IL-6 release to prevent viral spread [34]. TLR expression is highest in microglia and astrocytes. The innate immune response of producing IFN-α/β restricts viral tropism, perhaps directly suppressing viral replication, increases antigen presentation, and regulates lymphocyte function [35]. IFN-α/β also induces glial activation which effects the blood brain barrier (BBB) and proinflammatory cytokines (IL-6). Matrix metalloproteinases (MMP) are released and function to remodel the extracellular matrix and BBB breakdown allowing T-cell entry to the CNS [36]. Astrocytes release chemokines, such as CCL5, that allow virus-specific T cells to assist in the response to viral infection. The viral-specific response of the adaptive immune system is crucial to repelling the infection. The activity of the T cells is dependent on the ability of major histocompatibility complex (MHCII) antigen recognition, which is expressed on microglia. However, if chemokines persist with a prolonged infection, the subsequent macrophage recruitment may lead to increased demyelination and neurological deficits [36]. The ultimate outcome is dependent on viral dose versus the innate and adaptive immune systems ability to control and clear the infection without destructive consequences.

Herpes Simplex Virus

The most common viral agent causing sporadic encephalitis in an immuno-competent patient is herpes simplex virus-1 (HSV-1). HSV-1 can occur at any age, but HSV-2 is more often seen in neonates due to transmission during delivery. HSV-1 may cause infection through an invasion of trigeminal or olfactory routes, viremia, or reactivation. The onset of encephalitis is acute progressing over several days. Symptoms of personality change, anomia, and memory loss can occur but are not sensitive clinical signs. To establish the diagnosis, CSF is obtained for PCR testing (96–98% sensitive and 95–99% specific) [33]. False-negative PCR results can occur within the first 72 h of illness. Treatment does not lead to false negatives in the first few days, but most patients will be PCR negative after 14 days of therapy [37]. In 90% of PCR positive HSV, MRI will show focal edema in the medial temporal lobes, orbital surfaces, insular cortex, cingulate gyrus, and occasionally hemorrhage [38]. However, MRI findings are not specific enough to diagnose HSV and may be a late finding. The Infectious Disease Society of America recommends starting empirical treatment of children and adults suspected of meningoencephalitis with acyclovir 10 mg/kg IV every 8 h, neonates are dosed 20 mg/kg IV every 8 h [33]. Despite therapy, there is still a high morbidity and mortality (28% at 18 months). Poor predictors of outcome are age greater than 30, Glasgow coma score less than six, and symptoms 4 days prior to starting therapy [39].

West Nile Virus

West Nile virus (WNV) is a new seasonal arbovirus to the western hemisphere first appearing in 1999. During 2002–2003, an epidemic of WNV meningoencephalitis occurred. In 2009, a total of 720 cases were reported, 54% had nervous system involvement. WNV is now the leading arboviral cause of encephalitis [40]. The virus vector is the Culex mosquito and birds serve as the reservoir. Most (89%) of people develop an asymptomatic infection that is only found with screening blood bank donations [41]. Only about 1 in 150 people infected develop the neuroinvasive disease, which include meningitis, encephalitis, and acute flaccid paralysis [42]. Patients typically develop fever, headache, fatigue, and less commonly a generalized maculopapular rash. Cranial nerves may be involved in, as many as 10–20% of cases, most commonly the ophthalmic or facial nerve [41, 42]. Initial CSF results are typical of viral meningitis mentioned above. The diagnosis is found by CSF IgM antibodies using ELISA with confirmatory titer comparisons because of cross-reacting antibodies to yellow fever and Japanese encephalitis. False-negative testing is possible early and clinical suspicion should prompt repeat testing in 3 days [41]. MRI of the brain is abnormal in 50% of patients with the thalamus, basal ganglia, and upper brainstem typically demonstrating hyperintensities on T2 and FLAIR sequences [42]. There is no approved therapy for WNV except supportive management; however, promising results were seen in a small group of patients treated with IVIG (intravenous immune gammaglobin) [43]. A larger randomized placebo-controlled trial of IVIG is completed, but results are not yet published. Additional therapies involving humanized monoclonal antibody and interferon-γ are undergoing trials [42]. WNV encephalitis has a 20% mortality rate and about 50% experience residual cognitive difficulties. Other post-infectious complications of WNV may include tremors, myoclonus, and parkinsonism [41].

Enterovirus

Other common causes of seasonal meningioencephalitis include enteroviruses (e.g., coxsackie and echovirus). Enteroviruses are often included in the term aseptic meningitis that refers to meningeal inflammation without evidence of bacterial infection. About 90% of viral meningitis is caused by enteroviruses, especially in children and in the summer to fall months. Humans are the only natural reservoir and it is transmitted by the fecal-oral route or less frequently in respiratory secretions. The virus crosses the gut wall and travels to lymphoid tissue where replication occurs leading to viremia. Mononuclear cells that cross the choroid plexus lead to meningoencephalitis [44]. The common clinical presentation is the meningeal pattern described above. However, patients may present with seizures and those who are immunocompromised by congenital hypo or agammaglobulinemia are unable to clear the infection and may develop meningioencephalitis [45]. Enterovirus 71 outbreaks in immunocompetent children have caused a rhomboencephalitis (myoclonus, tremors, ataxia, and cranial nerve deficits) [43]. Other symptoms may include respiratory symptoms, diarrhea and rash. CSF studies are consistent with viral meningitis and PCR testing will yield the diagnosis. The MRI pattern with enterovirus 71 infection demonstrates hyperintense T2/FLAIR brainstem lesions [43]. Treatment is generally supportive with fluid and electrolyte management. However, patients who are immunocompromised or are suffering from chronic/severe infection, IVIG may be used [33, 45, 46].

Varicella Zoster Virus

VZV is a common viral infection of the nervous system with an incidence of three to five cases per 1,000 people per year [32]. A reactive CSF pleocytosis can occur in 40–50% of cases, with a lesser number of immunocompetent patients developing clinical signs of meningitis. An epidemiological study conducted in Finland found that VZV accounted for 8% of the aseptic meningitis cases and 12% of the encephalitis cases [46]. VZV is initially contracted through respiratory aerosol in the winter and spring months and manifests as chickenpox. The virus may then migrate to the sensory nerve ganglion and becomes latent. Reactivation of the virus results in herpes zoster. This reemergence usually occurs later in life, likely due to waning immunity and is associated with other immunocompromised states. The infection may initially manifest as itching or burning sensation in a dermatome that days later exhibits a vesicular skin eruptions. Pain in this area may last for weeks but can continue for months to years. Other complications are cranial nerve herpetic lesions that may involve the first division of the trigeminal nerve (ophthalmic herpes), the facial nerve (Ramsay Hunt syndrome), or the vagus and glossopharyngeal nerves (herpes occipitocollaris). In children, VZV may present as a cerebellar ataxia. Occasionally, seizures and delirium are also associated with herpes zoster. However, the most concerning complication is a delayed granulomatous arteritis that can lead to infarction and focal neurologic deficits such as hemiparesis. CSF PCR for VZV (80–95% sensitive, more than 95% specific) and IgM antibody can help make the diagnosis. An MRA of the brain may show arteritis. The MRI can reveal ischemic or hemorrhagic infarcts, demyelinating lesions, and enhancement around the ventricles. The recommended treatment of VZV infection is acyclovir. Less evidence supports using ganciclovir and adjunctive corticosteroids, but they remain possible treatment options [33].

JC Virus

Similar to VZV encephalitis, which is due to reactivation of a latent infection, the JC virus is also opportunistic. Almost 80% of adults are seropositive for the JC virus. After the primary infection, the virus becomes latent in the kidney, bone marrow, and lymphoid organs [47]. The JC virus is reactivated during immunodeficient states such as AIDS, hematologic malignancies, and immunomodulating therapies. The virus migrates from the bloodstream to infect the CNS and cause oligodendrocyte lysis with resulting demyelination [48]. This demyelinating disease is called progressive multifocal leukoencephalopathy (PML) and before combination anti-retroviral therapy (CART) was associated with 90% mortality in 1 year [48]. Since CART therapy has become routine, the incidence and mortality of PML has fallen significantly. This improvement is likely attributable to CART preventing patients' CD4 counts from falling below 200/mm³, which is associated with a 50-fold increased incidence of PML [48]. Immunotherapy with rituximab and natalizumab has also caused PML. These therapeutic agents are monoclonal antibodies, rituximab targets B cells, and natalizumab inhibits leukocyte migration. Natalizumab was marketed for the treatment of relapsing remitting multiple sclerosis and in post-marketing surveillance was associated with an increased incidence of PML. The risk of developing PML is 1 in 1,000 for patients on therapy for 18 months [49]. Patient with PML exhibit coordination disturbance, cognitive deficits, vision loss, and paresis [33, 49]. The JC virus is detected by CSF PCR (50–75% sensitive and 98–100% specific). MRI of the brain shows confluent nonenhancing white matter lesions. The treatment is to stop immunosuppressant medications and if the patient has HIV/AIDS to begin CART [33].

Human Immunodeficiency Virus

HIV is a worldwide pandemic that affects about one million people in the USA and around 40 million worldwide. The number of people infected is increasing among women, ethnic minorities, people over 50 years old [50]. The neurologic manifestations of HIV are diverse and include AIDS dementia complex, acute HIV-related encephalitis, cerebrovascular disorders, vacuolar myelopathy, aseptic meningitis, acute, and chronic inflammatory HIV polyneuritis, mononeuritis multiplex, and sensorimotor demyelinating polyneuropathy. In addition to the direct effects of HIV, the eventual loss of immune system integrity in AIDS leads to opportunistic neurologic diseases such as cytomegalovirus, varicella zoster virus, herpes virus, toxoplasmosis, crytococcus, neurosyphilis, PML, and primary CNS lymphoma [32]. With the highly effective combination antiretroviral therapy, HIV has turned from a uniformly fatal disease to a chronic disease. Therefore, the prevalence of opportunistic disease has decreased and the neurocognitive consequences of prolonged HIV are now more appreciated.

HIV is an RNA retrovirus in the category of lentiviruses. Lentiviruses have neurotropism and neurovirulence. HIV uses CXCR4, CD4, and CCR5 receptors to enter macrophage cells that cross the BBB. The pathological effect of this infection is white matter pallor, microglial nodules, multinucleated giant cells, gliosis, neuronal loss, damage to dendrites, and synapses [51]. The greatest viral burden is in the basal ganglia, subcortical white matter, and frontal cortex. As one might predict the synaptic loss may lead to disabling dementia that clinically manifests as distractability, ataxia, dysdiadochokinesia, hyperreflexia, spasticity, and the inability to learn new information [52]. The prevalence of HIV-associated dementia has declined with CART, but shifted the burden to milder cases of neuropsychologically impairment and minor cognitive motor disorder. MRI of the brain shows cerebral atrophy with ventricular enlargement and FLAIR patchy hyperintensities in the white matter which spares the U fibers [52]. The diagnosis of HIV is based on serum testing of ELISA and confirmatory western blot test. Treatment with CART consists of three or four drugs including a reverse transcriptase inhibitors (e.g., lamivudine) and protease inhibitors (e.g., indinavir). Further investigation is required to clarify the extent of BBB penetration of CART, and methods to increase concentration of the drugs in the CNS by blocking efflux transporters. The ultimate goal is to help improve the functional outcomes of patients who suffer from chronic HIV infection.

Fungal and Parasitic Infections

Fungal and parasitic infections of the CNS are relatively rare and may occur in the setting of diminished or suppressed immunity and/or unusual exposure. Susceptibility to an infection and morbidity is related to both the pathogen's virulence and tissue tropism as well as the host genetic variability and the breakdown of natural defense mechanisms. The sequestered yet vulnerable tissues of the CNS and protective meninges may be exposed to pathogens via several routes including as follows. (1) Contiguous spread from structures such as the inner ear, mastoid cells, or sinuses or rarely via dental infections. (2) Hematogenous spread-original site of exposure/infection for most fungi are lungs after inhalation of spores. (3) Traumatic infections may be accidental-by skull fractures or iatrogenic by surgery or insertion of devices such as shunts. (4) Intracellular transport (axonal transmission) is usually rare and more often used by viruses such as the Rabies virus.

Mechanism of Injury

Fungi and parasites such as any other invading microorganism infect the host after a continuum of interactions with the host's defense mechanisms. They initially breech nonspecific natural barriers such as the respiratory mucus membranes or less often the skin and may be further impeded by antimicrobial peptides or proteins produced by glands in these barriers. The innate immune system is the second line of defense and its pattern recognition receptors (PRRs), toll-like receptors (TLRs) bind to specific structural motifs common to fungi and parasites and trigger immune mediators, such as cytokines and chemokines. An example is zymosan, a yeast cell wall component [53]. Its major polysaccharide constituents: Beta-glucan and mannan are the main ligands for the extracellular domain of TLR-2. This reaction triggers a chain of signal transduction, via a complex cascade of adapter molecules and kinases culminating in the induction of nuclear factor kappa B transcription factor (NF-kB)-dependent gene expression and the induction of proinflammatory cytokines. Three of the major proinflammatory cytokines, IL-1, TNF-α, and IL-6, are induced through similar signaling mechanisms. This initial innate inflammatory response thus provoked has an essential role in focusing and directing the final interaction of the host with the invading organism – the adaptive immune response which confers microbial-specific long-lasting immune memory.

Skin, a natural barrier to infection may lose natural defenses in atopy, dryness, or malnutrition leading to colonization and invasion. Natural barriers such as mucus membranes and skin may be weakened by stress and malnutrition. Altering symbiotic normal microflora, such as with broad-spectrum antibiotics, can lead to overgrowth and superinfection with ordinarily commensals such as *Candida albicans*.

Other forms of immunity can be perturbed by infections such as T-cell depletion in HIV, but by far the most common etiology of immune suppression is

Table 14.1 Opportunistic fungal pathogens and possible mechanisms of immune dysfunction.

Immune compromise	Examples	Mechanism of decreased immunity	Opportunistic pathogens
Disruption of barriers function	Burns	Loss of beta-defensins with antifungal properties	Candidal colonization and infections
	Chemotherapy-induced ulcers		
	Intravenous catheters surgery	Replacement of normal flora	
	Use of antibiotics		
Neutropenia or neutrophil dysfunction	Solid organ or bone marrow transplant recipient	Immunosuppression	Invasive aspergillosis and zygomyces
	Chronic granulomatous disease, leukocyte adhesion deficiency		Candidal infection
	Diabetes and hyperglycemia		
	Adrenal corticosteroids		
Interferon γ/IL-12 pathway defects	Tumor necrosis factor-α (TNF-α) inhibitors or other anti-interleukin biological modulators	Monocyte dysfunction	*H. capsulatum, C. immitis*
		Phagocyte dysfunction	
Lymphocyte (T cell) deficiency	Severe combined immunodeficiency, acquired immunodeficiency syndrome (AIDS)	CD4 T (helper/suppressor) lymphocyte deficiency	*Pneumocystis (carinii) jirovecii, Cryptococcus neoformans*

iatrogenic. Surgery, modern medical technologies and devices, and antibiotics all play a role in the breakdown of natural barriers to infection. Immune modulating drugs, steroids, and biologic agents such as anti-TNF agents may produce breakdown of the innate and adaptive immune responses (Tables 14.1 and 14.2).

Clinical Features of Fungal Infection

Pathogenic fungi studied under medical mycology may be yeasts or molds or dimorphic. Infections caused by molds in tissues are rare and typically occur in the severely immunocompromised [54]. These are aggressive filamentous growths that are angioinvasive and through infarction and obstruction of blood vessels produce necrotizing disease. CNS infections by yeasts present typically as chronic meningitis or abscesses. *Cryptococcus* and *Candida* are monomorphic and exist only as yeasts. Other pathogenic fungi are dimorphic existing as molds in the environment.

Most fungi enter the body inhaled as spores and the lungs are typically infected first. CNS infection is generally secondary after hematogenous spread. Hematogenous seeding of infection in the CNS is hampered by an intact blood–brain barrier. Beyond this barrier, local opsonization is deficient and organisms may escape efficient phagocytosis in the brain parenchyma. Infection once established may thus be inadequately controlled by immune defenses.

Cryptococcal meningitis, the most common of these infections, presents as a chronic meningitis [55]. The enzyme phenoloxidase is a virulence factor in this fungus and not only protects against oxidants in phagocytes but is also responsible for the characteristic melanin production on culture plates using dopamine as substrate [56]. The tropism of Cryptococci for the brain may be explained by the presence of this enzyme.

Table 14.2 Typical fungal pathogens and disease.

Mycoses	Epidemiology	Clinical presentation and pathophysiology	Host factors
Cryptococcus neoformans	Monomorphic yeast associated with	Mild respiratory illness and self-limited infection in the normal host	Chronic meningitis is the primary systemic manifestation in typically immunocompromised host
	Bird or pigeon dropping. Ubiquitous presence	Fungus is CNS tropic as its virulence factor phenoloxidase uses dopamine as substrate	AIDS defining illness with CD4 counts <100
Histoplasma capsulatum	North and Latin America, Ohio, Mississippi rivers	Systemic infection may manifest as chronic granulomatous meningitis	Severe fulminant disease in immune compromised and AIDS
	Caribbean, Africa		Predilection for HIV
	Moist soil near river		Rate is 2–5% in HIV patients and up to 25% in high endemic areas in patients with low CD4 counts
	Bat, caves, and birds		
Coccidioides immitis	Dry sand-deserts American SW; Arizona, CA, NM, Mex	Eosinophilic meningitis. Estradiol binding proteins on surface. Meningitis common if systemic spread with facial involvement	May affect immune-competent. This pathogen virulent to women and in pregnancy. Severe disease in dark skinned races and Asians of Filipino descent
	Central/S America		
Blastomycosis	Moist soil near river beds-similar to Histoplasmosis area but includes Canada	Rare infection; usually associated microabscesses not typical meningitis	Juvenile and adult males affected usually with intact immunity
	South, SE, SC Mississippi, Ohio Rivers AND the great Lakes and St. Lawrence River		
Paracoccidioides brasiliensis	SC America	Estradiol inhibits conversion of mycelial to yeast form and adult females are thus somewhat protected	Juvenile and adult males affected usually with intact immunity
	Brazil>Columbia>Venezuela		
Penicillium marneffei	Presumptive soil organism. South East Asia, Southern China	Rare in immunocompetent	Predilection in HIV
		Brain infection is rare	Opportunistic infection (OI) in HIV CD4<100
			4th common OI in Thailand in HIV
Candidiasis	Ubiquitous yeast which is a part of normal body flora	Fungal brain abscesses, microabscesses, and rarely acute meningitis	Underweight premature neonates, catheter-related infection, postneurosurgery or hyperglycemia. Parenteral nutrition
Sporothrix schenckii (rare)	Soil organism, inoculation by skin prick	Fungal brain abscesses very rare	Alcoholism
		Initial infection is the skin after transcutaneous inoculation	DM
			Anti-TNF therapy

(continued)

Table 14.2 (continued)

Mycoses	Epidemiology	Clinical presentation and pathophysiology	Host factors
Mucormycosis (zygomycosis)	Ubiquitous environmental molds	Invasive fulminant infection – angioinvasive and typically produce hemorrhage and space occupying destructive lesions	Diabetes mellitus with acidosis, acidemia from profound systemic illnesses (sepsis, severe dehydration, severe diarrhea, and chronic renal failure), hematologic neoplasms, renal transplantation, injection drug use, and deferoxamine
			Less than 5% of hosts are normal
Molds (rare): Scedosporium, Aspergillus, Cladophialophora and other dark-walled molds	Ubiquitous environmental fungi	Locally invasive disease or angioinvasion with hemorrhagic infarction, chronic meningitis is rare	Usually in severely immunocompromised
			Hematogenous dissemination from a pulmonary route, by the way of an intravenous catheter or by direct extension from infected sinuses

In the immunocompetent host, there is an indolent onset of symptoms for at least 4 weeks and have signs of chronic inflammation in the cerebrospinal fluid. These symptoms may wax and wane over weeks and months. While there may be systemic features of illness such as fevers or rashes, often patients are afebrile with a normal physical examination. Nonspecific neurologic signs may be the most frequent abnormality, with decreased recent and remote memory, confusion, apathy, papilledema, and cranial nerve palsies, particularly sixth nerve palsy. Skin lesions if present may help with diagnosis by biopsy.

CNS abscesses may cause local symptoms such as pressure effects and focal neurological deficits. These are typically seen in patients dying of systemic candidiasis which rarely also produces meningitis. When a brain abscess ruptures into the ventricular system, a rapidly progressive purulent meningitis results with a strong tendency to obstruct the aqueduct of Sylvius, accelerating the progression to coma. Cerebral edema occurs more often with more invasive disease and late stage large abscesses.

Patients with aspergillosis and mucormycosis in the CNS most commonly present with angioinvasion and hemorrhagic infarction, not chronic meningitis [57]. Dark-walled molds have a predisposition for spread to the brain, causing a brain abscess, meningitis, or both.

Clinical Features of Parasitic Infections

Parasites that infect the CNS can be separated into two broad categories: natural CNS parasites and opportunistic CNS parasites. Natural CNS parasites can infiltrate and infect the CNS of a healthy individual. This usually involves the targeted attacking of the blood–brain barrier's endothelial cells to access CNS tissue. On the other hand, opportunistic CNS parasites do not characteristically infect the CNS except in immunocompromised patients; this is usually due to the body's inability to effectively resolve inflammation of the BBB's endothelial cells, which increases the permeability of the barrier and allows larger molecules and parasites to enter the CNS capillaries from the bloodstream. CNS infections are much more common in the immunocompromised host.

Parasites and helminths generally cause eosinophilic meningitis. *Angiostrongylus cantonensis* is the most common parasitic cause of eosinophilic meningitis outside Europe and North America [58]. Cysticercosis and hydtid cause space occupying lesions in the brain [59, 60].

Naegleria fowleri, is the main protozoan causing *Primary Amebic Meningoencephalitis* (PAM) in humans and has been recovered in soil and collections of fresh water from puddles to lakes [61]. The amoeba produces enzymes which have a highly cytopathic effects on the host's cells, and this likely not only contributes to the virulence but also its ability to successfully infiltrate the host by damaging impeding cells. PAM occurs in two forms. The acute form is usually indistinguishable from acute bacterial meningitis with an incubation period, 3–8 days followed by sudden onset of high fever, photophobia, bifrontal or bitemporal headache, nuchal rigidity, and progression to stupor or coma. Death in untreated patients generally occurs within 2–3 days from the onset of symptoms. The subacute or chronic form of PAM is manifested more insidiously by low-grade fever, headache, and focal signs (e.g., hemiparesis, aphasia, cranial nerve palsies, visual-field disturbances, diplopia, ataxia, and seizures). Deterioration occurs over a period of 2–4 weeks until death. Longer durations of illness have also been reported (range, 5–18 months).

Most infections by *Toxoplasma gondii* are asymptomatic, but the risk of CNS infection is increased drastically in immunocompromised patients, young children, and cases of congenital transmissions. Pathogenic infection by this opportunistic CNS parasite can cause encephalitis and other neurological syndromes [62]. One of the more common causes of pathogenic infection is the reactivation of a latent infection as a result of the immunosuppressant effect of AIDS in comorbid patients. The lack of antibodies in the brain due to the blood–brain barrier makes it more likely for cysts in the CNS to have persisted and not be cleared as the protozoa in other tissues might have been. As a result, a strong reinfection in an immunocompromised state is often centralized in the CNS and can lead to the severe pathogenesis associated with toxoplasmosis.

The development and persistence of living fluid-cysts of *Taenia solium* within the CNS is known as active *neurocystercosis* and is the most common parasitic CNS infection worldwide [63]. Once formed into cysts within the CNS, the metacestodes are significantly more shielded from the immune response than when in their egg or larval stages. Neurocysticercosis behaves as a space occupying lesion in the brain and occasionally can cause meningitis. It is also one of the most common causes of seizures in the world [64].

Cerebral malaria is an encephalopathy associated with infection by *Plasmodium falciparum*. Is most often characterized by unarousable coma and high risk of death if left untreated. Cognitive deficits may persist even after adequate treatment [65]. Only *P. falciparum* is currently thought to cause cerebral malaria; though rare cases of unarousable coma have been associated with infections of *P. malariae* and *P. vivax*, it is suspected that coinfection by *P. falciparum* was present. The mechanical sequestration of erythrocytes in cerebral capillaries was once thought to be the primary cause of cerebral malaria, but recent studies have suggested an alternative mechanism involving the host inflammatory response [66]. It is now believed that schizonts bind to endothelial cells and subsequently rupture, releasing toxins that are thought to be responsible for malarial paroxysm. However, the released toxins also upregulate TNF production in leukocytes, which stimulates increased expression of intercellular adhesion molecule-1 (ICAM-1) and possibly the cytoadherence receptor E-selectin. Additional parasitized cells can subsequently adhere to endothelium more readily, obstructing small vessels, and causing pathology through a purely mechanical mechanism.

Diagnosis

While *Candida albicans* is ubiquitous and disease usually signifies immune barrier breach a history of travel and exposure may be helpful in the diagnosis of certain other fungal and parasitic infections. Coccidioidomycosis, common to southwestern USA or northern Mexico, is rare in people who have never been there. Histoplasmosis is common in the Midwest USA and rarer in the Pacific Northwest and Rocky Mountain states. Neurocysticercosis occurs mostly residents of endemic countries. AIDS and corticosteroid therapy are major predisposing factors to cryptococcal infection.

Hilar lymphadenopathy on chest radiographs is seen with *Histoplasma capsulatum* and *Coccicoides immitis*. Cavitary lesions may be present in blastomyces and paracoccidioides. MRI is the preferred test for imaging the brain and may show intracranial mass lesions, hydrocephalus, or parameningeal foci. Flattening of the sulci over the cerebral convexities may indicate increased intracranial pressure. Increased width of the optic sheath may indicate papilledema or cerebral edema. Granulomas may be seen within the brain in cryptococcal or Histoplasma meningitis.

CSF opening pressure is generally elevated >120 mm. Glucose may be very low and sometimes profound hypoglycorrhachia can occur in cryptococcal meningitis. Glucose values are generally inversely related to protein levels and cell count. There is lymphocytic pleocytosis, although cell count and cell type are variable. Eosinophilic meningitis is defined as the presence of 10 eosinophils/μL in CSF or at least 10% eosinophils in the total CSF leukocyte count. High-grade peripheral eosinophilia is common in parasitic diseases. Culture on standard media is usually possible from CSF for most yeast. Acanthamoeba can also be cultured on special media.

Specific tests such as cryptococcal antigen test, complement fixation antibody to coccidioides species, urine histoplasma antigen, and aspergillus galactomannan are useful for earlier diagnosis. Serological test are also available for cysticercosis and other parasitic infections.

Treatment

Detailed discussion of treatment of fungal and parasitic infections is beyond the scope of this book. In general, antifungal treatment for CNS fungal infections typically requires a prolonged period, often several months to years; thus, it is imperative to define the etiological agent and treat accordingly. If noninvasive methods of diagnosis are unsuccessful, the risks and benefits of brain biopsy should be weighed against the advantages of empiric antifungal treatment. Specific agents commonly used are amphotericin B, flucytosine, and azole derivatives. Rifampicin given with amphotericin B potentiates the activity. Surgical therapy for abscess, hydrocephalus, or parameningeal foci may be indicated. Spinal decompression may be required at times. Intraventricular chemotherapy through ommaya reservoir may be tried.

Treatment of CNS parasitic infections may involve the use of anti-helminthes. The use of anti-parasitic agents in the treatment of neurocysticercosis remains controversial [67]. Surgery may be required in cases involving brain mass lesions (cysticercosis and hydatid cyst). Occasionally, corticosteroids are used to reduce an acute inflammatory response to the dying cysticerci.

Conclusion

Fungal and parasitic infections of the CNS occur due to uncommon exposure or immune suppression. Current era of exotic travel, cuisine and ecotourism, and iatrogenic immune modulation by novel biological agents is producing new avenues of interaction between the various innate and adaptive immune barriers and a variety of potential pathogens. Early diagnosis and aggressive treatment can prevent substantial morbidity and mortality associated with these infections.

References

1. Scheld WM, Koedel U, Nathan B, Pfister HW. Pathophysiology of bacterial meningitis: mechanism(s) of neuronal injury. J Infect Dis. 2002;186 Suppl 2:S225–33.
2. De Gans J, van de Beek D. Dexamethasone in adults with bacterial meningitis. N Engl J Med. 2002;347(20):1549–56.

3. Sinner SW, Tunkel AR. Antimicrobial agents in the treatment of bacterial meningitis. Infect Dis Clin North Am. 2004;18:581.

4. Tunkel AR, Hartman BJ, Kaplan SL, et al. Practice guidelines for the management of bacterial meningitis. Clin Infect Dis. 2004;39:1267.

5. Schmidt H, Heimann B, Djukic M, et al. Neuropsychological sequelae of bacterial and viral meningitis. Brain. 2006;129:333–45.

6. Gerber J, Nau R. Mechanisms of injury in bacterial meningitis. Curr Opin Neurol. 2010;23:312–8.

7. Rosenstein NE, Perkins BA, Stephens DS, et al. Meningococcal disease. N Engl J Med. 2001;344:1378–88.

8. Join-Lambert O, Morand PC, Carbonnelle E, et al. Mechanisms of meningeal invasion by a bacterial extracellular pathogen, the example of Neisseria meningitidis. Prog Neurobiol. 2010;91(2):130–9.

9. Klaschik S, Tross D, Shirota H, Klinman DM. Short- and long-term changes in gene expression mediated by the activation of TLR9. Mol Immunol. 2010;47:1317–24.

10. Srivastava A, Henneke P, Visintin A, Morse SC, et al. The apoptotic response to pneumolysin is Toll-like receptor 4 Dependent and protects against pneumococcal disease. Infect Immun. 2005;73:6479–87.

11. Stringaris AK, Geisenhainer J, Bergmann F, et al. Neurotoxicity of pneumolysin, a major pneumococcal virulence factor, involves calcium influx and depends on activation of p38 mitogen-activated protein kinase. Neurobiol Dis. 2002;11:355–68.

12. Braun JS, Hoffmann O, Schickhaus M, et al. Pneumolysin causes neuronal cell death through mitochondrial damage. Infect Immun. 2007;75:4245–54.

13. Akira S, Sato S. Toll-like receptors and their signaling mechanisms. Scand J Infect Dis. 2003;35:555–62.

14. Krieg AM, Yi AK, Matson S, Waldschmidt TJ, Bishop GA, Teasdale R, et al. CpG motifs in bacterial DNA trigger direct B-cell activation. Nature. 1995;374:546–9.

15. Underhill DM. Toll-like receptors: networking for success. Eur J Immunol. 2003;33:1767–75.

16. von Bernuth H, Picard C, Jin C, Pankla R, et al. Pygenic bacterial infections in humans with MyD88 deficiency. Science. 2008;321:691–6.

17. Grandgirard D, Schurch C, Cottagnoud P, et al. Prevention of brain injury by the nonbacteriolytic antibiotic daptomycin in experimental pneumococcal meningitis. Antimicrob Agents Chemother. 2007;51:2173–8.

18. Spreer A, Lugert R, Stoltefaut V, et al. Short-term rifampicin pretreatment reduces inflammation and neuronal cell death in a rabbit model of bacterial meningitis. Crit Care Med. 2009;37:2253–8.

19. Kornelisse RF, Savelkoul HFJ, Mulder PHG, et al. Interleukin-10 and soluble tumor necrosis factor receptors in cerebrospinal fluid of children with bacterial meningitis. J Infect Dis. 1996;173:1498–502.

20. Brouwer MC, McIntyre P, de Gans J, Prasad K, van de Beek D. Corticosteroids for acute bacterial meningitis. Cochrane Database Syst Rev. 2010;(9):CD004405.

21. Steere AC. Lyme disease. N Engl J Med. 1989;321:586–96.

22. Reik L, Steere AC, Bartenhagen NH, Shope RE, Malawista SE. Neurologic abnormalities of Lyme disease. Medicine. 1979;58:281–94.

23. Halperin J, Luft BJ, Volkman DJ, Dattwyler RJ. Lyme neuroborreliosis: peripheral nervous system manifestations. Brain. 1990;113:1207–21.

24. Garcia-Monco JC, Fernandez Villar B, et al. Lyme borreliosis: neurologic manifestations. Neurologia. 1990;5(9):315–22.

25. Wormser GP et al. The clinical assessment, treatment, and prevention of lyme disease, human granulocytic anaplasmosis, and babesiosis: clinical practice guidelines by the Infectious Diseases Society of America. Clin Infect Dis. 2006;43(9):1089–134.

26. Wile UJ, Hasley CK. Involvement of nervous system during primary stage of syphilis. JAMA. 1921;76:8–9.

27. Golden M et al. Update on syphilis. JAMA. 2003;290(11):1510–4.

28. Burke JM, Schaberg DR. Neurosyphilis in the antibiotic era. Neurology. 1985;35:1368–71.

29. Flood JM, Weinstock HS, Guroy ME, Bayne L, Simon RP, Bolan G. Neurosyphilis during the AIDS epidemic, San Francisco, 1985–1992. J Infect Dis. 1998;177:931–40.

30. Workowski K, Berman S, Centers for Disease Control and Prevention (CDC). Sexually transmitted diseases treatment guidelines, 2010. MMWR Recomm Rep. 2010;59(RR12):1–110.

31. Granerod J, Tam CC, Crowcroft NS, et al. Challenge of the unknown. A systematic review of acute encephalitis in non-outbreak situations. Neurology. 2010; 75(10):924–32.

32. Ropper AH, Brown RH. Viral infections of the nervous system, chronic meningitis, and prion diseases. Adam and Victor's principles of neurology. 8th ed. New York: McGraw-Hill; 2005. p. 636–43.

33. Tunkel AR, Glaser CA, Bloch KC, et al. The management of encephalitis: clinical practice guidelines by the Infectious Disease Society of America. Clin Infect Dis. 2008;47:303–27.

34. Kawai T, Akira S. Antiviral signaling through pattern recognition receptors. J Biochem. 2007;141(2):137–45.

35. Thompson JM, Iwasaki A. Toll-like receptors regulation of viral infection and disease. Adv Drug Deliv Rev. 2008;60(7):786–94.

36. Savarin C, Bergmann CC. Neuroimmunology of central nervous system viral infections: the cells, molecules, and mechanisms involved. Curr Opin Pharmacol. 2008;8:472–9.

37. Tyler KL. Update on herpes simplex encephalitis. Rev Neurol Dis. 2004;1(4):169–78.

38. Domingues RB, Fink MC, Tsanaclis AMC, et al. Diagnosis of herpes simplex encephalitis by magnetic resonance imaging and polymerase chain reaction assay of cerebrospinal fluid. J Neruol Sci. 1998;157:148–53.

39. Taira N, Kamei S, Morita A, et al. Predictors of a prolonged clinical course in adult patients with herpes simplex virus encephalitis. Inter Med. 2009;48:89–94.

40. Centers for Disease Control and Prevention. West Nile virus activity – United States, 2009. MMWR Morb Mortal Wkly Rep. 2010;59(25):769–72.

41. Davis LE, Beckham JD, Tyler KL. North American encephalitic arbovirus. Neurol Clin. 2008;26:727–57.

42. Tyler KL. Emerging viral infections of the central nervous system. Arch Neurol. 2009;66(8):939–48.

43. Makhoul B, Braun E, Herskovitz M, et al. Hyperimmune gammaglobin for the treatment of West Nile virus encephalitis. Isr Med Assoc J. 2009;11:151–3.

44. Irani DN. Aseptic meningitis and viral myelitis. Neurol Clin. 2008;26(3):635–55.

45. McKinney Jr RE, Katz SL, Wilfert CM. Chronic enteroviral meningoencephalitis in agammaglobulinemic patients. Rev Infect Dis. 1987;9(2):334–56.

46. Kupila L, Vuorinen T, Vainionp R, et al. Etiology of aseptic meningitis and encephalitis in an adult population. Neurology. 2006;66(1):75–80.

47. Tyler KL. Emerging viral infections of the central nervous system part 2. Arch Neurol. 2009;66(9):1065–74.

48. Engsig FN, Hansen AB, Omland LH, et al. Incidence, clinical presentation, and outcome of progressive multifocal leukoencephalopathy in HIV-infected patients during the highly active antiretroviral therapy era: a nationwide cohort study. J Infect Dis. 2009;199(1):77–83.

49. Yousry TA, Major EO, Ryschkewitsch C, et al. Evaluation of patients treated with natalizumab for progressive multifocal leukoencephalopathy. N Engl J Med. 2006;354(9):924–33.

50. Lindl KA, Marks DR, Kolson DL, et al. HIV-associated neurocognitive disorder: pathogenesis and therapeutic opportunities. J Neuroimmune Pharmacol. 2001;5(3): 294–309.

51. Ances BM, Ellis RJ. Dementia and neurocognitive disorders due to HIV-1 infection. Semin Neurol. 2007;27(1):86–92.
52. Heaton RK, Clifford DB, Franklin DR. HIV-associated neurocognitive disorders persist in the era of potent antiretroviral therapy. Neurology. 2010;75(23):2087–96.
53. Sato M, Sano H, Iwaki D, et al. Direct binding of toll-like receptor 2 to zymosan, and zymosan-induced NF-κB activation and TNF-α secretion are down-regulated by lung collectin surfactant protein A. J Immunol. 2003;171(1):417–25.
54. Clark TA, Hajjeh RA. Recent trends in the epidemiology of invasive mycoses. Curr Opin Infect Dis. 2002;15:569–74.
55. Khanna N, Chandramuki A, Desai A, Ravi V. Cryptococcal infection of the central nervous system: an analysis of predisposing factors, laboratory findings and outcome in patients from South India with special reference to HIV infection. J Med Microbiol. 1996;45:376–9.
56. Rhodes JC, Polacheck I, Kwon-Chung KJ. Phenoloxidase activity and virulence in isogenic strains of Cryptococcus neoformans. Infect Immun. 1982;36:1175–84.
57. Sundaram C, Mhadevan A, Laxmi V, Yasha TC, Santosh V, Murthy JM, et al. Cerebral zygomycosis. Mycoses. 2005;48:396–407.
58. Ramirez-Avila L, Slome S, Schuster FL, et al. Eosinophilic meningitis due to Angiostrongylus and Gnathostoma species. Clin Infect Dis. 2009;48(3):322–7.
59. Kerstein AH, Massey AD. Neurocysticercosis. Kans J Med. 2010;3(4):52–4.
60. Altinors N, Senveli E, Donmez T, Bavbek M, Kars Z, Sanli M. Management of problematic intracranial hydatid cysts. Infection. 1995;23:283–7.
61. Cabanes PA, Wallet F, Pringuez E, Pernin P. Assessing the risk of primary amoebic meningoencephalitis from swimming in the presence of environmental Naegleria fowleri. Appl Environ Microbiol. 2001;67(7):2927–31.
62. Ramsey RG, Gean AD. Neuroimaging of AIDS. I. Central nervous system toxoplasmosis. Neuroimaging Clin N Am. 1997;7(2):171–86.
63. Grcia HH, Del Brutto OH. Neurocysticercosis: updated concepts about an old disease. Lancet Neurol. 2005;4:653–61.
64. Del Brutto OH, Santibanez R, Noboa CA, Aguirre R, Diaz E, Alarcon TA. Epilepsy due to neurocysticercosis: analysis of 203 patients. Neurology. 1992;42:389–92.
65. Fernando SD et al. The 'hidden' burden of malaria: cognitive impairment following infection. Malar J. 2010;9:366.
66. Idro R et al. Cerebral malaria: mechanisms of brain injury and strategies for improved neurocognitive outcome. Pediatr Res. 2010;68(4):267–74.
67. Carpio A, Santillan F, Leon P, Flores C, Hauser WA. Is the course of neurocysticercosis modified by treatment with antihelminthic agents? Arch Intern Med. 1995;155:1982–8.

15

The Neuroimmunology of Cortical Disease (Dementia, Epilepsy, and Autoimmune Encephalopathies)

Julie L. Roth, Brian R. Ott, John N. Gaitanis, and Andrew S. Blum

Keywords: Dementia, Neuritic plaques, Immunotherapy, Limbic encephalitis, Neuromyotonia

Dementia: Immunologic Aspects of Alzheimer's Disease

Introduction

Alzheimer's disease (AD) is a neurodegenerative disorder characterized pathologically by large numbers of extracellular neuritic plaques containing a core of amyloid Aβ fibrils as well as intracellular neurofibrillary tangles containing hyperphosphorylated tau protein filaments in the neurons of the cerebral cortex. Other features include reactive gliosis, synaptic loss, neuronal death, and mitochondrial dysfunction. A small percentage of cases are due to genetic mutations of the amyloid precursor gene on chromosome 21 and mutations in presenilin 1 and 2 genes on chromosomes 2 and 14, respectively [1]. These presenilin proteins are inherent to secretase enzymes involved with cleavage of the amyloid Aβ precursor protein into amyloidogenic A fragments, particularly Aβ42 [2]. Apolipoprotein E4 is an important risk factor allele for other cases [3]. The molecular underpinnings for the common form of AD occurring sporadically in older patients remain largely to be elucidated.

In this way, different genetic factors, as well as age-related processes, interact to produce a clinically recognizable phenotype marked by gradual loss of global cognitive functions starting with memory, as pathology typically spreads from entorhinal cortex to heteromodal association areas in the temporal, parietal, and frontal lobes. A primary immunologic etiology has not been implicated in this disease; however, there is evidence of inflammation in neuritic plaques. Recent experimental approaches to treatment of the disease have focused on manipulation of this inflammatory response and the use of immune modulation to prevent or remove amyloid β deposits from the brain.

From: *Clinical Neuroimmunology: Multiple Sclerosis and Related Disorders*, Current Clinical Neurology,
Edited by: S.A. Rizvi and P.K. Coyle, DOI 10.1007/978-1-60327-860-7_15,
© Springer Science+Business Media, LLC 2011

Inflammation in AD

Examination of neuritic plaques has revealed important signs of inflammation, including activated complement factors and clusters of activated microglia [4]. The presence of such inflammation and the association of reduced risk for developing AD seen in users of anti-inflammatory medications in numerous epidemiologic studies [5–8] have led to primary treatment as well as prevention trials. Unfortunately, these trials have not succeeded, and the anti-inflammatory approach has largely been abandoned [9].

One early controlled trial of indomethacin showed beneficial effects on cognition among the 28 subjects with AD who were able to tolerate the treatment [10]. Subsequent randomized controlled trials of diclofenac [11], rofecoxib [12], naproxen and rofecoxib [13], and prednisone [14] all failed to show efficacy in subjects with AD. A randomized controlled primary prevention trial in 2,528 subjects, using naproxen and celecoxib, failed to show benefit for either treatment arm; however, the study was terminated early due to safety concerns about the cardiovascular risk of nonsteroidal anti-inflammatory drugs [15].

These clinical trial results suggest that inflammation in AD may be a disease-ameliorating factor in pathogenesis or a non-etiologic consequence of a previous cascade of injurious events, rather than a primary cause [16]. Further support for a secondary role of inflammation in the pathogenesis comes from postmortem studies. One postmortem study of normal elders showed less microglial activation in nonsteroidal anti-inflammatory drug users compared with nonusers, but no differences in plaques or tangles [17]. Furthermore, a postmortem examination of AD users of anti-inflammatory drugs showed no difference in the amount of inflammatory glia, plaques, or tangles compared with AD nonusers [18].

Hopes for a role of anti-inflammatory therapy for AD have recently been rekindled by a controversial study of etanercept, an inhibitor of tumor necrosis factor-α, used in the treatment of rheumatoid arthritis. A 6-month open-label pilot study was conducted in 15 AD subjects with moderate-to-severe dementia, who were injected weekly by the perispinal route with etanercept. Rapid improvements in cognition were noticed [19, 20], leading to speculation that the mechanism of action in AD could have been through augmentation of gliotransmission as well as interference with proinflammatory cytokines [21, 22].

Immunotherapy in AD

The two pathological hallmarks of AD, plaques and tangles, are currently the main targets of experimental therapeutic intervention. While the role of neurofibrillary tangles should not be discounted or underestimated, the currently prevailing theory of pathogenesis has been called the amyloid cascade. Consequently, immunologic approaches to interrupt this cascade and reduce amyloid burden in the brain are currently underway.

The Amyloid Hypothesis

As previously mentioned, genetic mutations of the amyloid precursor and the presenilin genes provide causative evidence that amyloid deposition is an early and key factor to the pathogenesis of AD in hereditary, autosomal dominant, early-onset cases [23].

Further genetic evidence in support of the amyloid hypothesis comes from observations of brain pathology in patients with Down's syndrome, which is due to trisomy 21. The gene coding for the amyloid precursor protein is located on chromosome 21. Nearly all patients with Down's syndrome develop AD pathology in their fourth decade, and many go on to develop cognitive and behavioral changes of dementia in later decades [24–26].

The amyloid protein in the plaques of inherited genetic mutation cases, Down's syndrome, and late-onset sporadic and hereditary cases is the same. The protein, called Aβ, arises from amyloidogenic fragments, cleaved enzymatically from the precursor protein. The most amyloidogenic fragment is Aβ42. Brain Aβ42 levels correlate with disease severity, and transgenic mice producing Aβ42 show impaired learning and memory. It appears that the soluble oligomers of Aβ participate at an early stage of disease in a cascade of pathogenic events eventually leading to the β pleated sheets in the core of the neuritic plaque, and that these are the most neurotoxic forms of amyloid [2, 27]. If so, then these oligomers may serve as a primary target of immunotherapy to facilitate their removal from the brain and slow or stop disease progression [28].

Active Immunization

The development of transgenic mice that overexpress the human amyloid precursor protein gene via mutations linked to familial AD has enabled investigators to test the effect of active and passive immunotherapy in vivo. In a series of experiments using such transgenic mice, Schenk and colleagues injected aggregated Aβ42 either before the onset of AD-like pathology (6 weeks) or at an older age (11 months), when amyloid had already been deposited. They demonstrated that mice injected very early were relatively devoid of amyloid plaques after 18 months, compared with mice injected with a buffer vehicle. Among older mice that were injected at a late time, cells resembling activated microglial cells and monocytes were observed, presumably clearing amyloid by phagocytosis [29].

A Phase I study of 20 AD subjects established the immunogenicity of a synthetic, human aggregated Aβ42 (AN1792). One patient developed meningoencephalitis, diagnosed after death and 219 days after discontinuing the study [30]. Subsequently, a Phase II clinical trial was undertaken in the USA and Europe. A majority (274/300) of patients received two injections. Dosing was suspended after reports of meningoencephalitis, which ultimately developed in 18 of the immunized patients [31]. Post hoc analyses showed treatment signals among those with a predefined responder antibody titer, including memory improvement [32, 33], activities of daily living improvement [32, 33], plaque clearance at autopsy [34, 35], reduction in brain volume by MRI [36], and lowering of spinal fluid total tau levels [33]. The development of meningoencephalitis has been attributed to the stimulation of an anti-Aβ T-cell response [37], and alternative safer methods of immunotherapy are being explored.

Passive Immunization

Specific monoclonal antibodies against Aβ have been developed with the goal of clearing Aβ, without activating a T-cell response and triggering meningoencephalitis. This could be accomplished by at least two possible mechanisms.

If the antibodies cross the blood–brain barrier and attach to Aβ, the protein can then be removed by activated microglia. An alternative mechanism is the "sink" hypothesis, in which circulating antibodies serve as a sponge to draw Aβ out of the brain compartment into the circulation where it can then be cleared [37].

To this end, a large world-wide multicenter clinical trial is underway using bapineuzumab/AAB-001 (Janssen), an antibody directed against the N-terminus of Aβ to determine whether this approach is safe as well as effective in slowing the progression of AD in patients with mild-to-moderate disease [38] A phase II controlled trial of bapineuzumab in 28 patients showed that 78 weeks of treatment was associated with reduced brain amyloid burden on ^{11}C-PiB positron emission tomography scans compared with both baseline and placebo [39, 40]. Passive immunization with a monoclonal antibody against the mid-domain of Aβ is also under development in phase II clinical trials [41].

Another approach under development is to use intravenous immunoglobulin (IVIG), which contains antibodies against monomeric as well as aggregated forms of Aβ [39]. In an open-label 6-month study of five patients with mild-to-moderate AD, monthly injections of IVIG were associated with stabilization of cognitive function and reduction in levels of cerebrospinal fluid Aβ [42]. More recently, a double-blind, placebo-controlled trial of 24 AD subjects confirmed symptomatic benefits, including improved cognition [43]. A larger Phase II study is underway that will look at this agent's safety and effectiveness in 360 patients.

Challenges to the Immunotherapeutic Approach

As previously mentioned, the development of encephalomyelitis in some cases of patients actively immunized with injections of Aβ has significantly tempered enthusiasm for this approach. While passive immunotherapy may address this risk, and still result in the reduction of amyloid deposits, it remains unproven whether or not such alterations in brain pathology will provide clinically relevant symptomatic or disease altering benefits. The initial results from Phase III clinical trials of agents, such as tarenflurbil and transiposate, aimed at reducing amyloid burden, so far have been disappointing, causing some investigators to speculate that targeting tau as well as other targets may be more effective [44]. Also, since the amyloid cascade begins many years before the symptoms of dementia, current anti-amyloid trials may be targeted at a stage of disease that is too advanced for effective remediation.

In terms of toxicity, there are concerns about the risk of passive immunization producing microhemorrhages and brain edema as a result of amyloid removal from vessel walls and disruption of vascular integrity [45]. This may be a particular hazard for those with already established amyloid angiopathy.

In summary, immunotherapy has been shown to alter the amyloid pathology of AD and holds promise as a potential disease modifying approach that could significantly enhance the results obtained with current symptomatic therapies aimed at the downstream effects of the disease. The ideal methods to achieve this result and the full-safety profile of this therapeutic approach remain to be elucidated by current and future clinical trials.

Immunological Aspects of Epilepsy and Autoimmune Encephalopathies

Introduction

Seizures are felt to represent a transient imbalance of excitation and inhibition in the brain, leading to spontaneous, hypersynchronous neuronal activity in the cerebral cortex. The pathophysiological states that result in this final common pathway are diverse and include both inborn and acquired conditions. Within these broad categories are genetic and congenital factors, vascular factors, trauma, prior or active inflammation and infection, toxic and metabolic disturbances, neoplasm, and immunological factors. Several immune-mediated conditions are highly associated with seizures and epilepsy, often with other features – including focal neurological deficits and decline, alterations of mental status, and systemic symptoms. This section focuses on those immune-mediated conditions in which seizures and epilepsy are the primary clinical symptom; a large number of conditions exist in which seizures are one of many features, and these are discussed elsewhere in this text.

Rasmussen's Encephalitis

Rasmussen's encephalitis is a rare condition that affects primarily children, characterized by the progression of severe, intractable partial epilepsy affecting one hemisphere, often with concurrent cognitive and motor decline. The syndrome was first described by Rasmussen in his 1958 case report of three patients with intractable focal motor seizures and progressive hemiparesis. They had histopathological evidence of chronic focal encephalitis, specifically perivascular inflammation and glial nodules [46]. Although children are most often affected, adolescents and adults can rarely develop the disease; an earlier age of onset (less than 2 years of age) is associated with a poorer neurological prognosis. Rasmussen's encephalitis is often seen as the prototype of an immune-mediated, progressive epileptic syndrome. The pharmacoresistant nature of seizures in Rasmussen's encephalitis and its inflammatory pathology have prompted new exploration of immunological strategies for its treatment.

The pathophysiology of this disorder is presumed to be autoimmune, although the precise mechanism remains unknown. In the 1990s, a potential autoimmune explanation emerged after the discovery that rabbits immunized with a glutamate (AMPA) receptor protein fragment (GluR3) developed a clinical syndrome similar to Rasmussen's encephalitis, with progressive, intractable seizures and similar histopathological changes [47]. GluR3 antibodies have been demonstrated experimentally to activate cortical neurons and induce cytotoxicity [48]. Additional theories for the mechanism of Rasmussen's encephalitis suggest a role for the activation of complement pathways, activation of T-cells, microglial response, and ultimate breakdown of the blood–brain barrier to allow antibodies to pass [49].

Clinically, the utility of testing for GluR3 antibodies has not been demonstrated [50]. Antibodies to GluR3 have been found in some patients with known Rasmussen's encephalitis, but the antibody has demonstrated neither specificity nor sensitivity for the disease. Antibodies to GluR3, among other antibodies directed against other glutamate receptor subunits, have been demonstrated in patients with epilepsy without Rasmussen's encephalitis, when compared with healthy controls. A number of patients with Rasmussen's encephalitis do not demonstrate positivity for GluR3 antibodies [51]. Antibodies to the NMDA GluR epsilon 2 subunit have also been found in patients with Rasmussen's encephalitis and unexplained epilepsia partialis continua (continuous focal motor seizures), suggesting that patients with Rasmussen's encephalitis may have autoantibodies against a number of different neural proteins [52].

Definitive treatment for Rasmussen's encephalitis is hemispherectomy, although partial cortical resection can be beneficial for some patients. Immunotherapeutic treatments have been explored in Rasmussen's encephalitis, and these include corticosteroids (or ACTH), IVIG, plasmapheresis, selective immunoadsorbtion, immunosuppressive drugs such as cyclophosphamide, tacrolimus and azathioprine, and other therapies including interferon-α and antiviral treatments [53]. Of these options, corticosteroids are the most commonly used in the clinical setting; regimens include long-term immunosuppression with ACTH, hydrocortisone, methylprednisolone, or dexamethasone. Intravenous immunoglobulin and plasmapheresis have also shown benefit in small series of patients [54–56]. No randomized controlled trials exist for these treatments, in part due to the low incidence of the disease. Immunotherapy is felt to improve seizure frequency and neurological deficits, and possibly to slow the course of the disease; however, patients tend to progress to hemispherectomy despite treatment. Nonetheless, immunotherapy can be useful in patients with late-onset of disease, a slower clinical course, dominant or bilateral hemisphere involvement, or other cases in which delay of surgical intervention is preferable [53, 54].

Management of the seizures in Rasmussen's encephalitis, and in particular the occurrence of epilepsia partialis continua, can be difficult. No current guidelines exist on anticonvulsant therapy in the disease, thus medications are chosen based on side effect profiles. Levetiracetam and topiramate have shown some anecdotal benefit in patients with the disease, possibly due to levetiracetam's utility in treating cortical myoclonus and epilepsia partialis continua, and topiramate's effect as an agonist of inhibitory GABA receptors. Intravenous steroid bolus has also been used anecdotally in some instances in acute management of status epilepticus [53].

Hashimoto's Encephalopathy (Steroid-Responsive Encephalopathy)

Hashimoto's encephalopathy is a rare disease that is characterized clinically by cognitive and behavioral abnormalities and seizures. Tremulousness, transient aphasia, psychotic symptoms, myoclonus, gait ataxia, sleep abnormalities, and extrapyramidal signs can be prominent, and stroke-like episodes of sudden deterioration can also occur [57]. The disease typically affects middle-aged women, although children can also be affected; the disease course is typically relapsing–remitting, with progression if not treated. Patients with Hashimoto's encephalopathy have high titers of antithyroid antibodies, including anti-thyroglobulin and anti-thyroperoxidase, which can exist independently of abnormal thyroid function studies. The CSF in patients with Hashimoto's encephalopathy typically demonstrates high protein, sometimes with a pleocytosis and oligoclonal bands. EEG is most often abnormal, demonstrating generalized slowing, occasionally with focal slowing, triphasic waves, or epileptiform features. Although brain MRI tends to show diffuse atrophy or white matter signal abnormalities including ischemic changes, in many cases it is normal [57].

First described by Brain and colleagues in 1966 in a middle-aged man with episodic confusion, seizures and fluctuating hemiparesis, there are now a number of cases reported in the literature, many with differing neurological features [58–60]. As the disorder commonly presents as a rapidly progressive dementia (RPD), it is often mistaken for prion diseases such as Creutzfeldt–Jakob disease (CJD), neurodegenerative conditions, and other autoimmune or paraneoplastic syndromes (discussed elsewhere in this chapter) [61, 62]. Proposed criteria in one review by Chong et al. suggested three findings necessary for diagnosis of Hashimoto's encephalopathy: impaired consciousness, lack of CSF evidence of infection, and elevation of at least one of the aforementioned antithyroid antibodies in the serum [59]. The syndrome's characteristic response to corticosteroids, along with the presence of antibodies, suggests that the underlying mechanism is autoimmune. In fact, immunotherapy can be curative in many cases [57].

Despite knowledge of treatment and diagnosis, the mechanism remains unknown. The antibodies in Hashimoto's encephalopathy are not thought to be causative of the central nervous systems symptoms, as many patients with elevated thyroid autoantibodies do not have the disorder. However, it is possible that a shared antigen between thyroid and brain exists, as is thought to be the case with many autoimmune and paraneoplastic syndromes. Other possible mechanisms include central nervous system autoimmune vasculitis, global cerebral hypoperfusion, humoral factors, and immune complex deposition [60, 63–67]. Controversy has existed over whether the entire clinical picture might be caused by the hypothyroidism itself; however, the lack of response of symptomatic patients to levothyroxine, and the dramatic and consistent response to corticosteroids argues against this [59].

Although no randomized controlled trials exist for treatment, patients typically receive high-dose intravenous pulse steroids for 3–5 days for flares, sometimes with immunomodulatory therapy between flares to maintain remission. Oral steroids are typically tapered over 6–12 months, with eventual withdrawal of the medication based on clinical response. In addition to oral steroids, azathioprine, methotrexate, cyclophosphamide, IVIG, and plasmapheresis have been used anecdotally, with inconsistent success [55, 66]. For patients who cannot tolerate steroids, plasmapheresis has been shown in one small study to improve cognitive symptoms [68]. Titers of antithyroid antibodies can be used as a marker of treatment response.

Limbic Encephalitis

Paraneoplastic syndromes associated with systemic malignancies can cause dysfunction of the central nervous system, resulting in seizures. The neurological dysfunction in paraneoplastic syndromes is thought to result from production of a neuronal protein by a tumor, which precipitates an immune-mediated reaction against both the tumor and the central nervous system itself [69–71]. Among the majority of patients with malignancy-associated paraneoplastic syndromes, the neurological dysfunction precedes the diagnosis of cancer. Limbic encephalitis is a cortical syndrome that consists of seizures (often complex partial in nature), within the context of subacute to chronic confusion, depression, anxiety, behavioral changes, sleep disturbances, and progressive memory loss. The majority of patients with limbic encephalitis have abnormalities on MRI, including T2 and FLAIR hyperintensities in one or both medial temporal lobes [69]. Unilateral or bilateral temporal epileptiform activity, with or without focal or generalized slowing is frequently observed on EEG. Analysis of CSF most often demonstrates a pleocytosis with lymphocytic predominance, elevated protein, and a normal glucose, frequently with elevated IgG index and oligoclonal bands; in a minority of cases the CSF can be normal. In general, treatment is aimed at discovery and treatment of the underlying malignancy; however, frequently, there is no underlying malignancy, and limbic encephalitis can, in fact, be either paraneoplastic or nonparaneoplastic (autoimmune) [70].

The first described autoantibodies associated with paraneoplastic encephalomyelitis (and by extension limbic encephalitis) included anti-Hu (ANNA-1), anti-CV2 (CRMP5), and anti-Ma antibodies [69]. Anti-Hu is a nonspecific antibody seen in a variety of central and peripheral neurological syndromes. While not felt to be epileptogenic in itself, it is often regarded as a marker for a possible underlying malignancy, prompting further workup. Both anti-Hu and anti-CV2 are frequently associated with small cell lung cancer among other malignancies. Anti-Ma antibodies have been linked with germ cell tumors of the testis and ovary. The recently described anti-NMDA receptor antibodies, discussed below, are associated with ovarian teratomas, while anti-AMPA receptor antibodies have been linked with breast cancer in case reports [72–74]. A positive test for a specific autoantibody, while potentially useful in the identification of an underlying malignancy, rarely predicts the specific neurological syndrome observed [71, 75].

Limbic encephalitis, such as Hashimoto's encephalopathy, often presents as an RPD prior to the onset of seizures. Among 67 cases of RPD that were not related to prion disease seen at the University of California, San Francisco between 1995 and 2001, 8.4% were due to immune-mediated conditions such as limbic encephalitis and Hashimoto's encephalopathy. Of the limbic encephalitis cases in which an antibody was discovered, two were due to antibodies to voltage-gated potassium channels (discussed below), and one each to antibodies to each of the following: Yo and Hu, Ma, CV2, GAD65, neuropil, adenylate kinase 5, and glial cells [61].

In most cases of limbic encephalitis, the mechanism of central nervous system dysfunction is unclear, and the presence of these antibodies as markers versus direct pathogens has been debated. Some evidence exists for a T-cell-mediated immune response, directed against the same antigens recognized by the antibodies [75, 76]. Immune-mediated mechanisms and possible novel treatments of limbic encephalitis have been advanced recently by the discovery of antibodies against specific cell membrane proteins that play a role in epilepsy, including receptors and ion channels, involved in neuronal excitation and inhibition. One proposed algorithm for treatment divides paraneoplastic syndromes into two categories: "classic" antibodies to intracellular antigens (including anti-Hu, anti-Ma, and anti-CV2) and antibodies to cell membrane antigens (VGKC, NMDA, and AMPA), with the hypothesis being that the "classic" syndromes are likely T-cell mediated, and may respond to directed therapy (cyclophosphamide, for example), while the cell membrane syndromes likely involve antibodies that are directly involved in pathogenesis, and thus more likely to respond to immunotherapy with IVIG, plasma exchange, corticosteroids, among other treatments [70, 76]. In clinical practice, the latter group appears significantly more responsive to immune-based treatment [76].

Voltage-Gated Potassium Channel Antibodies

Some patients diagnosed with limbic encephalitis have been found to have elevated titers of voltage-gated potassium channel (VGKC) antibodies. VGKC antibody syndrome is a rare condition characterized by global memory impairment, seizures, confusion, and other neuropsychiatric symptoms, commonly accompanied by sleep disturbances such as insomnia. MRI can demonstrate T2 and FLAIR hyperintensity in the medial temporal lobes or hippocampi, and PET scan may show hypermetabolism in these regions. Patients respond to IVIG, steroids, and plasmapheresis in many case reports, with normalization of the VGKC antibody levels and subjective improvement in sleep, autonomic, psychiatric, and memory symptoms. Although the typical clinical course of VGKC antibody syndrome is marked by relapses and remissions, the overall prognosis – in particular when compared with other antibody-mediated encephalopathies and paraneoplastic syndromes – is good [77]. VGKC antibodies are associated with neuromyotonia as well as Morvan's syndrome, which is characterized by peripheral nerve abnormalities, autonomic dysfunction, as well as central nervous system dysfunction including sleep disturbances and confusion. Very high titers of VGKC are most associated with the symptoms of seizure and encephalopathy. Although more often seen as an isolated autoimmune disorder with no underlying malignancy, VGKC antibodies can be identified in paraneoplastic syndromes associated with small-cell lung cancer and thymoma (20% of cases) [69]. Central nervous system manifestations of VGKC antibody syndromes can mimic Hashimoto's disease as well as Creutzfeldt–Jakob disease [78–80].

N-Methyl-D-Aspartate Receptor Antibodies

Anti-N-methyl-D-aspartate (NMDA) receptor syndrome is a recently described antibody-associated disorder associated with prominent seizures and psychiatric symptoms, usually after a prodrome of fever or headache, and followed by progression to unresponsiveness, central hypoventilation, autonomic instability, and extrapyramidal signs. Anti-NMDA receptor antibodies are present in paraneoplastic syndromes that usually affect young women with ovarian teratoma, which is often mistaken for a benign cyst on imaging [69, 74]. Although typically felt to be a disease of young women, there have been rare cases of men with the disease [81]. Examination of the CSF demonstrates immunoreactivity to NR1/NR2 heteromers of the NMDA receptor. The disease demonstrates good response to treatment with tumor resection, and immunotherapy that includes corticosteroids, plasma exchange, and IVIG [74, 82]. Antibodies to the NMDA receptor and its subunits can be nonspecific and have been demonstrated in Rasmussen's encephalitis [52] and psychotic disorders [83], among other central nervous system syndromes.

Glutamic Acid Decarboxylase Antibodies

Antibodies to glutamic acid decarboxylase (GAD), the enzyme that converts glutamate to GABA, can be seen in patients with type I diabetes mellitus, among other autoimmune disorders, as well as a number of central nervous system disorders, including cerebellar, brainstem, extrapyramidal, and spinal cord dysfunction [84–88]. The antibodies are frequently seen in the neurological condition known as stiff person syndrome, a presumed central nervous system disorder characterized by muscle pain, spasm, and rigidity [88]. Stiff person syndrome is managed with GABA agonists such as benzodiazepine and baclofen, as well as anticonvulsants in some cases, and exacerbations are typically treated with IVIG or plasmapheresis. Among patients with stiff person syndrome and anti-GAD antibodies, the prevalence of epilepsy is around 10–20% [89, 90]. A role for anti-GAD antibodies in patients with epilepsy has been postulated, given the role of the enzyme in limiting neuronal excitation. High titers of the antibody have been found in patients with pharmacoresistant epilepsy [91]. There is growing recognition of anti-GAD antibodies in paraneoplastic syndromes such as limbic encephalitis, and anecdotal evidence exists that immunotherapy may be useful in the treatment of the disorder [92–94] – for example, methylprednisolone, azathioprine, cyclophosphamide, and IVIG have tried [95–99]. The most frequently encountered epilepsy type among these patients appears to be complex partial epilepsy [95–99].

Other Antibody-Associated Epilepsy Syndromes

Some serum autoantibodies directed against those receptors and channels that play a role in neuronal excitation and inhibition, as discussed above, are felt to be epileptogenic. The role of autoantibodies in epilepsy outside the context of paraneoplastic or known autoimmune disorders is less clear. In one study, serum antibodies against gangliosides such as GM1 have been demonstrated in several patients with pharmacoresistant complex partial epilepsy with secondary generalization, concurrent psychiatric symptoms, and normal imaging [100]. Gangliosides are important in the structure of synaptic membranes, the disruption of which could provide a possible mechanism for epilepsy.

Antibodies against brain endothelial cells and neuronal nuclear proteins have been reported in cases of Landau–Kleffner syndrome, a childhood epilepsy syndrome characterized by progressive aphasia, seizures, and behavioral problems [101]. Autoantibodies associated with coagulopathies, specifically anticardiolipin antibody, lupus anticoagulant, and the antiphospholipid syndrome, have a high clinical association with epilepsy, although their specific role in the disorder is unknown [67].

Seizures and Systemic Disease

Several inflammatory and autoimmune systemic disorders can be accompanied by seizures in certain clinical settings. These disorders are covered more in depth in another chapter of this textbook. Among the many central nervous system complications of sarcoidosis, for example, seizures can result from either diffuse involvement of the meninges or brain parenchyma or through an isolated granuloma that mimics a tumor. In the case of diffuse involvement, cognitive and mood changes can accompany the seizures, often resulting in an encephalopathy; in the case of granuloma formation, focal neurological deficits can accompany the seizures. Neurosarcoidosis can remit spontaneously, but progression can be seen in up to 30% of cases; treatment generally includes corticosteroids, although both cyclosporine or irradiation of a focal lesion can be useful in some cases [102]. Systemic lupus erythematosis, Sjogren's syndrome and rheumatoid arthritis can also be associated with seizures, although often in the context of other neuropsychiatric symptoms, such as mood changes, psychosis, anxiety, confusion, disorientation, amnesia, and dementia [61, 102].

Chronic gluten enteropathy, seen in celiac disease, can be associated with severe central nervous system dysfunction, including encephalopathy, myelopathy, cerebellar dysfunction, and peripheral neuropathy. Seizures are a common neurological manifestation of the disorder, and EEG may show the characteristic pattern of bilateral or unilateral occipital spikes. Radiographic imaging findings can demonstrate occipital calcifications. Diagnosis of the disease is made in part through the detection of elevated antiendomysial or antigliadin antibodies, as well as anti-tissue tranglutaminase; and treatment with a gluten-free diet can lead to resolution of symptoms [61, 103, 104].

Conclusion

A number of proposed immunological mechanisms for seizures and epileptogenesis exist. Among the most well-studied are autoantibodies, and their effect on the central nervous system, both directly, when targeted against receptors, ion channels, and enzymes, and indirectly with various intracellular targets, in association with T-cell and humeral factors and immune complex formation [105]. Rasmussen's encephalitis is an example of an autoimmune epilepsy syndrome in which a possibly pathogenic antibody against GluR3 has been investigated, although the clinical utility of this association has yet to be demonstrated. In Hashimoto's encephalopathy, a recognized clinical syndrome correlates with high titers of anti-thyroid antibodies, but their role in the disease process is unclear. Limbic encephalitis represents a spectrum of disease, including paraneoplastic and autoimmune, in which identifying the specific antibody and its target might influence the treatment and the prognosis for response and recovery. Newly discovered antibodies, and antibodies known for their association with other diseases might be important in epilepsy, although further work is necessary on this front. In addition to the direct antibody-mediated mechanisms, deposition of immune complexes in vessel walls and other forms of vasculitis, hypoperfusion, and coagulopathies that result in cerebral ischemia may play a role in some autoimmune disorders, particularly those that are systemic in nature [63–67, 106]. Future research on the immunological basis of seizures and epilepsy will broaden the horizon for treatment of these conditions.

References

1. Bird TD. Genetic aspects of Alzheimer disease. Genet Med. 2008;10(4):231–9.
2. Selkoe DJ. Alzheimer's disease results from the cerebral accumulation and cytotoxicity of amyloid beta-protein. J Alzheimers Dis. 2001;3(1):75–80.
3. Jofre-Monseny L, Minihane AM, Rimbach G. Impact of apoE genotype on oxidative stress, inflammation and disease risk. Mol Nutr Food Res. 2008;52(1): 131–45.
4. Eikelenboom P, Rozemuller AJ, Hoozemans JJ, Veerhuis R, van Gool WA. Neuroinflammation and Alzheimer disease: clinical and therapeutic implications. Alzheimer Dis Assoc Disord. 2000;14 Suppl 1:S54–61.
5. McGeer PL, McGeer EG. NSAIDs and Alzheimer disease: epidemiological, animal model and clinical studies. Neurobiol Aging. 2007;28(5):639–47.
6. Etminan M, Gill S, Samii A. Effect of non-steroidal anti-inflammatory drugs on risk of Alzheimer's disease: systematic review and meta-analysis of observational studies. BMJ. 2003;327(7407):128.

7. Hayden KM, Zandi PP, Khachaturian AS, et al. Does NSAID use modify cognitive trajectories in the elderly? The Cache County study. Neurology. 2007;69(3): 275–82.

8. Int V, Ruitenberg A, Hofman A, et al. Nonsteroidal antiinflammatory drugs and the risk of Alzheimer's disease. N Engl J Med. 2001;345(21):1515–21.

9. Firuzi O, Pratico D. Coxibs and Alzheimer's disease: should they stay or should they go? Ann Neurol. 2006;59(2):219–28.

10. Rogers J, Kirby LC, Hempelman SR, et al. Clinical trial of indomethacin in Alzheimer's disease. Neurology. 1993;43(8):1609–11.

11. Scharf JM, Daffner KR. NSAIDs in the prevention of dementia: a Cache-22? Neurology. 2007;69(3):235–6.

12. Reines SA, Block GA, Morris JC, et al. Rofecoxib: no effect on Alzheimer's disease in a 1-year, randomized, blinded, controlled study. Neurology. 2004;62(1):66–71.

13. Aisen PS, Schafer KA, Grundman M, et al. Effects of rofecoxib or naproxen vs placebo on Alzheimer disease progression: a randomized controlled trial. JAMA. 2003;289(21):2819–26.

14. Aisen PS, Davis KL, Berg JD, et al. A randomized controlled trial of prednisone in Alzheimer's disease. Alzheimer's Disease Cooperative Study. Neurology. 2000;54(3):588–93.

15. Lyketsos CG, Breitner JC, et al. ADAPT Research Group. Naproxen and celecoxib do not prevent AD in early results from a randomized controlled trial. Neurology. 2007;68(21):1800–8.

16. Honig LS. Inflammation in neurodegenerative disease: good, bad, or irrelevant? Arch Neurol. 2000;57(6):786–8.

17. Mackenzie IR, Munoz DG. Nonsteroidal anti-inflammatory drug use and Alzheimer-type pathology in aging. Neurology. 1998;50(4):986–90.

18. Halliday GM, Shepherd CE, McCann H, et al. Effect of anti-inflammatory medications on neuropathological findings in Alzheimer disease. Arch Neurol. 2000;57(6):831–6.

19. Tobinick EL, Gross H. Rapid cognitive improvement in Alzheimer's disease following perispinal etanercept administration. J Neuroinflammation. 2008;5:2.

20. Tobinick E, Gross H, Weinberger A, Cohen H. TNF-alpha modulation for treatment of Alzheimer's disease: a 6-month pilot study. MedGenMed. 2006;8(2):25.

21. Griffin WS. Perispinal etanercept: potential as an Alzheimer therapeutic. J Neuroinflammation. 2008;5:3.

22. Tobinick E. Perispinal etanercept for treatment of Alzheimer's disease. Curr Alzheimer Res. 2007;4(5):550–2.

23. Serretti A, Olgiati P, De RD. Genetics of Alzheimer's disease. A rapidly evolving field. J Alzheimers Dis. 2007;12(1):73–92.

24. Crawford FC, Wood M, Ferguson S, et al. Genomic analysis of response to traumatic brain injury in a mouse model of Alzheimer's disease (APPsw). Brain Res. 2007;1185:45–58.

25. Ozturk C, Ozge A, Yalin OO, et al. The diagnostic role of serum inflammatory and soluble proteins on dementia subtypes: correlation with cognitive and functional decline. Behav Neurol. 2007;18(4):207–15.

26. Shah RS, Lee HG, Xiongwei Z, Perry G, Smith MA, Castellani RJ. Current approaches in the treatment of Alzheimer's disease. Biomed Pharmacother. 2008;62(4):199–207.

27. Andreasen N, Zetterberg H. Amyloid-related biomarkers for Alzheimer's disease. Curr Med Chem. 2008;15(8):766–71.

28. McLean CA, Cherny RA, Fraser FW, et al. Soluble pool of Abeta amyloid as a determinant of severity of neurodegeneration in Alzheimer's disease. Ann Neurol. 1999;46(6):860–6.

29. Schenk D, Barbour R, Dunn W, et al. Immunization with amyloid-beta attenuates Alzheimer-disease-like pathology in the PDAPP mouse. Nature. 1999; 400(6740):173–7.

30. Bayer AJ, Bullock R, Jones RW, et al. Evaluation of the safety and immunogenicity of synthetic Abeta42 (AN1792) in patients with AD. Neurology. 2005;64(1):94–101.
31. Orgogozo JM, Gilman S, Dartigues JF, et al. Subacute meningoencephalitis in a subset of patients with AD after Abeta42 immunization. Neurology. 2003;61(1):46–54.
32. Hock C, Konietzko U, Streffer JR, et al. Antibodies against beta-amyloid slow cognitive decline in Alzheimer's disease. Neuron. 2003;38(4):547–54.
33. Gilman S, Koller M, Black RS, et al. Clinical effects of Abeta immunization (AN1792) in patients with AD in an interrupted trial. Neurology. 2005;64(9):1553–62.
34. Holmes C, Boche D, Wilkinson D, et al. Long-term effects of Abeta42 immunisation in Alzheimer's disease: follow-up of a randomised, placebo-controlled phase I trial. Lancet. 2008;372(9634):216–23.
35. Masliah E, Hansen L, Adame A, et al. Abeta vaccination effects on plaque pathology in the absence of encephalitis in Alzheimer disease. Neurology. 2005;64(1):129–31.
36. Fox NC, Black RS, Gilman S, et al. Effects of Abeta immunization (AN1792) on MRI measures of cerebral volume in Alzheimer disease. Neurology. 2005;64(9):1563–72.
37. Relkin NR. Current state of immunotherapy for Alzheimer's disease. CNS Spectr. 2008;13(10 Suppl 16):39–41.
38. Grundman M, Black R. Clinical trials of bapineuzumab, a beta-amyloid-targeted immunotherapy in patients with mild to moderate Alzheimer's disease. Alzheimers Dement. 2008;4 Suppl 2:T166.
39. Rinne JO, Brooks DJ, Rossor MN, et al. 11C-PiB PET assessment of change in fibrillar amyloid-β load in patients with Alzheimer's disease treated with bapineuzumab: a phase 2, double-blind, placebo-controlled, ascending-dose study. Lancet Neurol. 2010;9(4):363–72.
40. Gandy S. Testing the amyloid hypothesis of Alzheimer's disease in vivo. Lancet Neurol. 2010;9(4):333–5.
41. Siemers ER, Friedrich S, Dean RA, et al. Safety, tolerability and biomarker effects of an abeta monoclonal antibody administered to patients with Alzheimer's disease. Alzheimers Dement. 2008;4 Suppl 4:T774.
42. Dodel RC, Du Y, Depboylu C, et al. Intravenous immunoglobulins containing antibodies against beta-amyloid for the treatment of Alzheimer's disease. J Neurol Neurosurg Psychiatry. 2004;75(10):1472–4.
43. Relkin N, Tsakanikas DI, Adamiak B, et al. A double-blind, placebo-controlled, phase II clinical trial of intravenous immunoglobulin (IVIG) for treatment of Alzheimer's disease. In: Meeting of the American Academy of Neurology, 12–19 April 2008, Chicago, IL. Session S41.007.
44. Hampton T. Studies probe potential of experimental therapies for Alzheimer disease. JAMA. 2008;300(11):1287–9.
45. Pfeifer M, Boncristiano S, Bondolfi L, et al. Cerebral hemorrhage after passive anti-Abeta immunotherapy. Science. 2002;298(5597):1379.
46. Rasmussen T, Olszewski J, Lloyd-Smith D. Focal seizures due to chronic localized encephalitis. Neurology. 1958;8:435–45.
47. Rogers SW, Andrews PI, Gahring LC, et al. Autoantibodies to glutamate receptor GluR3 in Rasmussen's encephalitis. Science. 1994;265:648–51.
48. He XP, Patel M, Whitney KD, et al. Glutamate receptor GluR3 antibodies and death of cortical cells. Neuron. 1998;20:153–63.
49. Aarli JA. Rasmussen's encephalitis: a challenge to neuroimmunology. Curr Opin Neurol. 2000;13:297–9.
50. Pleasure D. Diagnostic and pathogenic significance of glutamate receptor autoantibodies. Arch Neuorl. 2008;65(5):589–92.
51. Wiendl H, Bien CG, Bernasconi P, et al. GluR3 antibodies: prevalence in focal epilepsy but no specificity for Rasmussen's encephalitis. Neurology. 2001;57(8):1511–4.

52. Takahashi Y, Mori H, Mishina M, et al. Autoantibodies to NMDA receptor in patients with chronic forms of epilepsia partialis continua. Neurology. 2003;61:891–6.

53. Granata T, Fusco L, et al. Experience with immunomodulatory treatments in Rasmussen's encephalitis. Neurology. 2003;61(12):1807–10.

54. Leach JP, Chadwick DW, Miles JB, Hart IK. Improvement in adult-onset Rasmussen's encephalitis with long-term immunomodulatory therapy. Neurology. 1999;52:738–42.

55. Hart YM, Cortez M, Andermann F, et al. The medical treatment of Rasmussen's syndrome (Chronic encephalitis and epilepsy): effect of high dose steroids and/or immunoglobulins in 19 patients. Neurology. 1994;44:1030–6.

56. Andrews PI, Dichter MA, Berkovic SF, Newton MR, McNamara JO. Plasmapheresis in Rasmussen's encephalitis. Neurology. 1996;46:242–6.

57. Castillo P, Woodruff B, Caselli R, et al. Steroid-responsive encephalopathy associated with autoimmune thyroiditis. Arch Neurol. 2006;63:197–202.

58. Brain L, Jellinek E, Ball K. Hashimoto's disease and encephalopathy. Lancet. 1966;2:512–4.

59. Chong J, Rowland L, Utiger R. Hashimoto encephalopathy: syndrome or myth? Arch Neurol. 2003;60:164–71.

60. Shaw P, Walls T, Newman P, et al. Hashimoto's encephalopathy: a steroid-responsive disorder associated with high anti-thyroid antibody titers – report of 5 cases. Neurology. 1991;41:228–33.

61. Geschwind MD, Shu H, Haman A, et al. Rapidly progressive dementia. Ann Neurol. 2008;64(1):97–108.

62. Seipelt M, Zerr I, Nau R, et al. Hashimoto's encephalitis as a differential diagnosis of Creutzfeldt-Jakob disease. J Neurol Neurosurg Psychiatry. 1999;66:172–6.

63. Ferracci F, Moretto G, Candeago RM, et al. Antithyroid antibodies in the CSF: their role in the pathogenesis of Hashimoto's encephalopathy. Neurology. 2003; 60(4):712–4.

64. Forchetti CM, Katsamakis G, Garron DC. Autoimmune thyroiditis and a rapidly progressive dementia: global hypoperfusion on SPECT scanning suggests a possible mechanism. Neurology. 1997;49:623–6.

65. Mocellin R, Walterfang M, Velakoulis D. Hashimoto's encephalopathy: epidemiology, pathogenesis and management. CNS Drugs. 2007;21(10):799–811.

66. Nolte KW, Unbehaun A, Sieker H, et al. Hashimoto encephalopathy: a brainstem vasculitis? Neurology. 2000;54:769–70.

67. Palace J, Lang B. Epilepsy: an autoimmune disease? J Neurol Neurosurg Psychiatry. 2000;69:711–4.

68. Hussain NS, Rumbaugh J, Kerr D, et al. Effects of prednisone and plasma exchange on cognitive impairment in Hashimoto encephalopathy. Neurology. 2005;64(1):165–6.

69. Graus F, Dalmau J. Paraneoplastic neurological syndromes: diagnosis and treatment. Curr Opin Neurol. 2007;20:732–7.

70. Tuzun E, Dalmau J. Limbic encephalitis and variants: classification, diagnosis and treatment. Neurologist. 2007;13:261–71.

71. Pittock SJ, Kryzer TJ, Lennon VA. Paraneoplastic antibodies coexist and predict cancer, not neurological syndrome. Ann Neurol. 2004;56:715–9.

72. Bataller L, Galiano R, Garcia-Escrig M. Reversible paraneoplastic limbic encephalitis associated with antibodies to the AMPA receptor. Neurology. 2010;74(3): 265–7.

73. Voltz R, Gultekin SH, Rosenfeld MR, et al. A serological marker of paraneoplastic limbic and brain-stem encephalitis in patients with testicular cancer. N Engl J Med. 1999;340:1788–95.

74. Dalmau J, Tuzun E, Wu H-Y, et al. Paraneoplastic anti-N-methyl-D-aspartate receptor encephalitis associated with ovarian teratoma. Ann Neurol. 2007; 61(1):25–36.

75. Gulekin SH, Rosenfeld MR, Voltz R, et al. Paraneoplastic limbic encephalitis: neurological symptoms, immunological findings and tumour association in 50 patients. Brain. 2000;123:1481–94.
76. Graus F, Saiz A, Lai M, et al. Neuronal surface antigen antibodies in limbic encephalitis: clinical-immunologic associations. Neurology. 2008;7:1930–6.
77. Vincent A, Buckley C, Schott JM, et al. Potassium channel antibody-associated encephalopathy: a potentially immunotherapy-responsive form of limbic encephalitis. Brain. 2004;127(3):701–12.
78. Tan KM, Lennon VA, Klein CJ, et al. Clinical spectrum of voltage-gated potassium channel autoimmunity. Neurology. 2008;70:1883–90.
79. Rueff L, Graber JJ, Bernbaum M, Kuzniecky RI. Voltage-gated potassium channel antibody-mediated syndromes: a spectrum of clinical manifestations. Rev Neurol Dis. 2008;5(2):65–72.
80. Geschwind MD, Tan KM, Lennon VA, et al. Voltage-gated potassium channel autoimmunity mimicking Creutzfeldt-Jakob disease. Arch Neurol. 2008;65(10):1341–6.
81. Novillo-Lopez ME, Rossi JE, Dalmau J, Masjuan J. Treatment-responsive subacute limbic encephalitis and NMDA receptor antibodies in a man. Neurology. 2008;70(9):728–9.
82. Iizuka T, Sakai F, Ide T, et al. Anti-NMDA receptor encephalitis in Japan: long-term outcome without tumor removal. Neurology. 2008;70:504–11.
83. Nasky KM, Knittel DR, Manos GH. Psychosis associated with anti-N-methyl-D-aspartate receptor antibodies. CNS Spectr. 2008;13(8):699–702.
84. Pittock SJ, Yoshikawa H, Ahlskog JE, et al. Glutamic acid decarboxylase autoimmunity with brainstem, extrapyramidal, and spinal cord dysfunction. Mayo Clin Proc. 2006;81(9):1207–14.
85. Honnorat J, Saiz A, Giometto B, et al. Cerebellar ataxia with anti-glutamic acid decarboxylase antibodies: study of 14 patients. Arch Neurol. 2001;58:225–30.
86. Reetz A, Solimena M, Matteoli M, et al. GABA and pancreatic beta-cells: colocalization of glutamic acid decarboxylase (GAD) and GABA with synaptic-like microvesicles suggests their role in GABA storage and secretion. EMBO J. 1991;10:1275–84.
87. Zimmet PZ, Shaten BJ, Kuller LH, et al. Antibodies to glutamic acid decarboxylase and diabetes mellitus in the multiple risk factor intervention trial. Am J Epidemiol. 1994;140:683–90.
88. Darnell RB, Victor J, Rubin M, et al. A novel antineuronal antibody in stiff-man syndrome. Neurology. 1993;43(1):114–20.
89. Solimena M, Folli F, Aparisi R, et al. Auto-antibodies to GABAergic neurons and pancreatic beta cells in stiff-man syndrome. N Engl J Med. 1990;322:1555–60.
90. Meinck HM, Thompson PD. Research review: stiff man syndrome and related conditions. Mov Disord. 2002;17(5):853–66.
91. Peltola J, Kulmala P, Isojarvi J, et al. Autoantibodies to glutamic acid decarboxylase in patients with therapy-resistant epilepsy. Neurology. 2000;55:46–50.
92. Mazzi G, DeRoia D, Cruciatti B, et al. Plasma exchange for anti GAD associated non paraneoplastic limbic encephalitis. Transfus Apher Sci. 2008;39(3):229–33.
93. Saiz Al, Blanco Y, Sabater L, et al. Spectrum of neurological syndromes associated with glutamic acid decarboxylase antibodies: diagnostic clues for this association. Brain. 2008;131(10):2553–63.
94. Mata S, Muscas GC, Naldi I, et al. Non-paraneoplastic limbic encephalitis associated with anti-glutamic acid decarboxylase antibodies. J Neuroimmunol. 2008;199:155–9.
95. Nemni R, Braghi S, Natali-Sora MG, et al. Autoantibodies to glutamic acid decarboxylase in palatal myoclonus and epilepsy. Ann Neurol. 1994;36:665–7.
96. Giomotto B, Nicolao P, Macucci M, et al. Temporal-lobe epilepsy associated with glutamic-acid-decarboxylase autoantibodies. Lancet. 1998;352:457.

97. Yoshimoto T, Doi M, Fukai N, et al. Type I diabetes mellitus and drug-resistant epilepsy: presence of high titer of anti-glutamic acid decarboxylase autoantibodies in serum and cerebrospinal fluid. Intern Med. 2005;44:1174–7.

98. Vulliemoz S, Vanini G, Truffert A, et al. Epilepsy and cerebellar ataxia associated with anti-glutamic acid decarboxylase antibodies. J Neurol Neurosurg Psychiatry. 2007;78:187–9.

99. Kanter IC, Huttner HB, Staykov D, et al. Cyclophosphamide for anti-GAD antibody-positive refractory status epilepticus. Epilepsia. 2007;49:914–20.

100. Bartolomei F, Boucraut J, Barrie M, et al. Cryptogenic partial epilepsy's with anti-GM1 antibodies: a new form of immune-mediated epilepsy? Epilepsia. 1996;37:922–6.

101. Connolly AM, Chez MG, Pestronk A, et al. Serum antibodies to brain in Laundau-Kleffner variant, autism and other neurological disorders. J Pediatr. 1999;134:607–13.

102. Bradley WG, Daroff RB, Fenichel GM, Jankovic J. Neurology in clinical practice. 4th ed. Philadelphia: Elsevier; 2004.

103. Gobbi G, Bouquet F, Greco L, et al. Coeliac disease, epilepsy and cerebral calcifications: The Italian working group on celiac disease and epilepsy. Lancet. 1992;340(8817):439–43.

104. Ebersole JS, Pedley TA. Current practice of clinical electroencephalography. Philadelphia: Lippincott Williams and Wilkins; 2003.

105. Ransohoff R. Immunology: barrier to electrical storms: epilepsy is characterized by repetitive seizures due to abnormal electrical activity in the brain. Immune cells promote development of this disorder by mediating the breakdown of the blood-brain barrier. Nature. 2009;457(7226):155–6.

106. Tamagno G, Federspil G, Murialdo G. Clinical and diagnostic aspects of encephalopathy associated with autoimmune thyroid disease (or Hashimoto's encephalopathy). Intern Emerg Med. 2006;1(1):15–23.

16

Autoimmune Movement Disorders

Victoria C. Chang

Keywords: Ataxia, Chorea, Paraneoplastic syndromes, Parkinsonism, Tremor, Neuromyotonia

Introduction

Neurologic movement disorders caused by an autoimmune system response phenomenologically span all categories of abnormal movements, but consist mostly of hyperkinetic movement conditions such as chorea, stiffening syndromes, myoclonus, tics, and ataxias. A growing subset of immune-mediated movement disorders is the post-streptococcal neuropsychiatric disorders, some of which remain controversial and many of which remain to be more clearly defined. Paraneoplastic disorders, including anti-NMDA receptor encephalitis, have been covered in another chapter and will only be briefly discussed in this review.

As a whole, the incidence and prevalence of autoimmune movement disorders are difficult to ascertain due to the lack of epidemiological studies. With the exception of Sydenham's chorea, this is most likely a product of this being a continually evolving group of disorders that are still developing specific definitions with ongoing investigations into their immunological mechanisms.

Classification

The autoimmune-mediated neurological movement disorders can be classified most easily by known and currently proposed etiologies. They can be also delineated by phenomenology for those that appear to encompass one particular type of movement or whose immunological mechanisms are less clearly defined (Tables 16.1 and 16.2). The emergence of movement disorders other than Sydenham's chorea felt to be associated with streptococcal infections in the last two decades of literature has made it necessary to mention this as a manner of classification as well. For clarity, we will discuss conditions first in

From: *Clinical Neuroimmunology: Multiple Sclerosis and Related Disorders*, Current Clinical Neurology,
Edited by: S.A. Rizvi and P.K. Coyle, DOI 10.1007/978-1-60327-860-7_16,
© Springer Science+Business Media, LLC 2011

Table 16.1 Autoimmune etiologies of movement disorders.

Paraneoplastic syndromes

Post-infectious

    Bacterial (a β-hemolytic group A streptococci)

      Sydenham's chorea, PANDAS

Systemic autoimmune disorders

    SLE, anti-phospholipid Ab syndrome

Channelopathies (anti-VGKC)

    Neuromyotonia

Unknown or idiopathic

    Encephalitis lethargica, ADEM

Table 16.2 Phenomenology of movement disorders.

Stiffness/rigidity

Tics

Ataxia

Parkinsonism

Tremors

Chorea/ballism

Dyskinesias

Dystonia

Myoclonus

Opsoclonus-myoclonus

Catatonia

the context of post-streptococcal neuropsychiatric disorders, then followed by those not necessarily preceded by or associated with streptococcal infections.

Post-streptococcal Neuropsychiatric Movement Disorders

To date Sydenham's chorea is the only movement disorder that has been confirmed as a consequence of Group Aβ-hemolytic streptococcal infection and serves as the prototype for those movement disorders that have been subsequently described. The evidence available for the other conditions felt induced by streptococcal infections is not yet definitive. They include tics [1], paroxysmal dystonic choreoathetosis [2], dystonia [3], tremor [4], parkinsonism [5], myoclonus [6], opsoclonus myoclonus [7], as well as a post-streptococcal form of encephalitis lethargica and ADEM [8, 9]. Many of these illnesses have been predominantly found in the pediatric population, but there have been some adult cases also described.

Sydenham's Chorea

Sydenham's chorea has been accepted as being a consequence of group Aβ-hemolytic streptococcal infection and is one of the major criterion of diagnosis of rheumatic fever in the Jones Criteria [10]. It can occur in 10–30% of patients who contract acute rheumatic fever, is more common in females and predominantly affects the pediatric population between ages 5 and 15. Motor characteristics include generalized, though often asymmetric, random, rapid, jerky movements (chorea) that can range from mild distal chorea to more proximal larger amplitude chorea (ballism), decreased muscle tone, difficulty with speech, ocular motion abnormalities, and impairment of gait and balance [11]. Chorea is the most well-known abnormal movement manifestation, but in some opinions it is felt to encompass other phenomenologies, mainly tics, thus proposing the condition be termed Sydenham's disease [12]. Neuropsychiatric issues were described as well early on in the twentieth century and have been more closely examined in recent years. They can include attentional problems, obsessive compulsive traits, irritability, emotional lability, anxiety, and oppositional behavior [13, 14]. The appearance of both motor and behavioral components is latent, can occur up to 6 months after the acute infection and resolve in 3–4 months, though they can persist up to 2 years in some observations [15]. Sometimes Sydenham's chorea is the only manifestation of acute rheumatic fever.

The established mechanism is of antibody cross-reactivity where anti-streptococcal antibodies produced in response to an infection also affect normal structures in the skin, heart, joints, and brain [16–18]. It has been shown that antibodies react with the subthalamic and caudate nuclei neurons in patients with chorea and acute rheumatic fever [19]. Standard treatment involves antibiotic administration to target the underlying streptococcal infection for the prevention of acute rheumatic fever and its cardiac sequelae. Steroid therapy is sometimes necessary though has variable results [20, 21]. If the chorea is mild and non-bothersome, no symptomatic treatment is necessary, but for more troublesome movements, valproic acid is the treatment of choice. Neuroleptics should be used only if symptoms are severe given the risk of acute or chronic abnormal movement reactions associated with these medications. Intravenous immunoglobulin treatment and plasma exchange have been used with some success, although evidence for a significant response is lacking [22]. Further studies are required to see if these immunomodulatory measures should become part of routine management.

PANDAS

Pediatric autoimmune neuropsychiatric disorders associated with streptococcal infections (PANDAS) was first introduced into the literature in 1998 by Swedo and colleagues. The diagnostic criteria include as follows.

- Presence of obsessive–compulsive disorder (OCD) and/or tic disorder (either or both meeting their DSM-IV diagnostic criteria).
- Pediatric onset (between 3 years and onset of puberty).
- Abrupt onset or dramatic exacerbations with episodic course of symptoms.
- Temporal relation between GAS infection and onset and/or exacerbation by positive throat culture or elevated anti-GABHS antibody titers.
- Neurologic abnormalities on exam, such as motoric hyperactivity (including choreiform movements and tics) [23].

Since its appearance, it has remained a controversial topic in the movement disorders community given the common occurrences of tic disorders and streptococcal infections in the pediatric population. It is known that tic disorders typically wax and wane and are often worsened in the setting of an acute infection [24]. There is also debate regarding the types of movements seen in the condition and how they are specifically defined (i.e., "choreiform" movements versus "frank" chorea). In addition to these issues, the indistinct temporal window between GAS infection and symptom onset have also caused difficulty in making accurate diagnoses. Given the perspective that Sydenham's may at times include other type of movements, mainly tics, as well as the inclusion of choreiform movements in the PANDAS criteria, one could argue that these two conditions might be variants of the same disease, but this remains to be more rigorously delineated [25].

At this time treatment for PANDAS focuses mainly on symptomatic treatment for movement and behavioral issues, much like the management of all other tic disorders. Antimicrobial administration [26–29] remains inconclusive, and immunomodulatory treatments that have been explored, while showing some promise for improvement in symptoms, have some methodological criticisms [30–32] and are still felt to be investigational. Though it continues to be disputed whether this is truly a distinct entity, PANDAS has established itself enough in the literature and neurological parlance to warrant continued discussion and clarification. Identification of this particular category as a clinically useful construct will require further standardization of evaluations for the movements observed, preferably by pediatric movement disorders specialists, methods of investigation, and treatment response outcomes [33].

Other Post-streptococcal Movement Disorders

Some studies have proposed that encephalitis lethargica and acute disseminated encephalomyelitis (ADEM) may be included in the spectra of Sydenham's chorea and PANDAS. Dale and colleagues have described 20 modern cases of encephalitis lethargica many with elevated anti-streptolysin-O titers and autoantibodies against basal ganglia antigens. The movements found in these patients included parkinsonism, dystonia, chorea/hemiballism, tics, stereotypies, facial grimacing, blepharospasm, and oculogyric crises [9]. ADEM has likewise been studied by this group with similar laboratory findings and included the addition of abnormal imaging in contrast to ADEM cases not associated with streptococcal infections. Movements described in this chapter which looked at ten children from ages 3 to 14 included hemidystonia and parkinsonism where the dystonic presentation was found in 50% and was accompanied quite commonly with behavioral disturbances such as emotional lability, inappropriate laughter, anxiety, and confusion [8]. Another case described choreiform movements and elevated ASO titers, but negative anti-DNAse B [34] ADEM not associated after streptococcal infections have not been characteristically associated with abnormal movements, though there is one case that has described segmental myoclonus [35]. The clinical descriptions of the post-streptococcal ADEM patients appear to closely resemble some of the original descriptions of encephalitis lethargica which will be discussed in more detail below.

Non-post-streptococcal Autoimmune Movement Disorders

The movement disorders described in this section are felt not to be a result of post-streptococcal infections, and most have been described to occur at times within the context of paraneoplastic syndromes. These conditions often encompass more than one phenomenology, though there are some that exhibit certain predominant types of movement.

Stiff and Rigid Syndromes

Stiff-person syndrome is a disorder that involves fluctuating muscular rigidity and spasms affecting primarily the axial muscles of the back and abdomen as well as the hips and shoulders [36]. It affects males and females equally and normally begins in the 4th to 5th decades. Often it can lead to slowly progressive hyperlordosis of the back due to continual contraction of the paraspinals and abdomen and, along with proximal limb involvement, results in a stiff appearing gait and sometimes frequent falls. At times, stiffness can spread to the thoracic area affecting respirations. Muscle spasms can occur often triggered by high-emotional states including anxiety and excitement, noise, or other external stimuli and there can be an exaggerated startle reflex. It is often associated with insulin-dependent diabetes in 30% and epilepsy in 10% of patients that can create additional complications in the patient's clinical course. Anti-glutamic acid decarboxylase (GAD) antibodies are found in both serum and CSF in more than 60% of patients [37]. There is some evidence that these play a pathogenic role in destroying GABAergic inhibitory mechanisms in the spinal cord, and along with impairment of intracortical inhibitory neurons creates the characteristic muscle stiffness [38, 39]. Electrophysiology reveals continuous motor unit activity that can be abolished by agents that increase GABA neurotransmission. Other movements that have been seen in the clinical presentation primarily consist of cerebellar ataxia [40, 41]. A smaller subset of stiff-person syndrome can also be seen in association with antiamphiphysin I antibodies in breast cancer patients [42, 43]. A variant of stiff-person syndrome is stiff-leg syndrome which is similar in symptomatology and antibody workup, with the exception of presenting asymmetrically in one leg, and may be a focal presentation of the condition. Treatment includes medications that enhance GABA neurotransmission such as benzodiazepines, baclofen, depakote, and vigabitran. Tizanidine has also been found to be helpful in the management of spasms and sometimes intrathecal baclofen is necessary for symptom control. Of the immunomodulatory treatments, intravenous immunoglobulin [44] has been the most promising and rituximab is being further studied for refractory cases [45].

Progressive encephalomyelitis and rigidity, formerly known as spinal interneuronitis, is a condition that is characterized by a relentless course of painful irritable muscles and is now felt to be a severe form of stiff-person syndrome. Patients develop a relentless and progressive course that includes pain, dysesthesia, weakness, stiffness, clumsiness, and rigidity. Eventually bulbar control is affected, along with cognitive impairment, autonomic involvement, long tract signs, myoclonus, and extensor trunk spasm. It has a much poorer prognosis compared with stiff-person syndrome as symptoms progress to death within 3 years [46–48]. There is some speculation of association with glycine receptor antibodies [49]. Clinical improvement has been reported in cases treated with corticosteroids [50, 51], IVIg [52], and rituximab [53].

Neuromyotonia, the most well-known form being Isaacs' syndrome, is a type of peripheral nerve hyperexcitability that causes spontaneous muscular activity. It is classified as one of the autoimmune neurological channelopathies, which are disorders of muscle or nerve function caused by aberrant membrane excitability due to functional disturbances of ion channels. Eighty percent of all cases are acquired and is suspected to be autoimmune mediated, possibly involving antibodies against voltage-gated potassium channels affecting the neuromuscular junction [54]. The resultant gain-of-function causes prolonged action potentials and repetitive discharges. Presentation can be variable and fluctuating, but include generalized muscle cramps, stiffness, fasciculations, and pseudomyotonia, and predominantly affect the limbs and trunk. Diagnosis is clinical and workup should include electroneurophysiology testing that reveals spontaneous, continuous, doublet, or multiplet single motor unit discharges, firing irregularly at a high intraburst frequencies of up to 190 Hz [55]. Prognosis is good and symptoms are typically manageable. Often immunomodulatory management is not necessary and anticonvulsant medications such as phenytoin and carbamazepine provide adequate relief of symptoms. In more severe cases, plasma exchange and IVIg treatment in some cases have shown short-term improvement, and immunosuppressants, such as prednisone may provide longer-term relief [55, 56].

Encephalitis Lethargica

Between the years of 1916 and 1927, an epidemic encephalitis occurred predominantly throughout western Europe and North America which left survivors with a variety of movement disorders. First described by Constantin von Economo in 1917, it was termed encephalitis lethargica due a characteristic aspect of its acute phase where patients presented with progressive somnolence and lethargy [57]. Common accompanying symptoms included fever, ophthalmoplegia, pharyngitis, headache, fatigue, parkinsonism, and confusion. CSF lymphocytic pleiocytosis [50–100] was often found, and in more serious presentations, patients succumbed to a prolonged coma-like state after which 40% died. Varied presentations have been categorized into several subtypes with the most common being a clinical picture of somnolence, ophthalmoplegia, and parkinsonism, though a hyperkinetic form was also recognized [58]. If they survived the acute phase, recovery involved a spectrum from complete return to baseline to a host of residual behavioral, respiratory, sleep, and movement disorders sometimes appearing after months or years [59, 60]. Fifty percent of survivors became parkinsonian in 5 years and 80% in 10 years. Many of those who contracted the encephalitis were children and youths with the average age of parkinsonism developing in their late 1920s. Epidemiologic observations noted that post-encephalitic parkinsonism from encephalitis lethargica was one of the most common forms of parkinsonism in the first half of the twentieth century [61, 62]. While parkinsonism appears to be the most well-known movement sequelae from encephalitis lethargica, other abnormal movements found in both the acute and latent forms included oculogyric crises, catatonia, blepharospasm, palilalia, dystonia, tics, hiccups, akinetic mutism, chorea, and myoclonus [63, 64]. Cases continued to be reported in large numbers during and following the initial epidemic, peaking in the mid-1920s but then disappeared from the literature for 10 years after the start of World War II. Sparse reports began appearing from 1949 on with isolated cases less severe than the original descriptions. A recurrence of epidemic proportions has not been described since.

Its course and clinical findings suggested an infective cause, and given the concomitant H1N1 influenza pandemic (the Spanish influenza) of approximately the same time period, much speculation occurred throughout the years regarding a possible connection; however, modern postmortem studies failed to find evidence of the virus [65, 66]. It still remains a possibility for some investigators [67] as mechanisms other than direct invasion of the CNS involving more acute on chronic activation of the immune system are postulated where future damage is done by a subsequent insult triggering an overwhelming autoimmune response [68]. A recent mouse model showing destruction of dopaminergic neurons after infection by an H5N1 bird flu strain which can invade the CNS suggests that this might be a possibility in humans [69]. Evidence with western immunoblotting has revealed 95% (19 out of 20) patients had autoantibodies against human basal ganglia antigens as opposed to 2–4% of controls that included both children and adults [9]. Apart from purported mechanisms, acute pathological findings appear to involve more cortical and meningeal damage with inflammation, hyperemia, and congestion [70], whereas the later stages have a predilection for neuronal loss and gliosis to the brainstem and basal ganglia structures with neurofibrillary tau pathology and absence of α-synuclein [71].

In reviewing some of the historical cases, it is interesting to compare their descriptions with observations of the currently reported encephalitides that have abnormal movements. The similarities that appear bring up the possibility that some of the initial cases of encephalitis lethargica described could have been consistent with ADEM or NMDAR encephalitis or perhaps vice versa; the latter being at a disadvantage without the benefit of further characterization through imaging and modern laboratory and antibody studies.

The treatment of encephalitis lethargica at initial presentation is supportive for any cardiopulmonary complications and symptomatic for the movement and neuropsychiatric manifestations, though there may be some benefit to steroid therapy or IVIg administration [72, 73]. For the acute phase, tetrabenazine, a VMAT inhibitor and monoamine depletor, has been found to have some benefit. For presentations that have myoclonus agents such as clonazepam may also be helpful [74]. In the later phase, levodopa can be useful to manage the parkinsonism and can provide dramatic improvement at times, though with variable results [75, 76].

Autoimmune Movement Disorders Associated with Systemic Inflammatory Conditions

Antiphospholipid syndrome (APS) is an autoimmune hematologic disorder that impairs coagulation leading to vascular and arterial thrombosis throughout the body. Abnormal movements, primarily chorea, occur in approximately

2% of patients. Systemic lupus erythematosus (SLE) is closely associated with APS and has a similar occurrence. Other movements that have been described include dystonia, oral dyskinesias, paroxysmal dyskinesias, myoclonus, tics, tremor, and parkinsonism [77–79]. While a proportion of neurological manifestations from these conditions can be localized to thrombotic sequelae, there have been a number of reports of abnormal movements in the absence of cerebral infarcts [80]. Functional neuroimaging cases in patients with transient chorea without stroke show that there are changes in striatal metabolism that may suggest inflammatory activity [81, 82].

An interesting observation in these patients as well as those without APS or SLE has been the descriptions of chorea induced by either pregnancy (chorea gravidarum) or oral contraceptive medicines. While this phenomenon has been described in the presence of autoantibodies to the basal ganglia [83], it has not been proven to have an autoimmune mechanism. Rather, it seems, those with previous subclinical damage to the striatum via rheumatic fever, infarction, or in the setting of SLE or APS may be more susceptible to developing chorea. It is thought that the hormonal changes that occur affects dopaminergic action directly or does so by binding to catechol-O-methyltransferase resulting in an accumulation of cerebral dopamine [84].

Paraneoplastic Syndromes

There have been a variety of abnormal movements seen in the setting of paraneoplastic syndromes including opsoclonus myoclonus (associated with neuroblastoma in children or breast cancer in adults) and ataxia (with or without other neurological symptoms) which have been well-described. Other movements observed include chorea, dyskinesia, dystonia, stiffening and hyperexcitable syndromes, and rarely parkinsonism [85]. A relatively newly described condition is N-methyl-D-aspartate receptor (NMDAR) encephalitis which appeared in the clinical literature in 2007 and is characterized by psychosis, cognitive deficits, seizures, unresponsiveness, abnormal movements, and autonomic dysfunction [86]. The variety of movements observed include restlessness, chorea and choreoathetoid movements (including ballism), dystonia (including oculogyric crises), myoclonus, catatonia-like states, and opisthotonic posturing, with the most classic movements being oral-lingual-facial dyskinesias [87]. Though a malignancy is not always found, approximately 60% of NMDAR encephalitis cases have been associated with ovarian teratomas [88]. Paraneoplastic disorders are discussed in more detail in a separate chapter.

Speculations on Other Phenomenologies

Tic Disorders

Much of the interest into tic disorders and a potential autoimmune mechanism is tied closely to the post-streptococcal investigations. Anti-basal ganglia antibodies have been found in various tic disorders and seem to be associated with higher anti-streptolysin-O titers [89]. Their presence in Tourette's syndrome (TS) has been somewhat controversial and other studies that have sought to induce tic-like symptoms in mouse and rat models with sera from patients with TS and PANDAS have been inconsistent [90, 91].

Ataxia

Autoimmune ataxias have been largely described in the context of paraneoplastic disorders, but are commonly observed in other settings. Monosymptomatic postinfectious illnesses have been associated with acute cerebellar ataxia in the pediatric population with varicella infection being the most common antecedent, though Epstein–Barr virus, influenza, HSV, among others have been identified [92–94]. Proposed pathophysiology involves cross-reactivity between antibodies against these infectious agents and cerebellar epitopes resulting in demyelination [95]. A study looking at idiopathic sporadic ataxia reveals that many cases had a higher prevalence of autoimmune disorders and anti-cerebellar antibodies than those with genetic ataxia suggesting that some ataxias of unknown etiology may actually have an immune-mediated pathology [96]. One of the proposed conditions is with gluten-sensitive diseases and their associated antibodies, but this connection remains uncertain [97].

Parkinsonism

Parkinsonism has been discussed above within encephalitis lethargica and mentioned as an uncommon post-streptococcal phenomenon, but the etiology of classic Parkinson's disease (PD) remains elusive. While there has been some conjecture of PD having an immune-mediated etiology given the presence of some inflammatory markers, it remains unclear if these reflect primary or secondary changes in nigral degeneration. The inflammation found is likely only one of many components involved in the general process of neurodegeneration. These changes appear to be nonspecific to PD and with the additional lack of HLA association an autoimmune mechanism is not supported at this time.

Antibodies in Autoimmune Movement Disorders

Antineuronal antibodies including anti-basal ganglia antibodies have been increasingly looked at in conditions with abnormal movements felt to have an autoimmune mechanism. Anti-basal ganglia Abs (ABGA) were first described by Husby in 1976 in patients with chorea and acute rheumatic fever and have been subsequently described in various other movement disorders. In the setting of streptococcal infections, antineuronal antibodies were higher in frequency in children with acute movement disorders than in those without [98], and they may have some specificity to post-streptococcal neuropsychiatric disorders and potential sensitivity in diagnosing Sydenham's chorea in particular [99, 100]. Having said this, the correlation between PSNDs and ABGAs, including Sydenham's chorea, and its significance are still being defined. Other non-paraneoplastic neuronal antibodies include those against, glutamic acid decarboxylase (anti-GAD), phospholipid antibodies (including lupus anticoagulant and anti-cardiolipin antibodies), and voltage-gated potassium channel (anti-VGKC). Paraneoplastic syndromes are associated with a variety of serum antibodies, some that are well-characterized than others [101].

The main antibodies that have described in association with movement disorders have been summarized in Tables 16.3 and 16.4 with respect to general

Table 16.3 Paraneoplastic movement disorders antibodies.

	Yo (PCA1)	Ri (ANNA-2)	Hu (ANNA-1)	Tr	Ma (2)	Ta	CV2 (CRMP5)	NMDA	PCA2	ANNA-3	VGCCA	MGluR1	Purkinje	Amphiphysin	P/Q type Ca channels
Opsoclonus-myoclonus		X	X										X		
Oro-facial/lingual dyskinesias								X							
Chorea	X		X				X	X							
Tics/OCD															
Stiff person														X	
Neuromyotonia															
Progressive encephalomyelitis and rigidity		X													
Ataxia	X	X	X				X				X	X			X
Dystonia								X							
Myoclonus								X						X	
Other tremor															
Parkinsonism					X	X									
Catatonia								X							

Table 16.4 Non-paraneoplastic movement disorders antibodies.

	Anti-BG	Anti-GAD	Anti-glycine receptor	Anti-phospholipid Abs (lupus anticoagulant anti-cardiolipin β-2-glycoprotein I)	Anti-VGKC	Homer 3
Opsoclonus-myoclonus						
Oro-facial/lingual dyskinesias						
Chorea	X			X		
Tics/OCD	X					
Stiff person		X	X			
Neuromyotonia					X	
Progressive encephalomyelitis and rigidity			X			
Ataxia		X	X			X
Dystonia	X	X				
Myoclonus						
Other tremor		X (palatal)				
Parkinsonism	X					
Catatonia						

etiology (i.e., paraneoplastic versus non-paraneoplastic) and phenomenology [19, 85, 98, 101, 102]. When viewing these tables, for all the newer antibodies, the specificity and sensitivity of the immunohistochemistry methods used are still being improved. Also, with respect to those movements dealing with ABGA's, one must keep in mind that many of these investigations were done in selected populations who also had streptococcal infections and presence of other antibodies cannot be ruled out. The specific involvement of these antibodies in inducing abnormal movements remains unclear. Some are thought to impart pathogenesis more than others, and some may be simply a result of local damage. Further delineation of their clinical role is ongoing.

Conclusion

Autoimmune -mediated movement disorders remain an evolving category in the field of neuroimmunology. Of the post-streptococcal disorders only Sydenham's chorea has been shown to have benefit from antibiotic prophylaxis and is mainly guided by the prevention of rheumatic fever and its possible cardiac manifestations. The remainder, including PANDAS, should focus on symptomatic treatment for both the abnormal movements and neuropsychiatric manifestations. In these conditions, yet to be further defined, antibiotic treatment and immunomodulatory regimens remain investigational and are not recommended as standard of therapy until further evidence emerges. The role of immune system modifying agents is sound in the established autoimmune conditions and in those with significant morbidity and mortality refractory to symptomatic treatments. In the case of suspected paraneoplastic syndromes, investigation and treatment of any underlying malignancy should be done promptly.

The varied presentations of both hypokinetic and hyperkinetic movements in these disorders, sometimes within the same patient, speaks to the complexity of the basal ganglia, midbrain, cerebellum, and their connections with each other and the cortex. With further characterization of the autoimmune movement disorders, and improving potential biomarker methods, the phenomenology of these conditions can be better utilized to recognize particular syndromes and guide workup, diagnosis, and management.

References

1. Mercadante MT, Campos MC, Marques-Dias MJ, Miguel EC, Leckman J. Vocal tics in Sydenham's chorea. J Am Acad Child Adolesc Psychiatry. 1997;36(3):305–6.
2. Dale RC, Church AJ, Surtees RA, Thompson EJ, Giovannoni G, Neville BG. Post-streptococcal autoimmune neuropsychiatric disease presenting as paroxysmal dystonic choreoathetosis. Mov Disord. 2002;17(4):817–20.
3. Dale RC, Church AJ, Benton S, et al. Post-streptococcal autoimmune dystonia with isolated bilateral striatal necrosis. Dev Med Child Neurol. 2002;44(7):485–9.
4. Dale RC, Heyman I, Surtees RA, et al. Dyskinesias and associated psychiatric disorders following streptococcal infections. Arch Dis Child. 2004;89(7):604–10.
5. McKee DH, Sussman JD. Case report: severe acute Parkinsonism associated with streptococcal infection and antibasal ganglia antibodies. Mov Disord. 2005;20(12):1661–3.
6. DiFazio MP, Morales J, Davis R. Acute myoclonus secondary to group A beta-hemolytic streptococcus infection: a PANDAS variant. J Child Neurol. 1998;13(10):516–8.
7. Dassan P, Clarke C, Sharp DJ. A case of poststreptococcal opsoclonus-myoclonus syndrome. Mov Disord. 2007;22(10):1490–1.
8. Dale RC, Church AJ, Cardoso F, et al. Poststreptococcal acute disseminated encephalomyelitis with basal ganglia involvement and auto-reactive antibasal ganglia antibodies. Ann Neurol. 2001;50(5):588–95.
9. Dale RC, Church AJ, Surtees RA, et al. Encephalitis lethargica syndrome: 20 new cases and evidence of basal ganglia autoimmunity. Brain. 2004;127(Pt 1):21–33.
10. Gerber MA, Baltimore RS, Eaton CB, et al. Prevention of rheumatic fever and diagnosis and treatment of acute Streptococcal pharyngitis: a scientific statement from the American Heart Association Rheumatic Fever, Endocarditis, and Kawasaki Disease Committee of the Council on Cardiovascular Disease in the Young, the Interdisciplinary Council on Functional Genomics and Translational Biology, and the Interdisciplinary Council on Quality of Care and Outcomes Research: endorsed by the American Academy of Pediatrics. Circulation. 2009;119(11):1541–51.
11. Cardoso F, Eduardo C, Silva AP, Mota CCC. Chorea in fifty consecutive patients with rheumatic fever. Mov Disord. 1997;12(5):701–3.
12. Fahn S, Jankovic J, Hallet M, Jenner P. Principles and practice of movement disorders. Philadelphia: Churchill Livingstone Elsevier; 2007.
13. Swedo SE, Leonard HL, Schapiro MB, et al. Sydenham's chorea: physical and psychological symptoms of St Vitus dance. Pediatrics. 1993;91(4):706–13.
14. Moore DP. Neuropsychiatric aspects of Sydenham's chorea: a comprehensive review. J Clin Psychiatry. 1996;57(9):407–14.
15. Cardoso F, Vargas AP, Oliveira LD, Guerra AA, Amaral SV. Persistent Sydenham's chorea. Mov Disord. 1999;14(5):805–7.
16. Kingston D, Glynn LE. A cross-reaction between Str. pyogenes and human fibroblasts, endothelial cells and astrocytes. Immunology. 1971;21(6):1003–16.

17. Dorling J, Kingston D, Webb JA. Anti-streptococcal antibodies reacting with brain tissue. II. Ultrastructural studies. Br J Exp Pathol. 1976;57(3):255–65.
18. Kingston D, Glynn LE. Anti-streptococcal antibodies reacting with brain tissue. I. Immunofluourescent studies. Br J Exp Pathol. 1976;57(1):114–28.
19. Husby G, Van De Rijn I, Zabriskie JB, Abdin ZH, Williams RC. Antibodies reacting with cytoplasm of subthalamic and caudate nuclei neurons in chorea and acute rheumatic fever. J Exp Med. 1976;144(4):1094–110.
20. Green LN. Corticosteroids in the treatement of Sydenham's chorea. Arch Neurol. 1978;35:53–4.
21. Cardoso F, Maia D, Cunningham MC, Valenca G. Treatment of Sydenham chorea with corticosteroids. Mov Disord. 2003;18(11):1374–7.
22. Garvey MA, Snider LA, Leitman SF, Werden R, Swedo SE. Treatment of Sydenham's chorea with intravenous immunoglobulin, plasma exchange, or prednisone. J Child Neurol. 2005;20(5):424–9.
23. Swedo SE, Leonard HL, Garvey M, et al. Pediatric autoimmune neuropsychiatric disorders associated with streptococcal infections: clinical description of the first 50 cases. Am J Psychiatry. 1998;155(2):264–71.
24. Singer HS, Giuliano JD, Zimmerman AM, Walkup JT. Infection: a stimulus for tic disorders. Pediatr Neurol. 2000;22(5):380–3.
25. Murphy TK, Goodman WK, Ayoub EM, Voeller KK. On defining Sydenham's chorea: where do we draw the line? Biol Psychiatry. 2000;47(10):851–7.
26. Garvey MA, Perlmutter SJ, Allen AJ, et al. A pilot study of penicillin prophylaxis for neuropsychiatric exacerbations triggered by streptococcal infections. Biol Psychiatry. 1999;45(12):1564–71.
27. Snider LA, Lougee L, Slattery M, Grant P, Swedo SE. Antibiotic prophylaxis with azithromycin or penicillin for childhood-onset neuropsychiatric disorders. Biol Psychiatry. 2005;57(7):788–92.
28. Gilbert D, Gerber MA. Regarding "antibiotic prophylaxis with azithromycin or penicillin for childhood-onset neuropsychiatric disorders." Biol Psychiatry. 2005;58(11):916.
29. Budman C, Coffey B, Dure L, et al. Regarding "antibiotic prophylaxis with azithromycin or penicillin for childhood-onset neuropsychiatric disorders". Biol Psychiatry. 2005;58(11):917. author reply 918–919.
30. Allen AJ, Leonard HL, Swedo SE. Case study: a new infection-triggered, autoimmune subtype of pediatric OCD and Tourette's syndrome. J Am Acad Child Adolesc Psychiatry. 1995;34(3):307–11.
31. Perlmutter SJ, Leitman SF, Garvey MA, et al. Therapeutic plasma exchange and intravenous immunoglobulin for obsessive-compulsive disorder and tic disorders in childhood. Lancet. 1999;354(9185):1153–8.
32. Singer HS. PANDAS and immunomodulatory therapy. Lancet. 1999;354(9185):1137–8.
33. Mink J, Kurlan R. Acute postinfectious movement and psychiatric disorders in children and adolescents. J Child Neurol. 2011;26(2):214–7.
34. Ha AD, Sue C. ADEM presenting as a movement disorder. Mov Disord. 2010;25(14):2464–6.
35. Kabakus N, Taskin E, Aydin M. Segmental myoclonus as the presenting symptom of an acute disseminated encephalomyelitis: a case report. Eur J Paediatr Neurol. 2006;10(1):45–8.
36. Moersch FP, Woltman HW. Progressive fluctuating muscular rigidity and spasm ("stiff-man" syndrome); report of a case and some observations in 13 other cases. Proc Staff Meet Mayo Clin. 1956;31(15):421–7.
37. Solimena M, Folli F, Denis-Donini S, et al. Autoantibodies to glutamic acid decarboxylase in a patient with stiff-man syndrome, epilepsy, and type I diabetes mellitus. N Engl J Med. 1988;318(16):1012–20.

38. Raju R, Foote J, Banga JP, et al. Analysis of GAD65 autoantibodies in Stiff-Person syndrome patients. J Immunol. 2005;175(11):7755–62.

39. Levy LM, Dalakas MC, Floeter MK. The stiff-person syndrome: an autoimmune disorder affecting neurotransmission of gamma-aminobutyric acid. Ann Intern Med. 1999;131(7):522–30.

40. Rakocevic G, Raju R, Semino-Mora C, Dalakas MC. Stiff person syndrome with cerebellar disease and high-titer anti-GAD antibodies. Neurology. 2006;67(6):1068–70.

41. Saiz A, Blanco Y, Sabater L, et al. Spectrum of neurological syndromes associated with glutamic acid decarboxylase antibodies: diagnostic clues for this association. Brain. 2008;131(10):2553–63.

42. Saiz A, Minguez A, Graus F, Marin C, Tolosa E, Cruz-Sanchez F. Stiff-man syndrome with vacuolar degeneration of anterior horn motor neurons. J Neurol. 1999;246(9):858–60.

43. Wessig C, Klein R, Schneider MF, Toyka KV, Naumann M, Sommer C. Neuropathology and binding studies in anti-amphiphysin-associated stiff-person syndrome. Neurology. 2003;61(2):195–8.

44. Karlson EW, Sudarsky L, Ruderman E, Pierson S, Scott M, Helfgott SM. Treatment of stiff-man syndrome with intravenous immune globulin. Arthritis Rheum. 1994;37(6):915–8.

45. Baker MR, Das M, Isaacs J, Fawcett PR, Bates D. Treatment of stiff person syndrome with rituximab. J Neurol Neurosurg Psychiatry. 2005;76(7):999–1001.

46. Whiteley AM, Swash M, Urich H. Progressive encephalomyelitis with rigidity. Brain. 1976;99(1):27–42.

47. Brown P, Marsden CD. The stiff man and stiff man plus syndromes. J Neurol. 1999;246(8):648–52.

48. Gouider-Khouja N, Mekaouar A, Larnaout A, Miladi N, Ben Khelifa F, Hentati F. Progressive encephalomyelitis with rigidity presenting as a stiff-person syndrome. Parkinsonism Relat Disord. 2002;8(4):285–8.

49. Hutchinson M, Waters P, McHugh J, et al. Progressive encephalomyelitis, rigidity, and myoclonus: a novel glycine receptor antibody. Neurology. 2008;71(16):1291–2.

50. McCombe PA, Chalk JB, Searle JW, Tannenberg AE, Smith JJ, Pender MP. Progressive encephalomyelitis with rigidity: a case report with magnetic resonance imaging findings. J Neurol Neurosurg Psychiatry. 1989;52(12):1429–31.

51. Baraba R, Jusic A, Sruk A. Progressive encephalomyelitis with rigidity: a case report. J Spinal Cord Med. 2010;33(1):73–6.

52. Molina JA, Porta J, Garcia-Morales I, Bermejo PF, Jimenez-Jimenez FJ. Treatment with intravenous prednisone and immunoglobin in a case of progressive encephalomyelitis with rigidity. J Neurol Neurosurg Psychiatry. 2000;68(3):395–6.

53. Saidha S, Elamin M, Mullins G, Chaila E, Tormey VJ, Hennessy MJ. Treatment of progressive encephalomyelitis with rigidity and myoclonic jerks with rituximab: a case report. Eur J Neurol. 2008;15(5):e33.

54. Irani SR, Alexander S, Waters P, et al. Antibodies to Kv1 potassium channel-complex proteins leucine-rich, glioma inactivated 1 protein and contactin-associated protein-2 in limbic encephalitis, Morvan's syndrome and acquired neuromyotonia. Brain. 2010;133(9):2734–48.

55. Newsom-Davis J, Mills KR. Immunological associations of acquired neuromyotonia (Isaacs' syndrome). Report of five cases and literature review. Brain. 1993;116(Pt 2):453–69.

56. Merchut MP. Management of voltage-gated potassium channel antibody disorders. Neurol Clin. 2010;28(4):941–59.

57. Wilkins RH, Brody IA. Neurological classics IV. Encephalitis lethargica. Arch Neurol. 1968;18(3):324–8.

58. Gullan AG. A clinical study of encephalitis lethargica, based on sixty-two cases. Br Med J. 1925;1(3364):1120–4.

59. Smith CM. Sequelae of encephalitis lethargica: notes on 128 cases. Br Med J. 1927;1(3462):872–3.
60. Hunter C. The late sequelae of encephalitis lethargica and of influenza. Can Med Assoc J. 1931;24(6):828–30.
61. Hoehn MM, Yahr MD. Parkinsonism: onset, progression and mortality. Neurology. 1967;17(5):427–42.
62. Hoehn MM. Age distribution of patients with Parkinsonism. J Am Geriatr Soc. 1976;24(2):79–85.
63. Krusz JC, Koller WC, Ziegler DK. Historical review: abnormal movements associated with epidemic encephalitis lethargica. Mov Disord. 1987;2(3):137–41.
64. Vilensky JA, Goetz CG, Gilman S. Movement disorders associated with encephalitis lethargica: a video compilation. Mov Disord. 2006;21(1):1–8.
65. McCall S, Henry JM, Reid AH, Taubenberger JK. Influenza RNA not detected in archival brain tissues from acute encephalitis lethargica cases or in postencephalitic Parkinson cases. J Neuropathol Exp Neurol. 2001;60(7):696–704.
66. Lo KC, Geddes JF, Daniels RS, Oxford JS. Lack of detection of influenza genes in archived formalin-fixed, paraffin wax-embedded brain samples of encephalitis lethargica patients from 1916 to 1920. Virchows Arch. 2003;442(6):591–6.
67. Maurizi CP. Influenza caused epidemic encephalitis (encephalitis lethargica): the circumstantial evidence and a challenge to the nonbelievers. Med Hypotheses. 2010;74(5):798–801.
68. Henry J, Smeyne RJ, Jang H, Miller B, Okun MS. Parkinsonism and neurological manifestations of influenza throughout the 20th and 21st centuries. Parkinsonism Relat Disord. 2010;16(9):566–71.
69. Jang H, Boltz D, Sturm-Ramirez K, et al. Highly pathogenic H5N1 influenza virus can enter the central nervous system and induce neuroinflammation and neurodegeneration. Proc Natl Acad Sci USA. 2009;106(33):14063–8.
70. Anderson LL, Vilensky JA, Duvoisin RC. Review: neuropathology of acute phase encephalitis lethargica: a review of cases from the epidemic period. Neuropathol Appl Neurobiol. 2009;35(5):462–72.
71. Jellinger KA. Absence of alpha-synuclein pathology in postencephalitic parkinsonism. Acta Neuropathol. 2009;118(3):371–9.
72. Blunt SB, Lane RJ, Turjanski N, Perkin GD. Clinical features and management of two cases of encephalitis lethargica. Mov Disord. 1997;12(3):354–9.
73. Maranis S, Tsouli S, Kyritsis AP. Encephalitis lethargica with quick response to immunoglobulin. Clin Neuropharmacol. 2010;33(6):323–4.
74. Lopez-Alberola R, Georgiou M, Sfakianakis GN, Singer C, Papapetropoulos S. Contemporary encephalitis lethargica: phenotype, laboratory findings and treatment outcomes. J Neurol. 2009;256(3):396–404.
75. McAuley J, Shahmanesh M, Swash M. Dopaminergic therapy in acute encephalitis lethargica. Eur J Neurol. 1999;6(2):235–7.
76. Raghav S, Seneviratne J, McKelvie PA, Chapman C, Talman PS, Kempster PA. Sporadic encephalitis lethargica. J Clin Neurosci. 2007;14(7):696–700.
77. Carecchio M, Comi C, Varrasi C, et al. Complex movement disorders in primary antiphospholipid syndrome: a case report. J Neurol Sci. 2009;281(1–2):101–3.
78. Engelen M, Tijssen MAJ. Paroxysmal non-kinesigenic dyskinesia in antiphospholipid antibody syndrome. Mov Disord. 2005;20(1):111–3.
79. Martino D, Chew NK, Mir P, Edwards MJ, Quinn NP, Bhatia K. Atypical movement disorders in antiphospholipid syndrome. Mov Disord. 2006;21(7):944–9.
80. Cervera R, Asherson RA, Font J, et al. Chorea in the antiphospholipid syndrome. Clinical, radiologic, and immunologic characteristics of 50 patients from our clinics and the recent literature. Medicine (Baltimore). 1997;76(3):203–12.
81. Furie R, Ishikawa T, Dhawan V, Eidelberg D. Alternating hemichorea in primary antiphospholipid syndrome: evidence for contralateral striatal hypermetabolism. Neurology. 1994;44(11):2197–9.

82. Krakauer M, Law I. FDG PET brain imaging in neuropsychiatric systemic lupus erythematosis with choreic symptoms. Clin Nucl Med. 2009;34(2):122–3.

83. Miranda M, Cardoso F, Giovannoni G, Church A. Oral contraceptive induced chorea: another condition associated with anti-basal ganglia antibodies. J Neurol Neurosurg Psychiatry. 2004;75(2):327–8.

84. Schipper HM. Sex hormones in stroke, chorea, and anticonvulsant therapy. Semin Neurol. 1988;8(3):181–6.

85. Grant R, Graus F. Paraneoplastic movement disorders. Mov Disord. 2009;24(12):1715–24.

86. Dalmau J, Lancaster E, Martinez-Hernandez E, Rosenfeld MR, Balice-Gordon R. Clinical experience and laboratory investigations in patients with anti-NMDAR encephalitis. Lancet Neurol. 2010;10(1):63–74.

87. Dalmau J, Tuzun E, Wu HY, et al. Paraneoplastic anti-N-methyl-D-aspartate receptor encephalitis associated with ovarian teratoma. Ann Neurol. 2007;61(1): 25–36.

88. Dalmau J, Gleichman AJ, Hughes EG, et al. Anti-NMDA-receptor encephalitis: case series and analysis of the effects of antibodies. Lancet Neurol. 2008;7(12):1091–8.

89. Church A, Dale R, Giovannoni G. Anti-basal ganglia antibodies: a possible diagnostic utility in idiopathic movement disorders? Arch Dis Child. 2004;89(7):611–4.

90. Hallett JJ, Harling-Berg CJ, Knopf PM, Stopa EG, Kiessling LS. Anti-striatal antibodies in Tourette syndrome cause neuronal dysfunction. J Neuroimmunol. 2000;111(1–2):195–202.

91. Loiselle CR, Lee O, Moran TH, Singer HS. Striatal microinfusion of Tourette syndrome and PANDAS sera: failure to induce behavioral changes. Mov Disord. 2004;19(4):390–6.

92. Uchibori A, Sakuta M, Kusunoki S, Chiba A. Autoantibodies in postinfectious acute cerebellar ataxia. Neurology. 2005;65(7):1114–6.

93. Saito H, Yanagisawa T. Acute cerebellar ataxia after influenza vaccination with recurrence and marked cerebellar atrophy. Tohoku J Exp Med. 1989;158(1): 95–103.

94. Dano G. Acute cerebellar ataxia associated with herpes simplex virus infection. Acta Paediatr Scand. 1968;57(2):151–2.

95. Hayakawa H, Katoh T. Severe cerebellar atrophy following acute cerebellitis. Pediatr Neurol. 1995;12(2):159–61.

96. Hadjivassiliou M, Boscolo S, Tongiorgi E, et al. Cerebellar ataxia as a possible organ-specific autoimmune disease. Mov Disord. 2008;23(10):1370–7.

97. Green PH, Alaedini A, Sander HW, Brannagan 3rd TH, Latov N, Chin RL. Mechanisms underlying celiac disease and its neurologic manifestations. Cell Mol Life Sci. 2005;62(7–8):791–9.

98. Kiessling LS, Marcotte AC, Culpepper L. Antineuronal antibodies in movement disorders. Pediatrics. 1993;92(1):39–43.

99. Martino D, Giovannoni G. Antibasal ganglia antibodies and their relevance to movement disorders. Curr Opin Neurol. 2004;17(4):425–32.

100. Church AJ, Dale RC, Cardoso F, et al. CSF and serum immune parameters in Sydenham's chorea: evidence of an autoimmune syndrome? J Neuroimmunol. 2003;136(1–2):149–53.

101. Graus F, Saiz A, Dalmau J. Antibodies and neuronal autoimmune disorders of the CNS. J Neurol. 2009;257(4):509–17.

102. Valldeoriola F. Movement disorders of autoimmune origin. J Neurol. 1999;246(6): 423–31.

CNS Vasculitis

David S. Younger and Adam P.J. Younger

Keywords: Arteritis, Urticarial, Postmortem, Blood vessels, Arthralgia

Introduction

Vasculitis, defined by inflammation of arteries and veins of varying caliber, results in a variety of clinical neurologic manifestations and neuropathologic changes of the central and peripheral nervous system (CNS and PNS). Unrecognized and therefore untreated, vasculitis leads to ischemia and injury of the involved tissues. Remarkable progress has been achieved in the pathogenesis, diagnosis, and treatment of vasculitis of the CNS, making it an important topic for all practicing clinicians. Several excellent reviews of this topic have been published [1, 2].

Classification

Vasculitis in its various forms affects blood vessels of varying caliber from the aorta to capillaries and veins (Figure 17.1). The diverse forms of vasculitis and autoimmune diseases are summarized in Table 17.1.

Systemic Necrotizing Arteritis

The group of systemic necrotizing arteritis includes polyarteritis nodosa (PAN), Kawasaki disease (KD), microscopic polyangiitis (MPA) syndrome, and Churg–Strauss syndrome.

Polyarteritis Nodosa

The first American patient with PAN was described at the turn of the twentieth century [3], a 35-year-old man with constitutional symptoms and subacute leg pains. Postmortem examination showed widespread necrotizing arteritis and nodules along small-and medium-sized vessels of the heart, liver, kidney,

From: *Clinical Neuroimmunology: Multiple Sclerosis and Related Disorders*, Current Clinical Neurology,
Edited by: S.A. Rizvi and P.K. Coyle, DOI 10.1007/978-1-60327-860-7_17,
© Springer Science+Business Media, LLC 2011

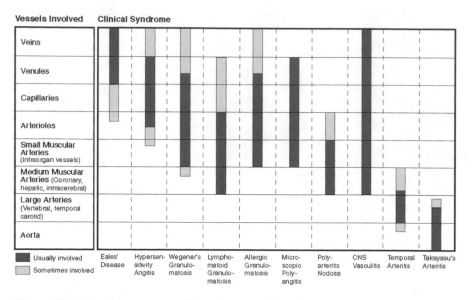

Figure 17.1 Pathologic spectrum of the major vasculitides (from Younger DS. Vasculitis and connective tissue disorders. In: Griggs R, Joynt R, editors. Baker and Joynt's clinical neurology on CD-ROM. Philadelphia: Lippincott Williams & Wilkins; 2003, with permission)

pancreas, testicles, brain, nerves, and skeletal muscles, sparing the lungs and spleen. The histologic lesions consisted of mononuclear cell infiltration, necrosis of internal and external elastic lamina of the media, fibrin deposition, aneurysmal dilatation, perivascular inflammation of the adventitia, and intimal proliferation resulting in narrowing of arterial lumina. Later investigators [4] summarized the clinical and pathologic aspects of PAN. The dominant neurologic picture was a peripheral neuritis that occurred in one-half of patients early in the illness, with a predilection for the legs. In PAN, as in the other systemic necrotizing arteritis, the vasculitic lesion proceeds in a characteristic manner (Figure 17.2), commencing with invasion of the intima, media, and adventitia by polymorphonuclear (PMN) cells, plasma cells, eosinophils, and lymphocytes and leading to swelling of the media and fibrinoid necrosis that clusters around the vasa vasorum, with fragmentation of the internal elastic lamina. Focal deposition of perivascular connective tissue, vascular necrosis, and denuding of the endothelium occur, followed by vascular thrombosis, ischemia, aneurysm formation, rupture, and hemorrhage. Healed lesions coexist with active lesions. Neuroimaging reveals areas of focal cerebral infarction (Figure 17.3). Arteriography and biopsy of involved vascular tissue are the only certain means of histologic diagnosis, but they are impractical or impossible in patients with isolated CNS involvement. Consideration should be given to obtaining a biopsy from potentially involved nerve and muscle biopsy tissue.

Kawasaki Disease

Kawasaki published the first report of KS in 1967; a decade later, the disorder was independently recognized in the USA [5, 6]. Kawasaki disease or mucocutaneous lymph node syndrome is an acute febrile illness of unknown etiology primarily affects children younger than 5 years, with worldwide occurrence, but highest incidence in Japan. The clinical diagnosis is suspected in children with fever for 5 days or more, with rash, cervical lymphadenopathy, conjunctival

Table 17.1 Classification of vasculitis.

Systemic necrotizing arteritis
Polyarteritis nodosa
Microscopic polyangiitis
Churg–Strauss syndrome
Kawasaki disease
Hypersensitivity vasculitis
Drug-related vasculitis
Serum sickness
Henoch–Schönlein purpura
Hypocomplementemic vasculitis
Cryoglobulinemia
Systemic granulomatous vasculitis
Wegener granulomatosis
Lymphomatoid granulomatosis, lethal midline granuloma
Giant cell arteritis, temporal arteritis, Takayasu arteritis
Granulomatous angiitis of the nervous system
Connective tissue disorders associated with vasculitis
Systemic lupus erythematosus
Scleroderma
Rheumatoid arthritis
Sjögren syndrome
Mixed connective tissue disease
Behçet disease
Infection-associated vasculitis
Bacterial meningitis
Mycobacterium tuberculosis
Spirochetes
Treponema pallidum, Borrelia burgdorferi
Varicella-zoster virus, fungi, human immunodeficiency virus type 1
Central nervous system vasculitis associated with amphetamine abuse

injection, oral mucosal, and peripheral extremity changes. Patients with fever and coronary artery abnormalities but lacking others clinical features are classified as atypical or incomplete KD. The vasculitic lesions in KD proceed in a systematic manner over a month in four stages as shown in postmortem cases of varied duration of illness before death. Stage 1 (0–9 days) includes perivasculitis of small arteries leading to pericarditis, myocarditis, AV node inflammation, endocarditis, and valvulitis. Stage 2 (12–25 days) is characterized by pan-vasculitis of medium-sized muscular arteries with aneurysm formation and thrombosis. Stage 3 (28–31 days) leads to myointimal proliferation with disappearance of acute inflammation. Stage 4 is characterized by vascular scarring and stenosis. Coronary artery aneurysms, the most common sequelae of KD, occur in up to a quarter of children. Remote areas of vasculitis beyond the heart rarely occur. Primary CNS involvement was argued in 6 of 21 (29%) patients with localized cerebral hypoperfusion on single photon emission-computed

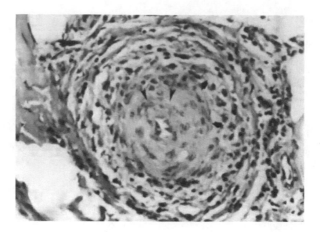

Figure 17.2 This small muscular artery from muscle is from a patient with polyarteritis nodosa. In the third, or proliferative, phase illustrated here, chronic inflammatory cells replace the neutrophils of the second phase; evidence of necrosis of the media (*arrows*), early intimal proliferation (*arrowheads*), and fibrosis is seen. The lumen is almost completely occluded. Ultimately, in the healing phase, this process is replaced by dense, organized connective tissue (hematoxylin and eosin stain; original magnification ×250) (from Younger DS. Vasculitis and connective tissue disorders. In: Griggs R, Joynt R, editors. Baker and Joynt's clinical neurology on CD-ROM. Philadelphia: Lippincott Williams & Wilkins; 2003, with permission)

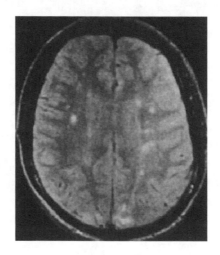

Figure 17.3 Magnetic resonance imaging scan of a patient with polyarteritis nodosa with cerebral involvement. Multiple small cortical and subcortical regions of increased signal on these proton density-weighted images reflect infarcts in the distribution of small, unnamed branch arteries (from Younger DS. Vasculitis and connective tissue disorders. In: Griggs R, Joynt R, editors. Baker and Joynt's clinical neurology on CD-ROM. Philadelphia: Lippincott Williams & Wilkins; 2003, with permission)

tomography (SPECT) during the acute illness [7]; and in another study that noted variable leptomeningeal thickening, endarteritis, and periarteritis of cerebral vessels [8]. CNS complications overall occur in less than 1% of cases including seizures, ataxia, aseptic meningitis, facial palsy, sensorineural hearing loss, acute hemiparesis, subdural effusion, and encephalopathy; and their relation to active vasculitis is speculative. Intravenous gamma globulin (IVIG) and aspirin administered early in the course of the acute illness is highly effective [9].

Microscopic Polyangiitis

At about the same time as the limits of PAN were being delineated, the essential features of MPA were being described [10]. This disorder differed from PAN in the affliction of small arterioles, capillaries, and venules of the lungs and kidney with necrotizing glomerulonephritis. Circulating antineutrophil cytoplasmic autoantibodies (ANCA), usually myeloperoxidase (MPO) or p-ANCA, are detected in up to 80% of patients, which is rarely, if ever, seen in PAN. Small vessel involvement is considered the definite diagnostic criterion of MPA and is of the caliber involved in epineurial arteries of the PNS, with rare CNS affliction.

Churg–Strauss Syndrome

Churg–Strauss syndrome, named in honor of the authors who first described the syndrome of asthma, eosinophilia, extravascular granulomas, and necrotizing vasculitis of small and medium arteries, arterioles, capillaries, and veins [11], has the essential lesions of angiitis and extravascular necrotizing granulomas with eosinophilic infiltrates. The vasculitis may be granulomatous or nongranulomatous and characteristically involves arteries and veins, as well as pulmonary and systemic vessels. The granulomas are located near small arteries and veins and are characterized by palisading epithelioid histiocytes arranged around central necrotic zones in which eosinophils predominate. Pulmonary lesions reflect the combination of necrotizing vasculitis and areas resembling eosinophilic pneumonia. The disease has three phases. The first is a prodromal period of constitutional symptoms that includes rhinitis and asthma. The second is peripheral blood and tissue eosinophilia. The third phase is a systemic vasculitis, wherein neurologic involvement occurs, including stroke and hemorrhage similar to PAN. The laboratory diagnosis is ascertained by serologic investigation, primarily ANCA MPO, MPO or p-ANCA, and tissue biopsy.

Hypersensitivity Vasculitis

The group of vasculitis with its unique predilection for the dermis [12] and has as its prototype hypersensitivity vasculitis (HSV) (Figure 17.4), which commences with extravasation of erythrocytes, pronounced endothelial swelling, and infiltration of PMN and later mononuclear cells, with fibrosis, typical involvement of arterioles, capillaries, and postcapillary venules. It results in nuclear fragments or leukocytoclasia with variable necrosis and fibrinoid material termed leukocytoclastic vasculitis (LCV) and circulating immune complexes that deposit in the skin and vasculitic lesions. In contrast to PAN, the lesions are all in the same stage of evolution. Rare CNS involvement can lead to microinfarction, and hemorrhage can occur. The group of HSV includes drug-related vasculitis, serum sickness, Henoch–Schönlein purpura, and hypocomplementemic and cryoglobulinemic vasculitis.

Drug-Related Vasculitis

Drug reactions are responsible for approximately 20% of cases of dermal vasculitis. The clinical spectrum ranges from urticaria, wheezing, rhinitis, rash, and serum sickness to laryngeal edema and hypotension, evolving over minutes, hours, or days. The rash is maculopapular or vesicular, less often palpable purpura that situates along the arms and legs and abates after drug withdrawal.

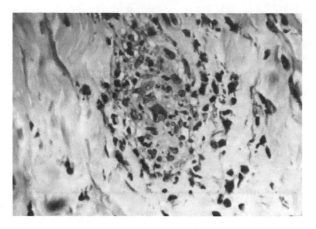

Figure 17.4 This arteriole from muscle is from a patient with leukocytoclastic vasculitis. The entire vessel and perivascular tissue are infiltrated with polymorphonuclear leukocytes and chronic inflammatory cells with necrosis and nuclear debris. The vascular lumen is nearly obliterated (hematoxylin and eosin stain; original magnification ×400) (from Younger DS. Vasculitis and connective tissue disorders. In: Griggs R, Joynt R, editors. Baker and Joynt's clinical neurology on CD-ROM. Philadelphia: Lippincott Williams & Wilkins; 2003, with permission)

More severe drug reactions develop multiple organ involvement, especially the heart, liver, kidneys, gastrointestinal tract, lungs, and CNS. This disorder results from the focal deposition of immune complexes, which are caused by the covalent binding of the offending drug, or its metabolites, with native or foreign proteins to produce hapten molecules. The latter form hapten-antibody complexes that deposit in the skin, eliciting the dermal vasculitic response.

Serum Sickness

The vasculitis of serum sickness consists of varying degrees of infiltration of arterioles, capillaries, and venules, with interstitial inflammation by PMN cells, eosinophils, and mononuclear inflammatory cells, with variable fibrinoid necrosis and perivascular granuloma formation. Urticaria, noted in the majority of patients, is followed by erythematous or maculopapular rash, petechiae, palpable purpura, and lymphadenopathy, first at the site of injection and later generalized, with arthralgia, edema, headache, and lethargy. CNS involvement includes blurring of vision, retinal and palpebral hemorrhages, meningismus, stroke, and myelopathy. The clinical presentation of serum sickness parallels the appearance of protein antigen and antibody excess and persists until immune complexes are eliminated. The reaction to injection of heterologous serum and many drugs is a complex one, and its multiple neurologic manifestations may be explainable on the basis of the immune complex disease with incipient cytotoxic and humoral and cell-mediated immune mechanisms.

Henoch–Schönlein Purpura

Henoch–Schönlein purpura is characterized by nonthrombocytopenic purpura, arthralgia, abdominal pain, and LCV of skin lesions in an affected child with fever, headache, and anorexia. Palpable purpuric lesions arise along extensor surfaces of the lower extremities and buttocks, sometimes in association with migratory angioneurotic edema of the hands, scalp, face, lower legs, and genitalia. The presence of LCV suggests an immune complex-mediated pathogenesis; in that regard, deposits of immunoglobulins, particularly IgA, and C3 have been demonstrated in the kidney and blood vessel walls, and some affected patients had hereditary C2 deficiency.

Hypocomplementemic Vasculitis

Hypocomplementemic or urticarial vasculitis is characterized by urticaria, migratory arthralgia, and persistent or intermittent hypocomplementemia. In affected patients, urticarial, bullous, and purpuric skin lesions develop and sometimes severe angioneurotic edema and life-threatening laryngeal edema, accompanied by arthralgia, conjunctivitis, episcleritis, uveitis, mild renal disease, pericarditis, abdominal pain, and splenomegaly. Pseudotumor cerebri is probably the most common associated CNS manifestation. Hypocomplementemic vasculitis resembles a forme fruste of systemic lupus erythematosus (SLE). Immunologic studies show a binding of IgG antibody to C1q along basement membranes, in which it activates the complement cascade. It is not known whether the autoantibody is more than a marker of the disease.

Cryoglobulinemia

Cryoglobulins reversibly precipitate at temperatures below 37°C. They are composed of IgG and IgM, complement, lipoprotein, and antigenic protein moieties. They are classified into three types with implications for clinical and etiologic specificity. Type I is composed of a single monoclonal IgM or IgG antibody; type II, mixed, has monoclonal IgM, possessing activity against polyclonal IgG; and type III has mixed polyclonal and nonimmunoglobulin molecules in the form of immunoglobulin–antiimmunoglobulin immune complexes. Types I and II cryoglobulins are associated with lymphoproliferative diseases, particularly multiple myeloma and Waldenström macroglobulinemia. Type III cryoglobulins are associated with infection and collagen vascular diseases. One subgroup, termed *essential mixed cryoglobulinemia* (*EMC*), harbors circulating hepatitis C virus (HCV) RNA and corresponding antibodies in the cryoprecipitate. Type I cryoglobulins cause the hyperviscosity syndrome. Four vascular lesions are noted in cryoglobulinemia: (1) occlusion of small and large vessels in those with high levels of cryoglobulins of type I or II; (2) bland thrombosis of small arteries and arterioles; (3) endothelial swelling, proliferation, and basement membrane thickening; and (4) LCV.

True vasculitis is occasionally seen, mainly in those with associated PAN. Dermatitis is the most conspicuous feature, accompanied by palpable purpura, which persists for a week to 10 days, heralded by a sharp or burning sensation. Purpura is noted in all types but is more common with type III and in EMC. PNS and CNS manifestations are more common with types II and III. Renal disease is a major feature of EMC. Hepatic disease is far more common with this syndrome by virtue of its association with HCV. The appearance of high levels of cryoglobulins in the blood in patients who reported cold sensitivity and vasomotor symptoms led to the presumption that cryoprecipitation was the cause of ischemia of arterioles and capillaries due to hyperviscosity and the direct plugging of small vessels. However, it is now known that the cryoprecipitate, when present, may be tangential to the pathogenesis of the clinical syndrome and even an artifact. CNS manifestations in types I and II disease are related to vascular occlusion with or without vasculitis. Cryoglobulinemia should be considered in patients with features of characteristic skin lesions, mononeuritis multiplex (MNM), hyperviscosity, easily coagulable blood, IgM monoclonal paraproteinemia, and risk factors for HCV infection. If found, the presence of cryoglobulinemia directs the performance of bone marrow studies, nerve biopsy, and studies for HCV and human immunodeficiency virus type 1 (HIV-1) infection, acquired immunodeficiency syndrome (AIDS), occult cancer, infection, plasma cell dyscrasia, and collagen vascular disease.

Systemic Granulomatous Vasculitis

The group of systemic granulomatous vasculitis includes Wegener granulomatosis (WG), lymphomatoid granulomatosis, and lethal midline granuloma.

Wegener Granulomatosis

Although first believed to be a form of PAN and later rhinogenic pneumogenic granulomatosis by the investigator for whom it was later named, WG differed from PAN in the triad of necrotizing granulomatous lesions of the sinuses and lower respiratory tract, systemic necrotizing vasculitis of small arteries and veins, and glomerulonephritis [13]. Nervous system involvement was appreciated almost a decade later [14]. The lesions of WG begin as minute foci of granular necrosis and fibrinoid degeneration with PMN cells followed by histiocytes and giant cells along the margins of granulomas of the upper airways and in renal glomeruli. Necrotizing granulomatous lesions secondarily involve small arteries, arterioles, capillaries, and venules with segmental fibrinoid necrosis in involved tissues. Affected patients present with multifocal pain, sensory loss, and weakness. Circulating c-ANCA directed against proteinase 3 (PR3) is predictive of the disease in the majority of patients even in the initial phase of illness. One-fourth of patients demonstrate CNS and PNS involvement due to direct destruction of brain and nerve tissue by necrotizing granulomas, locally or remote from upper or lower respiratory tract granulomas, and necrotizing arteritis of cerebral and arteriae nervorum of peripheral nerves. The CNS manifestations, include stroke, intracerebral lesions, subarachnoid hemorrhage, and optic neuritis, result from vasculitic involvement, as well as contiguous extension of granulomas.

Lymphomatoid Granulomatosis

Lymphomatoid granulomatosis is a malignant lymphoreticular disorder with a strong predilection for the CNS. Patients present with constitutional symptoms and skin lesions that resemble erythema nodosum. Focal neurologic involvement occurs early, including MNM, unilateral cranial nerve palsies, hemiparesis, ataxia, seizures, spinal and radicular syndromes, and even myopathy. CNS involvement, with invasion of unifocal and multifocal necrotizing angiocentric and angiodestructive lesions of small- and medium-sized muscular arteries and their endothelia by masses of T cells, plasma cells, histiocytes, and atypical lymphoreticular cells is accompanied by immunoblast formation in the cerebrum, brainstem, cerebellar parenchyma, and meninges (Figures 17.5 and 17.6).

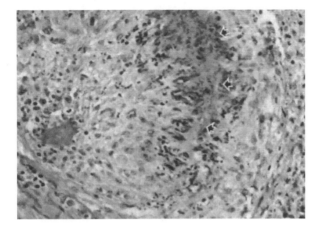

Figure 17.5 Wegener granulomatosis. This small muscular artery is nearly completely destroyed. A large confluent area of fibrinoid degradation (*arrows*) is surrounded by neutrophils, palisading histiocytes, lymphocytes, plasma cells, and some giant cells (hematoxylin and eosin stain; original magnification ×250) (from Younger DS. Vasculitis and connective tissue disorders. In: Griggs R, Joynt R, editors. Baker and Joynt's clinical neurology on CD-ROM. Philadelphia: Lippincott Williams & Wilkins; 2003, with permission)

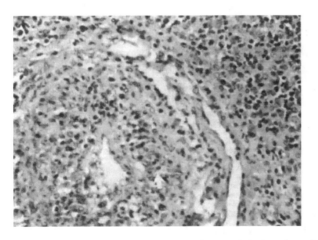

Figure 17.6 Lymphomatoid granulomatosis. The characteristic invasion of the vessel wall (*arrow*) and the perivascular tissue by a polymorphocellular infiltrate consists of lymphocytes, plasma cells, and atypical reticuloendothelial cells. The vessel lumen is markedly narrowed. Notice the absence of well-formed granulomas and fibrinoid necrosis (hematoxylin and eosin stain; original magnification ×250) (from Younger DS. Vasculitis and connective tissue disorders. In: Griggs R, Joynt R, editors. Baker and Joynt's clinical neurology on CD-ROM. Philadelphia: Lippincott Williams & Wilkins; 2003, with permission)

Lethal Midline Granuloma

Historically, this disorder was likened to WG, but systemic disease is not a major feature of lethal midline granuloma, and WG rarely, if ever, causes such extensive facial mutilation. It is now known to be a relentlessly invasive necrotizing process of the nose and palate that causes destruction of sinuses and all major midline structures of the head, producing grotesque facial mutilation and ultimately death. The CNS complications most often result from direct invasion of the orbit and face, jugular vein, sigmoid, and cavernous sinuses, leading to vascular thrombosis, sepsis, meningitis, and exsanguinations. The disorder is associated with idiopathic midline granuloma, poorly differentiated diffuse small or large B-cell lymphomas, plasmacytomas, and other polymorphic reticuloses that mediate the damage.

Giant Cell Arteritis

The concept of temporal arteritis was first described [15] and then named [16] for the site of granulomatous giant cell inflammation and vessel involvement. Patients with biopsy-proven temporal arteritis and associated blindness due to vasculitic involvement of ophthalmic and posterior ciliary vessels were originally classified as having cranial arteritis. Other patients had prominent constitutional and musculoskeletal complaints and typical polymyalgia rheumatica. The occasional finding of giant cell lesions along the aorta and its branches and in other medium- and large-sized arteries at autopsy in some cases warranted the diagnosis of generalized giant cell arteritis. The pathologic heterogeneity of temporal arteritis was further demonstrated by the finding of intracranial lesions in several patients, who also qualified for the diagnosis of granulomatous angiitis. The earliest lesions of giant cell arteritis consist of vacuolization of smooth muscle cells of the media, with enlargement of mitochondria and infiltration of lymphocytes, plasma cells, and histiocytes. With progression, there is extension inflammation into the intima and adventitia, leading to segmental fragmentation and necrosis of the elastic lamina, granuloma formation, and proliferation of connective tissue along the vessel wall. This eventuates in vascular thrombosis, intimal proliferation, and fibrosis (Figure 17.7).

Temporal Arteritis and Takayasu Arteritis

Two forms of giant cell arteritis, temporal arteritis and Takayasu arteritis, are of clinical importance to neurologists. They differ epidemiologically and in the size of vessels involved. Temporal arteritis occurs in elderly whites of either gender and involves medium and large arteries. Takayasu arteritis affects the aorta and its branches in young Asian women. The clinical manifestations of temporal arteritis, namely, headache, scalp tenderness, thickened nodular and pulseless superficial temporal artery, unilateral vision loss, and jaw claudication, are related primarily to disease along branches of the external carotid artery and arteritis of the vertebral and carotid arteries, typically at end points of dural investment. The characteristic involvement of obliterative lesions in large arteries such as the aorta and its major branches in Takayasu arteritis, especially late in the disease, leads to other symptoms not typically seen in temporal arteritis, including dizziness, syncope, subclavian steal, carotid sinus syndrome, stoke, amaurosis fugax, corneal opacification, cataracts, claudication and gangrene of the limbs, and chest and abdomen angina. Biopsy of the temporal artery for tissue diagnosis should be performed in all suspected patients before therapy is commenced with long-term corticosteroids or other immunosuppressive agents; arterial biopsy is impractical in Takayasu arteritis.

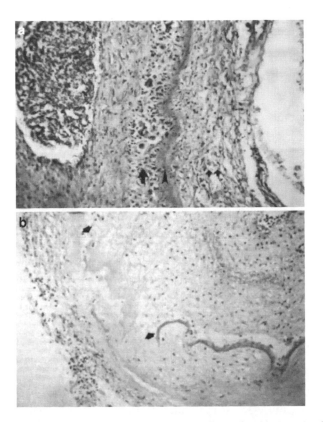

Figure 17.7 Temporal arteritis. (**a**) In an early lesion of a large muscular artery, necrosis, inflammation, and giant cell formation (*single arrow*) can be seen immediately adjacent to the internal elastic lamina (*arrowhead*), which is undergoing degenerative changes, and there is some intimal proliferation (*double arrows*) (hematoxylin and eosin stain; original magnification ×100). (**b**) This more advanced lesion has complete segmental destruction of the internal elastic lamina and virtually the entire media (*arrows*). Marked intimal proliferation has nearly occluded the lumen, and few inflammatory cells remain (hematoxylin and eosin stain; original magnification ×50) (from Younger DS. Vasculitis and connective tissue disorders. In: Griggs R, Joynt R, editors. Baker and Joynt's clinical neurology on CD-ROM. Philadelphia: Lippincott Williams & Wilkins; 2003, with permission)

Granulomatous Angiitis of the Nervous System

The first two patients with this disorder [17] had unrelenting progressive mental change culminating in stupor, coma, and death in less than a year. Postmortem examination showed granulomatous vasculitis of the meninges composed of lymphocytes, multinucleate giant cells, and epithelioid cells, with vessel necrosis and extension into the brain along involved veins and arteries of varying caliber. The clinicopathologic syndrome was later delineated and named for the distinctive pathology [18]. For two more decades, rare affected cases of so-called granulomatous angiitis of the nervous system (GANS) were reported in life, but there was no effective treatment. Investigators at the National Institutes of Health advocated clinical and angiographic criteria to establish the antemortem diagnosis while emphasizing the potentially restricted nature of the vasculitis rather than the granulomatous histology [19].

Enthusiasm for the empiric treatment of cerebral vasculitis based upon clinical and radiographic criteria alone has waned as a result of several influences. First, beading in a cerebral angiogram is an inconsistent finding is an inconsistent finding in histologically proven cases of granulomatous angiitis of the brain [20]. Second, the diagnosis of primary angiitis of the CNS based upon the presence of beading in many young women was later amended to benign angiopathy of the CNS which differed in frequent spontaneous resolution [21]. Third, permanent side effects occur in a significant number of patients treated with cyclophosphamide. Fourth, a historic analysis demonstrated an equivalent efficacy of corticosteroids and cyclophosphamide in the initial treatment of this disorder [22]. Current investigators still admix cases of primary CNS vasculitis, failing to discriminate between histologically confirmed cases from those defined clinically; as well as those with or without giant and epithelioid-related histology, and vascular necrosis, making comparisons of prognosis and treatment more challenging [23], prompting continuing debate [24].

Diagnostic biopsy of the brain and overlying meninges and postmortem examination shows granulomatous giant cell and epithelioid cell inflammation with necrotizing arteritis of cerebral vessels of all calibers from named cerebral vessels to medium and small leptomeningeal vessels (Figure 17.8). The disorder has nearly exclusive neurologic manifestations, including headache, mental change, and pleocytosis and elevated protein content in the CSF, with signs of angiographic beading that precedes focal seizure and stroke (Figure 17.9) and, if untreated, coma and death. The clinical heterogeneity is manifested by the occurrence of GANS in association with cell arteritis, sarcoidosis, varicella zoster virus, lymphoma, amyloid angiopathy, and HIV infection.

Collagen Vascular Diseases

The collagen vascular diseases associated with CNS vasculitis include SLE, scleroderma, rheumatoid arthritis, Sjögren syndrome, mixed connective tissue disease, and Behçet disease, each with recognizable clinical neurologic and histopathologic syndromes. This section discusses the various forms of vasculitis associated with these disorders and a separate chapter deals with other neurological complications.

Systemic Lupus Erythematosus

Once thought to be an important cause of cerebral lupus, true vasculitis occurs in only about 10% of patients at postmortem examination. The vasculitis of SLE shows fibrinoid necrosis of small arteries, arterioles, and capillaries (Figure 17.10). As collagen swells and fragments in the course of SLE, it dissolves to form a homogenous hyaline and granular periodic acid-Schiff-positive material. The fibrinoid material contains immunoglobulins, antigen–antibody complexes, complement, and fibrinogen. Major cerebral vessel occlusion in association with anticardiolipin and SLE is attributed to in situ thrombosis and vasculopathy (Figure 17.11) [25].

Scleroderma

Scleroderma or systemic sclerosis is characterized by widespread microvascular changes and diffuse fibrosis that affect first the skin and later systemic organs and the nervous system. Vascular lesions include increased collagen deposition, sclerosis, and hyalinization, followed by proliferation

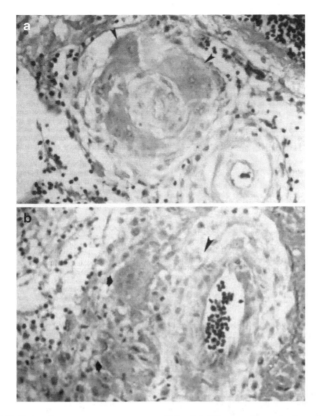

Figure 17.8 Central nervous system vasculitis. (**a**) The media and adventitia of this small leptomeningeal artery have been almost completely replaced by multinucleated giant cells (*arrowheads*). Intimal proliferation with obliteration of the vascular lumen and a dense, perivascular, mononuclear inflammatory infiltrate can be seen (hematoxylin and eosin stain; original magnification ×250). (**b**) A somewhat larger leptomeningeal vessel shows necrosis of the media and internal elastic lamina with multinucleated giant cell formation (*arrows*), intimal proliferation (*arrowhead*), and lymphocytic infiltration of the adventitia and neighboring meninges (hematoxylin and eosin stain; original magnification ×250) (from Younger DS. Vasculitis and connective tissue disorders. In: Griggs R, Joynt R, editors. Baker and Joynt's clinical neurology on CD-ROM. Philadelphia: Lippincott Williams & Wilkins; 2003, with permission)

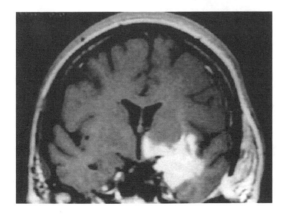

Figure 17.9 Magnetic resonance imaging (fluid-attenuated inversion recovery sequence) of a patient with biopsy-proven, unifocal central nervous system vasculitis that is largely confined to the left temporal and basal frontal regions (from Younger DS. Vasculitis and connective tissue disorders. In: Griggs R, Joynt R, editors. Baker and Joynt's clinical neurology on CD-ROM. Philadelphia: Lippincott Williams & Wilkins; 2003, with permission)

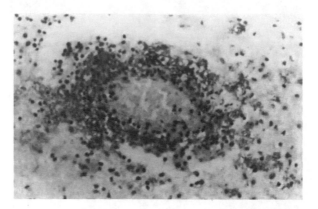

Figure 17.10 Systemic lupus erythematosus. This small vessel within brain parenchyma is largely necrotic. Abundant fibrin (*darkly* stained) is evident in vessel walls and surrounding tissues. A few chronic inflammatory cells are seen, indicating the presence of vasculitis, which may be found in 20% of patients (fibrin stain; original magnification ×250) (from Younger DS. Vasculitis and connective tissue disorders. In: Griggs R, Joynt R, editors. Baker and Joynt's clinical neurology on CD-ROM. Philadelphia: Lippincott Williams & Wilkins; 2003, with permission)

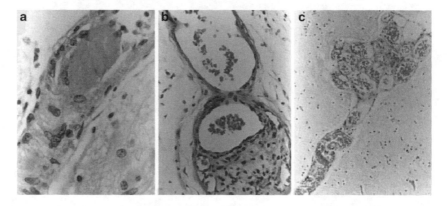

Figure 17.11 (**a–c**) Thrombotic–embolic cerebral microangiopathy in a patient with antiphospholipid antibody syndrome (see text for details) (from Younger DS. Vasculitis and connective tissue disorders. In: Griggs R, Joynt R, editors. Baker and Joynt's clinical neurology on CD-ROM. Philadelphia: Lippincott Williams & Wilkins; 2003, with permission)

of the endothelium, fibrosis of the adventitia and intima, and duplication and fraying of the internal elastic membrane, with progressive luminal obliteration (Figure 17.12). The microvascular lesions in scleroderma are mediated by the anticentromere, anti-SCL-70 or topoisomerase, and anti-RNA polymerase III antibodies, as well as the HLA-DQB1 haplotype, accompanied by autoreactive lymphocytes that produce interleukins (IL)-4 and -6, which are chemotactic for dermal fibroblasts and capable of inducing collagen synthesis. Necrotizing vasculitis with prominent neurologic involvement can be indolent or fulminant and even resemble PAN, with calcinosis, Raynaud phenomenon, esophageal dysmotility, sclerodactyly, and telangiectasia of the skin and face (CREST syndrome).

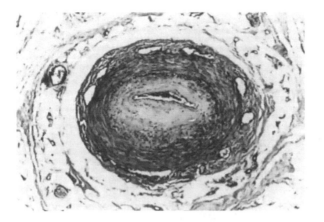

Figure 17.12 Progressive systemic sclerosis. This digital artery has severe intimal hyperplasia and greater than 90% luminal narrowing. Severe adventitial fibrosis and marked telangiectasia of the vasa vasorum are also present, but the media and internal elastic lamina are relatively spared (trichrome stain; original magnification ×60) (from Younger DS. Vasculitis and connective tissue disorders. In: Griggs R, Joynt R, editors. Baker and Joynt's clinical neurology on CD-ROM. Philadelphia: Lippincott Williams & Wilkins; 2003, with permission)

Rheumatoid Arthritis

Three forms of vasculitis occur in rheumatoid arthritis, with affliction of all calibers of blood vessels, from dermal postcapillary venules to the aorta, usually in association with circulating IgM and IgG rheumatoid factor as measured by the latex fixation test, decreased complement, and positive antinuclear antibody. The first is a proliferative endarteritis of a few organs, particularly the heart, muscle, and nerves, characterized by inflammatory infiltration of all layers of small arteries and arterioles, with intimal proliferation, necrosis, and thrombosis. The second is a fulminant vasculitis indistinguishable from PAN with less severe leukocytosis, myalgia, renal and gastrointestinal involvement, and bowel perforation, which can be accompanied by CNS sequelae. The third is an LCV with palpable purpura, arthritis, cryoglobulinemia, and low complement levels. Nonvasculitic spinal and epidural involvement leads to vertebral collapse, subluxation, and direct narrowing of the spinal canal due to rheumatoid pannus that leads to myelopathy, radiculopathy, and stenosis.

Sjögren Syndrome

Sjögren syndrome is recognized clinically by keratoconjunctivitis sicca and xerostomia. Two types of vasculitis occur: (1) LCV of the skin with palpable purpura, urticaria, erythematous macules, and papules and (2) another that resembles PAN with muscle, nerve, CNS, and visceral vascular involvement, without aneurysm formation. Humeral and cell-mediated mechanisms underlie hypergammaglobulinemia, CD4 infiltration of exocrine glands with blast transformation, and association with extractable RNA proteins Ro or Sjögren syndrome (SS)-A and intranuclear RNA-associated antigen La or SS-B. Vasculitis is best confirmed by skin, muscle, and sural nerve biopsy, as in PAN and HSV.

Mixed Connective Tissue Disease

Also known as an overlap syndrome, mixed connective tissue disease has clinical and histopathologic features of SLE, scleroderma, and polymyositis along with proliferative vascular changes, capillary involvement, and mild tissue fibrosis. Headache and encephalopathy are common neurologic symptoms due to CNS involvement.

Behçet Disease

Behçet disease is characterized by the trial of oral and genital ulcers and uveitis and is associated with cutaneous, retinal, and CNS vasculitis. Large artery involvement resulting from smoldering vasculitis along the carotid, radial, and subclavian arteries, and less commonly cerebral veins and arteries, without aneurysm formation leads to secondary vascular thrombosis and pseudotumor cerebri. Neurologic inflammatory involvement also results from direct inflammation of the neuraxis, for example, in the occurrence of focal brainstem meningoencephalitis.

Infection-Associated Vasculitis

The group of infection-related vasculitides include acute purulent meningitis, tuberculosis, syphilis, Lyme neuroborreliosis, varicella zoster virus, fungal infection, seropositivity to HIV-1 infection, and AIDS. Recognition of an infection is important because prompt treatment averts or lessens the severity of vasculitis.

Purulent bacterial meningitis causes arteritis and thrombophlebitis of vessels because of infiltration of blood vessels as they traverse sites of exudation at the base of the brain and across foci of cerebritis, leading to vascular narrowing, cerebral ischemia, infarction, hemorrhage, and abscess formation. Host and immune factors are equally important determinants of whether mycobacterial tubercles rupture in cisterns of the brain with a similar outcome of arteritis. *Treponema pallidum*, the agent of syphilis, and *Borrelia burgdorferi*, the agent of Lyme neuroborreliosis, have particular attraction for blood vessels. Untreated, acute syphilitic meningitis leads to arteritis and meningovascular disease, endarteritis, and, later, general paresis and tabes dorsalis. Like syphilis, the diagnosis of Lyme neuroborreliosis is made on clinical grounds and supported by compatible laboratory findings including serological assays performed on paired specimens of serum and CSF in suspected patients. Neuropathologic studies in two patients that underwent brain biopsy with active Lyme neuroborreliosis revealed nonnecrotizing mononuclear inflammatory cell vascular infiltration with endothelial swelling prompting aggressive salutary antibiotic therapy, as did a third patient studied at postmortem with severe widespread *Borrelia burgdorferi* infection [26]. CD8 suppressor T-cell perivasculitis was noted in femoral cutaneous nerve biopsy in a patient with acute inflammatory polyradiculoneuritis prompting a second month of intravenous antibiotics [27].

Cerebral vasculitis follows varicella zoster virus ophthalmicus with a characteristic syndrome of contralateral hemiplegia owing to ipsilateral vasculitis of the anterior and middle cerebral arteries. Pathologic studies of the vasculitic lesions show necrotizing granulomatous angiitis with demonstrable viral particles. Four fungal agents – *Aspergillus*, *Candida*, *Coccidioides*, and *Mucor* – lead to opportunistic infection in immunocompromised and severely disabled hosts and have the capacity to invade arteries of the CNS.

Vasculitis of the nervous system occurs in association with HIV-1 infection alone or with AIDS, including primary granulomatous angiitis of the brain, eosinophilic temporal arteritis, vasculitic meningoencephalitis, and MNM and myositis resembling PAN, although these are all rare occurrences. The pathogenesis of HIV-associated vasculitis appears to result from direct infection of VEC by HIV and other infectious agents, in association with immune complex deposition, upregulation of cytokine section, and adhesion molecules in native cerebral and peripheral nerve vessels.

Substance Abuse

Parenteral drug use as a cause of CNS vasculitis was first reported in 1970 among 14 drug addicts who experienced strokes and intracranial hemorrhage in association with multiple amphetamine and narcotic drug use [28]. Necrotizing arteritis of the polyarteritis type was found in cerebral arteries and arterioles (Figure 17.13). Many of the patients had complicating factors, including severe hypertension and hepatitis B antigenemia. Similar histologically proven cases have been described in other uses of amphetamine, cocaine, and opioids, alone or in combination. However, four observations cast doubt on the frequent association of substance abuse including amphetamine with true cerebral vasculitis. First, most cases have been diagnosed by beading alone on a cerebral angiogram, without pathologic verification. Second, the vascular insult associated with drug abuse is likely due to contributory factors, including HIV-1 and opportunistic bacterial, fungal, viral, and spirochete infection. That frequency accompanies potential drug abuse. Third, necrotizing arteritis

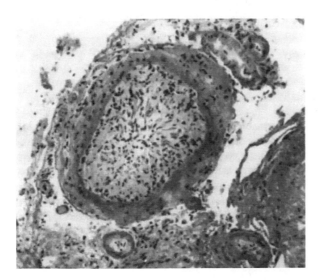

Figure 17.13 Cerebral vasculopathy in a case of intracerebral hemorrhage associated with the use of phenylpropanolamine as an aid to weight loss. The profound intimal hyperplasia all but obliterates the vascular lumen. Polymorphonuclear leukocytes are in all three vascular layers but particularly the intima. The media are remarkably well preserved compared with cases of polyarteritis nodosa and leukocytoclastic vasculitis (hematoxylin and eosin stain; original magnification ×100) (from Younger DS. Vasculitis and connective tissue disorders. In: Griggs R, Joynt R, editors. Baker and Joynt's clinical neurology on CD-ROM. Philadelphia: Lippincott Williams & Wilkins; 2003, with permission)

itself is not a feature of an experimental animal model in which vessel beading develops within 2 weeks of potential administration of amphetamine, postmortem examination of which shows perivascular cuffing, not arteritis.

Laboratory Diagnosis

General Principles

Four principles are generally agreed upon in the diagnosis of vasculitis: First, vasculitis is a potentially serious disorder with a propensity for permanent disability owing to tissue ischemia and infarction; recognition of the neurologic manifestations is important in developing a differential etiologic diagnosis. Second, undiagnosed and untreated, the outcome of vasculitis is potentially fatal. Third, a favorable response to an empiric course of immunosuppressive and immunomodulating therapy should never be considered a substitute for the absolute proof of the diagnosis of vasculitis. Fourth, histopathologic confirmation of vasculitis in the nervous system is essential for accurate diagnosis, such as by brain and meninges where there is CNS involvement and analysis of nerve and muscle biopsy tissue when PNS involvement is postulated.

Recommended Laboratory Evaluation

The laboratory evaluation of vasculitis of the CNS is summarized in Table 17.2. Serologically specific serum studies should be obtained in all patients guided by the clinical presentation and postulated etiologic diagnosis to avoid excessive cost and spurious results. Electrodiagnostic studies are useful in the initial investigation of systemic vasculitis because they can identify areas of asymptomatic involvement and sites for muscle and nerve biopsy and distinguish the various neuropathic syndromes associated with peripheral nerve and muscle involvement. A wide sampling of nerves and muscles should be examined, distal and proximal, using standard recording and needle electrodes for the performance of nerve conduction studies and needle electromyography, at skin temperatures of 34°C, with comparison to normative data. Most patients with peripheral nerve vasculitis show evidence of active

Table 17.2 Laboratory evaluation of vasculitis.

CBC, ESR, chemistries, CK, ANA, complement levels, RF, cryoglobulins, IFE, quantitative immunoglobulins, T and B cell subset panels, Ro (SS-A), La (SS-B), Sm, SCL-70, hepatitis B and C, HIV, *Borrelia burgdorferi* (enzyme-linked immunosorbent assay, and IgG and IgM Western blots), c- and p-antinuclear cytoplasmic autoantibodies (ANCA)

Magnetic resonance imaging (MRI), Magnetic resonance angiography and venography (MRA and MRV); single photon emission computed tomography (SPECT), systemic and cerebral angiography

Electroencephalography, electromyography and nerve conduction studies, lumbar puncture for cerebrospinal fluid analysis: protein, glucose, cell count, immunoglobulin G level, cytology, VDRL, Gram stain, culture, India ink; viral antigens, Lyme Ab, and polymerase chain reaction (PCR)

Biopsy of skin, muscle, and nerve; temporal artery, meninges, and cortex axonopathy acutely in an MNM pattern and over time in a distal symmetric or asymmetric pattern. Cerebrospinal fluid analysis, electroencephalography, and neuroimaging studies are integral to the diagnostic evaluation of most CNS disorders, including vasculitis. Properly performed, lumbar puncture carries minimal risk and provides potentially useful information regarding possible underlying vasculitis so suggested by pleocytosis in excess of five cells per mm^3, protein elevation greater than 100 mg/dL, and evidence of intrathecal synthesis of immunoglobulin and oligoclonal bands. Molecular genetic, immunoassay, and direct staining techniques to exclude spirochetal, fungal, mycobacterial, and viral infections, as well as cytospin examination of CSF for possible malignant cells, should be performed.

CNS vasculitis has no typical electroencephalographic findings but may be warranted if seizures occur. Magnetic resonance imaging is more sensitive than computed tomography, but both methods lack specificity in histologically confirmed cases. The most common magnetic resonance imaging findings are multiple bilateral cortical and deep white matter signal abnormalities and enhancement of the meninges after gadolinium. MR angiography and functional imaging of the brain provide complementary findings to conventional magnetic resonance imaging. The former is useful in the evaluation of medium and large vessel disease but misses fine vessel contours better seen on cut-film or digital subtraction angiography. The abnormal diffuse and focal perfusion patterns seen on single photon emission computed tomography do not always correlate with neurologic symptoms or distinguish vasculitic from nonvasculitic vasculopathy. Some authorities claimed that cerebral angiography showed diagnostic features, but that assertion was later modified. Beading of vessels is found in only about a third of patients with histologically proven CNS vasculitis, as well as in CNS infection, atherosclerosis, cerebral embolism, and vasospasm of diverse cause (Figure 17.14). Multiple microaneurysms, often seen on visceral angiography in systemic vasculitis, are distinctly rare in CNS vessels.

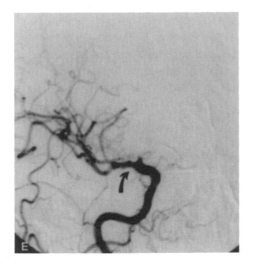

Figure 17.14 Radiographic features of cerebral vasculitis. Ectasia and beading in the M1 segment and lack of flow in the A1 segment of the right anterior cerebral artery (*arrow*) (from Younger DS. Vasculitis and the nervous system. Curr Opin Neurol 2004;17:317–36, with permission)

Brain and meningeal biopsy remain the gold standard for the diagnosis of CNS vasculitis, but false-negatives occur because of focal lesions and sampling errors. Radiographic studies that guide the biopsy site toward areas of abnormality probably improve the sensitivity, but this has not been formally studied. The risk of serious morbidity related to biopsy is less than 2% at most centers, which is probably less than the cumulative risk of an empiric course of long-term immunosuppressive therapy. No certain guidelines have been formulated as to when to proceed to brain and meningeal biopsy. However, it would certainly be warranted, if there were no other explanation for the progressive syndrome of fever, headache, encephalopathy, and focal cerebral signs, in association with CSF pleocytosis and protein content elevation greater than 100 mg/dL, which is suggestive of GANS.

The importance of nerve and muscle biopsy in the diagnosis of vasculitis cannot be overemphasized [29, 30]. The nerve and muscle should be clinically and electrophysiologically affected. A segment of the sural, superficial peroneal sensory, or femoral intermedius sensory nerve can be surgically removed without incurring a serious deficit, along with pieces of muscle tissue, respectively, from the soleus, peroneus brevis, or rectus femoris muscle, thereby providing potentially useful information regarding the severity of the underlying neuropathy and increasing the yield of vasculitic lesions.

Treatment

Neurologists treating vasculitis must choose the sequence and combination of available immunosuppressant and immunomodulating therapies, recognizing the possible beneficial and adverse effects while providing multidisciplinary rehabilitation, pain, and psychotropic therapy.

Immunosuppressant Therapy

The usefulness of corticosteroids in the treatment of systemic vasculitis has been appreciated for over 50 years. Untreated, patients with PAN had a 5-year survival rate of 10%; treatment with corticosteroids increased survival to 48% [31]. Although the effectiveness of corticosteroids is well established, there is uncertainty even among experts as to the optimal regimen. For example, in one analysis sustained benefit in PAN was obtained in patients with a minimum equivalent dosage of 31 mg prednisone daily for 7 months [32]. The beneficial effects of corticosteroids are attributed to a multiplicity of effects on the cell and humoral immune system, including inhibition of activated T and B cells, APC, and leukocytes at sites of inflammation, interferon-γ, induced MHC class II expression, macrophage differentiation, pathogenic cytokine expression, complement interactions, and immunomodulating CAM. Patients receiving long-term corticosteroid therapy for vasculitis should be monitored closely for hypertension, fluid retention, glucose intolerance, cataracts, myopathy, avascular necrosis, osteoporosis, infection, gastric and duodenal ulcers, and psychosis and followed empirically for the need of short-acting insulin coverage, physiotherapy, calcium supplementation, and bone densitometry.

The effectiveness of a daily oral regimen of cyclophosphamide and prednisone in WG served as a template for the treatment of virtually all types of systemic vasculitis for decades [33]. Its favorable affect on vasculitis derives from the preferential T-cell lysis resulting from the inhibition of hematopoietic precursors in the bone marrow, leaving stem cells unharmed. At high doses, this inhibition favors repopulation of the marrow and thus the cellular immune system. After an intravenous dose of cyclophosphamide, the nadir of peripheral leukopenia, which corresponds with peak marrow suppression, occurs in 7–18 days. Less than 20% of labeled cyclophosphamide is excreted unchanged in the urine, with the remainder metabolized to the active products phosphoramide mustard and acrolein, both of which are believed to exert toxic side effects, including hemorrhagic cystitis, bladder cancer, bone marrow suppression with risk of fatal infection, and gonadal toxicity. Bladder toxicity may be reduced by administration of the drug in a single daily oral morning dose followed by hydration and administration of the drug intravenously as pulse therapy, adjusting the dose to renal function. Monthly pulse intravenous cyclophosphamide at doses of 500–1,000 mg/m^2 body surface area, one-half the full-dose therapy for maximal marrow suppression in malignancy, probably achieves similar effectiveness in peripheral nerve vasculitis.

The purine analog azathioprine, which metabolizes to the cytotoxic derivative 6-mercaptopurine, exerts favorable action in vasculitis by the inhibition of T-cell activation and T-cell-dependent antibody-mediated responses. Azathioprine is generally considered a safe alternative to prednisone and cyclophosphamide in virtually all forms of vasculitis. However, there are three drawbacks to its use. First, idiosyncratic side effects, most often gastrointestinal and flu-like, occur in approximately 10% of patients and rarely necessitate permanent withdrawal of the medication. However, pancreatitis and gastritis that are severe enough to warrant hospitalization can occur. Second, bone marrow suppression occurs in nearly all patients, usually manifested by mild pancytopenia. Third, there is typically a long delay, 3 months or more, in the onset of the therapeutic effect. Taking all of these factors into account, most clinicians concur with the slow advancement of the dose over weeks, commencing with 50 mg/day and achieving maintenance levels of 2–3 mg/kg/day with careful monitoring of liver and marrow function.

Immunomodulating Therapy

High-dose intravenous immunoglobulin (IVIg) therapy is the most widely used immunomodulating agent for autoimmune neurologic disorders [34] and has applicability in the treatment of CNS and PNS vasculitis, as primary therapy in those who are not candidates for immunosuppressant therapy, and in others as adjunctive therapy. The immunomodulating and anti-inflammatory actions of IVIg are provided by monthly doses of 2,000 mg/kg/body weight given at 400 mg/kg/day for 5 days each month at a slow drip with acetaminophen and diphenhydramine pretreatment to prevent the commonest side effects, including fever, chills, rash, erythema, flushing, headache, nausea, myalgia, arthralgia, abdominal cramps, and chest and back pain. True anaphylactic reactions to IVIg can occur in recipients with documented prior allergies to immunoglobulins or antibodies, especially IgA type. Transient reversible renal insufficiency occurs in patients with preexisting renal disease. Susceptible individuals can be identified by less than normal expected 24-h creatinine clearance rates for age and abnormal vascular perfusion on radionuclide scans. Aseptic meningitis rarely occurs several hours after treatment and resolves over several days with discontinuation of therapy.

Supportive Therapy

A multidisciplinary approach to vasculitis requires the commitment of a team of health professionals and caregivers to optimize recovery while initiating immunotherapy. Physical therapy and orthosis may be warranted for disabling motor and cognitive disorder impairments to maintain range of motion and strength, to improve function status, and to maintain ambulation. Effective pain management may be an important aspect of their care, not only to provide overall well-being but also to permit more aggressive physiotherapy. Agents such as tricyclic antidepressants, gabapentin, mexiletine, opioids, clonazepam, and topical anesthetic creams have all been used with varying success. Finally, efforts should be made to limit ischemic-enhancing effects of other conditions, such as with diabetes mellitus through improved glycemic control and regulation of blood pressure.

Conclusions

Vasculitis involving the CNS and PNS can be seen in a variety of systemic disorders. True isolated CNS vasculitis seems to be rare but carries a relatively poor prognosis. Early diagnosis and appropriate treatment is key in preventing significant mortality and morbidity associated with this condition.

References

1. Younger DS. Vasculitis and connective tissue disorders. In: Griggs R, Joynt R, editors. Baker and Joynt's clinical neurology on CD-ROM. Philadelphia: Lippincott Williams &Wilkins; 2003.
2. Younger DS. Vasculitis and the nervous system. Curr Opin Neurol. 2004;17: 317–36.
3. Longcope WT. Periarteritis nodosa, with report of a case with autopsy. Bull Ayer Clin Lab Penn Hosp Phila. 1908;5:1.
4. Kernohan JW, Woltman HW. Periarteritis nodosa: a clinicopathologic study with special reference to the nervous system. Arch Neurol Psychiatry. 1938;39:655.
5. Kawasaki T. Pediatric acute mucocutaneous lymph node syndrome: clinical observation of 50 cases (in Japanese). Arerugi (Jpn J Allergy). 1967;16:178–222.
6. Melish ME, Hicks RM, Larson EJ. Mucocutaneous lymph node syndrome in the United States. Am J Dis Child. 1976;130:599–607.
7. Ichiyama T, Nishikawa M, Hayashi T, et al. Cerebral hypoperfusion during acute Kawasaki disease. Stroke. 1998;29:1320–1.
8. Amano S, Hazama F. Neural involvement in Kawasaki disease. Acta Pathol Jpn. 1980;30:365–73.
9. Newburger JW, Takahashi M, Burns JC, et al. The treatment of Kawasaki syndrome with intravenous immunoglobulin. NEJM. 1986;315:341–7.
10. Davson J, Ball J, Platt R. The kidney in periarteritis nodosa. QJM. 1948;17:175.
11. Churg J, Strauss L. Allergic granulomatosis, allergic angiitis, and periarteritis nodosa. Am J Pathol. 1951;27:277.
12. Zeek PM, Smith CC, Weeter JC. Studies on periarteritis nodosa, III: the differentiation between the vascular lesions of periarteritis nodosa and of hypersensitivity. Am J Pathol. 1948;24:889.
13. Godman GC, Churg J. Wegener's granulomatosis: pathology and review of the literature. Arch Pathol. 1954;58:533.
14. Drachman DA. Neurological complications of Wegener's granulomatosis. Arch Neurol. 1963;8:45.

15. Horton BT, Magath BT, Brown GE. Arteritis of temporal vessels: report of 7 cases. Proc Staff Meet Mayo Clin. 1937;12:548.
16. Jennings GH. Arteritis of the temporal vessels. Lancet. 1938;1:424.
17. Harbitz F. Unknown forms of arteritis with special reference to their relation to syphilitic arteritis and periarteritis nodosa. Am J Med Sci. 1922;163:250.
18. Cravioto H, Fegin I. Non-infectious granulomatous angiitis with a predilection for the nervous system. Neurology. 1959;9:599.
19. Cupps T, Moore P, Fauci A. Isolated angiitis of the central nervous system: prospective diagnostic and therapeutic experience. Am J Med. 1983;74:97.
20. Younger DS, Hays AP, Brust JCM, Rowland LP. Granulomatous angiitis of the brain: an inflammatory reaction of nonspecific etiology. Arch Neurol. 1988;45:514–8.
21. Calabrese LH, Graff LA, Furlan AJ. Benign angiopathy: a distinct subset of angiographically defined primary angiitis of the central nervous system. J Rheumatol. 1993;20:2046.
22. Younger DS, Calabrese LH, Hays AP. Granulomatous angiitis of the nervous system. Neurol Clin. 1997;15:821–34.
23. Salvarani C, Brown Jr RD, Calamia KT, et al. Primary CNS vasculitis with spinal cord involvement. Neurology. 2008;70:2394–400.
24. Younger DS. CNS vasculitis with spinal cord involvement. J Watch Neurol. 2008;10:76–7.
25. Younger DS, Sacco RL, Khandji AG, et al. Major cerebral vessel occlusion in SLE due to circulating anticardiolipin antibodies. Stroke. 1994;25:912–4.
26. Oksi J, Kalimo H, Martila RJ. Inflammatory brain changes in Lyme borreliosis. A report on three patients and review of the literature. Brain. 1996;119:2143–54.
27. Younger DS, Rosoklija G, Hays AP. Lyme polyradiculoneuritis: immunohistochemical findings in sural nerve. Muscle Nerve. 1995;18:359–60.
28. Citron BP, Halpern M, Mccarron M, et al. Necrotizing angiitis associated with drug abuse. N Engl J Med. 1970;283:1003.
29. Lovelace RE. Mononeuritis multiplex in polyarteritis nodosa. Neurology. 1964;14:434.
30. Wees SJ, Sunwood LN, Oh SJ. Sural nerve biopsy in systemic necrotizing vasculitis. Am J Med. 1981;71:525–32.
31. Frohnert PP, Sheps SG. Long-term follow-up study of periarteritis nodosa. Am J Med. 1967;43:8.
32. Leib ES, Restivo C, Paulus HE. Immunosuppressive and corticosteroid therapy of polyarteritis nodosa. Am J Med. 1979;67:941.
33. Fauci AS, Wolff SM, Johnson JS. Effect of cyclophosphamide upon the immune response in Wegener's granulomatosis. N Engl J Med. 1971;285:1493.
34. Dalakas MC. Intravenous immunoglobulin in autoimmune neuromuscular diseases. JAMA. 2004;291:2367–75.

Part III

Peripheral Nervous System Disorders

Immunologic Disorders of Neuromuscular Junction and Muscle

Kara A. Chisholm, James M. Gilchrist, and John E. Donahue

Keywords: Neuromuscular junction, Synapses, Weakness, Voltage-gated sodium channels, Electromyography

Introduction

A range of inherited and acquired processes can adversely affect the neuromuscular junction (NMJ) and muscle, many of which are not amenable to medical therapy, such as the muscular dystrophies. Autoimmune disorders of NMJ and muscle provide some of the limited number of peripheral neuromuscular diseases responsive to medical therapy and thus, are essential to recognize. Immune disorders account for the most common diseases of neuromuscular transmission and are very important to understand, not least because the autoimmune nature of disease provides opportunities for effective treatment. On the other hand, inflammatory disorders of muscle are a diverse group, some of which appear to have an immunologic basis, e.g., polymyositis and dermatomyositis, and possibly, inclusion body myositis (IBM).

Neuromuscular Junction Anatomy

The NMJ is a synapse which transmits signals between a motor nerve terminal and a muscle fiber, the pre- and postsynaptic areas, respectively. The motor axon terminal contains active zones of arranged P/Q-type voltage-gated calcium channels (VGCC). Acetylcholine (ACh)-filled synaptic vesicles collect at these active zones. The primary synaptic cleft which divides the pre- and postsynaptic areas is composed of a basal lamina which contains acetylcholinesterase, which catabolizes acetylcholine as it diffuses across the primary synaptic cleft. The postsynaptic membrane is composed of junctional folds containing nicotinic-acetylcholine receptors (AChR) with ligand-gated cation channels. At the base of the folds are voltage-gated sodium channels (VGSC). The adult AChR is a tetramer containing 2 α subunits, and one each of β, δ, and ε subunits.

From: *Clinical Neuroimmunology: Multiple Sclerosis and Related Disorders*, Current Clinical Neurology,
Edited by: S.A. Rizvi and P.K. Coyle, DOI 10.1007/978-1-60327-860-7_18,
© Springer Science+Business Media, LLC 2011

Fetal AChR contain a γ subunit in place of the ε subunit. Each α subunit contains a ligand site for ACh as well as a main immunogenic region (MIR). ACh must bind to both ligand sites to activate the receptor channel [1].

When an action potential reaches the motor nerve terminal, VGCC are activated allowing influx of calcium into the nerve terminal. The influx of calcium triggers exocytosis of the ACh-synaptic vesicles and ACh is released into the primary synaptic cleft. ACh passively diffuses across the synaptic cleft to bind to postsynaptic AChR. Once activated, AChR undergo a conformational change allowing the influx of sodium and efflux of potassium, causing a small depolarization in the adjacent muscle membrane. A miniature endplate potential (MEPP) is the potential generated by the release of a single quanta of ACh. Since many synaptic vesicles are released, many MEPPs temporally and spatially summate to form an endplate potential (EPP). If this EPP is sufficient to depolarize the membrane to threshold, an action potential is generated and propagated by way of VGSC leading to muscle fiber contraction [1].

Myasthenia Gravis

Clinical Description

Myasthenia gravis (MG) was first described by Thomas Willis in 1672. It is characterized by fatigable weakness and prior to the discovery of anticholinesterase inhibitors and mechanical ventilation, it was a frequently lethal disease. It is the most common disorder of neuromuscular transmission and the discovery of polyclonal auto-antibodies directed against the postsynaptic NMJ in 1970 revolutionized the treatment and prognosis of MG. The most common presentation involves ocular, bulbar, and limb muscles. Fifty to sixty percent of patients present with ocular muscle weakness manifesting as ptosis and diplopia. An additional 30% will eventually develop ocular symptoms. Up to 90% of ocular myasthenics will eventually have generalized disease, causing bulbar, limb, and respiratory weakness [2]. Bulbar symptoms such as dysarthria and dysphagia can result in weight loss and aspiration pneumonia. Myasthenic crisis is the most severe manifestation when respiratory muscle weakness leads to respiratory failure.

Infants have two unique varieties – juvenile and neonatal myasthenia. Neonatal myasthenia occurs in progeny of myasthenic mothers within hours to days of birth. Arthrogryposis, generalized weakness, poor suck and swallow, and respiratory dysfunction can occur. Disease results from placentally transmitted AChR auto-antibodies and can be fatal if there is antenatal involvement. If not, symptoms generally, fully resolve in a few weeks and the infants are not at further risk for myasthenia gravis. Juvenile myasthenia is similar to the adult variety with slower progression, more severe ophthalmoplegia, and a higher likelihood for remission [3].

Diagnosis

The diagnosis is suggested by fatigable weakness of ocular, bulbar, or limb skeletal muscles. The clinical suspicion can be confirmed with autoantibody testing, short-acting anticholinesterase inhibitors such as edrophonium and electrodiagnostic testing. Eighty percent of patients have antibodies against the acetylcholine receptor. These antibodies include binding, blocking, and modulating varieties, the former of which accounts for over 90% of acetylcholine receptor antibodies [1]. Seronegative myasthenia may be a manifestation of technical laboratory errors, antibodies with high affinity to their antigens, prolonged immunosuppression or unknown auto-antibodies [4]. Recently, up to 40% of seronegative myasthenic patients were found to have antibodies against muscle-specific kinase (MuSK). MuSK is a tyrosine kinase which regulates and maintains acetylcholine receptor clustering [5]. These antibodies effectively disrupt the structure and function of the postsynaptic NMJ and lead to loss of acetylcholine receptors. Anti-striated muscle antibodies directed against thymic myoid cells are present in 27% of myasthenic patients and up to 90% of myasthenic patients with thymoma [6].

Edrophonium testing allows for transient improvement of symptoms in a clinically weak, easily tested muscle such as the deltoid or a ptotic eyelid. Such testing is 90–95% sensitive for generalized myasthenia and 80–90% sensitive and specific for ocular myasthenia. Electrodiagnostic testing includes repetitive nerve stimulation and single fiber electromyography (EMG). Repetitive nerve stimulation tests for compound motor action potential decrement from baseline and transient postexercise facilitation. Single fiber EMG quantitatively assesses jitter, a manifestation of the variability in time it takes the EPP to reach threshold for action potential propagation at the NMJs of individual muscle fibers. In myasthenia gravis, there is increased jitter with intermittent neuromuscular transmission blocking, clinically manifesting as weakness [1].

Pathophysiology

Myasthenia gravis results from an antibody-mediated, T-cell-dependent autoimmune attack on the postsynaptic NMJ with associated damage to, and simplification of, the postsynaptic membrane and reduction in number of AChR. The autoimmune nature of MG is thought related to the loss of tolerance to self-antigens originating from thymic T cells. Up to 70% of myasthenics have thymic hyperplasia and another 15% have thymomas [1, 4]. The hyperplastic thymus has an increased number of myoid cells which produce AChR similar to endplate AChR. These myoid cells are in close proximity to MHC-II interdigitating cells, which function as antigen presenting cells, and are thought to present AChR fragments to auto-reactive T cells. These T-cells then aid AChR B-cells in producing autoantibodies through the production of cytokines. AChR-specific T-cells are also found in patients without MG, implying loss of tolerance or inhibitory control is necessary to lead to myasthenia gravis [4].

Antibodies in MG are heterogeneous with differing mechanisms, epitope recognition, and isotypes. This polyclonal expansion may explain the lack of correlation at times between symptoms and antibody titers. Most AChR antibodies bind to the α subunit, at the MIR. Antibodies may bind, block, or modulate the AChR. Binding antibodies crosslink two AChR, causing internalization and degradation, a process which is accelerated if more than one antibody binds. In this latter case, the clustered AChR are destroyed as well as VGSC, thereby increasing the depolarization threshold needed for generation of action potentials [4].

Complement also plays a major role in the destruction of the postsynaptic membrane. Lytic phase activation and membrane attack complex (MAC) deposition at the NMJ causes shedding of postsynaptic junctional folds and AChR. The combination of antibody degradation of AChR and MAC destruction of junctional folds limits the surface area and the number of AChR available at the postsynaptic NMJ [4].

Treatment

Treatment can be symptomatic in purely ocular disease, using a longer acting form of acetylcholinesterase inhibitor such as pyridostigmine. Pyridostigmine is also efficacious in quickly but transiently treating fatigable weakness in generalized myasthenia. Steroids are used as first-line immunomodulating therapy and can effectively induce clinical remission in up to 80% of patients, with sustained improvement beginning within 2 weeks. High-dose steroid induction can cause transient worsening of myasthenia and requires inpatient hospitalization to monitor for respiratory failure. Second-line therapies include azathioprine, which inhibits T-cell proliferation, and mycophenolate mofetil, which inhibits an enzyme crucial in purine synthesis and critical for B- and T-cell production. Cyclosporine was proven effective by a prospective, double-blind, placebo-controlled trial but is usually limited to patients who fail steroids and azathioprine, due to kidney and liver toxicity, and hypertension. Pulse cyclophosphamide has been shown to help refractory patients in a small open trial, but its use is limited by myelosuppression, malignancy, and hemorrhagic cystitis [7]. A Cochrane review of immunosuppressants in MG found improvement with cyclophosphamide or with cyclosporine with or without corticosteroids in small randomized control trials. Other small randomized control trials showed no improvement with azathioprine, mycophenolate mofetil, or tacrolimus [8].

Intravenous immunoglobulin (IVIG) causes transient improvement in 70% of myasthenic patients within 5 days, and can last for 8–12 weeks. A Cochrane review showed benefit of IVIg over placebo, but no difference between IVIG and plasma exchange. There was no difference between 1 and 2 g/kg of IVIG or between IVIG and oral methylprednisolone. Plasma exchange rapidly but temporarily reduces antibody titers and is a very important part of the treatment of myasthenic crisis [9]. It can also be useful in patients refractory to other treatments or in those needing immediate but transient improvement, such as prior to thymectomy. Thymectomy provides long-term benefit which may be delayed for 6–12 months or even, years, and is usually done in patients between 18 and 55 with generalized disease. It is essential in the 15% of myasthenic patients with thymomas. The goal of thymectomy is improved symptoms, decreased medication requirement, and an increased rate of remission postthymectomy. Recent small, open studies suggest rituximab, an anti-CD20+ monoclonal antibody, and etanercept, a tumor necrosis factor blocking agent, may be efficacious in myasthenia [10]. Eculizamab, an inhibitor of the C5 component of the complement cascade, therefore inhibiting the MAC, is also under investigation for MG.

Lambert–Eaton Myasthenic Syndrome

Clinical Description

Lambert–Eaton myasthenic syndrome (LEMS) was initially described in 1953, as potentially the first paraneoplastic disease. LEMS presents insidiously with symmetric weakness and fatigue in a proximal to distal gradient. Muscle aches and paresthesias are often present. Reflexes are characteristically absent, but return transiently following voluntary muscle contraction [11]. Seventy-five percent of patients with LEMS have dysautonomia manifesting as dry mouth, dry eyes, impotence, constipation, difficulty with micturation, decreased sweating, and pupillary abnormalities [1]. Unlike myasthenia gravis, oculomotor abnormalities and respiratory crises are uncommon.

While 50% of LEMS patients are associated with paraneoplastic syndrome, three-quarters of the neoplasm are not diagnosed until 1–5 years following neurological presentation. Paraneoplastic LEMS is often associated with other paraneoplastic syndromes such as cerebellar degeneration, sensorimotor polyneuropathy, and encephalomyelitis, which helps to distinguish this from the autoantibody variety [11–13].

One striking clinical feature pathognomonic to disorders of presynaptic NMJ transmission is facilitation. Muscles and reflexes that were once weak return to nearly normal strength after exercise.

Diagnosis

Diagnosis is based on a high-degree of clinical suspicion. Electrodiagnostic findings of reduced compound muscle action potentials (CMAP) with greater than 100% increment of CMAP amplitude following 10–30 s of exercise (postexercise facilitation) are diagnostic of a presynaptic disorder. Similar postexercise facilitation is seen following 20–50 Hz repetitive nerve stimulation, which is not recommended in the conscious patient due to its great discomfort. Slow repetitive nerve stimulation (2–5 Hz) reveals >10% decrement preexercise with repair of decrement and increase in CMAP amplitude immediately following exercise and subsequent decrement after 2–3 min. Single fiber EMG shows abnormal jitter with blocking, but jitter decreasing with an increase in firing rate. Electrodiagnostic testing cannot differentiate paraneoplastic from autoimmune LEMS [11, 13]. Serial CMAP amplitude measurements and single fiber EMG studies may correlate with treatment response [14].

Antibodies against P/Q-type VGCC are found in up to 85% of LEMS patients. High titers strongly support the diagnosis, whereas low titers can be seen in non-LEMS patients and absent titers do not rule out the diagnosis. Anti-Hu or other antinuclear neuronal antibodies are suggestive of paraneoplastic LEMS in association with small cell lung carcinoma [15].

Once the diagnosis is made, the search for neoplasm should focus on small cell lung carcinoma, the primary neoplasm implicated in paraneoplastic LEMS. Other neoplasms associated include T-cell leukemia, lymphoma, Castleman's syndrome, and reticulum-cell sarcoma [16].

Pathophysiology

LEMS is caused by a polyclonal antibody attack directed against the P/Q VGCC located on the presynaptic membrane of the NMJ. VGCCs contain $\alpha 1$, β, and $\alpha 2/\delta$ subunits, with the $\alpha 1$ subunit serving as the ligand-binding site as well as containing the calcium conductance channel. The autoimmune attack results in the loss of calcium channels and disorganization of the active zones, where exocytosis of acetylcholine-containing synaptic vesicles occurs. There is reduction in acetylcholine release into the NMJ, resulting in fewer MEPPs at the postsynaptic terminal, resulting in a decreased EPP. If the EPP is below threshold for action potential generation, then neuromuscular transmission is unsuccessful and weakness occurs. Exercise serves to increase ingress of calcium, allowing for increased synaptic vesicle release, increased numbers of MEPPs, and an EPP sufficient to reach threshold, thus explaining facilitation [1].

Treatment

In paraneoplastic LEMS, treatment is directed at the primary neoplasm, removal of which often reduces symptoms or allows remission [12]. Symptomatic treatments include pyridostigmine, guanidine, and 3,4-diaminopyridine (3,4 DAP). Pyridostigmine, an acetylcholinesterase inhibitor, inhibits the breakdown of acetylcholine, effectively enhancing the MEPP amplitudes allowing for increased EPP and successful neuromuscular transmission. Guanidine enhances synaptic vesicle release of acetylcholine from the presynaptic terminal, but is no longer available due to significant toxicity. Diaminopyridine inhibits voltage-gated potassium channels, which lengthens the action potential and prolongs calcium entry into the presynaptic terminal, thereby increasing acetylcholine release into the primary synaptic cleft. It is not approved by the FDA in the USA but may be obtained via a compassionate use Investigational New Drug (IND) [1].

Immunologic therapy is an important mainstay in patients not undergoing cancer treatment. Prednisone and azathioprine or their combination has been shown to be efficacious [17]. Plasma exchange and IVIG are used as in myasthenia to remove autoantibodies or suppress their production. A Cochrane review of treatments in LEMS showed improvement in strength in two studies of 3,4-DAP with 38 total patients and one study of nine patients using IVIg. Other LEMS treatments have not been studied in randomized, controlled trials [18].

Polymyositis

Clinical Description

Polymyositis (PM) presents insidiously in adults with progressive symmetrical proximal weakness. Symptoms include difficulty climbing stairs, getting out of a chair, and combing hair. Up to 50% have myalgias and tenderness to palpation. Atrophy occurs in severe weakness with associated reduced reflexes. Pharyngeal and neck extensor weakness may lead to dysphagia and head drop. In advanced cases, there may be involvement of respiratory muscles and distal hand muscles. Facial and extraocular muscles are typically spared. Other organ system involvement includes cardiac disease due to myocarditis and interstitial lung disease (ILD). ILD can be a result of methotrexate toxicity or in 10% of PM, seen in association with anti-Jo or ribonucleoprotein antibodies [19, 20].

Diagnosis

The diagnosis of PM is based on clinical suspicion, muscle enzyme testing, EMG, and muscle biopsy. Characteristically, creatine kinase can be up to 50 times the upper limit of normal. EMG findings include short-duration, low-amplitude polyphasic potentials with abnormal spontaneous activity which is

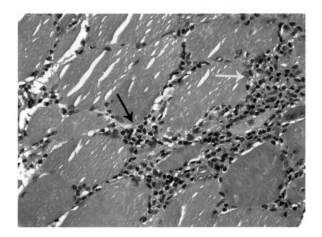

Figure 18.1 Polymyositis. Muscle fibers are surrounded by inflammatory cells, mainly lymphocytes (*black arrow*). At least one fiber in this figure is undergoing myophagocytosis (*white arrow*). H&E stain, ×400

characteristic of necrotic myopathies such as PM. Muscle biopsy is the most specific diagnostic test, revealing endomysial inflammation with muscle fiber necrosis (Figure 18.1). CD8+ T-cells invading non-necrotic muscle fibers expressing MHC-1 antigens are characteristic [20, 21].

Pathophysiology

PM is thought due to a T-cell-mediated attack on muscle fibers. Macrophages and cytotoxic CD8+ T-cells surround and eventually invade non-necrotic muscle tissue, eventually leading to muscle fiber destruction. These cytotoxic T-cells recognize an unknown antigenic target in association with MHC-1 antigens expressed by muscle fibers. T-cells induce muscle fiber necrosis via perforin, a membrane lytic molecule [20–22].

In up to 20% of inflammatory myopathies, there are autoantibodies against nuclear and cytoplasmic antigens (Table 18.1). Ribonucleoproteins are involved in translation and protein synthesis and are the target of several anti-cytoplasmic antibodies such as Jo-1, PL-7, PL-12, OJ, EJ, SRP, PMS1, and PMS2. Anti-Jo-1, directed against histidyl-transfer RNA synthetase, comprises up to 75% of the antisynthetase antibodies. These antibodies are not specific to PM as they are seen in both dermatomyositis (DM) and IBM, and occur in ILD in the absence of myositis [23, 24].

Antisynthetase syndrome is the most common syndrome with myositis and autoantibodies. The typical presentation is ILD and myositis, often with Raynaud's, fever, arthralgia, and thickened cracked fingers known as "mechanic's hands," often with a more acute, crescendo presentation. Anti-Jo-1, named for the first person in which the antibody was identified is found in 60–80% of patients, with PL-7, PL-12, EJ, OJ, or KS found in the remainder of patients. There is a threefold increase in mortality compared with PM, perhaps due to its association with ILD [23].

Overlap syndromes exist between connective tissue diseases and either PM or DM. Systemic lupus erythematosis has an associated myositis in 8% of patients. Of these patients, antinuclear antibodies directed against native DNA and anti-Sm

Table 18.1 Antibodies seen in inflammatory myopathies.

Autoantibody	Antigen target	Clinical presentation
Anti-Jo 1	Histidyl t-RNA synthetase	Antisynthetase syndrome
Anti-PL-7	Threonyl-t-RNA synthetase	Polyarthritis
Anti-PL-12	Alanyl-t-RNA synthetase	
Anti-EJ	Glycl-t-RNA synthetase	ILD
Anti-KS	Asparaginyl-t-RNA synthetase	"Mechanic" hands
Anti-OJ	Isoleucyl-t-RNA synthetase	Myositis
Anti-SRP	325-kDa ribonucleoprotein	Anti-SRP syndrome (muscle, cardiac involvement, steroid resistant)
Anti-Mi2	Transcription peptide complex	DM ± ILD
Anti-Scl-PM	Peptide complex	Scleroderma, myositis, scleroderma/PM or DM
Anti-Ku	Heterodimer associated with DNA-dependant protein kinase	Scleroderma/PM or DM overlap syndromes, SLE, scleroderma, MCTD, Sjogren's, thyroiditis, pulmonary hypertension
Anti-PMS	DNA binding protein complex	PM and DM
Anti-56 kDa	Ribonucleoprotein	PM and DM of childhood onset

ILD inflammatory lung disease, *SRP* signal recognition protein, *DM* dermatomyositis, *PM* polymyositis, *SLE* systemic lupus erythematosis, *MCTD* mixed connective tissue disease.

are specific to SLE-myositis patients. Other antibodies include anti-SSA (Ro), anti-SS-B (La), and anti-U1 ribonuclear protein, but are not specific to SLE-myositis patients. Myositis is rarely associated with Sjogren's syndrome with antibodies against the ribonucleoproteins SS-A and SS-B. Up to 13% of rheumatoid arthritis is associated with myositis. Scleroderma has myositis as a feature in 5–17%. In North America, 25% of patients with Scleroderma and myositis have anti-PM-Scl (anti-PM1) antibodies, while in Japan, anti-Ku antibodies are more common. Anti-U1 ribonuclear protein is seen in mixed connective tissue disease [24]. Anti-signal recognition particle antibodies were previously associated with PM, but recent studies have shown that they are part of a distinctive syndrome consisting of a steroid-resistant necrotizing myopathy with little inflammation, and MAC deposition and capillary loss [25, 26].

PM can be seen during the course of other autoimmune diseases such as Crohn's disease, vasculitis, sarcoidosis, celiac disease, primary biliary cirrhosis, Behcet's disease, and Hashimoto's disease, among others. Giant cell myositis is associated with thymomas and as such, can also be seen in patients with myasthenia gravis [21].

Treatment

Corticosteroids remain the mainstay of treatment for PM with more than 80% of patients responding to some degree. Noticeable clinical improvement occurs within 3–6 months. For patients who do not respond, or who relapse during prednisone therapy, second-line agents include azathioprine, methotrexate, cyclophosphamide, chlorambucil, cyclosporine, mycophenolate mofetil, IVIG, and plasmapheresis. Methotrexate is a folate antagonist used in patients who respond poorly to steroids or azathioprine [19]. Chlorambucil is an ankylating agent used in cancer treatment with variable response in inflammatory myopathies. Relapses should be differentiated from steroid myopathy, which has normal CK levels, no abnormal spontaneous activity on needle EMG, and type 2 fiber atrophy on muscle biopsy. The myositis, arthralgias, and systemic symptoms of antisynthetase syndrome tend to respond to steroids, while the ILD can be steroid responsive, depending on subset. Case reports have shown efficacy with cyclosporine, cyclophosphamide, and tacrolimus in the steroid-resistant cases. Undetectable antisynthetase antibodies after treatment predicts a favorable prognosis [23]. A Cochrane review of treatments for both PM and DM found equal efficacy with azathioprine and methotrexate, with the latter having a more favorable side-effect profile. Studies comparing cyclosporine and methotrexate as well as intramuscular methotrexate versus oral methotrexate and azathioprine found no differences [27].

Dermatomyositis

Clinical Description

Dermatomyositis (DM) occurs in children and adults and is characterized by skin changes which accompany or may precede weakness. An edematous bluish-purple discoloration of the upper eyelid, "heliotrope rash," flat erythematous rash of the face, chest and extensor surface dermatitis exacerbated by sun exposure, and Gottron's rash, a erythematous, scaly, violaceous rash on the knuckles, are all characteristic. Nail changes with dilated capillary loops, thickened cuticles and rough, cracked "mechanic hands" may occur. Subcutaneous calcifications occur more frequently in children and may cause ulcerations [19]. Weakness occurs subacutely with a proximal to distal gradient.

Cardiac manifestations include cardiomyopathy, conduction defects and tachyarrhythmia similar to polymyositis. Pulmonary symptoms are related to ILD, methotrexate toxicity, or thoracic muscle weakness. Gastrointestinal ulceration, joint contractures, and systemic symptoms occur. Rarely, renal failure and rhabdomyolysis may be seen in acute presentations. DM has an increased risk of malignancy which can precede the diagnosis, but usually occurs within 2 years of the myositis. Women over the age of 40 appear to be at greatest risk of associated neoplasm. Commonly associated cancers include breast, lung, ovarian, and gastrointestinal [19].

Diagnosis

Skin manifestations of dermatomyositis are pathognomonic. Clinical diagnosis can be confirmed with muscle enzyme testing, electrodiagnostic testing, and muscle biopsy. Creatine kinase often reflects disease severity and can be increased up to 50-fold. Electromyography reveals myopathic features interspersed with rare neurogenic motor unit potentials and abnormal spontaneous activity. Perifasicular inflammation, endothelial hyperplasia, and capillary loss are characteristic muscle biopsy features (Figures 18.2 and 18.3). Frequently, a high percentage of B cells and an increased CD4+/CD8+ ratio may be found on immunohistochemistry of muscle [19]. Perifasicular atrophy (Figure 18.3) results from watershed zone microinfarcts within muscle fascicules and is highly suggestive of DM.

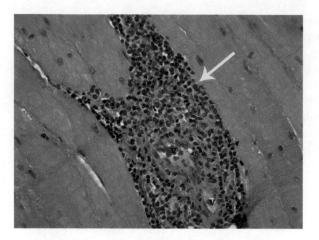

Figure 18.2 Dermatomyositis. Inflammatory cells, mainly lymphocytes (*arrow*) are seen completely surrounding and invading two small, interstitial blood vessels (V). H&E stain, ×400

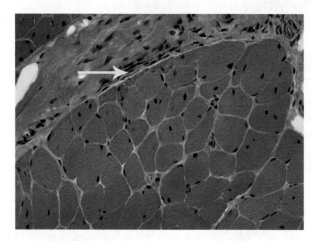

Figure 18.3 Dermatomyositis. Unlike polymyositis, dermatomyositis is a vasculitis, which leads to ischemic damage along the periphery of the muscle fascicles, resulting in "perifasicular atrophy" (*arrow*). H&E stain, ×400

Pathophysiology

Dermatomyositis is caused by antibody-mediated damage of muscle capillaries with subsequent necrosis, capillary loss, and focal muscle ischemia. While the antigen is unknown, it is thought to be a component of the endothelium of endomysial vessels. An antibody-mediated activation of complement C3 leads to the formation and deposition of C3bNEO and MAC deposition on endomysial capillaries. MAC deposition leads to endothelial damage and subsequent capillary necrosis [19]. The remaining capillaries dilate to compensate for the capillary loss, and perifasicular atrophy occurs as a result of hypoperfusion to this watershed area. Microinfarcts occur as a result of necrosis of larger intramuscular vessels. Muscle fiber damage also occurs from recruitment of macrophages and T-cells by chemotactic factors as a result of complement activation.

Treatment

The mainstay of treatment is corticosteroids in high doses. The mechanism of action is unclear but may involve inhibiting movement of lymphocytes to areas of muscle inflammation. Steroid-sparing medications include azathioprine, methotrexate, cyclophosphamide, and IVIg. Other treatments used with varying success include mycophenolate, rituximab, cyclosporine, and chlorambucil [19]. A Cochrane review of treatments showed benefit in DM with IVIg versus placebo in one small trial [27].

Inclusion Body Myositis

Clinical Description

IBM is the most common primary muscle disorder in people older than 50 years. There is a male predominance and IBM is usually sporadic with rare autosomal recessive inheritance. The course is one of indolent progression of asymmetric weakness affecting the legs before the arms. Patients often present with falling and tripping from quadriceps and foot plantar flexor weakness. Finger flexor weakness contributes to difficulty with fine motor skills such as buttoning and opening jars. The combination of quadriceps and finger flexor weakness and atrophy is characteristic of IBM. Weak quadriceps muscles contribute to depressed patellar reflex. Other muscles commonly affected include biceps, triceps, iliopsoas, and tibialis anterior. Dysphagia is a presenting feature in 30–40%. Facial weakness can occur along with other cranial nerves, but respiratory muscles are relatively spared [28].

Diagnosis

Diagnosis is based on clinical, laboratory, electrodiagnostic, and biopsy findings. Creatine kinase is often elevated two- to threefold but can be up tenfold or may be normal. Electrodiagnostic testing helps to exclude neurogenic conditions such as amyotrophic lateral sclerosis. Myopathic features are most commonly seen on needle electromyography though in 1/3 of patients neurogenic features may be interspersed with myopathic motor unit potentials [29]. Spontaneous activity is seen due to myonecrosis but may be underwhelming. Muscle biopsy (Figure 18.4) findings include rimmed vacuoles, endomysial inflammation, eosinophilic inclusions, swollen or vacuolated nuclei, and a combination of hypertrophic and atrophic fibers. Red-ragged fibers may be seen due to abnormal mitochondria after nuclear damage. Electron microscopy reveals intranuclear and intracytoplasmic filamentous inclusions, approximately 10–18 nm in diameter.

Pathophysiology

Muscle biopsy findings in IBM include significant endomysial inflammation similar to PM. Cytotoxic T-cells comprise 70% of the endomysial inflammatory

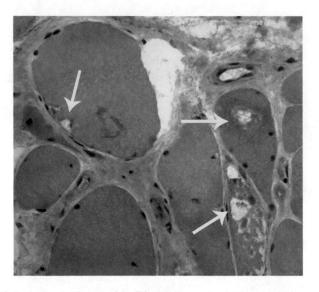

Figure 18.4 Inclusion body myositis. Rimmed vacuoles (*arrows*) within muscle fibers are a prominent part of the pathology of inclusion body myositis. Modified Gomori trichrome stain, ×400

cells and preferentially invade non-necrotic muscle, implicating inflammatory cells in muscle fiber necrosis. MHC-1 antigens have also been found surrounding these inflammatory cells, implicating a T-cell-mediated process similar to that in PM [22].

No specific antigen has been found in IBM, and the possibility that the presence of cytotoxic T-cells is a reactive rather than a primary autoimmune phenomenon, as seen in Duchenne muscular dystrophy, has been raised [30]. Amemiya et al. found that a limited number of T-cell receptor gene rearrangements persisted over time, implicating an immune process against a few specific antigens [31].

Treatment

Treatment in IBM is largely supportive as no effective pharmacologic treatment has been found. Steroids, azathioprine, cyclophosphamide, methotrexate, beta-interferon 1a, lymphoid irradiation, and IVIG have shown no benefit. Cricopharyngeal botulinum toxin may be beneficial in patients with severe dysphagia [32].

Other Myopathies

Eosinophilic myositis is a rare form of PM in which there is peripheral eosinophilia and eosinophilic infiltrates of the endomysium. The cytokine IL-5 is thought to activate eosinophils which invade muscle fibers (Figure 18.5), degranulate and release cytotoxic materials. Eosinophilic myositis has

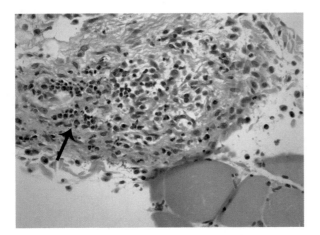

Figure 18.5 Eosinophilic myositis. A cluster of inflammatory cells with a prominent eosinophilic component (*arrow*) can be seen adjacent to a group of muscle fibers. The patient was thought to have Churg–Strauss syndrome. H&E stain, ×400

occurred as a consequence of calpain-3 mutations, which often causes adult-onset limb girdle muscular dystrophy (LGMD type 2A), in children under 10 years with elevated creatine kinase and peripheral eosinophilia [33, 34]. Laminin $\alpha 2$ (merosin) deficiency can have an associated perimysial, endomysial, and perivascular B- and T-cell infiltration with myofiber necrosis [35]. Macrophages and lymphocytes with MHC-I expression have been found in LGMD2L, Duchenne muscular dystrophy, Becker muscular dystrophy, and LGMD2B [36].

Inflammatory cells are found in 40–80% of biopsies in fascioscapulohumeral muscular dystrophy (FSHD). The absence of CD8+ T-cells and perforin implies that there is likely no cytotoxic T-cell-mediated muscle fiber damage. Like DM, there is a high CD4+ to CD8+ ratio and CD4+ cells are in close proximity to B cells, though there is no inflammatory invasion of non-necrotic muscle fibers nor capillary complement deposition. Perivascular T-cell accumulation with mononuclear vessel invasion (initiated by connective tissue signaling) has lead to the suggestion that FSHD may be a result of T-cell-mediated response to connective or vascular tissue [37].

While sarcoidosis may have a variety of neurologic presentations, 50–80% of patients with systemic sarcoid have muscle granulomas, 80% of which are asymptomatic. Sarcoid myositis thus uncommonly presents with proximal weakness, myalgias, muscle tenderness, and weight loss. Chronic sarcoid myopathy presents as proximal muscle wasting of limb, trunk, and neck muscles. Noncaseating granulomas form in the muscle (Figure 18.6) as a result of accumulation and aggregation of CD4+ helper T cells. The mainstay of treatment for systemic and symptomatic myopathic sarcoid is corticosteroids. Immunosuppressants such as methotrexate, azathioprine, cyclophosphamide, or irradiation are reserved for those patients who remain refractory or continue to progress despite treatment with corticosteroids [38].

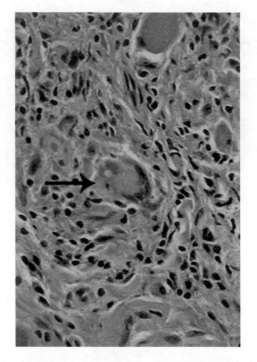

Figure 18.6 Sarcoid myopathy. A multinucleated giant cell (*arrow*) is seen within a non-caseating granuloma. H&E stain, ×400

Conclusion

The discovery in 1970 of antibodies directed against the acetylcholine receptor in patients with Myasthenia gravis finally provided a rationale for treatment directed at the underlying problem, and dramatically improved survival and quality of life. The discovery a couple of decades later of auto-antibodies in Lambert–Eaton myasthenic syndrome similarly provided treatment strategies beyond the merely symptomatic. Continued advances in immunologic knowledge have allowed for advances in diagnostic testing and new treatment options in the inflammatory diseases of muscle as well. IBM, however, remains stubbornly obdurate to our understanding and to effective treatment. Further randomized, placebo-controlled trials are important to best determine the most effective treatments for these immune-mediated disorders.

References

1. Gilchrist JM. Neurophysiology of neuromuscular transmission and its disorders. In: Blum AS, Rutkove SB, editors. The clinical neurophysiology primer. New Jersey: Humana; 2007. p. 353–68.
2. Grob D, Arsura EL, Brunner NG, Namba T. The course of myasthenia gravis and therapies affecting outcome. Ann NY Acad Sci. 1987;505:472.
3. Grob D. Natural history of myasthenia gravis. In: Engel AG, editor. Myasthenia gravis and myasthenic disorders. New York: Oxford University Press; 1999. p. 131–45.
4. Holhlfeld R, Wekerle H. The immunopathogenesis of myasthenia gravis. In: Engel AG, editor. Myasthenia gravis and myasthenic disorders. New York: Oxford University Press; 1999. p. 87–110.

5. Evoli A, Tonali PA, Padua L, et al. Clinical correlates with anti-MuSK antibodies in generalized seronegative myasthenia gravis. Brain. 2003;126:2304–11.
6. Limburg PC, The H, Hummel-Tappel E, Oosterhuis HJ. Anti-acetylcholine receptor antibodies in myasthenia gravis. Part I: Their relation to the clinical state and the effect of therapy. J Neurol Sci. 1983;58:357.
7. Seybold ME. Treatment of myasthenia gravis. In: Engel AG, editor. Myasthenia gravis and myasthenic disorders. New York: Oxford University Press; 1999. p. 167–204.
8. Hart IK, Sathasivam S, Sharshar T. Immunosuppressive agents for myasthenia gravis. Cochrane Database Syst Rev. 2007;(4):CD005224.
9. Gajdos P, Chevret S, Toyka K. Intravenous immunoglobulin for myasthenia gravis. Cochrane Database Syst Rev. 2008;(1):CD002277.
10. Rowin J, Meriggioli MN, Tüzün E, Leurgans S, Christadoss P. Etanercept treatment in corticosteroid-dependant myasthenia gravis. Neurology. 2004;63:2390–2.
11. O'Neill JH, Murray NM, Newsom-Davis J. The Lambert-Eaton myasthenic syndrome: a review of 50 cases. Brain. 1988;111:577–96.
12. Titulaer M, Wirtz PW, Kuks JB, et al. The Lambert-Eaton myasthenic syndrome 1988-2008: a clinical picture of 97 patients. J Neuroimmunol. 2008;201–202:153–8.
13. Comola M, Nemni R, Sher E, et al. Lambert-Eaton myasthenic syndrome and polyneuropathy in a patient with epidermoid carcinoma of the lung. Eur J Neurol. 1993;33:121–5.
14. Chalk CH, Murray NM, Newsom-Davis J, O'Neill JH, Spiro S. Response of the Lambert-Eaton myasthenic syndrome to treatment of associated small cell lung carcinoma. Neurology. 1990;40:1552–6.
15. Wirtz PW, Smallegange TM, Wintzen AR, Verschuuren JJ. Differences in clinical features between the Lambert-Eaton myasthenic syndrome with and without cancer: an analysis of 227 published cases. Clin Neurol Neurosurg. 2002;104:359–63.
16. Newsome-Davis J, Lang B. The Lambert-Eaton myasthenic syndrome. In: Engel AG, editor. Myasthenia gravis and myasthenic disorders. New York: Oxford University Press; 1999. p. 205–28.
17. Tim RW, Massey JM, Sanders DB. Lambert-Eaton myasthenic syndrome: electrodiagnostic findings and response to treatment. Neurology. 2000;54:2176–8.
18. Maddison P, Newsom-Davis J. Treatment for Lambert-Eaton myasthenic syndrome. Cochrane Database Syst Rev. 2005;(2):CD003279.
19. Dalakas MC, Hohlfeld R. Polymyositis and dermatomyositis. Lancet. 2003;362:971–82.
20. Dalakas MC. Therapeutic targets in patients with inflammatory myopathies: present approaches and a look to the future. Neuromuscul Disord. 2006;16:223–36.
21. Engel AG, Hohlfeld R, Banker BQ. The polymyositis and dermatomyositis syndrome. In: Engel AG, Franzini-Armstrong C, editors. Myology. New York: McGraw-Hill; 1994. p. 1335–83.
22. Arahata K, Engel AG. Monoclonal antibody analysis of mononuclear cells in myopathies. I: quantitation of subsets according to diagnosis and sites of accumulation and demonstration and counts of muscle fibers invaded by T cells. Ann Neurol. 1984;16:193–208.
23. Imbert-Massaeu A, Hamidou M, Agard C, Grolleau JY, Chérin P. Antisynthetase syndrome. Joint Bone Spine. 2003;70:161–8.
24. Sordet C, Goetz J, Sibilia J. Contribution of autoantibodies to the diagnosis and nosology of inflammatory muscle disease. Joint Bone Spine. 2006;73:646–54.
25. Miller T, Al-Lozi MT, Lopate G, Pestronk A. Myopathy with antibodies to the signal recognition particle: clinical and pathological features. J Neurol Neurosurg Psychiatry. 2002;73:420–8.
26. Dimitri D, Andre C, Roucoules J, Hosseini H, Humbel RL, Authier FJ. Myopathy associated with anti-signal recognition peptide antibodies: Clinical heterogeneity contrasts with stereotyped histopathology. Muscle Nerve. 2007;35:389–95.

27. Choy EHS, Hoogendijk JE, Lecky B, Winer JB. Immunosuppressant and immunomodulatory treatment for dermatomyositis and polymyositis. Cochrane Database Syst Rev. 2005;(3):CD003643.
28. Lotz BP, Engel AG, Nishino H, Stevens JC, Litchy WJ. Inclusion body myositis: observations in 40 patients. Brain. 1989;112:727–47.
29. Joy JL, Oh SJ, Baysal AI. Electrophysiological spectrum of inclusion body myositis. Muscle Nerve. 1990;13:949–51.
30. Arahata K, Engel AG. Monoclonal antibody analysis of mononuclear cells in myopathies. IV: cell-mediated cytotoxicity and muscle fiber necrosis. Ann Neurol. 1988;23:168–73.
31. Amemiya K, Granger RP, Dalakas MC. Clonal restriction of T-cell receptor expression by infiltrating lymphocytes in inclusion body myositis persists over time. Brain. 2000;123:2030–9.
32. Liu LW, Tarnopolsky M, Armstrong D. Injection of botulinum toxin A to the upper esophageal sphincter for oropharyngeal dysphagia in two patients with inclusion body myositis. Can J Gastroenterol. 2004;18:397–9.
33. Brown RH, Amato AA. Calpainopathy and eosinophilic myositis. Ann Neurol. 2006;59:875–7.
34. Krahn M, Lopez de Munain A, Streichenberger N, et al. CAPN3 mutations in patients with idiopathic eosinophilic myositis. Ann Neurol. 2006;59:905–11.
35. Pegoraro E, Mancias P, Swerdlow SH, et al. Congenital muscular dystrophy with primary laminin a2 (merosin) deficiency presenting as inflammatory myopathy. Ann Neurol. 1996;40:782–91.
36. McNally EM, Ly CT, Rosenmann H, et al. Splicing Mutation in Dysferlin produces limb-girdle muscular dystrophy with inflammation. Am J Med Genet. 2000;91:305–12.
37. Arahata K, Ishihara T, Fukunaga H, et al. Inflammatory response in fascioscapulohumeral muscular dystrophy (FSHD): Immunocytochemical and genetic analyses. Muscle Nerve. 1995;Suppl 2:S56–66.
38. Barnard J, Newman LS. Sarcoidosis: immunology, rheumatic involvement, and therapeutics. Curr Opin Rheumatol. 2001;13:84–91.

19

Autoimmune Neuropathies

George Sachs

Keywords: Guillain-Barre Syndrome, Inflammatory neuropathy, vasculitis, Monoclonal Gammopathy, CIDP

Introduction

Autoimmune neuropathies comprise a diverse array of disorders. Their temporal evolution may be acute and self-limited, relapsing–remitting or chronically progressive. Deficits and symptoms may be distal or proximal, in a symmetric or multifocal pattern. Within each temporospatial profile, pathophysiology may reflect demyelination or axonal degeneration. Rather than attempt an exhaustive catalog, this chapter addresses major, common autoimmune neuropathies. Their clinical presentation, laboratory evaluation, pathogenesis and therapeutic options are reviewed.

Guillain–Barre Syndrome

Historically, Guillain–Barre syndrome (GBS) represents the earliest description of an autoimmune neuropathy, though it was not recognized as such until nearly a century after Landry's initial case reports in 1859. The main contribution of Guillain, Barre, and Strohl in 1916 was the identification of an associated elevation of protein in an acellular CSF [1]. This finding of albuminocytologic dissociation served to distinguish GBS from the known infectious causes of ascending paralysis (i.e., polio and syphilis). Curiously, Guillain himself continued to favor an infectious etiology, rejecting proposals by Bannwarth and others that GBS was an allergic phenomenon [2]. The emergence of experimental allergic neuritis (EAN) as an animal model in the 1950s fostered acceptance of an immune-mediated pathogenesis for GBS [3, 4].

Pathologic and nerve conduction studies of GBS in Europe and North America revealed evidence of a primary demyelinating neuropathy similar to that found in the animal model of EAN [5]. As a result, the term acute inflammatory demyelinating polyneuropathy (AIDP) became synonymous with

From: *Clinical Neuroimmunology: Multiple Sclerosis and Related Disorders*, Current Clinical Neurology,
Edited by: S.A. Rizvi and P.K. Coyle, DOI 10.1007/978-1-60327-860-7_19,
© Springer Science+Business Media, LLC 2011

GBS. More recently, the study of GBS cases worldwide has emphasized its syndromic nature with different pathologic and physiologic processes leading to similar clinical presentations.

Clinical Features

GBS is defined as an acute neuropathic weakness with strength decreasing to a nadir within 4 weeks along with loss of deep tendon reflexes. Its course is most often ascending, beginning in the lower extremities. Weakness of the limbs is nearly always symmetric or becomes so as it progresses. Initial weakness may involve proximal or distal muscles. Over half of GBS cases show facial or bulbar weakness. Respiratory muscle weakness is common with approximately one quarter of patients requiring mechanical ventilation [6, 7].

Sensory symptoms often precede the onset of weakness. Over half of GBS cases begin with paresthesia in distal lower extremities; however, initial paresthesia may occur in any location. Sensory deficits tend to reflect preferential involvement of large caliber sensory axons and ataxia is common. The loss of tendon reflexes, even in relatively strong muscles, reflects conduction block or desynchronization in 1A afferents [6].

Autonomic dysfunction complicates nearly 2/3 of GBS cases. Alteration in blood pressure and cardiac arrhythmias predominate with hypertension and tachycardia being most common. Urinary incontinence occurs in roughly 25% of cases [6, 7].

Laboratory Investigations

Approximately 90% of GBS cases reveal elevated CSF protein without abnormal cell counts. Protein levels may not exceed normal range during the first weak of symptoms but usually peak by 2–3 weeks after onset. Thereafter, levels decline slowly for months. Cases with significant CSF pleocytosis can occur in the setting of HIV or possibly Lyme boreliosis [8].

Electrodiagnostic studies typically reveal a picture of AIDP with evidence of a demyelinating polyneuropathy affecting motor more than sensory fibers [9, 10]. In some cases, particularly early in the course, distal conduction studies will be normal since demyelination may be largely proximal. Abnormalities may be limited to F waves. As the disease progresses, various degrees of axonopathy may supervene reducing CMAP and SNAP potential amplitudes. This is accompanied by the evidence of ongoing denervation on EMG. Low CMAP amplitudes with denervation provide the most reliable prognosis for slow recovery [11]. Sensory nerve conduction studies may show demyelinative slowing or less-specific decrease in amplitude. One common feature of AIDP is preserved sural sensory conduction studies in the face of abnormal median and ulnar sensory studies [12]. This sural sparing may reflect the fact that this nerve is studied at a more proximal level than the nerves within the hand.

Sural nerve biopsy is not routinely performed in cases with typical presentation especially if CSF findings or nerve conduction studies support the diagnosis. Pathological studies of the AIDP form of GBS have shown changes similar to those found in experimental EAN [4]. There are areas of demyelination with variable lymphocytic infiltrates. Ultrastructural studies have revealed the invasion of intact myelin lamellae by macrophages [13] (Figure 19.1).

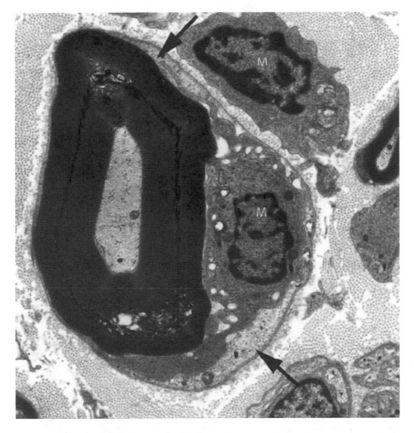

Figure 19.1 Electron micrograph from a case of AIDP demonstrating attack of myelin lamellae by macrophages (M). From: Hughes RAC. Guillain-Barre syndrome. Heidelberg: Springer; 1998

GBS Variants

In the USA, Canada, and Europe, over 90% of GBS cases show AIDP as their underlying pathophysiology. The remaining minority of patients present either as acute primary axonopathies, the Miller Fisher variant, or other regional variants. The existence of "axonal GBS" was long a matter of debate, until studies of GBS in China revealed that over 30% of cases could be classified as acute motor and sensory axonal neuropathy (AMSAN) or its pure motor counterpart AMAN [14]. These axonal subtypes show no evidence of demyelination on nerve conduction studies and typically present as quadriparesis with low amplitude or absent motor potentials and marked evidence of denervation on EMG. Pathologic studies confirm a primary axolemmal attack by macrophages [15]. An acute reversible pure motor syndrome marked by transient conduction block has been interpreted as a mild form of AMAN, where axolemmal attack may be limited to regions at nodes of Ranvier [16, 17] (Figure 19.2).

The Miller Fisher variant of GBS presents with ophthalmoparesis, ataxia, and areflexia [18]. It accounts for approximately 5% of all GBS cases. Given its rarity and generally benign course, pathologic investigations have been lacking and the pathophysiology remains poorly elucidated. There is general agreement that cranial and sensory peripheral nerves are the primary targets

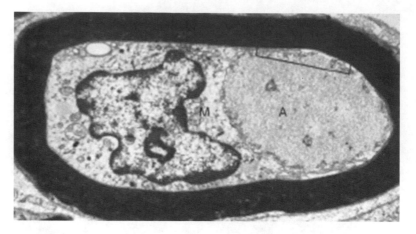

Figure 19.2 Electron micrograph from a case of AMAN demonstrating primary attack of a macrophage (M) on an axon (A) within an intact myelin sheath. From: Griffin JW, Li CY, Macko C, et al. Early nodal changes in the acute. motor axonal neuropathy pattern of the Guillain-Barré syndrome. J Neurocytol. 1996;25:33–51

of immune attack, though cases with accompanying limb weakness and CNS involvement have been described. Nerve conduction studies typically reveal low amplitude or absent sensory nerve action potentials. These improve rapidly during clinical recovery, suggesting reversible demyelination or nodal conduction block as the underlying process [19, 20].

Other variants of GBS are even more rare and include pure sensory, pure autonomic presentations, as well as regional weakness (e.g., oropharyngeal variant). The underlying pathophysiology in some of these appears similar to that in AIDP. In other instances, distinct antibody profiles suggest different immune processes (see below).

Immune Pathogenesis

The mechanisms of immune attack in GBS are complex, likely involving both cellular and humoral processes. Insights into cell-mediated hypersensitivity underlying AIDP have come from animal studies of EAN. Infiltrates of T-lymphocytes occur in areas of demyelination, in both AIDP and EAN [4]. Adoptive transfer studies in rats have demonstrated that injection of T-cells sensitized to myelin proteins is sufficient to induce demyelination in peripheral nerve of naïve animals [21]. To what extent T-cell-mediated hypersensitivity accounts for AIDP is not clear. For AIDP, the triggering mechanism related to prior infection has not been delineated and antigenic protein targets in peripheral nerve myelin remain unspecified.

A clearer picture is emerging for antibody-mediated mechanisms in GBS variants (Table 19.1). Support for post-infectious molecular mimicry has advanced through investigations of anti-glycolipid antibodies in AMAN and Miller Fisher variants. Antibodies to gangliosides GM1, GM1b, or GD1a occur in approximately 2/3 of AMAN cases [22, 23]. These gangliosides localize to the axolemma and paranodal myelin of motor and sensory axons. Interestingly, antibodies to GD1a seem to bind selectively to motor axons, perhaps due to slight differences in GD1a fatty acid configuration in sensory axons [24]. About one-third of patients with AMAN exhibit antibodies to a minor ganglioside (GalNAc-GD1a) found only on motor axons [25].

Table 19.1 Antiganglioside antibodies associated with different subtypes of Guillain–Barre syndrome (adapted from ref. [23]).

GBS subtype	Antibodies
Acute inflammatory demyelinating polyradiculoneuropathy (AIDP)	Unknown
Acute motor and sensory axonal neuropathy (AMSAN)	GM1, GM1b, GD1a
Acute motor axonal neuropathy (AMAN)	GM1, GM1b, GD1a, GalNac-GD1a
Fisher syndrome	GQ1b, GD1b, GT1a
Oculopharyngeal variant	GT1a

Cases of Miller Fisher variant exhibit antibodies to another set of gangliosides. GQ1b ganglioside antibodies occur in over 85% of such cases and, interestingly, also occur in "overlap" cases of AIDP with ophthalmoparesis [22]. Though widely distributed in the PNS and optic nerves, the highest concentrations of GQ1b ganglioside occur at nodes of Ranvier and paranodal myelin in oculomotor cranial nerves [26]. A smaller percentage of Miller Fisher cases exhibit antibodies to GD1b and GT1a gangliosides. Antibodies to GD1b bind specifically to large neurons in dorsal root ganglia [24]. This suggests an underlying mechanism for the sensory ataxia and hyporeflexia. Along these lines, antibodies to GD1b also occur in cases of acute sensory neuronopathy [27]. GT1a antibodies may preferentially target cranial nerves as they occur in the oropharyngeal regional variant of GBS as well as in Miller Fisher cases [28].

Experimental studies in animals as well as findings from human trials of ganglioside therapy support a true pathogenic role for anti-ganglioside antibodies. Rabbits immunized with GM1 developed high titers of IgG antibodies and degeneration of ventral roots with pathologic findings similar to those in AMAN [29, 30]. Therapeutic trials of mixed ganglioside therapy for various neurologic disorders conducted in the 1990s resulted in a small number of acute neuropathies which closely resembled AMAN [31]. Melanoma patients receiving experimental monoclonal anti-ganglioiside antibodies also developed an acute reversible neuropathy [32].

Campylobacter jejuni and Molecular Mimicry

Campylobacter enteritis is the most common infection preceding GBS worldwide [33]. Although recognized as a prodrome for AIDP, *Campylobacter* infections are most closely associated with AMAN [34]. Studies of antiganglioside antibodies in AMAN and Miller Fisher variants have generated a coherent picture of molecular mimicry as a mechanism of post-infectious GBS. Lipooligosaccharides (LOSs) from certain strains of *Campylobacter* are structurally similar to various gangliosides. Such analogy was first documented between GM1 ganglioside and LOSs from *Campylobacter* infecting a patient with AMAN [35]. Later experimental studies in animals have supported a causal role of *Campylobacter* via molecular mimicry. Injection of appropriate bacterial LOSs into rabbits induced both GM1 antibodies and neuropathy resembling AMAN [30]. Strains of *Campylobacter* which precipitate the Miller Fisher variant exhibit LOSs structurally similar to GQ1b and GT1a gangliosides [36].

Treatment

The most dramatic advances in the management of GBS have come with improvements in supportive ICU care. Vigilant monitoring and therapy for respiratory decompensation, cardiac arrhythmia, blood pressure changes, and infections have had significant impact. These, along with preventative measures against deep vein thrombosis and pulmonary embolus have reduced overall mortality to 3–10% [37].

Beyond this, randomized placebo-controlled clinical trials have confirmed the benefit of immunomodulating therapies in GBS. The largest early trials of plasma exchange revealed significantly greater improvement in a disability scale at 4 weeks and faster recovery of ambulation [38, 39]. Subsequent studies documented that four exchange sessions (of 1.5 plasma volumes each) accelerated recovery more than two sessions, but that recovery was no faster with six total sessions [40]. Data compiled from major plasma exchange trials indicates a higher rate of full recovery in strength compared with supportive treatment alone (relative rate of 1.24) [41].

Clinical trials have shown a comparable benefit from treatment with high-dose intravenous immune globulin (IVIG). Studies comparing IVIG to supportive treatment alone have been limited to small trials in children, and these indicated greater improvement in disability score and a higher rate of return to normal strength [42, 43]. Adult trials of IVIG have compared its effect to that of PE. The largest of these revealed equivalent improvement of a disability score at 4 weeks [44]. Smaller adult studies also failed to show significant differences between IVIG and PE in various outcome measures [45, 46].

Overall, trials of corticosteroids have not shown significant benefit. Two trials of intravenous methyl prednisolone produced no significant change in time to recovery or disability scores at 4 weeks to 6 months [47, 48]. Analysis of small trials using oral steroids indicated that they may have a negative effect at the 4-week mark [49, 50]. The combination of intravenous steroids and IVIG conferred no benefit over IVIG alone [51].

The choice between treatment with PE or IVIG usually depends on availability and side effect profile as their cost and efficacy are comparable. Since trials of IVIG have entered patients only within 2 weeks of symptom onset, some guidelines endorse PE more strongly for treatment at 2–4 weeks [37]. There is limited evidence that ambulatory patients with milder disease may benefit from PE, while the effects of IVIG have not been tested in this group [40]. Data on axonal variants such as AMSAN and AMAN is insufficient to draw conclusions about the relative efficacy of IVIG and PE in these subgroups. A retrospective study has suggested that IVIG may provide more benefit to GBS cases with GM1 antibodies [52], but this has not been rigorously proven and any practical utility would be limited by the time required for antibody testing in a clinical setting.

Both PE and IVIG treatment can be complicated by relapse within a few weeks of initial response [53]. In such cases, more sustained improvement usually follows a second course of the same treatment. Indications are less clear for patients that continue to deteriorate through their initial treatment. A large, controlled trial failed to show benefit from IVIG following a course of PE [44]. A very small observational study has suggested that patients continuing to worsen after initial IVIG treatment may benefit from a second course of IVIG [54].

CIDP

In its broadest definition, chronic inflammatory demyelinating polyradiculo-neuropathy (CIDP) encompasses a wide variety of clinical presentations. Many chronic neuropathies involve some degree of immune-mediated demyelination. It is difficult to decide which of these should be included under the umbrella of CIDP. There is reasonable agreement concerning characteristics of "classic CIDP," but the classification of variant presentations continues to stir debate. From a practical standpoint, differential response to therapy should be a primary consideration in distinguishing various clinical entities.

Clinical Features

Classic CIDP is often viewed as a chronic form of AIDP. As such, defining features include symmetric weakness of proximal and distal muscles, sensory disturbance involving large-fiber modalities more than small and generalized hyporeflexia. In contrast to AIDP, progression of symptoms must extend beyond 8 weeks. Temporal evolution may be chronically progressive, stepwise progressive or relapsing–remitting . There is a history of infection in the month preceding symptom onset in fewer than 20% of CIDP patients (as apposed to 70% of patients with AIDP) [55]. Involvement of cranial nerves occurs less frequently in CIDP than in AIDP (15% versus 50%) [56]. Respiratory decompensation and dysautonomia are far less prevalent in CIDP. Urinary dysfunction and ventilatory failure complicate less than 25 and 10% of patients [57, 58].

Estimates of prevalence for classic CIDP have ranged from one to four cases per 100,000 in most populations [59–61]. This rate increases in patients with chronic viral infections of Hepatitis B and C as well as HIV.

Lymphoproliferative disorders including lymphomas are also associated with higher rates of CIDP as are lupus and other collagen vascular diseases. The prevalence of CIDP in diabetics exceeds general population rates and may be underestimated, since neuropathies are less scrutinized within this group [62].

Monoclonal gammopathies are commonly associated with CIDP. Series collected within the last 25 years demonstrate paraprotcincmia in 20–45% of patients with CIDP [63]. Clinical features and differential response to therapy distinguish the demyelinating neuropathies seen with a subset of paraproteinemic disorders (including POEMS syndrome and IgM gammopathies with anti-MAG antibodies) and these will be discussed separately below. Apart from these, CIDP associated with MGUS is often viewed as similar to CIDP without paraproteinemia . However, the largest series comparing CIDP with and without MGUS noted that the MGUS cases were more indolent with less dramatic response to immunotherapy [64]. Some investigators have suggested that demyelinating neuropathies with IgM MGUS of any type are refractory to immunomodulating therapy [65, 66]. Other researchers have stressed that the high incidence of distally predominant weakness in IgM MGUS neuropathies accounts for this poor response. They advocate classifying such cases as "distal acquired demyelinating symmetric" (DADS) neuropathies, in contradistinction to CIDP [67].

Laboratory Studies

Most diagnostic criteria for CIDP require electrophysiological findings of demyelination. Elevated CSF protein is generally considered supportive rather than requisite evidence, though over 90% of CIDP cases show levels exceeding 45 mg/dl [68]. CSF usually reveals fewer than ten WBC cases of HIV-related CIDP often exhibit pleocytosis, but a WBC count exceeding 50 is extremely rare and excludes the diagnosis by some criteria [69]. Morphologic evaluation of autopsy material is limited and has shown abnormalities at the level of spinal roots and proximal nerve trunks. These include areas of segmental demyelination, remyelination, and onion bulb formation. In addition, studies have found variable degrees of edema and inflammatory infiltrates within epineurium and endoneurium [70, 71]. Less specific findings of axonal degeneration along with clusters of regenerating axons have also been noted. In general, sural nerve biopsies are less helpful than electrodiagnostic studies and CSF analysis. Biopsies may appear relatively unremarkable or show axonal degeneration without the specific diagnostic findings seen at more proximal levels.

Immune Pathogenesis

The immune mechanisms underlying CIDP are complex and only roughly delineated. As with AIDP, both cell-mediated and humorally mediated processes seem to contribute. There is evidence of T-cell activation and migration through the blood nerve barrier . T cells infiltrating nerves are of CD4 and CD8 subgroups and may directly attack myelin in addition to activating macrophage attack and phagocytosis [72, 73].

Humoral immune processes have been implicated in CIDP by the observation of immunoglobulin and complement deposition on myelinated nerve fibers [74] as well as oligoclonal IgG bands in the CSF [75]. The therapeutic effect of plasma exchange in CIDP supports a humoral process. Further evidence derives from passive transfer experiments where serum or IgG from patients with CIDP cause nerve demyelination in rats [76]. Antibody responses to a number of targets in peripheral myelin have been identified including GM1 and other glycolipids [77, 78] as well as peripheral myelin protein 22 [79, 80]. However, there is no predominant antigenic target yet identified to account for a major proportion of CIDP cases (Figure 19.3).

Treatment

Studies over the last 50 years have investigated response of CIDP to immunomodulating therapy. The benefit of ACTH and oral steroids was initially recognized in the 1950s [81]. In 1982, Dyck et al. evaluated 35 patients in the only randomized, controlled trial of corticosteroids to date [82] and demonstrated a positive effect of prednisone on disability scores over 3 months. Progressive and relapsing cases showed similar improvement. Several observational studies have also revealed benefit from corticosteroids. Overall, 60–75% of patients responded to treatment, though the first evidence of improvement occurred as late as 5 months in some cases [83].

Two randomized controlled trials of plasma exchange have demonstrated benefit in CIDP-related disability. The first compared 15 patients receiving six sessions of PE over 3 weeks with a parallel group receiving and sham exchange [84]. The second trial evaluated the effect of ten plasma exchange sessions over 4 weeks versus sham exchange in a crossover design [85]. Analysis of data combined from both trials revealed that approximately

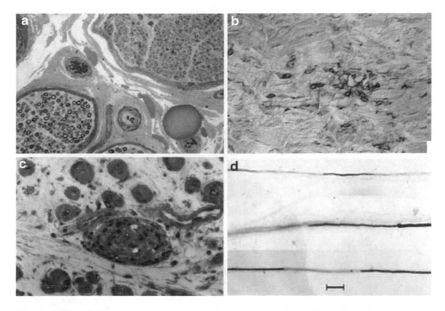

Figure 19.3 CIDP. (a) Semithin section demonstrating loss of myelinated axons, more pronounced in the *upper right* fascicle. (b) Immunohistological demonstration of lymphocytes within the endoneurium. (c) Higher power micrograph of a semithin section revealing endoneurial edema, perivascular inflammation, and early onion bulbing around myelinated axons. (d) Teased fiber preparation demonstrating demyelinated segments of individual axons. (a–c) From Rizzuto N, Morbin M, Cavallaro T, Ferrari S, Fallahi M, Galiazzo Rizzuto S. Focal lesions area feature of chronic inflammatory demyelinating polyneuropathy (CIDP). Acta Neuropathol. 1998;96:603–9. (d) From Pytel P, Rezania K, Soliven B, Frank J, Wollmann R. Chronic inflammatory demyelinating polyradiculoneuropathy (CIDP) with hypertrophic spinal radiculopathy mimicking neurofibromatosis. Acta Neuropathol. 2003;105:185–8

2/3 of patients responded to active treatment. Responders improved rapidly, but the effect was short lived and rebound worsening occurred in some cases once treatment ceased. There was a moderate incidence of adverse events including myocarditis and stroke.

A greater number of rigorous studies have investigated the effects of IVIG in CIDP. At least seven randomized, controlled trials have demonstrated benefit [86]. These have included various treatment schedules and most assessed change in disability within 1 month of treatment. The largest and most recent trial revealed sustained benefit from IVIG treatments (1 g/kg every 3 weeks) up to 24 weeks [87]. Studies comparing IVIG against corticosteroids [88] and plasma exchange [89] have demonstrated comparable benefits for these treatments.

With corticosteroids, PE and IVIG showing roughly equal efficacy, the choice of initial treatment for CIDP should weigh speed of response and side effect profile against convenience and cost. When available and affordable, IVIIG is an option which acts rapidly with relatively few adverse effects. Risk of stroke and renal failure are generally low, but may temper its use in patients with renal insufficiency and cerebrovascular disease. The main drawbacks to IVIG therapy are the cost and inconvenience of repeated treatments.

Plasma exchange remains an alternative treatment for rapidly progressive CIDP, but its invasive nature and lack of a home treatment option limit its suitability for long-term maintenance. Corticosteroid treatment is reasonable for debilitating but slowly progressive disease. Its advantages include low initial cost, ease of administration and greater chance of inducing remission. Adverse effects accrue with longer steroid treatment and their associated long-term cost needs to be considered in comparing the economics of different therapies.

Approximately two-thirds of the patients receiving any of the three major treatments will respond. Patients failing one of these treatments may show better response to either of the others [90]. For those refractory to all three, alternative immunosuppressants may prove beneficial. A number of series have demonstrated improvement with cyclophosphamide [91–95] or cyclosporine [96–100] and these are fairly frequently used in cases of debilitating refractory CIDP. However, there are no randomized controlled studies of these agents. A single controlled randomized trial evaluated azathioprine as add-on treatment to prednisone [101] but failed to show additional benefit. Since uncontrolled series have suggested a beneficial effect from azathioprine [68, 93], perhaps its slow onset of action may help explain negative results in relatively short trials.

After an open label study of interferon-beta [102] showed promise, it was evaluated as an IVIG sparing agent but the study failed to show a benefit of adding interferon-beta to IVIG. A slight benefit was noted in patients with severe disability and those requiring high doses of IVIG [103]. A recent prospective placebo-controlled study of methotrexate failed to show significant benefit in allowing reduction in IVIG or corticosteroid dosing for CIDP patients [104].

CIDP Variants

Multifocal Acquired Demyelinating Sensory and Motor Neuropathy

This disorder, also known as Lewis–Sumner syndrome, is a demyelinating mononeuropathy multiplex marked by areas of persistent conduction block that affect both sensory and motor axons [105]. It presents with pain, paresthesia, and weakness in the distribution of individual nerves. Aside from this multifocality, it shares characteristics with classic CIDP. In addition to conduction block, electrodiagnostic studies reveal other demyelinating features including segmental slowing and temporal dispersion of potentials. Pathologic abnormalities resemble CIDP with inflammation and onion-bulb formation. Spinal fluid protein levels are frequently elevated. Most importantly, multifocal acquired demyelinating sensory and motor neuropathy (MADSAM) and CIDP respond to the same range of immune therapies including corticosteroids, IVIG, and plasma exchange. There is general agreement that MADSAM represents a true variant form of CIDP, a fact underscored by the occasional evolution of multifocal cases into a more confluent picture of classic CIDP [106].

Pure Sensory CIDP

Cases presenting the clinical picture of chronic pure sensory polyneuropathy may infrequently show electrophysiologic or pathologic evidence of a primary demyelinating process. Two small series have described cases with pathological evidence of segmental demyelination on teased nerve preparations. However, one series revealed electrophysiologic evidence of demyelination in motor nerve fibers, [107] where the other showed normal motor conduction or only axonopathic changes [108]. A third series demonstrated that CIDP cases with initial pure sensory presentations later developed motor deficits [109]. Taken together, these studies suggest that "sensory CIDP" may be part of a spectrum that includes more typical motor-predominant cases, rather than an entirely distinct entity. Though only limited data exist, sensory CIDP appears responsive to a similar range of immunomodulating treatment including corticosteroids, IVIG, and plasma exchange.

Distal Acquired Demyelinating Symmetric Neuropathy

Some authors have drawn a distinction between chronic demyelinating neuropathies with limited, distal weakness, and more classic CIDP. The former group that they refer to as DADS has a higher association with IgM monoclonal gammopathy. Patients with DADS and monoclonal gammopathy are predominantly male and older than CIDP patients on the average. They show significantly less response to immunomodulating therapy [67]. The features of DADS patients without gammopathy are less consistent.

Multifocal Motor Neuropathy

This disorder presents as a chronic, motor-selective mononeuropathy multiplex. Although clinically it resembles motor neuron disease, its physiologic hallmark of motor conduction block has led many to classify it as a variant of CIDP [110]. Response to immunomodulating therapy has strengthened the association between MMN and CIDP. However, some investigators have emphasized the differences between these two disorders [111]. Conduction block in MMN may involve alterations in axolemmal properties rather than simple demyelination [112]. Moreover, the number of effective immunomodulating treatments is more limited for MMN than for CIDP.

Clinical Features
MNN is an uncommon disorder with a prevalence of one to two cases per 100,000. It usually begins in young adulthood or middle age and affects men at least twice as often as women. Presenting as weakness within the distribution of individual nerves, the lack of associated pain, and sensory deficit differentiates MMN from other inflammatory mononeuropathies and nerve entrapments. Initially, weakened muscles may retain their bulk, but atrophy supervenes with progressive axonal degeneration over time. Cramps and fasciculations are common symptoms. Upper motor neuron signs are not attributable to MMN and their presence would indicate an alternative or additional diagnosis.

The vast majority of patients with MMN suffer weakness in the distal upper extremities, but foot drop is not uncommon. Involvement of cranial and phrenic nerves has been reported but is rare. Slowly progressive weakness is the most common course, though spontaneous improvement is occasionally seen. Acute presentations of multifocal motor neuropathies with rapid resolution have been described, but these may be more closely related to GBS than MMN [16, 17].

Laboratory Studies
Motor conduction block is a defining characteristic of MMN. A particular feature of conduction block in MMN is its selectivity for motor axons with preserved conduction in sensory fibers through the same length of nerve. It is more commonly found in the forearm and calf than in more proximal segments of nerves or roots. This may, in part, reflect the technical difficulty

of demonstrating conduction block at proximal levels, but the distribution of weak muscles is at least consistent with a distal predominance. In contrast to many cases of MADSAM or CIDP, sensory conduction studies and motor conduction outside the regions of block reveal only mild abnormalities. EMG of weakened muscles shows evidence of ongoing and chronic denervation, especially in cases of longstanding weakness.

IgM antibodies to gangliosides (mostly GM1 and also GD1a and GM2) can be detected in approximately half of patients with MMN [113]. Estimates have ranged from 20 to 80% of MMN patients showing such antibodies with differences in assays likely accounting for much of this variation. Though GM1 antibodies are sometimes detected in disorders other than MMN, reviews have indicated that their specificity is sufficiently high to confer clinical utility in supporting the diagnosis [114]. Other blood testing is usually unremarkable in MMN. CSF protein is normal in approximately half of cases with mild elevation in most of the other half.

Sural nerve biopsies have generally not shown dramatic or specific abnormalities. Mild demyelinating features have been noted on some electron microscopic studies [115]. Motor nerve fascicular biopsies at confirmed sites of conduction block have shown loss of large-myelinated fibers without evidence of demyelination [116] (Figure 19.4).

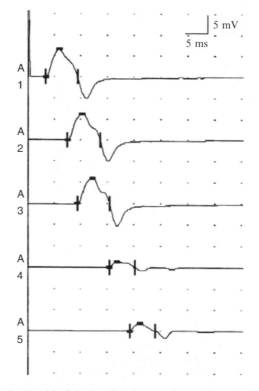

Figure 19.4 Conduction block in the ulnar nerve of a patient with MMN. Compound motor action potentials elicited from abductor digiti quinti by stimulation at the wrist (A1), below elbow (A2), above elbow (A3), axilla (A4), and Erb's point (A5). Reduction in amplitude by more than 50% demonstrates conduction block between the elbow and axilla. From: Van den berg-Vos RM, Van den berg LH, Visser J, de Visser M, Franssen H, Wokke JHJ. The spectrum of lower motor neuron disorders. J Neurol. 2003;250:1279–92

Immune Pathogenesis

Response to immunomodulating therapy and the frequent association of anti-ganglioside antibodies have fostered the notion that MMN is an autoimmune disorder. However, its pathogenesis remains largely unspecified. Disruption of paranodal myelin or axolemma mediated by GM1 antibodies is an attractive hypothesis yet not all experimental studies have supported this [117]. GM1 ganglioside is enriched at paranodal myelin and particularly on motor axons. Intraneural injection of serum from MMN patients has induced conduction block both in vivo [118] and in vitro [119]. However, similar experiments using purified GM1 antibodies failed to show conduction block [120]. Whether this reflects an artifact of the purification process or indicates a role for other components of the transferred serum is not clear. Although MMN is not typically recognized as a post-infectious disorder, a few case reports have described multifocal motor neuropathies with highly elevated levels of GM1 antibodies following *Campylobacter jejuni* enteritis [16, 17, 121]. These included acute, monophasic, and chronic relapsing presentations, raising the possibility that some cases of MMN may share the mechanism of molecular mimicry proposed for GBS following Campylobacter enteritis.

Treatment

Although cyclophosphamide was the earliest recognized treatment of MMN [122], there is now general agreement that IVIG should be offered as initial therapy. At least four randomized controlled trials have demonstrated significant benefit with IVIG [123–126]. Overall, 75–80% of patients treated with IVIG showed improvement in strength, and this effect was often rapid. No serious adverse effects were reported in randomized trials, though minor symptoms such as headache, rash, and fever were encountered in over half of participants.

Corticosteroids and plasma exchange have consistently proven ineffective in patients with MMN. Furthermore, there are reports of worsening deficits following treatment with these agents [113]. This contrasts with the beneficial effect seen in many cases of classic CIDP or MADSAM and supports the concept of MMN as a distinct disorder.

Patients unresponsive to IVIG, or in whom its effect wanes with repeated treatments, may benefit from cytotoxic agents. A number of reports have shown improvement with cyclophosphamide [122, 127, 128], but it should be considered only for patients with significant deficit since it may cause serious adverse effects. Experience with azathioprine, rituximab, and beta-interferon has been much more limited. A randomized controlled trial of mycophenolate mofetil failed to show benefit in reducing requirement for IVIG in 28 patients with MMN [129]. Given the long-term requirement for IVIG in most patients with MMN, continued efforts to identify more convenient and affordable treatments are warranted.

Neuropathies Associated with Monoclonal Gammopathy

An estimated 10% of otherwise idiopathic polyneuropathies are associated with monoclonal gammopathy [130, 131]. This includes neuropathy complicating malignant plasma cell dyscrasias and, more commonly, neuropathy seen in conjunction with monoclonal gammopathies of undetermined significance (MGUS). Neuropathic symptoms often lead to the initial recognition of a gammopathy.

Moreover, the existence of a neuropathy is of prognostic importance in MGUS, as it confers a greater risk of eventual transformation to a malignant gammopathy. This section describes the features of neuropathies associated with various malignant gammopathies and MGUS.

Malignant Gammopathies

Waldenstrom's macroglobulinemia (WM), a lymphoplasmacytic lymphoma with monoclonal IgM, is often complicated by neuropathy. When prospectively studied, nearly half of patients with WM develop neuropathic symptoms or signs [132]. Sensory deficits predominate, involving both large and small fiber modalities. When weakness occurs it is largely distal. Conduction studies show the evidence of demyelination in a number of cases with prolonged distal latencies, slow conduction velocities but little conduction block. In approximately half of the demyelinating neuropathies, the IgM paraprotein reacts against MAG. These patients resemble MGUS patients with anti-MAG antibodies described below. Less frequently, patients with WM will suffer mononeuropathy multiplex due to amyloid deposition. Neuropathy will often improve with alkylating agents used to treat WM. Rituximab in combination with cyclophosphamide or fludarabine can also improve neuropathy. However, there are reports of dramatic worsening of neuropathy with rituximab in some cases [133, 134].

Although patients with multiple myeloma (MM) frequently show abnormalities on nerve conduction studies, only about 10% suffer significant neuropathic symptoms [135]. Typically, the neuropathy is distal, symmetric and sensory-motor, with features of primary axonal degeneration. Pathological studies reveal perineural deposition of IgG and IgM. Less frequently, the presentation is one of mononeuropathy multiplex due to the infiltration of amyloid. Neuropathies associated with MM are generally refractory to treatment [132].

Osteosclerotic myeloma, as part of POEMS syndrome, occurs less frequently than MM but has a much higher rate of associated neuropathy [136]. The neuropathy commonly involves sensory loss in both small- and large-fiber modalities along with weakness. These symptoms begin distally but can advance to produce significant proximal weakness and loss of mobility. Nerve conduction studies show evidence of demyelination with prolonged distal latencies, slow conduction velocities, and temporal dispersion of motor potentials. Associated paraproteins are IgG or IgA with lambda light chains. Pathologic studies revealing endoneurial deposition of light chains argue that the paraproteins are pathogenic. Recent evidence has also implicated high-level production of VEGF and cytokines by the plasmacytomas [137]. The resultant proliferation of perineural vasculature and breakdown of the blood–nerve barrier lead to edema and demyelination. The marked increase in CSF protein seen in POEMS cases likely reflects these vascular changes. In cases with solitary or limited plasmacytomas, their irradiation or surgical excision can lead to resolution of the neuropathy along with skin and endocrinologic manifestations of POEMS syndrome.

Monoclonal Gammopathy of Undetermined Significance

Over two-thirds of monoclonal gammopathies fall into the category of MGUS. These are characterized by a low level of paraprotein (less than 3 g/dl) in serum,

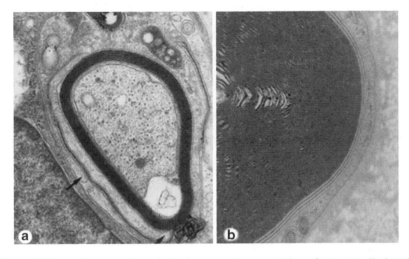

Figure 19.5 (**a**) Electron micrographs demonstrating separation of outer myelin lamellae (*arrow*) in a case of IgM MGUS neuropathy. (**b**) A higher power electron micrograph showing similar separation of outer lamellae from another case of IgM MGUS neuropathy. From: Vital A, Lagueny A, Julien J, et al. Chronic inflammatory demyelinating polyneuropathy with dysglobulinemia: a peripheral nerve biopsy study in 18 cases. Acta Neuropathol. 2000;100:63–8

little or no urinary paraprotein and less than 5% plasma cells in bone marrow. By definition, MGUS lacks features of malignant gammopathies such as anemia, renal failure, bone lesions, or amyloid deposition. The former designation of "benign monoclonal gammopathy" was abandoned as nearly one quarter of cases ultimately undergo malignant transformation.

Although most cases of MGUS involve IgG paraproteins, 60% of cases with neuropathy show an IgM paraprotein compared with 30% with IgG and 10% with IgA [138, 139]. A variety of neuropathies occur with MGUS of each type, but cases of IgM MGUS are associated with the most distinct forms of neuropathy. In approximately half of IgM MGUS-related neuropathies, antibodies react with myelin-associated glycoprotein (MAG) [140].

Anti MAG neuropathy most commonly afflicts older men. Their clinical presentation is marked by painless, gradual, distal loss of large fiber sensory modalities. This, along with distal weakness leads to a slowly progressive gait disorder. Nerve conduction studies reveal evidence of distal demyelination with disproportionate slowing of distal motor and sensory latencies. Nerve biopsies have shown separation of outer lamellae in myelin sheaths, a characteristic that anti-MAG cases may share with other IgM MGUS neuropathies (Figure 19.5).

Neuropathy in many patients with IgM MGUS but without specified autoantibodies, resembles the anti-MAG neuropathy described above. The category of distal acquired demyelinating sensorimotor (DADS) neuropathy is largely composed of IgM MGUS neuropathy. In general, their response to immunomodulating therapy is more modest than IgG and IgA MGUS neuropathies. Randomized controlled studies have shown short-term response to IVIG, but the overall benefit in these slowly progressive disorders is less clear. Small, uncontrolled series have reported benefit with fludarabine, cyclophosphamide, and rituximab. However, more systematic trials with long-term follow-up would be advisable for these potentially toxic treatments for a slowly progressive disorder.

Specific autoantibodies have not been identified for neuropathies in IgG and IgA MGUS. Therefore, a causal role for these paraproteins is less apparent. Associated neuropathies include CIDP which does not differ significantly from classic CIDP and generally shows similar response to treatment.

Vasculitic Neuropathy

Vasculitic neuropathy may arise in the context of systemic vasculitis or as a disorder limited to the peripheral nervous system (i.e., nonsystemic vasculitic neuropathy). Of the systemic vasculidites involving peripheral nerves, polyarteritis nodosa and rheumatoid vasculitis account for the majority of cases. Several other connective tissue disorders and infections comprise the remainder [141]. Clinical presentation, pathology, and electrophysiology are similar for neuropathies of systemic and nonsystemic vasculitis and have been discussed in detail in a separate chapter.

References

1. Guillain G, Barré JA, Strohl A. Sur un syndrome de radiculonévrite avec hyperalbuminose du liquide céphalo-rachidien sans réaction cellulaire. Remarques sur les caractéres cliniques et graphiques des réflexes tendineux. Bull Soc Méd Hôp Paris. 1916;40:1462–70.
2. Guillain G. Considerations sur le syndrome de Guillain-Barré. Ann Med Interne. 1953;54:81–149.
3. Waksman BH, Adams RD. Allergic neuritis: experimental disease of rabbits induced by the injection of peripheral nervous tissue and adjuvants. J Exp Med. 1955;102:213–21.
4. Asbury AK, Arnason BG, Adams RD. The inflammatory lesion in idiopathic polyneuritis. Its role in pathogenesis. Medicine. 1969;48:173–215.
5. Haymaker W, Kernohan JW. The Landry Guillain Barre syndrome: a clinicopathologic report of fifty fatal cases and a critique of the literature. Medicine. 1949;28:59–68.
6. Ropper AH. The Guillain-Barre syndrome. N Engl J Med. 1992;326:1130.
7. Gorson KC, Ropper AH. Guillain-Barre syndrome (acute inflammatory demyelinating polyneuropathy) and related disorders. In: Katirji B, Kaminski HJ, Preston DC, Ruff RL, Shapiro BE, editors. Neuromuscular disorders in clinical practice. Boston: Butterworth Heinemann; 2002. p. 544–66.
8. Thaisetthawatkul P, Logigian EL. Peripheral nervous system manifestations of lyme borreliosis. J Clin Neuromuscul Dis. 2002;3(4):165–71.
9. Albers JW, Donofrio PD, McGonagle TK. Sequential electrodiagnostic abnormalities in acute inflammatory demyelinating polyradiculoneuropathy. Muscle Nerve. 1985;6:504–9.
10. Cornblath DR. Electrophysiology in Guillain-Barré syndrome. Ann Neurol. 1990;27(Suppl):S17–20.
11. Cornblath MP, Mellits ED, Griffin JW, et al. Motor conduction studies in Guillain-Barre syndrome: description and prognostic value. Ann Neurol. 1988;23:354–9.
12. Deepak G, Muraleedharan N, Baheti NN, Sarma SP, Abraham K. Electrodiagnostic and clinical aspects of Guillain-Barré syndrome: an analysis of 142 cases. J Clin Neuromuscul Dis. 2008;10(2):42–51.
13. Prineas JW. Acute idiopathic polyneuritis. An electronmicroscope study. Lab Invest. 1972;26:133–47.
14. McKhann GM, Cornblath DR, Griffin JW, et al. Acute motor axonal neuropathy: a frequent cause of acute flaccid paralysis in China. Ann Neurol. 1993;33(4): 333–42.

15. Hafer-Macko C, Hsieh ST, Li CY, et al. Acute motor axonal neuropathy: an antibody-mediated attack on axolemma. Ann Neurol. 1996;40:635–44.
16. White JR, Sachs GM, Gilchrist J. Multifocal motor neuropathy with conduction block and Campylobacter jejuni. Neurology. 1996;46(2):562–3.
17. Abruzzese M, Reni L, Schenone A, Mancardi GL, Primavera A. Multifocal motor neuropathy with conduction block after Campylobacter jejuni enteritis. Neurology. 1997;48:544.
18. Fisher M. An unusual variant of acute immune polyneuritis (syndrome of ophthalmoplegia, ataxia, and areflexia). N Engl J Med. 1956;255:57–65.
19. Guiloff RJ. Peripheral nerve conduction in Miller Fisher syndrome. J Neurol Neurosurg Psychiatry. 1977;40:801–7.
20. Fross RD, Daube J. Neuropathy in the Miller-Fisher syndrome: clinical and electrophysiologic findings. Neurology. 1987;37:1493–8.
21. Wietholder H, Hulser PJ, Meier DH, Wessel K. Electrophysiological follow up of experimental allergic neuritis mediated by permanent T cell lines in rats. J Neurol Sci. 1988;83:1–12.
22. Hughes RA, Cornblath DR. Guillain Barre syndrome. Lancet. 2005;366: 1653–66.
23. Ogawara K, Kuwabara S, Mori M, et al. Axonal Guillain Barre syndrome: relation to antiganglioside antibodies and Campylobacter jejuni infection in Japan. Ann Neurol. 2000;48:624–31.
24. Gong Y, Tagawa Y, Lunn MP, et al. Localization of major gangliosides in the PNS. Brain. 2002;125:2491–9.
25. Yoshino H. Distribution of gangliosides in the nervous tissues recognized by axonal form of Guillain Barre syndrome. Neuroimmunology. 1997;5:174–82.
26. Chiba A, Kusunoki S, Obata H, Machinami R, Kanazawa I. Ganglioside composition of the human cranial nerves, with special reference to pathophysiology of Miller Fisher syndrome. Brain Res. 1997;745:32–6.
27. Notturno F, Caporale CM, Uncini A. Acute sensory ataxic neuropathy with antibodies to GD1b and GQ1b gangliosides and prompt recovery. Muscle Nerve. 2008;37:265–8.
28. Nagashima T, Koga M, Odaka M, Hirata K, Yuki N. Clinical correlates of Serum anti-GT1a IgG antibodies. J Neurol Sci. 2004;219:139–45.
29. Susuki K, Nishimoto Y, Yamada M, et al. Acute motor axonal neuropathy rabbit model: Immune attack on nerve root axons. Ann Neurol. 2003;54:383–8.
30. Yuki N, Yamada M, Koga M, et al. Animal model of axonal Guillain-Barré syndrome induced by sensitization with GM1 ganglioside. Ann Neurol. 2001; 49:712–20.
31. Illa I, Ortiz N, Gallard E, Juarez C, Grau JM, Dalakas MC. Acute axonal Guillain-Barré syndrome with IgG antibodies against motor axons following parenteral gangliosides. Ann Neurol. 1995;38:218–24.
32. Saleh MN, Khazaeli MB, Wheeler RH, et al. Phase I trial of the murine monoclonal anti-GD2 antibody 14G2a in metastatic melanoma. Cancer Res. 1992;52:4342–7.
33. Hughes RA, Hadden RD, Gregson NA, Smith KJ. Pathogenesis of Guillain Barre syndrome. J Neuroimmunol. 1999;100:74–97.
34. Kuwabara S, Ogawara K, Misawa S, et al. Does Campylobacter jejuni infection elicit "demyelinating" Guillain-Barré syndrome? Neurology. 2004;63:529–33.
35. Yuki N, Yoshino H, Sato S, et al. Acute axonal polyneuropathy associated with GM1 antibodies following Campylobacter jejuni enteritis. Neurology. 1990;40:1900–3.
36. Koga M, Gilbert M, Li J, et al. Antecedent infections in Fisher syndrome: a common pathogenesis of molecular mimicry. Neurology. 2005;64:1605–11.
37. Hughes RA, Wijdicks EF, Barohn R, et al. Quality Standards Subcommittee of the American Academy of Neurology. Practice parameter: immunotherapy for

Guillain-Barré syndrome: report of the Quality Standards Subcommittee of the American Academy of Neurology. Neurology. 2003;61(6):736–40.

38. The Guillain-Barré Syndrome Study Group. Plasmapheresis and acute Guillain-Barré syndrome. Neurology. 1985;35:1096–104.

39. French Cooperative Group on Plasma Exchange in Guillain-Barré Syndrome. Plasma exchange in Guillain-Barré syndrome: one-year follow-up. Ann Neurol. 1992;32:94–7.

40. French Cooperative Group on Plasma Exchange in Guillain-Barré Syndrome. Appropriate number of plasma exchanges in Guillain-Barré syndrome. Ann Neurol. 1997;41:298–306.

41. Hughes R, Swan A, Raphael J, Annane D, Van Koningsveld R, Van Doorn P. Immunotherapy for Guillain-Barré syndrome: a systematic review. Brain. 2007; 130:2245–57.

42. Gurses N, Uysal S, Cetinkaya F, Icslek I, Kalayci AG. Intravenous immunoglobulin treatment in children with Guillain-Barré syndrome. Scand J Infect Dis. 1995;27:241–3.

43. Korinthenberg R, Schessl J, Kirschner J, Möntning JS. Intravenous immunoglobulin in the treatment of childhood Guillain-Barré syndrome. Pediatrics. 2005;116:8–14.

44. Plasma Exchange/Sandoglobulin Guillain-Barré Syndrome Trial Group. Randomised trial of plasma exchange, intravenous immunoglobulin, and combined treatments in Guillain-Barré syndrome. Lancet. 1997;349:225–30.

45. Nomura T, Hamaguchi K, Hattori T, Satou T, Mannen T, et al. A randomized controlled trial comparing intravenous immunoglobulin and plasmapheresis in Guillain-Barré syndrome. Neurol Ther. 2000;18:69–81.

46. Diener HC, Haupt WF, Kloss TM, Rosenow F, Philipp T, Koeppon S, et al. A preliminary, randomized, multicenter study comparing intravenous immunoglobulin, plasma exchange, and immune adsorption in Guillain-Barré syndrome. Eur Neurol. 2001;46:107–9.

47. Guillain-Barré Syndrome Steroid Trial Group. Double-blind trial of intravenous methylprednisolone in Guillain-Barré syndrome. Lancet. 1993;341:586–90.

48. Garcıa AC, Vidal BE, Rebolledo A, Texeira F, Ordaz FA, Futrán YJ. Treatment of the acute phase of Guillain-Barré-Strohl syndrome with megadosis of methylprednisolone. Rev Invest Clin (Méx). 1985;37:119–24.

49. Shukla SK, Agarwal R, Gupta OP, Pande G, Mamta S. Double blind control trial of prednisolone in Guillain-Barré syndrome – a clinical study. Clin India. 1988; 52:128–34.

50. Singh NK, Gupta A. Do corticosteroids influence the disease course or mortality in Guillain-Barré syndrome. J Assoc Physicians India. 1996;44:22–4.

51. van Koningsveld R, Schmitz PIM. van der Meché FGA for the Dutch GBS Study Group. Effect of methylprednisolone when added to standard treatment with intravenous immunoglobulin for Guillain-Barré syndrome: randomised trial. Lancet. 2004;363:192–6.

52. Kuwabara S, Masahiro M, Ogawara K, et al. Intravenous immunoglobulin therapy for Guillain-Barre syndrome with IgG anti-GM1 antibody. Muscle Nerve. 2001;24(1):54–8.

53. Ropper AH, Albers JW, Addison R. Limited relapse in Guillain-Barre syndrome after plasma exchange. Arch Neurol. 1988;45(3):314–5.

54. Farcas P, Avnun L, Frisher S, Herishanu YO, Wirguin I. Efficacy of repeated intravenous immunoglobulin in severe unresponsive Guillain-Barré syndrome. Lancet. 1997;350:1747.

55. Bouchard C, Lacroix C, Plante V, et al. Clinicopathologic findings and prognosis of chronic inflammatory demyelinating polyneuropathy. Neurology. 1999;52:498–503.

56. Rotta FT, Sussman AT, Bradley WG, Ram Ayyar D, Sharma KR, Shebert RT. The spectrum of chronic inflammatory demyelinating polyneuropathy. J Neurol Sci. 2000;173:129–39.

57. Sakakibara R, Hattori T, Kuwabara S, et al. Micturitional disturbance in patients with chronic inflammatory demyelinating polyneuropathy. Neurology. 1998;50:1179–85.

58. Gorson KC, Ropper AH. Chronic Inflammatory Demyelinating Polyradiculoneuropathy (CIDP): a review of clinical syndromes and treatment approaches in clinical practice. J Clin Neuromuscul Dis. 2003;4(4):174–89.

59. Chio A, Cocito D, Bottacchi E, et al. Idiopathic chronic inflammatory demyelinating polyneuropathy: an epidemiological study in Italy. J Neurol Neurosurg Psychiatry. 2007;78:1349.

60. McCleod JG, Pollard JD, Macaskill P, Mohamed A, Spring P, Khurana V. Prevalence of chronic inflammatory demyelinating polyneuropathy in New South Wales, Australia. Ann Neurol. 1999;46:910–3.

61. Mygland A, Monstadt P. Chronic polyneuropathies in Vest-Agder, Norway. Eur J Neurol. 2001;8:157–65.

62. Stewart JD, McKelvey R, Durcan L, et al. Chronic inflammatory demyelinating polyneuropathy (CIDP) in diabetics. J Neurol Sci. 1996;142:59–64.

63. Cocito D, Durelli L, Isoardo G. Different clinical, electrophysiological and immunological features of CIDP associated with paraproteinemia. Acta Neurol Scand. 2003;108:274–80.

64. Simmons Z, Albers JW, Bromberg MB, Feldman EL. Presentation and initial clinical course in patients with chronic inflammatory demyelinating polyradiculoneuropathy: comparison of patients without and with monoclonal gammopathy. Neurology. 1993;43:2202–9.

65. Dyck PJ, Dyck PJB. Atypical varieties of chronic demyelinating neuropathies. Lancet. 2000;355(9212):1293–4.

66. Dyck PJ, Low PA, Windebank AJ, et al. Plasma exchange in polyneuropathy associated with monoclonal gammopathy of undetermined significance. N Engl J Med. 1991;325(21):1482–6.

67. Katz JS, Saperstein DS, Gronseth G, Amato AA, Barohn RJ. Distal acquired demyelinating symmetric neuropathy. Neurology. 2000;54(3):615–20.

68. Barohn RJ, Kissel JT, Warmolts JR, Mendell JR. Chronic inflammatory demyelinating polyradiculoneuropathy. Clinical characteristics, course, and recommendations for diagnostic criteria. Arch Neurol. 1989;46(8):878–84.

69. Research criteria for diagnosis of chronic inflammatory demyelinating polyneuropathy (CIDP). Report from an Ad Hoc Subcommittee of the American Academy of Neurology AIDS Task Force. Neurology. 1991;41:617.

70. Dyck PJ, Prineas J, Pollard J. Chronic inflammatory demyelinating polyneuropathy. In: Dyck PJ, Thomas PK, Griffin JW, et al., editors. Peripheral neuropathy. Philadelphia: WB Saunders; 1993. p. 1498–517.

71. Krendel DA, Parks HP, Anthony DA, et al. Sural nerve biopsy in chronic inflammatory demyelinating polyradiculoneuropathy. Muscle Nerve. 1989;12:257–64.

72. Kieseier BC, Dalakas MC, Hartung HP. Immune mechanisms in chronic inflammatory demyelinating neuropathy. Neurology. 2002;59:S7.

73. Kiefer R, Kieseier BC, Stoll G, Hartung HP. The role of macrophages in immune-mediated damage to the peripheral nervous system. Prog Neurobiol. 2001;64:109–14.

74. Dalakas MC, Engel WK. Immunoglobulin and complement deposits in nerves of patients with chronic relapsing polyneuropathy. Arch Neurol. 1980;37:637.

75. Dalakas MC, Houff SA, Engel WK, et al. CSF "monoclonal" bands in chronic relapsing polyneuropathy. Neurology. 1980;30:86.

76. Yan WX, Taylor J, Andrias-Kauba S, Pollard JD. Passive transfer of demyelination by serum or IgG from chronic inflammatory demyelinating polyneuropathy patients. Ann Neurol. 2000;47:765–70.

77. Ilyas AA, Mithen FA, Dalakas MC, et al. Antibodies to acidic glycolipids in Guillain-Barre syndrome and chronic inflammatory demyelinating polyneuropathy. J Neurol Sci. 1992;107:111–9.

78. Melendez-Vasquez C, Redford J, Choudary PP, et al. Immunological investigation of chronic inflammatory demyelinating polyneuropathy. J Neuroimmunol. 1997;73:124–31.

79. Gabriel CM, Gregson NA, Hughes RA. Anti-PMP22 antibodies in patients with inflammatory neuropathy. J Neuroimmunol. 2000;104:139–45.

80. Ritz MF, Lechner-Scott J, Scott RJ, et al. Characterization of autoantibodies to peripheral myelin protein 22 in patients with hereditary and acquired neuropathies. J Neuroimmunol. 2000;104:155–61.

81. Austin JH. Recurrent polyneuropathies and their corticosteroid treatment. With five-year observations of a placebo controlled case treated with corticotrophin, cortisone and prednisone. Brain. 1958;81(2):157.

82. Dyck PJ, O'Brien PC, Oviatt KF, Dinapoli RP, Daube JR, Bartleson JD, et al. Prednisone improves chronic inflammatory polyradiculoneuropathy more than no treatment. Ann Neurol. 1982;11:136–41.

83. Mehndiratta MM, Hughes RA. Corticosteroids for chronic inflammatory demyelinating polyradiculoneuropathy. Cochrane Database Syst Rev. 2002;(1):CD002062.

84. Dyck PJ, Daube J, O'Brien P, Pineda A, Low PA, Windebank AJ, et al. Plasma exchange in chronic inflammatory demyelinating polyradiculoneuropathy. N Engl J Med. 1986;314:461–5.

85. Hahn AF, Bolton CF, Pillay N, Chalk C, Benstead T, Bril V, et al. Plasma exchange in chronic inflammatory demyelinating polyradiculoneuropathy. A double blind, sham-controlled, crossover study. Brain. 1996;119(Pt 4):1055–66.

86. Eftimov F, Winer JB, Vermeulen M, de Haan R, van Schaik IN. Intravenous immunoglobulin for chronic inflammatory demyelinating polyradiculoneuropathy. Cochrane Database Syst Rev. 2009;(1):CD001797. doi:10.1002/14651858. CD001797.pub2.

87. Hughes RA, Donofrio P, Bril V, et al. Intravenous immune globulin (10% caprylate-chromatography purified) for the treatment of chronic inflammatory demyelinating polyradiculoneuropathy (ICE study): a randomised placebo-controlled trial. Lancet Neurol. 2008;7(2):136–44.

88. Hughes R, Bensa S, Willison H, et al. Randomized controlled trial of intravenous immunoglobulin versus oral prednisolone in chronic inflammatory demyelinating polyradiculoneuropathy. Ann Neurol. 2001;50(2):195–201.

89. Dyck PJ, Litchy WJ, Kratz KM, Suarez GA, Low PA, Pineda AA, et al. A plasma exchange versus immune globulin infusion trial in chronic inflammatory demyelinating polyradiculoneuropathy. Ann Neurol. 1994;36(6):838–45.

90. Gorson KC, Allam G, Ropper AH. Chronic inflammatory demyelinating polyneuropathy: clinical features and response to treatment in 67 consecutive patients with and without a monoclonal gammopathy. Neurology. 1997;48:321.

91. Dalakas MC, Engel WK. Chronic relapsing (dysimmune) polyneuropathy: pathogenesis and treatment. Ann Neurol. 1981;9(Suppl):134–45.

92. Brannagan TH, Pradhan A, Heiman-Patterson T, Winkelman AC, Styler MJ, Topolsky DL, et al. High-dose cyclophosphamide without stem-cell rescue for refractory CIDP. Neurology. 2002;58(12):1856–8.

93. McCombe PA, Pollard JD, McLeod JG. Chronic inflammatory demyelinating polyradiculoneuropathy. A clinical and electrophysiological study of 92 cases. Brain. 1987;110(Pt 6):1617–30.

94. Gladstone DE, Prestrud AA, Brannagan 3rd TH. High-dose cyclophosphamide results in long-term disease remission with restoration of a normal quality of life in patients with severe refractory chronic inflammatory demyelinating polyneuropathy. J Peripher Nerv Syst. 2005;10(1):11–6.

95. Good JL, Chehrenama M, Mayer RF, Koski CL. Pulse cyclophosphamide therapy in chronic inflammatory demyelinating polyneuropathy. Neurology. 1998;51(6):1735–8.

96. Barnett MH, Pollard JD, Davies L, McLeod JG. Cyclosporin A in resistant chronic inflammatory demyelinating polyradiculoneuropathy. Muscle Nerve. 1998;21(4):454–60.

97. Hodgkinson SJ, Pollard JD, McLeod JG. Cyclosporin A in the treatment of chronic demyelinating polyradiculoneuropathy. J Neurol Neurosurg Psychiatry. 1990;53(4):327–30.

98. Mahattanakul W, Crawford TO, Griffin JW, Goldstein JM, Cornblath DR. Treatment of chronic inflammatory demyelinating polyneuropathy with cyclosporin-A. J Neurol Neurosurg Psychiatry. 1996;60(2):185–7.

99. Matsuda M, Hoshi K, Gono T, Morita H, Ikeda S. Cyclosporin A in treatment of refractory patients with chronic inflammatory demyelinating polyradiculoneuropathy. J Neurol Sci. 2004;224(1–2):29–35.

100. Odaka M, Tatsumoto M, Susuki K, Hirata K, Yuki N. Intractable chronic inflammatory demyelinating polyneuropathy treated successfully with cyclosporin. J Neurol Neurosurg Psychiatry. 2005;76(8):1115–20.

101. Dyck PJ, O'Brien P, Swanson C, Low P, Daube J. Combined azathioprine and prednisone in chronic inflammatory demyelinating polyneuropathy. Neurology. 1985;35(8):1173–6.

102. Vallat JM, Hahn AF, Léger JM, Cros DP, Magy L, Tabaraud F, et al. Interferon beta-1a as an investigational treatment for CIDP. Neurology. 2003; 60(8 Suppl 3):23–8.

103. Hughes RAC, Gorson KC, Cros D, Griffin J, Pollard J, Vallat J-M, et al. Intramuscular interferon beta-1a in chronic inflammatory demyelinating polyradiculoneuropathy. Neurology. 2010;74:651–7.

104. RMC Trial Group. Randomised controlled trial of methotrexate for chronic inflammatory demyelinating polyradiculoneuropathy (RMC Trial): a pilot, multicentre study. Lancet Neurol. 2009;8(2):158–64.

105. Lewis R, Sumner A, Brown MJ, Asbury AK. Chronic multifocal demyelinative neuropathy: a unique disorder with persistent conduction block. Neurology. 1982;32:958–62.

106. Viala K, Renie L, Maisonobe T, et al. Follow-up study and response to treatment in 23 patients with Lewis-Sumner syndrome. Brain. 2004;127:2010–7.

107. Oh SJ, Joy JJ, Kuruoglu R. "Chronic sensory demyelinating neuropathy": chronic inflammatory demyelinating polyneruopathy presenting as a pure sensory neuropathy. J Neurol Neurosurg Psychiatry. 1992;55:677.

108. Chin RL, Latov N, Sander HW, et al. Sensory CIDP presenting as cryptogenic sensory polyneuropathy. J Peripher Nerv Syst. 2004;9:132–7.

109. Berger AR, Herskovitz S, Kaplan J. Late motor involvement in cases presenting as "chronic demyelinating polyneuropathy". Muscle Nerve. 1995;18(4):440–4.

110. Parry GJ, Clarke S. Multifocal acquired demyelinating neuropathy masquerading as motor neuron disease. Muscle Nerve. 1988;11:103–7.

111. Lewis R. Conduction block neuropathies. Curr Opin Neurol. 2007;20(5): 525–30.

112. Nobile-Orazio E. Multifocal motor neuropathy. J Neuroimmunol. 2001;115 (1–2):4–18.

113. Kornberg AJ, Pestronk A. The clinical and diagnostic role of anti-GM1 antibody testing. Muscle Nerve. 1994;17:100–4.

114. Taylor BV, Gross LA, Windebank AJ. The sensitivity and specificity of anti-GM1 antibody testing. Neurology. 1996;47:951–5.

115. Corse AM, Chaudry W, Crawford TO, Cornblath DR, Kuncl RW, Griffin JW. Sural nerve pathology in multifocal motor neuropathy. Ann Neurol. 1996;39: 319–25. Comment in: Ann Neurol. 1996;40:948–50.

116. Taylor BV, Dyck PJB, Engelstand J, Gruener G, Grant I, Dyck PJ. Multifocal motor neuropathy: pathologic alterations at the site of conduction block. J Neuropathol Exp Neurol. 2004;63:129–37.

117. Nobile-Orazio E, Cappellari A, Priori A. Multifocal motor neuropathy: current concepts and controversies. Muscle Nerve. 2005;31:663–80.

118. Santoro M, Uncini A, Corbo M, Staugaitis SM, Thomas FP, Hays AP, et al. Experimental conduction block induced by serum from a patient with anti-GM1 antibodies. Ann Neurol. 1992;31:385–90.

119. Arasaki K, Kusunoki S, Kudo N, Kanazawa I. Acute conduction block in vitro following exposure to anti-ganglioside sera. Muscle Nerve. 1993;16:587–93.

120. Harvey GK, Toyka KV, Zielasek J, Kiefer R, Simonis C, Hartung HP. Failure of anti-GM1 IgG or IgM to induce conduction block following intraneural transfer. Muscle Nerve. 1995;18:388–94.

121. Sugie K, Murataq K, Ikoma K, et al. A case of acute multifocal motor neuropathy wit conduction block after Campylobacter jejuni enteritis. Rinsho Shinkeigaku. 1998;38:436.

122. Pestronk A, Cornblath DR, Ilyas A, Baba H, Quarles RH, Griffin JW, et al. A treatable multifocal motor neuropathy with antibodies to GM1 ganglioside. Ann Neurol. 1988;24:73–8.

123. Azulay JP, Blin O, Pouget J, Boucraut J, Billé-Turc F, Carles G, et al. Intravenous immunoglobulin treatment in patients with motor neuron syndromes associated with anti-GM1 antibodies: a doubleblind, placebo-controlled study. Neurology. 1994;44(3 Pt 1):429–32.

124. Federico P, Zochodne DW, Hahn AF, Brown WF, Feasby TE. Multifocal motor neuropathy improved by IVIg: Randomized, doubleblind, placebo-controlled study. Neurology. 2000;55(9):1256–62.

125. Léger J-M, Chassande B, Musset L, Meininger V, Bouche P, Baumann N. Intravenous immunoglobulin therapy in multifocal motor neuropathy: A double-blind, placebo-controlled study. Brain. 2001;124(1):145–53.

126. Van den Berg LH, Kerkhoff H, Oey PL, Franssen H, Mollee I, Vermeulen M, et al. Treatment of multifocal motor neuropathy with high dose intravenous immunoglobulins: a double blind, placebo controlled study. J Neurol Neurosurg Psychiatry. 1995;59(3):248–52.

127. Pestronk A, Chaudhry V, Feldman EL, Griffin JW, Cornblath DR, Denys EH, et al. Lower motor neuron syndromes defined by patterns of weakness, nerve conduction abnormalities, and high titers of anti-glycolipid antibodies. Ann Neurol. 1990;27(3):316–26.

128. Feldman EL, Bromberg MB, Albers JW, Pestronk A. Immunosuppressive treatment in multifocal motor neuropathy. Ann Neurol. 1991;30(3):397–401.

129. Piepers S, Van den Berg-Vos R, Van der Pol WL, Franssen H, Wokke J, Van den Berg L. Mycophenolate mofetil as adjunctive therapy for MMN patients: a randomized, controlled trial. Brain. 2007;130(Pt 8):2004–10.

130. Kelly JJ, Kyle RA, O'Brien PC, Dyck PJ. Prevalence of monoclonal protein in peripheral neuropathy. Neurology. 1981;31(11):1480–3.

131. Ropper AH, Gorson KC. Neuropathies associated with paraproteinemia. N Engl J Med. 1998;338(22):1601–7.

132. Levine T, Pestronk A, Florence J, et al. Peripheral neuropathies in Waldenström's macroglobulinaemia. J Neurol Neurosurg Psychiatry. 2006;77:224–8. This report describes the symptoms and signs of peripheral neuropathy in a cohort of patients with Waldenström's macroglobulinaemia.

133. Noronha V, Fynan TM, Duffy T. Flare in neuropathy following rituximab therapy in Waldenstrom's macroglobulinemia. J Clin Oncol. 2006;24(1):e3.

134. Mauermann ML, Ryan ML, Moon JS, Klein CJ. Case of mononeuropathy multiplex onset with rituximab therapy for Waldenstrom's macroglobulinemia. J Neurol Sci. 2007;260:240–3.

135. Kelly Jr JJ, Kyle RA, Miles JM, O'Brien PC, Dyck PJ. The spectrum of peripheral neuropathy in myeloma. Neurology. 1981;31:24–31.

136. Drieger H, Pruzanski W. Plasma cell neoplasia with peripheral polyneuropathy. Medicine. 1988;59:301–10.

137. Watanabe O, Maruyama I, Arimura K, et al. Overproduction of vascular endothelial growth factor/vascular permeability factor is causative in Crow-Fukase (POEMS) syndrome. Muscle Nerve. 1998;21:1390–7.

138. Gosselin S, Kyle RA, Dyck PJ. Neuropathy associated with monoclonal gammopathies of undetermined significance. Ann Neurol. 1991;30:54–61.

139. Yeung KB, Thomas PK, King RHM, et al. The clinical spectrum of peripheral neuropathies associated with benign monoclonal IgM, IgG and IgA paraproteinemia: comparative clinical, immunological and nerve biopsy findings. J Neurol. 1991;238:383–91.

140. Latov N, Hays AP, Sherman WH. Peripheral neuropathy and anti-MAG antibodies. Crit Rev Neurobiol. 1988;3:301–32.

141. Kissel JT, Collins MP. Peripheral nerve vasculitis. In: Younger DS, editor. Motor disorders. Philadelphia: Lippincott Williams and Wilkins; 1999. p. 243–56.

Part IV

Systemic Disorders

20

Systemic Autoimmune Diseases with Neurological Manifestations

Richard Choi, Valarie Gendron, Mac McLaughlin, Jonathan Cahill,
Fathima Qadeer, and Syed A. Rizvi

Keywords: Immune mediated, Multifactorial, Antibodies, Remissions, Anticoagulation, Granuloma

Introduction

In this chapter, we discuss several systemic diseases that have an immune-mediated pathogenesis. Although most of these diseases are infrequent and seldom affect the neurological system, clinicians should always remain cognizant of their existence. Even though a detailed encounter with each of the following diseases is out of the scope of this chapter, we cover the most commonly encountered and the most prominent neurological and clinical manifestations to help guide the clinician into identifying, diagnosing, and treating these illnesses.

Systemic Lupus Erythematosus

Systemic Lupus Erythematosus (SLE) is an autoimmune disorder involving multiple organ systems that can have a widely variable presentation and clinical course. Women are affected nine times more than men. Life expectancy has dramatically increased from an approximate 4-year survival of 50% in the 1950s to a 15-year survival of 80% today [1].

Since the diagnosis of SLE can be quite challenging the American Academy of Rheumatology published consensus guidelines that consist of 11 categories of which four must be present, either serially or simultaneously, to make the diagnosis [2]. These categories include: malar rash, discoid rash, photosensitivity of the skin, oral ulcers, arthritis, serositis, renal disorder, hematologic disorder, immunologic disorder, antinuclear antibody, and neurologic disorder. Even though the category "neurologic" only includes seizures or psychosis, SLE can affect the nervous system in many capacities and at multiple levels.

Although there is no definite etiology, observations suggest a multi-factorial process for this disease with a role for genetic (particularly HLA-A1,

From: *Clinical Neuroimmunology: Multiple Sclerosis and Related Disorders*, Current Clinical Neurology,
Edited by: S.A. Rizvi and P.K. Coyle, DOI 10.1007/978-1-60327-860-7_20,
© Springer Science+Business Media, LLC 2011

B8, and DR3), hormonal (females compose 90% of patients affected by lupus), infectious (in one study, anti-EBV antibodies were present in 99% of patients and EBV DNA was present in 100% of patients) [3] and environmental factors.

Autoantibodies to double-stranded DNA are important in the pathogenesis of lupus and are present in over 70% of patients affected, but in only 0.5% of healthy controls or in patients with other autoimmune diseases [4].

How these autoantibodies develop is not well understood, but is felt to be secondary to exposure to cellular debris during apoptosis and exposure to nucleosomes, Ro 62, Ro 50, La, and anionic phospholipids as antibodies to these antigens are commonly found in patients with lupus. Although this debris is usually phagocytosed by macrophages, certain complement deficiencies such as C1q, C2, and C4 may lead to decreased phagocytosis [5]. Additionally, patients with lupus have been recognized to have elevated levels of interleukin-10, which is known to induce stimulation of B cells [6].

Even though various autoantibodies have been implicated in the neurological manifestations of lupus, there is no consistent evidence. Of particular interest to neurologists, however, is the anti-phospholipid autoantibody (aPL), a heterogeneous group of antibodies (including anti-cardiolipin [aCL] antibodies, lupus anticoagulant (LA), and the plasma protein beta-2 glycoprotein I antibody) that has been linked to thrombosis, recurrent fetal loss and various other manifestations in patients with and without lupus. Antiphospholipid antibodies have also been associated with other neurological manifestations of lupus, such as cognitive dysfunction [7, 8]. Another autoantibody of interest is anti-glutamate receptor antibody which may play a role in cognitive dysfunction and psychiatric manifestations, though the evidence is conflicting [9, 10].

Damage to the neurological system is believed to be due to a constellation of autoantibodies, microangiopathy, intrathecal production of proinflammatory cytokines, and premature atherosclerosis [11]. Even though this damage was originally thought to be secondary to antibody deposition, it is now suspected to arise from the activation of complement [12]. In postmortem histopathologic studies, a wide range of brain abnormalities was observed including cortical atrophy, gross infarcts, hemorrhage, ischemic demyelination, and patchy demyelination [13].

The pathophysiology of how lupus causes damage to the brain is unclear but is felt to be related to the blood–brain barrier, the interactions between endothelial cells, white blood cells, and adhesion proteins such as ICAM-1 as well as inflammatory cytokines and mediators [14].

Clinical Manifestations and Diagnosis

In 1999, The American College of Rheumatology published nomenclature and case definitions recommending that the term Neuropsychiatric SLE (NPSLE) be used to describe the constellation of 19 different potential neurologic manifestations of SLE (ACR). These are divided as follows.

1. PNS manifestations: (a) acute inflammatory demyelinating polyneuropathy (Guillain–Barré Syndrome); (b) autonomic disorder; (c) mononeuropathy (single/multiplex); (d) myasthenia gravis; (e) neuropathy (cranial); (f) plexopathy; and (g) peripheral neuropathy.

2. CNS manifestations: (a) acute confusional syndrome; (b) cerebrovascular disease; (c) cognitive dysfunction; (d) demyelinating syndrome; (e) headache; (f) movement disorder; (g) myelopathy; and (h) seizure.
3. Psychiatric manifestations: (a) anxiety disorder; (b) mood disorder; and (c) psychosis.

These symptoms have been estimated to occur in 10–80% of patients with SLE and can be present before or around the time of the diagnosis in 28–40% of patients. Afflictions of the nervous system are a major cause of mortality and morbidity and are associated with reduced quality of life and increased organ damage, irrespective of whether the manifestation is ultimately attributed to lupus or not [14].

Cognitive dysfunction, manifested by impairments in mental activities (e.g., memory, abstract thinking, and judgment) is the most common neurologic manifestation [15].

SLE may be associated with a significant increase in the risk of stroke and of premature death due to cerebrovascular disease. There is a strong association between anti-phospholipid antibodies (aPL) and stroke that has been observed in SLE patients. Furthermore, SLE patients with a positive LA or aCL test have been found to have an odds ratio for thrombosis ranging between 3.2 and 6.8 [16]. CNS vasculitis due to SLE typically presents with a distinct syndrome of fever, severe headaches, and confusional episodes, with rapid progression to psychotic symptoms, seizures, and coma.

The pathophysiology of seizures in SLE is not completely understood, though aPL antibodies and anti-ribosomal P protein antibodies have been implicated [17]. Patients can experience all seizure types, from generalized tonic–clonic seizures, simple partial seizures, and complex partial seizures to status epilepticus. These seizures can occur as single events or as part of epilepsy.

Patients with SLE can experience monophasic or recurrent attacks of inflammation that can resemble primary demyelinating disorders. Lupoid sclerosis is a term used to describe a clinical syndrome similar to multiple sclerosis (MS) in SLE patients. Patients with SLE are also at an increased risk of transverse myelitis. Aggressive immunosuppression (including cyclophosphamide) has been shown to be beneficial in these patients [18, 19]. Clinically, however, the disease course of these manifestations can be difficult to differentiate from multiple-sclerosis. Additional clinical criteria such as presence or absence of thrombi, miscarriages, livedo reticularis, thrombocytopenia, rashes, arthritis, peripheral nerve involvement in addition to laboratory, and imaging findings must then be examined to arrive at the correct diagnosis, though this can sometimes remain enigmatic [20].

Most headaches in patients with SLE fall under the categories of migraines with aura, migraines without aura, and tension-type headaches. Some studies have shown that an increase in the frequency of headaches implies a flare up of the disease. On the other hand, a recent meta-analysis has not verified an increased prevalence of headache among SLE patients or a unique headache phenotype among these patients in comparison with controls [21].

SLE less commonly presents with movement disorders (including chorea, hemiballismus, and parkinsonian features), an acute confusional state (most commonly associated with an underlying pathology), cranial neuropathies, and aseptic meningitis. Peripheral nervous system disorders are also seen, the most common of which is a symmetric, length-dependent polyneuropathy. The prevalence of PNS involvement has been estimated to be 20–30% but few of these studies required electrophysiologic evidence [22, 23]. Further complicating factors include the chronic use of corticosteroids in this population.

Treatment

There is no cure for SLE and sustained remissions are rare. The management of patients with NPSLE includes both symptomatic and immunosuppressive therapies, but evidence for the efficacy of these treatments is based on uncontrolled clinical trials and anecdotal experience. The key to treatment is to correctly diagnose the patient with NPSLE. The mainstay of treatment and the only FDA-approved medications to treat lupus currently are corticosteroids. Hydroxychloroquine also has a long-track record and is safe in pregnancy but is only effective in mild forms of the disease. Cyclophosphamide is another treatment option with documented benefits in the treatment of severe NPSLE unresponsive to other medications [24]. Other medications currently undergoing research as potential tools in our therapeutic arsenal against NPSLE include mycophenolate mofetil and rituximab.

Cognitive defects may respond to steroids, antidepressants, atypical antipsychotics, and/or anxiolytics. Unfortunately, most of these patients represent a therapeutic challenge and most remain impaired despite control of SLE symptoms.

Chronic anticoagulation therapy with warfarin or aspirin is indicated in most patients with stroke syndromes due to aPL or thrombosis once they are stable and if there is no evidence of hemorrhage. Current evidence suggests low-dose aspirin for patients with a positive antibody test and no history of thrombosis, whereas those with a history of stroke should receive aspirin or low-dose warfarin (with an INR titrated to 1.4–2.8). Patients with recurrent thrombosis despite this treatment should then have a higher target INR of 2–3 [25].

Neurosarcoidosis

Sarcoidosis is an inflammatory disease of multiple organs which is pathologically characterized by non-caseating granulomas. The pathogenesis of sarcoidosis is not known, but there is evidence for an underlying genetic predisposition and immune-mediated inflammation [26]. This rare disease affects women more often than men and is more prevalent among black populations than white. The lungs, lymphatic system, uvea, and skin are the most common organ systems affected by sarcoidosis, but in up to 5–10% of patients there is nervous system involvement [27–29]. Half of these patients present with neurological symptoms at the time of initial sarcoidosis diagnosis. The neurological manifestations of sarcoidosis, so-called neurosarcoidosis, can range from mild to severe and life-threatening and can affect all parts of the nervous system.

Clinical Manifestations and Diagnosis

Cranial neuropathies are the most common neurological signs in neurosarcoidosis, occurring in 22–72% of patients [30–32]. Facial nerve palsy is the most common, with 35% of facial nerve palsies being bilateral. Optic neuropathy and chronic optic nerve atrophy are also encountered frequently, but any cranial nerve can be affected in neurosarcoidosis. The cranial neuropathies may be caused by basal meningitis or by focal compressive lesions.

Because of the propensity for neurosarcoidosis to affect the base of the brain, hypothalamic dysfunction, and neuro-endocrine dysfunction are not uncommon [28, 30]. Diabetes insipidus, hypopituitarism, hypercalcemia, hypothyroidism, amenorrhea, and disorders of sleep are some of the conditions associated with hypothalamic neurosarcoidosis.

Meningitis affecting primarily the base of the brain is found in 3–26% of neurosarcoidosis patients [27, 30]. The clinical course of the meningitis can be either acute or a chronic, indolent meningitis. Cerebrospinal fluid (CSF) analysis demonstrates elevated protein with or without a lymphocytic pleocytosis and usually a low-CSF glucose. The meningitis commonly remits spontaneously or in response to steroid therapy, but can lead to obstructive hydrocephalus requiring mechanical CSF diversion such as a ventriculo-peritoneal or lumbo-peritoneal drain.

Focal granulomatous mass lesions can affect any part of the brain and can be symptomatic depending on the brain area affected. Epileptic seizures can occur as a result of focal cortical lesions. These seizures are typically easy to control with standard anti-epileptic medications, so long as the epileptogenic lesion is treated. Epileptic seizures have been thought to portend a worse prognosis in neurosarcoidosis, but recent case series do not support this theory.

The spinal cord including the conus medullaris and cauda equina are rare sites of neurosarcoidosis involvement, but disease in these areas can portend a poor prognosis. The lesions can be extradural or intradural and can present as myelopathy or radiculopathy.

Fifteen percent of neurosarcoidosis patients have a peripheral neuropathy which is usually axonal [30]. The prognosis of peripheral neuropathy is better than that of central nervous system disease.

The only definitive diagnostic test for neurosarcoidosis is biopsy revealing non-caseating granulomas. Because of difficulty biopsying nervous system tissue, and the risk involved with brain or meningeal biopsy, other diagnostic tests are generally used to make the diagnosis. The general approach is to rule out other conditions such as malignancy or infection and to look for other systemic manifestations of sarcoidosis. Radiologic studies such as contrast-enhanced MRI or fluorodeoxyglucose positron emission tomography (FDG-PET), neurophysiologic testing such as nerve conduction studies and electromyography (NCS/EMG), and CSF measures of lymphocytes, protein, and glucose can be helpful [32]. Contrast-enhanced MRI is the most commonly used diagnostic test for neurosarcoidosis and is also used to monitor response to therapy. Findings on MRI of leptomeningeal enhancement at the base of the brain can indicate inflammatory meningitis [32]. MRI also has high sensitivity for detecting parenchymal brain lesions. Approximately 40% of neurosarcoidosis patients have either basilar leptomeningeal enhancement or multiple white matter lesions on MRI. The pattern of white matter lesions often resembles the periventricular lesion pattern in multiple sclerosis.

NCS and EMG can demonstrate neuropathy when present in neurosarcoidosis, but there are no patterns specific for the disease. Axonal neuropathy is more common than demyelinating, but there are reports of an acute demyelinating neuropathy similar to Guillain–Barré Syndrome [30, 31].

CSF in neurosarcoidosis often demonstrates significantly elevated protein and a mild lymphocytic pleocytosis. Oligoclonal bands can be seen in 30–40% of neurosarcoidosis patients. Examination of the CSF for infectious etiologies or malignant cells is important to rule out mimicking diseases. Measurement of CSF angiotensin-converting enzyme (ACE) is often done, but elevations are not specific for neurosarcoidosis and can be elevated in other conditions such as infection or malignancy.

Other diagnostic tests to search for systemic sarcoidosis can be helpful in clinching the diagnosis in the absence of convincing findings on these tests of the nervous system. Chest X-ray, chest CT, serum ACE levels, skin biopsy, and muscle biopsy can all provide supportive evidence for the diagnosis.

Treatment

Although there have been no randomized, controlled trials of therapy for neurosarcoidosis, corticosteroids are the mainstay of treatment [31, 32]. Prednisone from 0.5 to 1 mg/kg daily is given and maintained depending on response to therapy. Many patients are maintained for long periods of time and have difficulty weaning below 10–20 mg of prednisone. Intravenous methyl-prednisolone is used for acute treatment for 3–5 days. Many other agents including methotrexate, azathioprine, cyclosporine, infliximab, hydroxychloroquine, and cladribine have all been used to avoid the long-term adverse effects of corticosteroids.

Sjogren's Syndrome

Sjogren's syndrome is a chronic autoimmune inflammatory condition which can be either primary or secondary to another rheumatologic condition, such as rheumatoid arthritis or SLE. It is primarily a disorder of the exocrine system leading to the destruction of the lacrimal and salivary glands (keratoconjunctivitis sicca and xerostomia).

Clinical Manifestations and Diagnosis

Peripheral neuropathy is the most common neurological manifestation of Sjogren's syndrome, occurring in 10–50% of patients. The pattern of neuropathy is most commonly a symmetric, sensorimotor polyneuropathy, but pure sensory neuropathy, mononeuropathy multiplex, autonomic neuropathy, and cranial neuropathies (especially trigeminal neuropathies) are also reported [33–36]. The pathophysiology of the varied neuropathies is not certain but there are reports of different pathological features depending on the pattern of neuropathy [33]. Lymphocytic infiltration of dorsal root ganglia (sensory neuropathy), vasculitis (mononeuropathy multiplex), and cryoglobulinemia (sensorimotor neuropathy) have all been reported.

Central nervous system effects of Sjogren's syndrome are difficult to study because of a lack of standardized diagnostic criteria. Estimates of the prevalence of CNS disease among patients with primary Sjogren's syndrome range from 0 to 48% [34]. Much like in neurosarcoidosis, the clinical presentation can be variable depending on the type of brain lesion noted: focal, multifocal or diffuse; brain or spinal cord; relapsing or progressive. The pathophysiology of CNS lesions in Sjogren's syndrome is not known but vasculitis or direct inflammatory cell infiltration of the brain is postulated. Making a diagnosis is further complicated by the fact that diagnostic tests, such as MRI and CSF evaluation can mimic other inflammatory neurological disease [37].

Treatment

The treatment of the neurological manifestations of Sjogren's syndrome is targeted toward the specific neurological manifestation of the disease, and also at the presumed underlying autoimmune reaction. For example, painful sensory neuropathy is usually treated with neuropathic pain agents such as gabapentin, whereas autonomic neuropathy associated with Sjogren's syndrome is treated with adrenocorticoids such as fludrocortisone. If vasculitis is suspected clinically, such as with an asymmetric neuropathy, or is present on nerve biopsy; often glucocorticoids will be used [33, 34].

Behçet's Disease

This disease, named after Huluci Behçet, a Turkish dermatologist who described three patients with oral and genital ulceration and hypopyon uveitis in 1937 [38]. Behçet is a relapsing inflammatory disorder of unknown cause affecting multiple organ systems. It is pathologically characterized by an inflammatory peri-vasculitis with a venous predominance. It is most prevalent in the Middle East, Far East and Mediterranean countries, or what is often referred to as the ancient "Silk Road" but has been reported all over the world. This disease affects young people with a mean age of onset between 20 and 35 years and is more prevalent in men. It is rare in patients older than 50 years and tends to be most severe in young men.

The usual course is characterized by exacerbations and remissions and there is usually complete remission, though sequelae have also been reported. The most common manifestations include oral and genital ulcers, ocular involvement (recurrent anterior uveitis with hypopyon formation or posterior uveitis associated with retinal involvement) and dermatologic manifestations (erythema nodosum-like lesions, folliculitis, pseudofolliculitis, acne-like lesions, superficial thrombophlebitis, cutaneous vasculitis, or papulopustular lesions) [39]. Vascular involvement can lead to superficial thrombo-phlebitis, superior vena cava syndrome, Budd–Chiari syndrome, Deep Vein Thrombosis and dural sinus thrombosis of the veins and occlusion and/or aneurysm formation of the pulmonary, renal, subclavian, femoral, or carotid arteries. Other manifestations include rheumatologic (non-deforming, non-erosive mono-, oligo-, or polyarthritis), pulmonary, cardiac, gastrointestinal, and urogenital presentations but are limited to case reports.

Neurologic involvement in Behçet's disease ranges from 1.3 to 59% in different studies [40]. It can present in any part of the nervous system, the muscles or the vasculature. Neurologic involvement is more common in men and usually presents after systemic manifestations, though has rarely been described to precede the other more common manifestations in up to 3% of patients [41]. Pathological findings of CNS involvement of Behçet's disease include peri-vascular cuffing with an intense inflammatory infiltrate composed of lymphocytes, neutrophils, eosinophils, and macrophages with areas of demyelination, necrosis and axonal loss most often encountered in the brainstem, thalamus, basal ganglia, and white matter [42].

Clinical Manifestations and Diagnosis

CNS manifestations of neuro-Behçet syndrome can be categorized into two main categories: Parenchymal manifestations, including brainstem, hemispheric, and spinal cord characterized by meningo-encephalitis and non-parenchymal CNS manifestations, with the involvement of large veins or arteries. Parenchymal manifestations are more common than non-parenchymal manifestations. Both presentations were thought to rarely coexist but recent studies suggest that both parenchymal and non-parenchymal presentations may coexist in up to 20% of patients [43].

Parenchymal CNS involvement presents with hemispheric manifestations such as hemiplegia/paresis, encephalopathy, hemisensory loss, visual-field defects, seizure (in up to 2–2.5%), psychosis, parkinsonism, chorea, and ataxia [39, 40] that are the direct effect of parenchymal or white matter lesions. Signs of involvement in the brainstem include ophthalmoparesis, cranial neuropathies, and cerebellar or pyramidal dysfunction. Pseudobulbar affect as an eventual consequence that has also been described [44]. Recurrent facial palsies, palatal myoclonus, paroxysmal dysarthria, intranuclear ophthalmoplegia, and isolated hypoglossal nerve palsy have also been reported [39]. Spinal manifestations can be seen in up to 30% of patients and include sensory level dysfunction and commonly sphincter dysfunction, but are rare in isolation of other parenchymal findings [45]. Optic neuritis and ischemic optic neuropathy have also been observed yet are rare (0.4%). Non-parenchymal CNS involvement of neuro-Behçet syndrome is also known as Neurovasculo-Behçet disease and can present with venous or arterial manifestations. Intracranial hypertension is a common manifestation of dural sinus thrombosis and presents as headache, papilledema, focal neurological deficits, seizures, sixth nerve palsy, or altered mental status [46]. Current opinion suggests that dural sinus thrombi are the result of vascular inflammation leading to endothelial cell activation with elevated activated protein C receptors, homocysteine, and serum markers of vascular endothelial cell injury such as Von Willebrand's factor, antithrombin III, or tissue plasminogen activator [40].

Arterial involvement is rare but can present as stenosis and/or aneurysm formation as well as dissection. These, in turn, can cause intracerebral or subarachnoid hemorrhages or arterial infarcts and have been documented to involve the common carotid, internal carotid, middle cerebral, anterior cerebral, anterior communicating, and vertebral arteries [39]. PNS involvement in neuro-Behçet syndrome is rare and can present as sensorimotor polyneuropathy, mononeuritis multiplex, or autonomic neuropathy and can rarely present with a picture similar to Guillain–Barré syndrome. It can also manifest in the muscles where it can cause necrotizing myositis with associated pain, swelling, and tenderness [47].

The diagnosis of non-neurologic Behçet's disease requires recurrent oral ulceration (at least three times in a 12-month period) in addition to two other manifestations including genital ulceration, eye (anterior or posterior uveitis, or cells in vitreous on slit lamp examination or retinal vasculitis), or skin lesions (erythema nodosum, pseudofolliculitis or papulopustular lesions, or acneiform nodules in postadolescent patients not on corticosteroids) and is necessary before the diagnosis of neuro-Behçet syndrome can be made [48]. There are no validated diagnostic criteria for neuro-Behçet disease which likely accounts for the wide range of neurological involvement in Behçet's disease. Neurological involvement is a poor prognosticating factor and has been reported to almost double the mortality rate (about 10%) when compared with non-neurologic Behçet disease [49].

An elevated erythrocyte sedimentation rate (ESR) has been shown to correlate with disease activity. HLA-B51 has been reported to be present in 60–70% of Japanese and Turkish patients, but in only 10–20% of European patients [40].

Common CSF findings include pleocytosis (initially neutrophilic and then lymphocytic) and elevated protein levels with normal glucose. Given the propensity for dural sinus thrombosis, an opening pressure should also be checked. There are reports of increased intrathecal beta-2 microglobulin synthesis as well as a few published studies demonstrating an elevation in cytokines 2, 8, and 10 as well as increased concentrations of interleukin 12 and 17, but this data is difficult to extrapolate clinically [50, 51]. There are also reports of increased immunoglobulin indices and oligoclonal bands, but these tend to be present only during acute attacks [52, 53].

In acute stages, MRI lesions can appear iso- or hypointense in T-1-weighted images and hyperintense in T-2-weighted or fluid-attenuated inversion recovery (FLAIR) images with enhancement. Diffusion-weighted imaging (DWI) will demonstrate increased diffusion coefficient but will not restrict unlike an acute ischemic infarct. These lesions are initially single and unilateral but over repeated attacks become scattered. The most common sites of involvement are the mesodiencephalic junction, cerebellar peduncles, pons and medulla, basal ganglia and internal capsule, cerebral hemispheres, and optic nerves with no predilection for the periventricular areas. These lesions become smaller and lose their contrast-enhancing properties after the disease state enters remission. With recurrent attacks, brainstem atrophy can develop. This can be helpful in later stages of the disease, when widespread lesions are present and other disease processes such as multiple sclerosis form part of the differential diagnosis. Patients with spinal cord involvement show a single lesion on MRI similar to transverse myelitis, though it often extends over two to three segments with evidence of enhancement and surrounding edema. Neurovasculo-Behçet's must be diagnosed using other imaging techniques such as magnetic resonance angiography (MRA), magnetic resonance venography (MRV), CT angiography, or conventional angiography. Positron emission tomography (PET) and sequential positron emission tomography (SPECT) can also show areas of decreased oxygen consumption and cerebral hypoperfusion and may be more sensitive than MRI for detecting brain lesions [54].

Treatment

There have not been any reported studies of prospective, double-blind, placebo-controlled studies for the treatment of neurological complications of Behçet's disease. Chlorambucil, methotrexate, interferon alpha, thalidomide, and cyclophosphamide have been successfully used in multiple studies and case reports. More recently, proinflammatory inhibitory immune mediators such as antitumor necrosis factor alpha and mycophenolate mofetil have been used and recommended [55].

In a recent paper, selection of treatment regimens has been proposed to be tailored to specific presentations and prognosis, with daily azathioprine or weekly methotrexate and corticosteroids as first-line therapy.

Methylprednisolone 1 g IV daily for up to 7 days followed by prednisone 0.5–1 mg/kg/day has been suggested for acute attacks, with a very gradual taper of 0.5 mg/day/week and over 2–3 months to prevent relapses [39, 56]. In high-risk groups of neuro-Behçet's disease patients (those of younger age, with multiple recurrent events, and with multiple areas of involvement), intravenous pulse cyclophosphamide, and corticosteroids are recommended. Should these regimens fail, agents such as infliximab or etanercept can be considered, with interferon alpha and chlorambucil reserved as a last resort. Corticosteroids and anticoagulants are suggested for the treatment of dural sinus thrombosis, with or without immunosupressants [56, 57].

Whipple's Disease

Whipple's disease is a rare, relapsing, slowly progressive systemic illness. It is caused by a gram-positive bacillus, *Tropheryma whippeli*. The initial systemic manifestations typically include fever of unknown origin, weight loss, polyarthralgias, and chronic diarrhea. The CNS, lungs, heart, eyes, and skin may also be involved. Gastrointestinal complaints typically precede neurologic complaints by several years. The high frequency of gastrointestinal symptoms and detection of the organism in feces of infected patients and in sewage water has led to the suggestion that oral ingestion is the likely mode of infection.

Whipple's disease is a rare disease, with only approximately 1,000 case reports in the medical literature to date [58]. Men account for approximately 80% of reported cases. The mean age at diagnosis is 50 years, but ages range from 3 months to 81 years. Most of the case reports have been from Europe and North America.

The prevalence of neurologic manifestations in Whipple's disease is estimated to be between 6 and 43% [59]. Neurologic symptoms tend to appear later in the clinical course and are often associated with disease relapse. The disease course can be fulminant with death in as little as 1 month. Gross pathological features include generalized cerebral atrophy and small chalky nodules or granulomas, 1–2 mm in size, scattered throughout the gray matter of the cerebral and cerebellar cortex, the hippocampus, the hypothalamus, and periaqueductal gray matter. Microscopic features of the granulomas include PAS staining macrophages surrounded by reactive astrocytes. As disease becomes more widespread, PAS positive cells infiltrate the white matter and can be associated with neuron death, vacuole formation, and demyelination.

Clinical Manifestations and Diagnosis

The classic triad of neurologic manifestations (found in 10% of patients) in Whipple's disease includes cognitive change, ophthalmoplegia, and myoclonus. The most common neurologic manifestation of Whipple's disease are cognitive changes (71%) and eye movement abnormalities (50%). Two findings felt to be pathognomonic for Whipple's disease include oculomasticatory myorhythmia (OMM) and oculofacial skeletal myorhythmia (OFSM). Oculomasticatory myorhythmia involves slow (1-Hz), pendular, convergent and divergent nystagmus that is synchronized with involuntary rhythmic contractions of muscles of mastication. Oculofacial skeletal myorhythmia is similar but involves nystagmus associated with myorhythmia of other skeletal muscles. In both cases, the myorhythmia occurs throughout the day, persists in sleep, and is unchanged by environmental stimuli. Despite their high specificity for Whipple's disease, these findings typically only occur in about 20% of patients [58, 59].

Neuroimaging with either CT or MRI is often normal. The most common abnormality is cerebral atrophy. Other findings on MRI include mass lesions with or without contrast enhancement, ring enhancing lesions, solitary tumors, multiple punctuate lesions, and hydrocephalus. Lesions on MRI will often show improvement after treatment [60].

A tissue-based diagnosis is important and can be established in many ways. In patients with gastrointestinal symptoms, endoscopically guided small bowel biopsy is the initial method of choice. Polymerase chain reaction (PCR) can also be performed not only on small bowel tissue, but also on lymph nodes, pericardium, lung, liver, and muscle. CSF cytology can show histiocytes with PAS-positive granular or sickle-shaped particles in the cytoplasm. PCR can be used in analysis of CSF which has increased the sensitivity over cytology alone. If required brain biopsy can be performed looking for characteristic pathologic features of granulomas with PAS-positive foamy macrophages surrounded by large, reactive astrocytes.

A guideline has been proposed regarding diagnosis. A diagnosis of definite CNS-Whipple's disease involves any one of the following three criteria: OMM or OFSM, positive tissue biopsy, or positive PCR. If the tissue biopsy or PCR was not performed on CNS tissue, the patient must have neurologic signs to make the diagnosis, but if positive result was on CNS tissue neurologic signs are not required. A diagnosis of possible CNS-Whipple's disease includes one of four systemic symptoms (fever of unknown origin, GI symptoms, chronic migratory arthralgias or polyarthralgias, or unexplained lymphadenopathy, night sweats, or malaise) and one of four neurologic signs (supranuclear vertical gaze palsy, rhythmic myoclonus, dementia with psychiatric symptoms, or hypothalamic manifestations) [60].

Treatment

In general, a long-term antibiotic course of 1–2 years is recommended. Shorted courses of antibiotics have been associated with higher relapse rates, and neurologic manifestations occur more frequently in patients with relapsed disease. The best approach to antibiotics involves a combination of parenteral antibiotics at initiation of therapy for 2–4 weeks followed by long-term treatment with oral antibiotic over the next 1–2 years. Initiation of treatment is often achieved with ceftriaxone 2 g/day. Alternatives to this include penicillin and streptomycin. After the initial 2–4 week period, long-term maintenance is most often achieved with TMP-SMX 160/800 mg twice a day for at least 1 year. Alternatives include cefixime 400 mg/day. Treatment should be continued until CSF PCR becomes negative [59].

Celiac Disease

Celiac disease, also called gluten-sensitive enteropathy, has been characterized as a small bowel disorder with an underlying immune-mediated and genetic predisposition. The pathogenesis is not completely understood but involves immune system activation by the gliadin component of gluten in genetically predisposed individuals. The classic histologic findings of the proximal small intestine include mucosal inflammation, crypt hyperplasia, and villous atrophy [61]. With the advent of sensitive and specific serologic testing came an increased awareness of subtle disease manifestations. With this recognition, prevalence ratios also increased to 1:300 to 1:500 in Caucasians of northern European ancestry [62]. This has also led to a shifting trend toward more patients presenting as asymptomatic or oligosymptomatic adults [63].

Clinical Manifestations and Diagnosis

Neurological manifestations are thought to occur in 6–10% of patients with celiac disease, although discrepancies (reflecting observational bias) exist when examining primary neurological patients versus primary celiac disease cohorts. The most commonly attributed neurological presentation is cerebellar ataxia [61]. While causality remains controversial; it has been accepted that patients with ataxia of unknown cause should be screened for celiac disease [64]. While some patients have low vitamin E levels, others have normal vitamin levels and the neurological symptoms may be attributed to celiac disease mechanisms rather than malabsorption.

Additionally, peripheral neuropathy has been recognized as a common neurological manifestation of celiac disease. It is usually described as a chronic symmetric distal predominantly sensory polyneuropathy and electrophysiologic studies range from normal or mildly abnormal to that of a sensorimotor axonal peripheral neuropathy. Reports also list a pure motor neuropathy, mononeuritis multiplex, Guillain–Barré-like syndrome, and autonomic neuropathy [64].

Several studies have demonstrated an association between celiac disease and seizures, both with an increase prevalence of epilepsy in patients diagnosed with celiac disease and a higher prevalence of celiac disease in patients with epilepsy. A specific but rare syndrome of bilateral occipital cerebral calcifications and seizures has been associated with celiac disease [64].

Treatment

Treatment of celiac disease involves life-long adherence to a gluten-free diet and recognition and treatment of nutritional deficiencies.

References

1. Rahman A, Iseberg DA. Mechanisms of disease: systemic lupus erythematosus. N Engl J Med. 2008;358:929–39.
2. Tan EM, Cohen AS, Fries JF, et al. The 1982 revised criteria for the classification of systemic lupus erythematosus. Arthritis Rheum. 1982;25:1271–7.
3. James JA, Kaufman KM, Farris AD, Taylor-Albert E, Lehman TJ, Harley JB. An increased prevalence of Epstein-Barr virus infection in young patients suggests a possible etiology for systemic lupus erythematosus. J Clin Invest. 1997;100: 3019–26.
4. Isenberg DA, Shoenfeld Y, Walport M, et al. Detection of cross-reactive anti-DNA antibody idiotypes in the serum of systemic lupus erythematosus patients and of their relatives. Arthritis Rheum. 1985;28:999–1007.
5. Walport M. Complement and systemic lupus erythematosus. Arthritis Res. 2002; 4 Suppl 3:S279–93.

6. Houssiau FA, Lefebvre C, Vanden Berghe M, Lambert M, Devogelaer JP, Renauld JC. Serum interleukin 10 titers in systemic lupus erythematosus reflect disease activity. Lupus. 1995;3:393–5.

7. Hanly JG, Hong C, Smith S, et al. A prospective analysis of cognitive function and anticardiolipin antibody levels and cognitive functioning in systemic lupus erythematosus. Arthritis Rheum. 1999;42:728–34.

8. Menon S, Jameson-Shortall E, Newman SP, Hall-Craggs MR, et al. A longitudinal study of anticardiolipin antibody levels and cognitive functioning in systemic lupus erythematosus. Arthritis Rheum. 1999;42:735–41.

9. Omdal R, Brokstad K, Waterloo K, et al. Neuropsychiatric disturbances in SLE are associated with antibodies against NMDA receptors. Eur J Neurol. 2005;12: 392–8.

10. Harrison M, Ravdin L, Volpe B, et al. Anti-NR2 antibody does not identify cognitive impairment in a general SLE population. Arthritis Rheum. 2004;50:S596.

11. Hanly JG. Neuropsychiatric lupus. Curr Rheumatol Rep. 2001;3:205–12.

12. Belmont HM, Abramson SB, Lie JT. Pathology and pathogenesis of vascular injury in systemic lupus erythematosus. Interactions of inflammatory cells and activated endothelium. Arthritis Rheum. 1996;39:9–22.

13. Hanly JG, Walsh NN, Sangalang V. Brain pathology in systemic lupus erythematosus. J Rheumatol. 1992;19:732–41.

14. Muscal E, Brey RL. Neurologic manifestations of systemic lupus erythematosus in children and adults. Neurol Clin. 2009;28:61–73.

15. Hanly JG, Urowitz MB, Sanchez-Guerrero J, et al. Neuropsychiatric events at the time of diagnosis of systemic lupus erythematosus: an international inception cohort study. Arthritis Rheum. 2007;56:265–73.

16. Petri M. Thrombosis and systemic lupus erythematosus: the Hopkins Lupus Cohort perspective. Scand J Rheumatol. 1996;25:191–3.

17. Yoshio T, Hirata D, Onda K, et al. Antiribosomal P protein antibodies in cerebrospinal fluid are associated with neuropsychiatric systemic lupus erythematosus. J Rheumatol. 2005;32:34–9.

18. Barile-Fabris L, Ariza-Andraca R, Olguin-Ortega L, et al. Controlled clinical trial of IV cyclophosphamide versus IV methylprednisolone in severe neurological manifestations in systemic lupus erythematosus. Ann Rheum Dis. 2005;64:620–5.

19. Greenberg BM, Thomas KP, Krishnan C, et al. Idiopathic transverse myelitis: corticosteroids, plasma exchange or cyclophosphamide. Neurology. 2007;68:1614–7.

20. Ferreira S, D'Cruz DP, Hughes GR. Multiple sclerosis, neuropsychiatric lupus and antiphospholipid syndrome: where do we stand? Rheumatology (Oxford). 2005;68:434–42.

21. Mitsikostas DD, Sfikakis PP, Goadsby PJ. A meta-analysis for headache in systemic lupus erythematosus: the evidence and the myth. Brain. 2004;127:1200–9.

22. Ainiala H, Loukkola J, Peltola J, et al. The prevalence of neuropsychiatric syndromes in systemic lupus erythematosus. Neurology. 2001;57:496–500.

23. Borchers AT, Aoki CA, Naguwa SM, et al. Neuropsychiatric features of systemic lupus erythematosus. Autoimmun Rev. 2005;4:329–44.

24. Petri M, Brodsky R. High-dose cyclophosphamide and stem cell transplantation for refractory systemic lupus erythematosus. JAMA. 2006;295:559–60.

25. Crowther MA, Ginsberg JS, Julian J, et al. A Comparison of two intensities of warfarin for the prevention of recurrent thrombosis in patients with the antiphospholipid antibody syndrome. N Engl J Med. 2003;349:1133–8.

26. Newman LS, Rose CS, Meier LA. Sarcoidosis. N Engl J Med. 1997;336: 1224–34.

27. Joseph FG, Scolding NJ. Neurosarcoidosis: a study of 30 new cases. J Neurol Neurosurg Psychiatry. 2009;80:297–304.

28. Joseph FG, Scolding NJ. Sarcoidosis of the nervous system. Pract Neurol. 2007;7:234–44.

29. Nowak DA, Widenka DC. Neurosarcoidosis: a review of its intracranial manifestation. J Neurol. 2001;248:363–72.
30. Delaney P. Neurologic manifestations in sarcoidosis: review of the literature with a report of 23 cases. Ann Int Med. 1977;87:336–45.
31. Sharma OP. Neurosarcoidosis: a personal perspective based on the study of 37 patients. Chest. 1997;112:220–8.
32. Zajicek JP, Scolding SN, Foster O, et al. Central nervous system sarcoidosis – diagnosis and management. Q J Med. 1999;92:103–17.
33. Delande S, de Seze J, Fauchais AL, et al. Neurologic manifestations in primary Sjogren syndrome: A study of 82 patients. Medicine. 2004;83(5):336–45.
34. Govini M, Padovan M, Rizzo N, Trotta F. CNS involvement in primary Sjogren's syndrome: prevalence, clinical aspects, diagnostic assessment and therapeutic approach. CNS Drugs. 2001;15(8):597–607.
35. Mellgren SI, Conn DL, Stevens JC, Dyck PJ. Peripheral neuropathy in primary Sjogren's syndrome. Neurology. 1989;39:390–4.
36. Chai J, Herrmann D, Stanton M, Barbano RL, Logigian EL. Painful small-fiber neuropathy in Sjogren syndrome. Neurology. 2005;65:925–7.
37. Reske D, Petereit HF, Heiss WD. Difficulties in the differentiation of chronic inflammatory diseases of the central nervous system – value of cerebrospinal fluid analysis and immunological abnormalities in the diagnosis. Acta Neurol. 2005;112:207–13.
38. Behçet H. Über rezidivierende, aphthöse, durch ein Virus verursachte Geschwüre am Mund, am Auge und an den Genitalien. Dermatol Wochr. 1937;105:1152–7.
39. Borhani Haghighi A, Pourmand R, Nikseresht AR. Neuro-Behçet disease – a review. Neurologist. 2005;11:80–9.
40. Al-Araji A, Kidd DP. Neuro-Behçet's disease: epidemiology, clinical characteristics and management. Lancet Neurol. 2009;8:192–204.
41. Akman-Demir G, Serdaroglu P, Tasci B, the Neuro-Behçet Study Group. Clinical patterns of neurological involvement in Behçet's disease: evaluation of 200 patients. Brain. 1999;170:105–11.
42. Borhani Haghighi A, Sharifzad HR, Matin S, Rezaee S. The pathological presentations of Neuro-Behçet's disease: a case report and review of the literature. Neurologist. 2007;13:209–14.
43. Houman MH, Neffati H, Braham A, et al. Behçet's disease in Tunisia. Demographic, clinical and genetic aspects in 260 patients. Clin Exp Rheumatol. 2007;25: S58–64.
44. Ashjazadeh N, Borhani Haghighi A, Samangooei Sh, et al. Neuro-Behçet's Disease: a masquerader of multiple sclerosis. Exp Mol Pathol. 2003;73:17–22.
45. Shakir RA, Sulaiman K, Lahn RA, et al. Neurological presentation of neuro-Behçet syndrome: clinical categories. Eur J Neurol. 1990;30:249–53.
46. Wechesler B, Vidailhet M, Piette JC, et al. Cerebral venous thrombosis in Behçet's disease: clinical study and long-term follow-up of 25 cases. Neurology. 1992;42:614–8.
47. Worthmann F, Bruns J, Turker T, et al. Muscular involvement in Behçet's disease: case report and review of the literature. Neuromuscul Disord. 1996;6:247–53.
48. International Study Group for Behçet's Disease. Criteria for diagnosis of Behçet disease. Lancet. 1990;335:1078–80.
49. Yazici H, Basaran G, Hamuryudan V, et al. The ten-year mortality in Behçet's syndrome a report of 24 cases. Br J Rheumatol. 1996;35:139–41.
50. Kawai M, Hirohata S. Cerebrospinal fluid beta-2 microglobulin in neuro-Behçet's syndrome. Folia Psychiatr Neurol Jpn. 1984;38:65–79.
51. Saruhan-Direskeneli G, Yentür SP, Akman-Demir G, Isik N, Serdaroglu P. Cytokines and chemokines in neuro-Behçet's disease compared to multiple sclerosis and other neurological diseases. J Neuroimmunol. 2003;145:127–34.

52. Sharief MB, Hentges R, Thomas E. Significance of CSF immunoglobulins in monitoring neurologic disease activity in Behçet's disease. Neurology. 1991;41: 1398–401.

53. Jongen PJ, Daelmans HE, Bruneel B, et al. Humoral and cellular immunologic study of cerebrospinal fluid in a patient with Behçet encephalitis. Arch Neurol. 1992;49:1075–8.

54. Kao CH, Lan JL, ChangLai SP, et al. Technetium-99m-HMPAO SPECT and MRI of brain in patients with neuro-Behçet's syndrome. J Nucl Med. 1998;39: 1707–10.

55. Hatemi G, Silman A, Bang D, et al. EULAR recommendations for the management of Behçet's disease: report of a task force of the European Standing Committee for International Clinical Studies Including Therapeutics (ESCISIT). Ann Rheum Dis. 2008;67:1656–62.

56. Borhani Haghighi A, Safari A. Proposing an algorithm for treatment of different manifestations of neuro-Behçet's disease. Clin Rheumatol. 2010;29:683–6.

57. Bank I, Weart C. Dural sinus thrombosis in Behçet's disease. Arthritis Rheum. 1984;27:816–8.

58. Anderson M. Neurology of Whipple's disease. J Neurol Neurosurg Psychiatry. 2000;68:2–5.

59. Lugassy MM, Louis ED. Neurologic manifestations of Whipple's disease. Curr Infect Dis Rep. 2006;8:301–6.

60. Louis ED, Lynch T, Kauffman P, Fahn S, Odel J. Diagnostic guidelines in central nervous system Whipple's disease. Ann Neurol. 1996;40:561–8.

61. Burk K, Farecki ML, Lamprecht G, Roth G, Decker P, Weller M, et al. Neurological symptoms in patients with biopsy proven celiac disease. Mov Disord. 2009;24:2358–62.

62. Fasano A. Where have all the American celiacs gone? Acta Paediatr Suppl. 1996;412:20–4.

63. Rampertab SD, Pooran N, Brar P, Singh P, Green PH. Trends in the presentation of celiac disease. Am J Med. 2006;119:355.

64. Bushara KO. Neurologic presentation of celiac disease. Gastroenterology. 2005;128:S92–7.

Index

A

"Acute black holes", 114
Acute disseminated encephalomyelitis (ADEM)
   clinical features, 204–205
   description, 203
   diagnosis
      adults, 206
      contrast enhancement, 207
      CSF, 207–208
      differential, 208
      MRI techniques, 207
      neuroimaging, 206–207
      pediatric, 205–206
   encephalitis lethargica, 297
   etiology
      CNS, 212
      cytokines, 213
      IgG antibodies, 212
      leucocyte antigen, 213
   management, 209
   pathology, 203–204
   pediatrics
      brain, 162
      CNS, 162
      demyelinating process, 161
      distinction, 162–163
      vs. MS, 161, 162
      multifocal lesions, 162
      pathological process, 161–162
      viral illness, 162
   prognosis, 209
   spectrum overlap disorders
      acute necrotizing encephalopathy, 210–211
      AHLE, 210
      Bickerstaff brainstem, 211
      CNS disorders, 209–210
      MS, 211–212

   streptococcal infections, 294
   triggering events, 203, 204
Acute hemorrhagic leukoencephalitis (AHLE)
   description, 210
   management, 210
   necrotizing encephalopathy, 211
Acute inflammatory demyelinating polyneuropathy
      (AIDP)
   vs. CIDP, 355
   electrodiagnostic studies, 350
   immune pathogenesis, GBS, 352–353
AD. *See* Alzheimer's disease
ADEM. *See* Acute disseminated encephalomyelitis
AHLE. *See* Acute hemorrhagic leukoencephalitis (AHLE)
AIDP. *See* Acute inflammatory demyelinating polyneuropathy
Alemtuzumab, 143
Alzheimer's disease (AD)
   amyloid hypothesis, 276–277
   description, 275
   immunization
      active, 277
      passive, 277–278
   immunotherapeutic approach, 278
   immunotherapy, 276
   inflammation, 276
Angioplasty
   central venous stenosis, 184
   focal jugular stenosis, 183
   stent placement, 184
   venous pressures reduction, 184
Antibodies
   anti-EBV, 376
   anti-phospholipid antibodies (aPL), 377
   autoantibodies, 376
Anticoagulation
   chronic anticoagulation therapy, SLE, 378
   dural sinus thrombosis, 384

From: *Clinical Neuroimmunology: Multiple Sclerosis and Related Disorders*, Current Clinical Neurology,
Edited by: S.A. Rizvi and P.K. Coyle, DOI 10.1007/978-1-60327-860-7,
© Springer Science+Business Media, LLC 2011

Anti-glial nuclear antibody (AGNA), 245
Approved agents
    fingolimod, 134–135
    GA, 132
    interferons (IFN), 131–132
    mitoxantrone binds, 135
    natalizumab and PML, 133–134
Aquaporin–4
    anti-aquaporin–4, 226
    brain lesions, 224
    MS and neuromyelitis optica, 226
    NMO-IgG
        discovery, 226
        target, 220
Area postrema, lesions, 221, 226
Arteritis
    giant cell, 316
    systemic necrotizing
        Churg–Strauss syndrome, 311
        HSV, 311
        KD, 308–310
        MPA, 311
        PAN, 307–308
    temporal and Takayasu, 316–317
Arthralgia
    hypocomplementemic vasculitis, 313
    immunomodulating therapy, 327
    serum sickness and Henoch–Schönlein purpura, 312
Astrocytes
    activation, 10
    CNS
        inflammation, 7
        innate immune responses, 4
        repair mechanisms, 8
    description, 7
    MMP–2, 10
    role, 7, 8
Ataxia
    autoimmune, 299
    cerebellar, 295
Autoantibody signatures, 193
Autoimmune movement disorders
    antibodies
        anti-basal ganglia Abs (ABGA), 299, 301
        non-paraneoplastic movement disorders, 301
        paraneoplastic movement disorders, 300
    ataxia, 299
    classification
        etiologies, 292
        immunological mechanisms, 291
        phenomenology, 292
    encephalitis lethargica
        H1N1 influenza, 297
        Parkinsonism, 296–297
        symptoms, 296
        treatment, 297
    neuromyotonia, 296
    non-post-streptococcal, 295
    PANDAS
        diagnostic criteria, 293
        tic disorders and streptococcal infections, 294

    treatment, 294
    paraneoplastic syndromes, 298
    Parkinsonism, 299
    post-streptococcal
        ADEM, 294
        neuropsychiatric, 292
    progressive encephalomyelitis and rigidity, 295–296
    stiff-person syndrome, 295
    Sydenham's chorea
        anti-streptococcal antibodies, 293
        characteristics, 293
        rheumatic fever, 292–293
    systemic inflammatory conditions
        APS, 297
        systemic lupus erythematosus (SLE), 298
    tic disorders, 298
Autoimmune neuropathies
    CIDP
        clinical features, 355
        immune pathogenesis, 356
        laboratory studies, 355–356
        treatment, 356–358
        variants, 358–361
    GBS
        Campylobacter jejeuni and molecular mimicry, 353
        clinical features, 350
        immune pathogenesis, 352–353
        laboratory investigations, 350–351
        pathologic and nerve conduction, 349–350
        protein elevation, acellular CSF, 349
        treatment, 354
        variants, 351–352
    monoclonal gammopathy
        idiopathic polyneuropathies, 361–362
        malignant gammopathies, 362
        MGUS, 362–364
        vasculitic neuropathy, 364
Autoimmunity
    adaptive immune activation, 16–17
    central and peripheral tolerance, 15
    clinical outcome, 16
    damage cells and tissue, 15
    disorders, 16
    environmental variables and infection, 15–16
    homeostatic balance, 16
    relapsing–remitting course, 16
Azathioprine, 139

B
Bacterial infections, CNS
    meningitis, 255–258
    neuroborreliosis, 258–259
    syphilis, 259–260
BBB. See Blood–brain barrier
B-cell-activating factor (BAFF-R) receptor, 23
B cells
    autoantibodies, 23
    B lymphocytes, 24
    cytokine production, 25
    depletion and chemoablative techniques, 25

development, 22
disorders, 24
follicular dendritic cells (FDCs), 26
formation, 26
functions, 24
immature, 22
lymphocytes, 21
lymphoid structures, 24, 26
lymphotoxins and TNFα, 26
maturation and humoral immune response, 21–22
memory, 25
MS, 54–55
naïve B cells, 25
neutrophils, 22–23
receptors
    BAFF-R, 23
    TNF-R/TNF, 22–23
    toll-like receptors (TLR), 23
regulation, 25
T-cell, divergence, 23
therapy targets, 26
T lymphocyte, 25
Behçet's disease
characteristics, 322
clinical manifestations and diagnosis
    arterial involvement, 382
    DWI, 383
    erythrocyte sedimentation rate (ESR), 383
    MRI lesion, 383
    non-neurologic form, 382
    parenchymal CNS involvement, 382
course, 381
description, 381
neurologic involvement, 381
treatment, 383–384
Biomarkers
future development, 192
immune, 193–194
MRI
    cellular imaging, 193
    double inversion-recovery imaging, 193
    drug development, 192
    gray matter atrophy, 192
    spinal cord dysfunction, 193
Blood–brain barrier (BBB)
leukocyte transmigration, 26, 27
vascular system, 60
Blood vessel
infiltration, 322
vasculitis, 307
Brain abscess
bacterial infections, 256
rupture, 269

C
Cancer neuroimmunology
active immunotherapy
    active-specific, 239–240
    nonspecific, 239
description, 233–234
glioma, 234–237
immune surveillance, 233
paraneoplastic neurologic syndromes
    cerebellar degeneration, 243–244
    encephalomyelitis, 244–245
    Lambert–Eaton myasthenic syndrome, 245
    opsoclonus/myoclonus, 245
    treatment, 246
paraneoplastic syndromes
    CNS, 241–242
    humoral-mediated, 242
    T-cell-mediated, 243
passive immunotherapy
    adoptive transfer, 238–239
    antibody, 238
treatment, 246
Celiac disease
clinical manifestations and diagnosis, 386
pathogenesis, 385–386
treatment, 386
Central nervous system (CNS)
ADEM, 203
APCs, 239
cells and components
    astrocytes, 7–8, 59
    BBB and vascular system, 60
    endothelial cells, 9
    excitotoxins, 60
    microglia, 6–7, 57
    mitochondria, 61
    neuotrophic factors, 61
    neurons/axons, 9, 59–60
    nitric oxide (NO), 60–61
    oligodendrocytes, 8–9
    oligodendrocytes and myelination, 57–58
disorders, 209–210
EAE, 51–52
infections
    bacterial, 255–260
    description, 255
    fungal and parasitic, 265–271
    viral, 260–265
MHC-I expression, 236
MS, 211
paraneoplastic syndromes, 241–242
repair and regeneration, 57
stem cells, 34
tissue damage, 53
transient infection, 212
Cerebral blood flow (CBF), 180, 181
Cerebral blood volume (CBV), 180
Cerebrospinal fluid (CSF)
barriers, 3
chemokines, 213
cytoalbuminologic dissociation, 211
evaluation, 205
MS, 211
pleocytosis, 210
Chemokines
activation
    immune, 17
    integrins, 27

Chemokines (*cont.*)
  autoimmune disorders, 29
  BBB transmigration, 28
  cytokines function, 32
  dendritic cells and maturation, 31
  leukocyte
    rolling, 27, 28
    transmigration, 27
Chorea
  ABGA, 299
  Sydenham's chorea, 292–293
  transient, 298
Chronic cerebrospinal venous insufficiency (CCSVI)
  angioplasty, RRMS, 183
  autoimmune and inflammatory, 182, 184
  extracranial venous stenosis, 182
  jugular vein, high-grade stenosis, 183
  parameters and abnormal ultrasound, 181
  PTA, 184
  sonographer scan, 182
  TCD techniques, 181
  venography, 181–182
  venous pressures reduction, 184
Chronic inflammatory demyelinating polyradiculoneu-
      ropathy (CIDP)
  clinical features, 355
  immune pathogenesis, 356
  laboratory studies, 355–356
  treatment
    corticosteroids, 356
    cyclophosphamide/cyclosporine, 358
    IVIG therapy *vs.* corticosteroids, 357–358
    plasma exchange, 356–357
  variants
    DADS neuropathy, 359
    MADSAM, 358
    MMN, 359–361
    pure sensory, 358–359
CIDP. *See* Chronic inflammatory demyelinating polyra-
      diculoneuropathy
CIS. *See* Clinically isolated syndrome
Cladribine, 144
Clinically isolated syndrome (CIS)
  CDMS, 90
  cortical lesions, 116
  disease-modifying therapies (DMT), 101
  MS, 101, 181
  treatment, 136
CNS. *See* Central nervous system
CNS vasculitis
  classification
    collagen vascular diseases, 318–322
    HSV, 311–314
    infection-associated, 322–323
    substance abuse, 323–324
    systemic granulomatous, 314–318
    systemic necrotizing arteritis, 307–311
  laboratory diagnosis
    brain and meningeal biopsy, 326

    electrodiagnostic studies, 324–325
    principles, 324
    radiographic features, cerebral vasculitis, 325
  treatment
    immunomodulating therapy, 327
    immunosuppressant therapy, 326–327
    supportive therapy, 328
Cognition, 170
Collagen vascular diseases
  Behçet disease, 322
  mixed connective tissue, 322
  rheumatoid arthritis, 321
  scleroderma
    necrotizing vasculitis, 320
    progressive systemic sclerosis, 320, 321
    vascular lesions, 318, 320
  Sjögren syndrome, 321
  SLE, 309, 318
Collapsin response-mediator brain protein (CRMP), 244
Combination antiretroviral therapy (CART), 264–265
Conventional MRI technique
  advanced sequences and contrast agents
    3D FLAIR, 116
    DIR, 116–117
  axial T1-WI postcontrast scans, 112
  brain atrophy
    BV loss, 119–120
    CNS, WM and GM atrophy, 120
  CNS, 114–115
  demyelinated lesions, 112–113
  DWI and DTI, 122–123
  functional MRI
    brain function, 123
    neuronal tissue, 123–124
  Gd-enhancing lesion, 112
  high field strength
    diagnosis, 118
    type III cortical lesions, 118–119
  high-resolution microautoradiography, 117–118
  hyperintense lesions, 115
  limitation, 112
  MRS, 122, 123
  MTI
    MTR, 121
    NAWM, 121–122
    TFCE, 122
  neuronal damage and repair, 119
  neuroprotective immunity/remyelination, 115
  remyelinated lesions, 113–114
  spinal cord lesion, 114
  T2 lesion, 115
  T1-WI/T2-WI, 114
  voxel-wise techniques, 115
  white matter lesions, 113
Corticosteroids, 139
CRMP. *See* Collapsin response-mediator brain protein
CSF. *See* Cerebrospinal fluid
Curing multiple sclerosis
  definitions, 196

immunotherapy, 197
    repairing damaged nervous system, 197–198
Cyclophosphamide, 139
Cytokines
    astrocytes, 7
    immunologic factors, 10
    immunotherapy
        autoimmune process, 31–32
        endogenous T1IFN, 33
        function, 32
        interferon (IFN), 33
        interleukins, 32
        receptors, 32–33
    proinflammatory, 6, 7, 9
    TNFα, 9, 10
Cytotoxic neurodegeneration, 195, 198

D
Daclizumab, 143–144
Dementia
    AD (*see* Alzheimer's disease)
    rapidly progressive dementia (RPD), 281
Demographic differences, 157–158
Demyelination
    axons, 49
    cortical, 48, 54
    gray matter, 48
Dendritic cells, 55
Dermatomyositis (DM)
    clinical description, 341
    diagnosis
        creatine kinase and electromyography, 341
        inflammatory cells, 342
        "perifasicular atrophy", 341, 342
    pathophysiology, 342–343
    treatment, 343
Disability
    depression, 95
    EDSS, 89
    progression, 133
    scores, 354
Disease modifying agents and treatment
    approved agents
        fingolimod, 134–135
        GA, 132
        interferons (IFN), 131–132
        mitoxantrone binds, 135
        natalizumab and PML, 133–134
    beneficial effect, 131
    clinically isolated syndrome, 136
    drugs
        efficacy, side effects and compliance, 140
        emerging diseases and modifying agents, 142
        evidence-based data, 140
        putative targets and modalities, 140
    GA and IFN, 137
    MCA
        alemtuzumab, B-cell lymphoma, 143
        daclizumab, binds CD25, 143–144

responses, 141
    rituximab, non-Hodgkin's lymphoma, 141, 143
    multiple disease-modifying agents, 146
    off-label agents, 139–140
    oral agents, 144–145
    radiologically isolated syndrome (RIS), 135
    reducing relapses and MRI activity, 131
    SPMS, 138
    therapeutic efficacy and safety, 146
    worse RRMS, 137–138
Disease modifying therapy (DMT)
    cognitive ability, 160
    pediatric
        efficacy, 166
        glatiramer acetate (GA) dosing, 168–169
        IFN β–1a intramuscular (IM) injection, 167
        IFN β–1a subcutaneous (SC) injection, 167–168
        IFN β–1b, 168
        natalizumab, 169
Distal acquired demyelinating symmetric (DADS)
        neuropathy, 359
Double-inversion recovery (DIR), 116–117
Drug development
    efficacy, side effects and compliance, 140
    emerging diseases and modifying agents, 142
    evidence-based data, 140
    putative targets and modalities, 140

E
EAE. *See* Experimental autoimmune encephalomyelitis
Electromyography (EMG)
    myopathic features, 341, 343
    single fiber, 335, 337
Encephalitis
    clinical features, 260
    diagnosis, 260–261
    immune response, 261
    WNV, 262
Endothelial progenitor cells (EPCs), 33
Epilepsy and encephalopathies
    antibody-associated syndromes, 284
    GAD, 283–284
    Hashimoto encephalopathy
        description, 280
        treatment and diagnosis, 281
    limbic encephalitis, 281–282
    NMDA, 283
    Rasmussen's encephalitis
        description, 279
        GluR3, 279–280
        treatment and management, 280
    seizures, 279
    systemic disease and seizures, 284–285
    VGKC, 283
Epstein–Barr virus (EBV)
    HLA DRB1, 76
    pathogen, 73
Experimental autoimmune encephalomyelitis
        (EAE), 51–52

F

Fatigue
    low T2 lesion load, 94–95
    MS-related, 170
    pharmacologic intervention, 95
    scale, 160
    therapies, 170
Follicular dendritic cells (FDCs), 26
Fungal and parasitic infections, CNS
    clinical features
        aspergillosis and mucormycosis, 269
        cerebral malaria, 270
        cryptococcal meningitis, 266
        neurocystercosis, 270
        PAM, 269
        Toxoplasma gondii, 270
        yeasts/molds, 266
    diagnosis, 270–271
    injury mechanism
        disease and pathogens, 267–268
        pathogens and immune dysfunction, 266
        skin, 265
    routes, 265
    treatment, 271

G

GAD. *See* Glutamic acid decarboxylase
GANS. *See* Granulomatous angiitis of the nervous
        system
GBS. *See* Guillain–Barre syndrome
Genetics
    cystic fibrosis and sickle cell anemia, 77
    histocompatibility complex, 77–78
    inflammatory/autoimmune diseases, 81, 82
    influence, MS, 80
    mapping and risk alleles
        GWAS, 78–79
        linkage approach, 78
Genome-wide association scan (GWAS)
    IMSGC, 77
    performance, 77
    SNP, 79
    use, 78
Glatiramer acetate (GA), 132
Glioma
    classification, 234–235
    immune defects
        MHC-I expression, 236
        T-cells, 237
        TGF-β and IL–10, 236
    immune therapy, 237
    molecular immunobiology, 235
Glutamic acid decarboxylase (GAD) antibodies,
        283–284
Gluten-sensitive enteropathy. *See* Celiac disease
GM. *See* Gray matter
G-protein-coupled receptor (GPCR), 17
Granuloma
    brain biopsy, 385
    focal granulomatous mass lesions, 379

    microscopic features, 384
    non-caseating, 378, 379
Granulomatous angiitis of the nervous system (GANS)
    CNS vasculitis and MRI, 318, 319
    postmortem examination, 317
Gray matter (GM)
    atrophy, 120
    demyelination, MS, 119
    3D-T1 image, tissue segmentation, 120
    lesions, 117–119
    MRI
        conventional, 114
        single-slab 3D, 117
    superior delineation, 116, 117
    tissue damage, 111
Guillain–Barre syndrome (GBS)
    Campylobacter jejeuni and molecular mimicry, 353
    clinical features, 350
    immune pathogenesis
        antiganglioside antibodies, 352–353
        Miller Fisher variant, 353
    laboratory investigations
        CSF protein level, 350
        myelin lamellae, 350–351
    pathologic and nerve conduction, 349–350
    protein elevation, acellular CSF, 349
    treatment, 354
    variants
        axonal, 351, 352
        Miller Fisher, 351–352

H

HAART. *See* Highly active antiretroviral therapy
Haplotype
    HLA-DRB1*1501, 76, 77, 80
    MHC/HLA, 15
Hematopoietic stem cell transplantation (HSCT), 33–34
Herpes simplex virus (HSV), 261–262
Heterogeneity, MS
    benign *vs.* early relapsing remitting, 192
    clinical and pathologic, 191
    disease susceptibility, 192
    syndrome, 191
    Th1 type MS *vs.* Th17 type, 191–192
Highly active antiretroviral therapy (HAART), 263–264
HIV. *See* Human immunodeficiency virus
HPA. *See* Hypothalamic-pituitary-adrenal gland
HSV. *See* Herpes simplex virus; Hypersensitivity vas-
        culitis
Human immunodeficiency virus (HIV)
    CART, 264–265
    description, 264
    encephalomyelitis, 163
    neurosyphilis, 260
    serologic test, 261
Human leukocyte antigen (HLA), 77
Hyper reflexia, 90, 92
Hypersensitivity vasculitis (HSV)
    arteriole, 311, 312
    cryoglobulinemia

classification, 313
  clinical features, 313–314
drug-related, 311–312
Henoch–Schönlein purpura, 312–313
hypocomplementemic/urticarial, 313
serum sickness, 312
Hypothalamic-pituitary-adrenal gland (HPA) axis, 11

I
IBM. *See* Inclusion body myositis
Idiopathic thrombocytopenic purpura (ITP), 169
Immune biomarkers, 193–194
Immune mediated
celiac disease, 385–386
inflammation, neurosarcoidosis, 378
pathogenesis, 375
proinflammatory inhibitory, 383
Immune system
cells
  B cells, 54–55
  dendritic, 55
  mast, 56
  monocytes/macrophages, 55
  natural killer (NK), 55–56
  plasma, 55
  T cells, 53–54
factors
  adhesion molecules, 57
  chemokines, 56
  cytokines, 56
  matrix metalloproteinases, 57
  osteopontin, 56
Immunity, CNS
dendritic cells, 4
microglia and astrocytes, 4
surveillance, 5
T cells, 5
Immunologic disorders, NMJ and muscle
autoimmune disorders, 333
DM (*see* Dermatomyositis)
eosinophilic myositis, 344–345
fascioscapulo-humeral muscular dystrophy (FSHD), 345
IBM, 343–344
LEMS (*see* Lambert–Eaton myasthenic syndrome)
myasthenia gravis, 334–336
noncaseating granulomas, 345
polymyositis, 338–341
sarcoidosis, 345, 346
Immunology, 51. *See also* Cancer neuroimmunology
Immunotherapy
active and passive, 277
AD, 276
amyloid pathology, AD, 278
autoimmunity, 15–17
B cells (*see* B cells)
clinical research, 35
cytokines (*see* Cytokines)
dendritic cells, maturation and subtypes, 30–31
halting disease activity and progression, 197

homeostasis and tolerance, 35
NK cells, 20–21
NKT cells, 21
S1P1, 29–30
stem cells
  embryonic cells, 33
  genomic integrity, 33
  HSCT and EPCs, 33–34
  MSCs and CNS, 34
  niche, 33
  populations, 33
  remyelination, 34–35
  therapeutic plasticity, 35
subtypes, DCs, 31
T cells
  cell polarization, 17–18
  control, 19–20
  definition, 18
  immunoglobulin (Ig) production, 18
  mutations, 19
  naive CD4+ lineage, 17, 18
  production and signature, 17
  subpopulation, lymphocytes, 18–19
  T_{reg} cell functions, 19
trafficking molecules
  BBB transmigration, 28
  chemokines, 28–29
  CNS, 26
  description, BBB, 26–27
  glia limitans, 29
  G-protein, 27
  integrins, 27
  interendothelial tight junctions, 28
  leukocyte transmigration, 27
  MMPs, 29
  TIMP control, 29
Inclusion body myositis (IBM)
description and diagnosis, 343
pathophysiology, 343–344
treatment, 344
Infection-associated vasculitis
bacterial meningitis, 322
HIV-1, 323
Treponema pallidum and *Borrelia burgdorferi*, 322
varicella zoster virus, 322
Inflammation
astrocytes, 7–8
CNS, 7
TLR, 10
Initial demyelinating event (IDE)
encephalopathy, 159
features, 158
self-limited disorder, 158
Innate immune system
described, 195, 196
pattern recognition receptors, 265
TLR, 10
Intravenous immunoglobulin (IVIG)
Bickerstaff brainstem encephalitis, 211
immunomodulating therapy, 327

Intravenous immunoglobulin (IVIG) (*cont.*)
    myasthenic patients, 336
    passive immunization, 278
    plasmapheresis, 140
    steroid resistant patients, 209
    treatment
        CIDP, 357–358
        GBS, 354
        MMN, 361
IVIG. *See* Intravenous immunoglobulin

K
Kawasaki disease (KD)
    diagnosis, 308–309
    SPECT and IVIG, 309–310
    stages, postmortem cases, 309
KD. *See* Kawasaki disease

L
Lambert–Eaton myasthenic syndrome (LEMS)
    clinical description
        paraneoplastic, 337
        symmetric weakness and fatigue, 336
    diagnosis, 337
    MG, 242
    pathophysiology, 337–338
    remissions, 246
    SCLC, 242, 245
    symptoms, 245
    treatment, 246, 338
Laquinamod
    derive roquinimex, 144
    fumaric acid, 145
    initial testing, 144–145
    neuroprotection, 145–146
    PPMS treatment, 146
    stem cell transplantation, 145
LEMS. *See* Lambert–Eaton myasthenic syndrome
Lesions
    MRI
        detect cortical, 193
        gadolinium enhancing, 192
    MS project, 48–49
    type III cortical, 118–119
LETM. *See* Longitudinally extensive transverse myelitis
Leukodystrophies, 164
Leukoencephalitis. *See* Acute hemorrhagic leukoen-
        cephalitis (AHLE)
Limbic encephalitis
    description, 281
    Hashimoto's encephalopathy, 282
    reversible, 242
    VGKC, 283
Longitudinally extensive transverse myelitis (LETM)
    lesion, spinal cord, 221
    NMO-IgG seropositivity, 224
Lymphocytes
    adoptive transfer, 238–239
    clonal expansion, 236
    fingolimod, 134

immunotherapy
    autoimmune diseases, 15–16
    B cells, 21
    B lymphocytes, 24
    CD4+, thymus, 18
    CSF across, 27
    dendritic cells, 30–31, 32
    interactions, 26
    interferon, 33
    matrix metalloproteinases, 29
    maturation, 22
    migration, 29
    NK cells, 20
    NKT cells, 21
    regulation, 16
    self-reactive, 34
    S1P1, 29
    stem cells, 33
    subpopulation, 18
    tissue destruction, 26

M
MADSAM. *See* Multifocal acquired demyelinating
        sensory and motor neuropathy
Magnetic resonance imaging (MRI). *See also* Biomark-
        ers; Conventional MRI technique
    brain and spinal cord, 206–207
    functional, 123–124
    high field strength, 118–119
    MTI, 111
    spin-echo T2-weighted imaging, 111
Magnetization transfer imaging (MTI)
    histopathologic analysis, 121–122
    MS lesions evolution, 111
    MTR, 121
    TFCE, 122
Magnetization transfer ratio (MTR), 121–122
Mast cells, 56
Matrix metalloproteinases (MMPs), 10, 28, 29
Meningitis
    brain injury mechanisms
        bacterial components, 257
        CNS invasion, 256
        immune system role, 257
        inflammation and neurology, 257–258
    clinical features, 256
    description, 255–256
    treatment, 256
Mesenchymal stem/stromal cells (MSCs), 33
Methotrexate, 140
MGUS. *See* Monoclonal gammopathy of undertermined
        significance
Microglia
    activated products, 7
    activation, 45, 46
    astrocytes, 4
    CNS cells and components, 57
    description, 6
    MMP, 10
    products, 7

role, 7
T cell, 9
TLRs, 10
Microscopic polyangiitis (MPA), 311
Mitochondrial disorders, 164
MMN. *See* Multifocal motor neuropathy
MMPs. *See* Matrix metalloproteinases
Monoclonal antibodies (MCA)
 alemtuzumab, B-cell lymphoma, 143
 daclizumab, binds CD25, 143–144
 responses, 141
 rituximab, non-Hodgkin's lymphoma, 141, 143
Monoclonal gammopathy of undertermined significance
  (MGUS)
 anti MAG neuropathy, 363
 characteristics, 362–363
 IgM and IgA, 363–364
Motor problems, 172
MPA. *See* Microscopic polyangiitis
MS. *See* Multiple sclerosis
MS hug, 98
MTR. *See* Magnetization transfer ratio
Multifactorial, 375
Multifocal acquired demyelinating sensory and motor
  neuropathy (MADSAM), 358
Multifocal motor neuropathy (MMN)
 clinical features, 359
 immune pathogenesis and treatment, 361
 laboratory studies
  conduction block, 359–360
  ulnar nerve block, 360
Multiple sclerosis (MS)
 CNS cells and components, 57–61
 curing
  definitions, 196
  immunotherapy, halting disease activity, 197
  meaning and goal, 196
  nervous system damage, 197–198
  prevention, 198
 description, 71
 diagnosis, 98–106
 diet, neuro-endocrine and factors, 75
 distribution
  human populations, 71
  migration, 72
 environmental and genetic risk
  HLA DRB1*1501, 76
  vitamin D, 76–77
 etiologic factors, 43
 genetics, 77–81
 immune system
  cells, 53–56
  factors, 56–57
 immunology
  animal models, 51–52
  inside-out hypothesis, 53
  outside-in hypothesis, 52
  systemic autoreactive CD4+ T cells, 51
  vascular disorder, 53
 infectious agents

 EBV, 73–74
 virus, 73
 MRI (*see* Magnetic resonance imaging)
 pathology
  autopsy specimens, 46–47
  axon, 49–50
  Balo concentric and myelinoclastic diffuse sclerosis,
   50–51
  cortical/gray matter, 50
  focal inflammation and neurodegeneration, 43–44
  lesion project, 48–49
  macroscopic injury, 45
  microscopic injury, 45
  plaque, 45–46
  progressive, 47–48
  remyelination, 49
  tumefactive and marburg variants, 50
 smoking, 74–75
 sunlight and vitamin D
  environmental agents, 72–73
  latitude rule, 73
 symptoms
  signs and, 90–94
  subjective/ "invisible", 94–98
 vitamin D, 61
Multiple sclerosis, next 20 years
 biomarkers development
  autoantibody immune signatures, 194
  immune measures, 193–194
  MRI, 192–193
 curing (*see* Curing multiple sclerosis)
 FDA-approved anti-inflammatory drugs, 198
 heterogeneity, 191–192
 immune system, 1970–1990, 198
 increments, 198
 prevent progressive forms, 2010–2030, 198
 prevent trials, 2030–2050, 198
 progressive and relapsing remitting
  early stages, 194–195
  immune status and disease course, 195
  innate immune system, 195
  neurodegeneration, 195–196
  primary and secondary, 194–195
Myasthenia gravis (MG)
 clinical description, 334
 diagnosis
  edrophonium testing, 335
  electrodiagnostic testing, 334
  muscle-specific kinase (MuSK), 335
 pathophysiology
  complement, 335–336
  polyclonal expansion, 335
  thymic T cells, 335
 treatment
  cyclosporine, 336
  intravenous immunoglobulin (IVIG), 336
Mycophenolate mofetil, 140
Myelin
 Balo concentric sclerosis, 50–51
 laden macrophage, 46

Myelin (*cont.*)
  oligodendrocytes, 57–58
  phagocytosis, 45, 46
Myelitis
  attack, 221, 222
  LETM, 221, 223–225
  plasmapheresis therapy, 227

N
National Multiple Sclerosis Society (NMSS), 172
Natural killer (NK) cells, 20–21, 55–56
Natural killer T (NKT) cells, 21
Neoplasms, 163
Nervous, immune and endocrine system network
  brain, 11
  description, 10
  HPA, 11
  neurotransmitters, 10
  psychoneuroimmunology, 11
Nervous system
  cancer, 233
  CNS (*see* Central nervous system (CNS))
  MHC-I expression, 236
  systemic cancer, 241
Neuritic plaques
  Aβ fibrils, 275, 277
  inflammation, 275, 276
Neuritis
  optic
    acute, 98
    relative afferent pupillary defect (RAPD), 90
    VEPs, 91
  optic neuritis treatment trial (ONTT), 89, 90
  retrobulbar, 99
Neuroborreliosis, 258
Neurocysticercosis
  anti-parasitic agents, 271
  occurence, 270
Neurodegeneration, 145–146
Neuroimmunology
  anatomy, 1–3
  blood–brain and blood–CSF barriers, 3
  CNS
    cell components, 6–11
    immunity, 4–5
    lymphatics, 3–4
  description, 1
  disorders, 1, 2
  MHC expression, 5
Neuromuscular junction (NMJ)
  anatomy
    acetylcholine (ACh)-filled synaptic vesicles, 333
    calcium influx, 334
    MEPPs, 334
    nicotinic-acetylcholine receptors (AChR), 333–334
  in neuroimmune disorders, 2
Neuromyelitis optica (NMO)
  attacks treatment, 227
  clinical course, 225
  defined, 219

definition
  diagnostic criteria, 222–223
  National Multiple Sclerosis Society task force, 223
epidemiology and clinical features
  diagnosis, 220
  longitudinally extensive transverse myelitis (LETM), 221
  myelitis, 220–221
investigations, 222
NMO-IgG
  anti-aquaporin–4, 226
  target, 220
nosology, 219
pathology
  aquaporin–4, 226
  evaluation, immunopathological, 225
  lesions, 225
spectrum disorders
  brain lesions, 224
  NMO-IgG discovery, 223–224
  SLE and Sjögren's syndrome, 224–225
therapy, 227
therapy, attack prevention
  immunopathological features, 228
  immunosuppressive approaches, 229
  patients, 227–228
  preventative approach, 228
  rituximab, 228–229
Neuromyotonia, 283, 296
Neurosarcoidosis, 378–380
Neurovasculo-Behçet disease, 382
N-methyl-D-aspartate (NMDA)
  paraneoplastic syndromes, 282
  syndrome, 283
NMO. *See* Neuromyelitis optica
Non-conventional MRI technique. *See* Susceptibility-weighted imaging
Non-Hodgkin's lymphoma, 141, 143

O
Off-label agents
  azathioprine, 139
  corticosteroids, 139
  cyclophosphamide, 139
  methotrexate, 140
  mycophenolate mofetil, 140
  plasmapheresis and IVIG, 140
Oligodendrocyte
  apoptosis, 50
  myelination, 57–58
  regeneration, 46
Omega3-fatty acids, 75
Optic neuritis (ON)
  diagnosis, 220
  effects, 227
  recurrent, 224
  treatment, 227
Oral agents
  cladribine, reduce lymphocyte counts, 144
  laquinamod

BG12 (fumaric acid), 145
    derive roquinimex, 144
    initial testing, 144–145
    neuroprotection, 145–146
    PPMS treatment, 146
    stem cell transplantation, 145
    teriflunomide, mitochondrial dehydrogenase, 144

P
PAM. *See* Primary Amebic Meningoencephalitis
PAN. *See* Polyarteritis nodosa
Paraneoplastic cerebellar degeneration (PCD)
    cerebrospinal fluid analysis, 244
    immune treatments, 246
    MRI scan, 244
    pathologic feature, 244
    symptoms, 243
    T-cells, cdr2-specific, 243
Paraneoplastic syndromes
    and CNS, 241–242
    humoral-mediated
        LEMS and MG, 242
        voltage-gated potassium channels (VGKC) anti-
            bodies, 242
    neurology
        encephalomyelitis, 244–245
        LEMS, 245
        opsoclonus/myoclonus, 245
        PCD, 243–244
        treatment, 246
    NMDAR encephalitis, 298
    T-cell-mediated, 243
Parkinsonism
    inflammation, 299
    levodopa, 297
    post-encephalitic, 296
PCD. *See* Paraneoplastic cerebellar degeneration
Pediatric autoimmune neuropsychiatric disorders associ-
        ated with streptococcal infections (PANDAS),
        293–294
Pediatrics
    ADEM (*see* Acute disseminated encephalomyelitis
        (ADEM))
    adherence, 169–170
    chronic disorder, 172
    clinical features
        brainstem, 160
        cognitive disability, 160
        fatigue and mood disorders, 160
        isolated transverse myelitis and ADEM, 159
        symptoms, 159
        verbalizing and neutrophils, 160
    cognitive dysfunction, 157
    demographic profile, 157–158
    diagnostic challenges, 157
    DMT (*see* Disease modifying therapy (DMT))
    EBV infection, 157
    family support, 172
    first-line treatments, 169
    infection, 163
    ITP, 169

leukodystrophies, 164
management, 157
mitochondrial disorders, 164
neoplasms, 163
NMO, 163
origination and development, disease, 165
prognosis, 161
risks
    Barkhof and Callen criteria, 159
    IDE features, 158–159
    IgG index *vs.* CSF, 159
    MRI, 159
    self-limited disorder, 158
symptom management
    adult and anecdotal reports, 170
    cognition, 170
    depression, 170–171
    fatigue, 170
    motor problems, 172
    paroxysmal spasms, 171
    spasticity, 171
    urinary/bowel dysfunction, 171
testing, 164–165
treatment
    acute relapse, 166
    communication, 165–166
    therapy, 166
vaccination, 165
vascular and inflammatory disorders, 163
viral infection role, 165
Percutaneous transluminal angioplasty (PTA), 184
Perivenous
    demyelination, 203
    inflammation, 203
    lesions, 203–204
Permeability factor is causative in Crow-Fukase
        (POEMS) syndrome, 362
Plaques
    brain, 50
    macroscopic, 49, 60
    pathology
        active lesions, 46
        myelin-laden macrophage, 46
        oligodendrocyte loss, 45
Plasma cells
    accumulation, 47
    described, 55
    location, 47
Plasmapheresis, 140
PML. *See* Progressive multifocal leukoencephalopathy
Polyarteritis nodosa (PAN)
    vs. MPA, 311
    muscular artery, 308, 310
    postmortem examination, 307–308
    survival rate, 326
    vs. WG, 314
Polymyositis (PM)
    clinical description, 338
    diagnosis, 338–339
    pathophysiology
        antibodies, inflammatory myopathies, 339, 340

Polymyositis (PM) (*cont.*)
    antisynthetase syndrome, 339
    ribonucleoproteins, 339
    scleroderma, 340
    systemic lupus erythematosis, 339–340
    treatment
        chlorambucil, 341
        Cochrane review, 341
        corticosteroids, 340
Postinfectious encephalitis/encephalomyelitis. *See* Acute
        disseminated encephalomyelitis (ADEM)
Postmortem
    Borrelia burgdorferi infection, 322
    examination
        GANS, 317, 318
        PAN, 307–308
        SLE, 318
Prevalence
    hygiene hypothesis, 73
    latitude gradient, 72
    MS, 71
Primary amebic meningoencephalitis (PAM), 269
Prognosis, 161
Progressive multifocal leukoencephalopathy (PML)
    and HAART therapy, 263–264
    immunotherapy, 264

R
Rapidly progressive dementia (RPD), 281, 282
Receptors
    antigen and cell surface, 20, 24
    BAFF binds, 23
    B cell and maturation, 17, 22, 25
    CD28 and CD40, 17
    chemokine, 28, 29
    cytokines, 32, 33
    dendritic cells maturation, 31
    Fc and IL–15, 20
    GPCR and IL–6R, 17
    G-protein, 27, 28
    interleukin (IL)–2, 19
    ligand pairs, tumor necrosis, 22
    NKT cells, 21
    roles, 29
    S1P1, 29
    T-cell, 17
    toll-like receptor (TLR), 23
Relapse rate
    alemtuzumab, 143
    CIS, 136
    cladribine, 144
    fingolimod, 135
    fumaric acid, 145
    glatiramer acetate, 132
    IFN –1b subcutaneous, 132
    interferons, 137
    natalizumab, 133
    rituximab, 143
    treatment
        induction, 138
        SPMS, 138

Relapsing–remitting MS (RRMS)
    CCSVI hypothesis, 182–184
    developing, treatment, 195
    early stages, 194–195
    immune biomarkers, 193
    immune status and disease course, 195
    innate immune system, 195
    neurodegeneration, 195–196
    vs. SPMS, 194
    vascular and perfusion abnormalities, 180–181
Remissions, 378, 381
Rituximab, 141, 143
RPD. *See* Rapidly progressive dementia

S
SCLC. *See* Small-cell lung cancer
Secondary progressive MS (SPMS), 193, 194
Seizures
    bacterial infections, 256
    herpes zoster, 263
    neurocystercosis, 270
Side effects
    alemtuzumab, 143
    azathioprine, 139
    cladribine, 144
    corticosteroids, 139
    cyclophosphamide, 139
    fingolimod, 135
    interferons, 132
    laquinamod, 144, 145
    natalizumab, 134
    rituximab, 143
    worsening RRMS, 137, 138
Single photon emission-computed tomography
        (SPECT), 309–310
Sjogren's syndrome
    clinical manifestations and diagnosis
        CNS, 380–381
        peripheral neuropathy, 380
    description, 380
    treatment, 381
SLE. *See* Systemic lupus erythematosus
Small-cell lung cancer (SCLC)
    CRMP, 244
    LEMS, 245
    paraneoplastic encephalomyelitis, 244
Spanish influenza, 297
Spasticity
    autonomic nervous system involvement, 97
    bowel issues, 97
    medication, 93
    muscle weakness, 93
    progressive MS forms, 92
    symptoms, 93
SPECT. *See* Single photon emission-computed tomography
Sphingosine 1-phosphate (S1P), 29–30
Standard diagnostic evaluation, 164–165
Stem cells, 145
Steroids
    corticosteroids, 210, 211
    unresponsive patients, 209

Superior sagittal sinus (SSS), 180
Susceptibility-weighted imaging (SWI)
    brain structures, 124–125
    magnitude and phase images, 124
    tissue damage, 125
    vein abnormalities and iron deposition, brain, 125
Symptom management, pediatrics
    adult and anecdotal reports, 170
    cognition, 170
    depression, 170–171
    fatigue, 170
    motor problems, 172
    paroxysmal spasms, 171
    spasticity, 171
    urinary/bowel dysfunction, 171
Symptoms, MS
    ambulatory difficulties, 94
    CIS, 90
    cranial nerves
        demyelinating disease, 90
        facial palsy, 91–92
        olfactory, 91
        spastic dysarthria, 92
        vestibular-cochlear system, 92
    eye movement abnormalities, 91
    hyperreflexia, 92
    incoordination and tremor
        "target seeking", cerebellar, 93
        therapeutic benefits, 93–94
    optic neuritis
        VEPs, 91
        visual acuity, 90–91
    sensory loss, 94
    spasticity, 93
    subjective/"invisible"
        bladder, and sexual dysfunction, 96–98
        cognitive dysfunction, 95–96
        depression, 95
        fatigue, 94–95
        pain, 96
        paroxysmal, 98
        seizures, 98
        sleep difficulties, 98
    weakness, 92
Synapses, 11, 264, 333
Syphilis
    classifications, 259
    meningovascular, 259
    neurosyphilis, 259–260
Systemic autoimmune diseases, neurological manifestations
    Behçet's, 381–384
    Celiac disease, 385–386
    neurosarcoidosis, 378–380
    Sjogren's syndrome, 380–381
    SLE (see Systemic lupus erythematosus)
    Whipple's disease, 384–385
Systemic granulomatous vasculitis
    GANS, 317–318
    giant cell arteritis, 316, 317
    lethal midline granuloma, 315–316
    lymphomatoid granulomatosis, 314, 315

    temporal and Takayasu arteritis, 316–317
    WG, 314
Systemic lupus erythematosus (SLE), 318, 320
Systemic necrotizing arteritis
    Churg–Strauss syndrome, 311
    KD, 308–310
    MPA, 311
    PAN, 307–308, 310

T
T cells
    CD4+, 53
    CD8+, 54
    Foxp3, 53
    receptor, 54
Teriflunomide, 144
Three-dimensional fluid-attenuated inversion recovery
        (3D FLAIR), 115–116
Tissue inhibitor of metalloproteinases (TIMP) control, 29
Toll-like receptors (TLRs)
    microglia, 6–7
    roles, 10
Transcranial Doppler (TCD) techniques, 181
Tremor, 93–94, 292, 298
Tumor necrosis factor (TNF)-α, 26

U
Urticarial vasculitis, 313

V
Varicella zoster virus (VZV)
    AIDS, 264
    description, 263
Vascular disease, MS
    abnormalities, 186
    CCSVI hypothesis, 181–184
    description, 179
    "double hit" model, 186
    historical perspectives, 179
    MR techniques, 186
    parallels, cerebrovascular diseases, 184–186
    and perfusion abnormalities, 180–181
    RRMS vs. PPMS, 186
    venous drainage, brain and spinal cord, 179–180
Vasculitic neuropathy, 364
Venous congestion
    brain and spinal cord, 179–180
    CNS, 186
    intracranial venous drainage, 180
    postural changes, hypertension, 185
    retrograde cortical, 185
Venous congestion, brain and spinal cord, 179–180
VGKC. See Voltage-gated potassium channel
Viral infections, CNS
    encephalitis, 260–261
    enterovirus, 262–263
    herpes simplex virus, 261–262
    HIV, 264–265
    JC virus, 263–264
    VZV, 263
    WNV, 262

Voltage-gated potassium channel (VGKC), 283
Voltage-gated sodium channels (VGSC)
    action potential, 334
    NMJ, 333
VZV. *See* Varicella zoster virus

W
Waldenstrom's macroglobulinemia (WM), 362
Weakness
    asymmetric, 343
    atrophy, 338
    facial, 343
    finger flexor, 343
    ocular muscle, 334
    sarcoid myositis, 345
    symmetric, 336
Wegener granulomatosis (WG)
    described, 314
    lethal midline granuloma, 315
West Nile virus (WNV), 262

WG. *See* Wegener granulomatosis
Whipple's disease
    clinical manifestations and diagnosis
        cognitive changes, 384
        diagnosis, 385
        neuroimaging, CT/MRI, 385
    neurologic symptoms, 384
    treatment, 385
White matter (WM)
    atrophy, 120
    conventional MRI techniques, 114
    3D-T1 image, tissue segmentation, 120
    FLAIR image, 113
    inflammatory damage, 119
    NAWM, 121–123
    single-slab 3D MRI, 117
    tissue damage, 111
WM. *See* Waldenstrom's macroglobulinemia;
        White matter
WNV. *See* West Nile virus